Textbook of Hemophilia

Textbook of Hemophilia

Edited by

Christine A. Lee, MA, MD, DSc, FRCP, FRCPath, FRCOG
Emeritus Professor of Haemophilia
University of London
London, UK

Erik E. Berntorp, MD, PhD
Professor of Coagulation Medicine
Lund University
Malmö Centre for Thrombosis and Haemostasis
Skåne University Hospital
Malmö, Sweden

W. Keith Hoots, MD
Director, Division of Blood Diseases and Resources
National Heart, Lung, and Blood Institute
National Institutes of Health
Bethesda, MD;
Professor of Pediatrics and Internal Medicine
University of Texas Medical School at Houston
Houston, TX, USA

THIRD EDITION

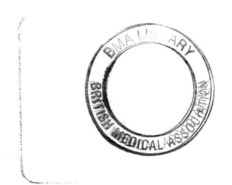

WILEY Blackwell

Library of Congress Cataloging-in-Publication Data

Textbook of hemophilia / edited by Christine A. Lee, Erik E. Berntorp, W. Keith Hoots. – Third edition.
  p. ; cm.
  Includes bibliographical references and index.
  ISBN 978-1-118-39824-1 (cloth)
  I. Lee, Christine A., editor of compilation.   II. Berntorp, Erik, editor of compilation.   III. Hoots, Keith, editor of compilation.
  [DNLM: 1. Hemophilia A–physiopathology.   2. Coagulation Protein Disorders–physiopathology.   3. Factor IX–physiology.   4. Factor VIII–physiology.   5. Hemophilia B–physiopathology.   WH 325]
  RC642
  616.1′572–dc23
                        2013049544

Cover image: Courtesy of Professor G.D. Tuddenham
Cover design by OptaDesign.co.uk

Set in 9.5/12 pt MinionPro-Regular by Toppan Best-set Premedia Limited
Printed and bound in Singapore by Markono Print Media Pte Ltd

1   2014

Contents

Contributors

Jan Astermark, MD, PhD
Associate Professor
Department for Hematology and Vascular Disorders
Malmö Centre for Thrombosis and Haemostasis
Skåne University Hospital
Malmö, Sweden

Trevor W. Barrowcliffe, MA, PhD
Retired from
Haemostasis Section
National Institute for Biological Standards and Control (NIBSC)
South Mimms, Potters Bar
Hertfordshire, UK

Angelika Batorova, MD, PhD
Associate Professor
Director of the National Hemophilia Center
Department of Hematology & Transfusion Medicine
Medical School of Comenius University, University Hospital
Bratislava, Slovakia

H. Marijke van den Berg, MD, PhD
Pediatric Hematologist
Julius Center for Health Sciences and Primary Care
University Medical Center
Utrecht, the Netherlands

Erik E. Berntorp, MD, PhD
Professor of Coagulation Medicine
Lund University
Malmö Centre for Thrombosis and Haemostasis
Skåne University Hospital
Malmö, Sweden

Sven Björkman, PhD (deceased)
Professor of Pharmacokinetics
Department of Pharmaceutical Biosciences
Uppsala University
Uppsala, Sweden

Victor S. Blanchette, FRCP
Professor of Paediatrics
Medical Director, Paediatric Thrombosis and Haemostasis Program
Division of Hematology/Oncology
The Hospital for Sick Children
University of Toronto
Toronto, ON, Canada

Paula H.B. Bolton-Maggs, DM, FRCP, FRCPath
Consultant Haematologist, Manchester Blood Centre and Honorary Senior Lecturer
University of Manchester;
Medical Director, Serious Hazards of Transfusion Haemovigilance Scheme
Manchester Blood Centre
Plymouth Grove
Manchester, UK

Kathleen Brummel Ziedins, PhD
Associate Professor
Department of Biochemistry
University of Vermont
College of Medicine
Colchester, VT, USA

Michael U. Callaghan, MD
Assistant Professor of Pediatrics
Children's Hospital of Michigan
Wayne State University
Department of Pediatrics
Detroit, MI, USA

Manuel D. Carcao, MD, FRCP(C), MSc
Associate Professor of Paediatrics
Division of Haematology/Oncology and Child Health Evaluative Sciences
The Hospital for Sick Children
University of Toronto
Toronto, ON, Canada

Giancarlo Castaman, MD
Consultant Haematologist
Department of Cell Therapy and Hematology
Hemophilia and Thrombosis Center
San Bortolo Hospital
Vicenza, Italy

Elizabeth A. Chalmers, MB, ChB, MD, MRCP(UK), FRCPath
Consultant Paediatric Haematologist
Royal Hospital for Sick Children
Yorkhill
Glasgow, Scotland

Meera B. Chitlur, MD
Associate Professor of Pediatrics
Wayne State University School of Medicine;
Barnhart-Lusher Hemostasis Research
Endowed Chair
Director, Hemophilia Treatment Center and Hemostasis Program
Division of Hematology/Oncology
Children's Hospital of Michigan
Detroit, MI, USA

Pratima Chowdary
Consultant Haematologist
Katharine Dormandy Haemophilia Centre and Thrombosis Unit
Royal Free Hospital
London, UK

Peter W. Collins, MB, BS, MD, FRCP, FRCPath
Professor and Consultant Haematologist
Arthur Bloom Haemophilia Centre
University Hospital of Wales
School of Medicine
Cardiff University
Cardiff, UK

Donna M. DiMichele, MD
Deputy Director, Division of Blood Diseases and Resources
National Heart, Lung, and Blood Institute
National Institutes of Health
Bethesda, MD, USA

Sharyne M. Donfield, PhD
Senior Research Scientist
Rho, Inc.
Chapel Hill, NC, USA

Andrea S. Doria, MD, PhD, MSc
Associate Professor of Radiology
University of Toronto;
Research Director
Department of Diagnostic Imaging
The Hospital for Sick Children
Toronto, ON, Canada

Geoffrey Dusheiko, MB, BCh, FCP (SA), FRCP
Professor of Hepatology
Centre for Hepatology
Royal Free Hospital
London, UK

Miguel A. Escobar, MD
Associate Professor of Medicine and Pediatrics
Division of Hematology
University of Texas Health Science Center;
Director
Gulf States Hemophilia and Thrombophilia Center
Houston, TX, USA

Albert Farrugia, PhD
Centre for Orthopaedic Research
Department of Surgery
Faculty of Medicine and Surgery
University of Western Australia
WA, Australia

Augusto B. Federici, MD
Associate Professor of Hematology
Hematology and Transfusion Medicine
L. Sacco University Hospital
Department of Clinical Sciences and Community Health
University of Milan
Milan, Italy

Kathelijn Fischer, MD, PhD, MSc
Pediatric Hematologist
Van Creveldkliniek
Department of Haematology
Julius Center for Health Sciences and Primary Care
University Medical Centre Utrecht
Utrecht, the Netherlands

Veronica H. Flood, MD
Associate Professor of Pediatrics
Medical College of Wisconsin
Milwaukee, WI, USA

Paul L.F. Giangrande, BSc, MD, FRCP, FRCPath, FRCPCH
Oxford Haemophilia & Thrombosis Centre
Churchill Hospital
Oxford, UK

Nicholas Goddard, MB, FRCS
Consultant Orthopaedic Surgeon
Royal Free Hospital and School of Medicine
London, UK

Keith Gomez, PhD, MRCP, FRCPath
Consultant Haematologist
Katharine Dormandy Haemophilia Centre and Thrombosis Unit
Royal Free Hospital
London, UK

Anne Goodeve, PhD
Professor of Molecular Medicine and Principal Clinical Scientist
Haemostasis Research Group
Department of Cardiovascular Science
University of Sheffield School of Medicine, Dentistry and Health;
Sheffield Diagnostic Genetics Service
Sheffield Children's NHS Foundation Trust
Sheffield, UK

Alessandro Gringeri, MD, MSc
Baxter Innovations GmbH
Vienna, Austria

Daniel Hampshire, PhD
Postdoctoral Research Fellow
Haemostasis Research Group
Department of Cardiovascular Science
University of Sheffield School of Medicine, Dentistry and Health
Sheffield, UK

Charles R.M. Hay, MD, FRCP, FRCPath
Honorary Clinical Professor of Haemostasis and Thrombosis
Consultant Haematologist
Manchester University Department of Haematology
Manchester Royal Infirmary
Manchester, UK

Michael Heim, MB, ChB
Professor of Orthopedic Surgery
University of Tel Aviv
Tel Aviv, Israel

Cedric R.J.R. Hermans, MD, PhD, FRCP(Lon), FRCP(Edin)
Professor
Head, Division of Haematology
Haemostasis and Thrombosis Unit
Haemophilia Clinic
St-Luc University Hospital
Brussels, Belgium

Katherine A. High, MD
William H. Bennett Professor of Pediatrics
Perelman School of Medicine at the University of Pennsylvania
Investigator, Howard Hughes Medical Institute;
Director, Center for Cellular and Molecular Therapeutics
The Children's Hospital of Philadelphia
Philadelphia, PA, USA

Pål Andrè Holme, MD, PhD
Associate Professor
Department of Haematology
Oslo University Hospital
Oslo, Norway

W. Keith Hoots, MD
Director, Division of Blood Diseases and Resources
National Heart, Lung, and Blood Institute
National Institutes of Health
Bethesda, MD;
Professor of Pediatrics and Internal Medicine
University of Texas Medical School at Houston
Houston, TX, USA

Loan Hsieh, MD
Children's Hospital of Orange County
Orange, CA, USA

Alfonso Iorio, MD, PhD, FRCPC
Departments of Clinical Epidemiology & Biostatistics and Medicine
McMaster University
Hamilton, ON, Canada

Marc G. Jacquemin, MD, PhD
Associate Professor
Center for Molecular and Vascular Biology and Haemophilia Center
University of Leuven
Leuven, Belgium

Rezan A. Kadir, MD, FRCS (Ed), MRCOG
Consultant Obstetrician and Gynaecologist
Honorary Clinical reader
The Royal Free Hospital / University College London
London, UK

Randal J. Kaufman, PhD
Sanford Burnham Medical Research Institute
Neuroscience, Aging, and Stem Cell Research Center
La Jolla, CA, USA

Geoffrey Kemball-Cook, PhD
University College London
London, UK

Craig M. Kessler, MD, MACP
Professor of Medicine and Pathology
Director, Division of Coagulation
Director, Comprehensive Hemophilia and Thrombosis Care Center
Lombardi Comprehensive Cancer Center
Georgetown University Medical Center
Washington, DC, USA

Steve Kitchen, PhD
Clinical Scientist, Sheffield Hemophilia and Thrombosis Centre
Royal Hallamshire Hospital
Sheffield, UK;
Scientific Director, UK National External Quality Assessment Scheme (NEQAS) for Blood Coagulation
Director, WFH International External Quality Assessment Program for Blood Coagulation
Sheffield, UK

Peter A. Kouides, MD
Medical and Research Director
Mary M. Gooley Hemophilia Center, Inc.;
Clinical Professor of Medicine
University of Rochester School of Medicine
Rochester, NY, USA

Thomas R. Kreil, PhD
Associate Professor of Virology
Senior Director, Global Pathogen Safety (GPS)
Baxter BioScience
Vienna, Austria

Rebecca Kruse-Jarres, MD, MPH
Associate Professor of Medicine
Section of Hematology/Oncology
Tulane University School of Medicine
New Orleans, LA, USA

Michael Laffan, DM, FRCP, FRCPath
Professor of Haemostasis and Thrombosis
Honorary Consultant in Haematology
Faculty of Medicine
Imperial College
Hammersmith Hospital
London, UK

Alice E. Lail, MPH
Senior Biostatistician
Rho, Inc.
Chapel Hill, NC, USA

Christine A. Lee, MA, MD, DSc, FRCP, FRCPath, FRCOG
Emeritus Professor of Haemophilia
University of London
London, UK

Cindy Leissinger, MD
Professor of Medicine and Pediatrics
Chief, Section of Hematology/Oncology
Director, Louisiana Center for Bleeding and Clotting Disorders
Tulane University School of Medicine
New Orleans, LA, USA

David Lillicrap, MD
Professor
Department of Pathology and Molecular Medicine
Richardson Laboratory
Queen's University
Kingston, ON, Canada

Rolf C.R. Ljung, MD, PhD
Professor of Pediatrics, Lund University
Departments of Paediatrics and Coagulation Disorders;
Paediatric Clinic
Skåne University Hospital
Malmö, Sweden

Sébastien Lobet, PhD, PT
Haemostasis and Thrombosis Unit
Haemophilia Clinic
St-Luc University Hospital
Brussels, Belgium

Christopher A. Ludlam, PhD, FRCP, FRCPath
Emeritus Professor of Haematology and Coagulation Medicine
University of Edinburgh;
Former Director, Haemophilia and Thrombosis Comprehensive Care Centre
Royal Infirmary
Edinburgh, Scotland

Björn Lundin, MD, PhD
Senior Consultant Radiologist
Center for Medical Imaging and Physiology
Department of Radiology
Skåne University Hospital, Lund
Lund University
Lund, Sweden

Jeanne M. Lusher, MD
Distinguished Professor Emeritus
Wayne State University
Detroit, MI, USA

Sylvia von Mackensen, PhD
Senior Scientist
Institute for Medical Psychology and Policlinics
University Medical Centre of Hamburg-Eppendorf
Hamburg, Germany

Michael Makris, MD
Professor of Haemostasis and Thrombosis
University of Sheffield
Sheffield Haemophilia and Thrombosis Centre
Royal Hallamshire Hospital
Sheffield, UK

Kenneth G. Mann, PhD
Emeritus Professor of Biochemistry and Medicine
University of Vermont
College of Medicine
Colchester, VT, USA

Pier M. Mannucci, MD
Professor of Medicine
Scientific Director
IRCCS Ca' Granda Maggiore Policlinico Hospital Foundation
Milan, Italy

Uri Martinowitz, MD
Director of the Institute of Thrombosis and Hemostasis and the National Hemophilia Center;
Ministry of Health
The Chaim Sheba Medical Center
Tel Hashomer, Israel;
Sackler School of Medicine
Tel Aviv, Israel

Eveline P. Mauser-Bunschoten, MD, PhD
Hemophilia Specialist
Center for Benign Hematology
Van Creveldkliniek
Department of Haematology
University Medical Center Utrecht
Utrecht, the Netherlands

Marzia Menegatti, PhD
Post-doctoral Fellow
Department of Pathophysiology and Transplantation
University of Milan
Milan, Italy

Carolyn M. Millar, MD, FRCP, FRCPath
Clinical Senior Lecturer
Honorary Consultant in Haematology
Faculty of Medicine
Imperial College
Hammersmith Hospital
London, UK

Robert R. Montgomery, MD
Professor of Pediatric Hematology
Medical College of Wisconsin;
Senior Investigator
Blood Research Institute
Milwaukee, WI, USA

Claude Negrier, MD, PhD
Professor of Haematology
Division of Haematology and Haemophilia Comprehensive Care Center
Edouard Herriot Hospital
University of Lyon
Lyon, France

Diane Nugent, MD
Division of Hematology
Children's Hospital of Orange County
Orange, CA, USA

Kathelijne Peerlinck, MD, PhD
Professor
Center for Molecular and Vascular Biology
Division of Cardiovascular Medicine and Haemophilia Center
KULeuven and University Hospitals
Leuven, Belgium

David J. Perry, MD, PhD, FRCPEdin, FRCPLond, FRCPath
Consultant Haematologist
Department of Haematology
Cambridge University Hospital NHS Foundation Trust
Cambridge, UK

Pia Petrini, MD
Assistant Professor
Centre of Paediatric Haemostasis and Bleeding Disorders
Karolinska University Hospital, Solna
Stockholm, Sweden

Flora Peyvandi, MD, PhD
Associate Professor of Internal Medicine
Angelo Bianchi Bonomi Hemophilia and Thrombosis Center
Fondazione IRCCS Ca' Granda Ospedale
Maggiore Policlinico and
Department of Pathophysiology and Transplantation
University of Milan
Milan, Italy

Steven W. Pipe, MD
Professor
Department of Pediatrics and Communicable Diseases
University of Michigan
Ann Arbor, MI, USA

Pradeep M. Poonnoose, MS, DNB Orth, DNB PMR
Professor
Department of Orthopaedics
Christian Medical College
Vellore, Tamil Nadu, India

Sanj Raut, PhD
Principal Scientist
Study Director for Haemophilia Therapeutics
Haemostasis Section
Biotherapeutics Group
National Institute for Biological Standards and Control (NIBSC)
South Mimms, Potters Bar
Hertfordshire, UK

Francesco Rodeghiero, MD
Director
Department of Cell Therapy and Hematology
Hemophilia and Thrombosis Center
San Bortolo Hospital
Vicenza, Italy

E. Carlos Rodriguez-Merchan, MD, PhD
Consultant Orthopaedic Surgeon
Department of Orthopaedic Surgery
La Paz University Hospital
Madrid, Spain;
Associate Professor of Orthopaedic Surgery
Autonoma University
Madrid, Spain

Jean-Marie R. Saint-Remy, MD, PhD
Professor
Center for Molecular and Vascular Biology
University of Leuven
Leuven, Belgium

Roger E.G. Schutgens, MD, PhD
Consultant Haematologist
Director Van Creveldkliniek
Head of Department
Department of Haematology
University Medical Center Utrecht
Utrecht, the Netherlands

Uri Seligsohn, MD
Head, Amalia Biron Research Institute of Thrombosis and Hemostasis
Sheba Medical Center and Sackler Faculty of Medicine
Tel Aviv University
Tel Hashomer, Israel

Sundar R. Selvaraj, PhD
Research Investigator
University of Michigan
Ann Arbor, MI, USA

Amy D. Shapiro, MD
Medical Director
Indiana Hemophilia and Thrombosis Center
Indianapolis, IN, USA

Midori Shima
Professor
Department of Pediatrics
Nara Medical University
Kashihara, Nara, Japan

Mark W. Skinner, JD
Institute for Policy Advancement
Washington, DC, USA

Benny Sørensen, MD, PhD
Medical Director
Alnylam Pharmaceuticals
Massachusetts, USA

Alok Srivastava, MD, FRACP, FRCPA, FRCP
Professor of Medicine
Head, Department of Haematology
Christian Medical College
Vellore, Tamil Nadu, India

Katarina Steen Carlsson, PhD
Researcher, Project Leader
Department of Clinical Sciences, Malmö, Lund University
Malmö, Sweden;
The Swedish Institute for Health Economics, IHE
Lund, Sweden

David Stephensen, PhD, PT
Kent Haemophilia Centre
East Kent Hospitals University Foundation Trust
Canterbury, UK

Alison M. Street, MB BS, FRACP
Department of Pathology and Immunology
Monash University
Melbourne, Australia

Anand Tandra, MD
Adult Hematologist
Indiana Hemophilia and Thrombosis Center
Indianapolis, IN, USA

Angela E. Thomas, MB BS, PhD, FRCPE, FRCPath, FRCPCH
Consultant Paediatric Haematologist
Royal Hospital for Sick Children
Edinburgh, Scotland

Leonard A. Valentino, MD
Professor of Pediatrics, Internal Medicine and Biochemistry
Director, Hemophilia and Thrombophilia Center
Rush University Medical Center
Chicago, IL, USA

Auro Viswabandya, MD, DM
Professor
Department of Clinical Haematology
Christian Medical College
Vellore, Tamil Nadu, India

Frederico Xavier, MD
Pediatric Hematologist
Indiana Hemophilia and Thrombosis Center
Indianapolis, IN, USA

Akira Yoshioka, MD, PhD
President
Nara Medical University
Kashihara
Nara, Japan

Guy Young, MD
Director, Hemostasis and Thrombosis Center
Children's Hospital Los Angeles;
Associate Professor of Pediatrics
University of Southern California Keck School of Medicine
Los Angeles, CA, USA

Historical introduction

Christine A. Lee

Emeritus Professor of Haemophilia, University College London, University of London, UK

"The history of haemophilia shows the human mind attempting to define and encompass a mysterious yet fascinating phenomenon; and also the human heart responding to the challenge of repeated adversity."
G.I.C. Ingram, Opening lecture to the World Federation of Hemophilia *(1976)*

Early history

Jewish writings of the second century AD are the earliest written references about hemophilia and a ruling of Rabbi Judah the Patriarch exempted a woman's third son from being circumcised if two elder brothers had died of bleeding after circumcision [1].

The first article written in America about hemophilia entitled "An account of a hemorrhagic disposition existing in certain families" was published in the *Medical Repository* in 1803 by Dr John Otto, a physician in the New York Hospital [2,3]. This was a case of a woman carrier, and the sex-linked inheritance was noted as well as the occurrence of premature death:

> "About seventy or eighty years ago, a woman by the name of Smith, settled in the vicinity of Plymouth, New-Hampshire, and transmitted the following idiosyncrasy to her descendants. It is one, she observed, to which her family is unfortunately subject, and had been the source not only of great solitude, but frequently the cause of death."

Many people became aware of this rare sex-linked disorder because Queen Victoria of the UK, who reigned from 1837 to 1901, was a carrier [1] (Figure 1). She had two carrier daughters, Alice and Beatrice [4], and a son with hemophilia, Leopold [5]. Alice was the grandmother of Alexis, the Tsarevich, whose repeated hemophilic bleedings resulted in his mother, Alexandra, coming under the influence of Rasputin, and it has been suggested that hemophilia may have had a profound effect on the course of Russian history [6]. Beatrice, born in 1856, was the last child of Victoria and Albert; her daughter Ena became Queen of Spain and had two hemophilic sons, Alphonso and Gonzalo [4]. It is now known, following forensic DNA examination of bones from the murdered Russian Royal family, recovered from graves near Yekaterinburg, that the royal disease was hemophilia B. [7]

The *Treasury of Human Inheritance*, published in 1911 by Bulloch and Fildes, described "for students of haemophilia . . . [their] Shakespeare for its drama and human warmth and their bible for its towering authority" contains 1000 references and case reports and 200 pedigrees of hemophilic families [1,8]. It includes a description of seven generations of the Appleton-Swain family, originating from a small town near Boston, USA, from the early part of the 18th century to the later years of the 19th century. This family was first described by Hay who noted, "None but males are bleeders . . . whose daughters only have sons thus disposed." William Osler reinvestigated the kindred in 1885 and recorded that many of the hemophilic males died an early death from bleeding [8].

The severe morbidity and early mortality of hemophilia without treatment was reported in great detail in a monograph published by Carol Birch in 1937 from the USA [9] and later summarized by Biggs [10]. The cause of death in 113 patients was recorded—many died from very trivial injury—82 died before 15 years of age and only eight survived beyond 40 years (Table 1).

Treatment

The first transfusion treatment for hemophilia was reported in 1840 in *The Lancet* [11]. George Firmin, an 11-year-old boy, bled after surgery for squint. Using the syringe recently developed by Dr Blundell (Figure 2), blood from "a stout woman" was directly transfused and the child survived. The paper describes the inheritance of hemophilia in the family.

Fractionation of human plasma was developed in response to the challenges of World War II. Cohn pioneered the fractionation of the major components of plasma using ethanol and by controlling the variables salt, protein, alcohol, pH, and temperature [12]. Cohn's fraction 1 was rich in factor VIII (FVIII) and fibrinogen.

McMillan was the first to use human FVIII in the USA, and in 1961 he published his experience [13]. Replacement therapy with Cohn's fraction 1 was used in 15 hemophilic patients presenting with a variety of hemorrhagic and surgical conditions. There was effective hemostasis in all patients. However, mild and transient hepatitis developed in one patient 35 days after infusion; this was most likely hepatitis C virus (HCV).

In 1954, in the UK, Macfarlane speculated that:

> ". . . maintenance therapy would be impracticable if only human AHG [FVIII] were available, since it would need a special panel of about 500,000 donors to treat the 500 haemophiliacs estimated to exist in the country [the UK] . . . Bovine blood has 16 times the anti haemophilic activity [FVIII] of human blood and enough would be

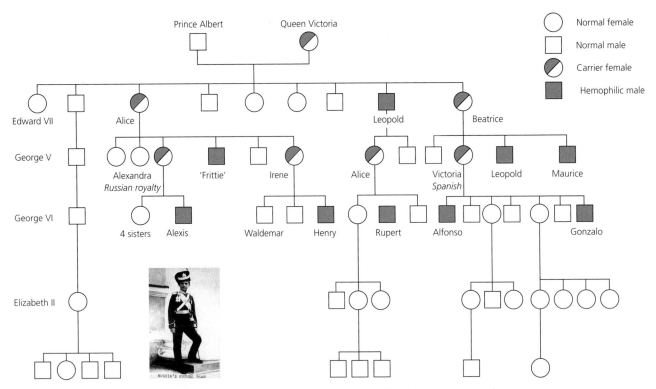

Figure 1 The family tree of Queen Victoria. Reproduced from [1]. With permission of British Publishing Group Ltd.

Table 1 Cause of death for 113 cases of hemophilia by Carroll Birch. Reproduced from [10]. With permission of John Wiley and Sons.

Cause of death	No. of cases	Notes	
Operations	25	Circumcision	15
		Tooth extraction	6
		Vaccination	1
		Lanced hematomas	2
		Tonsillectomy	1
Trivial injuries	23	Cut lip, bitten tongue, injuries to forehead, finger, scalp	
Epistaxis	6		
Hematuria	4		
Throat bleeding	3		
Cutting first tooth	1		
Fracture of leg	1		
Internal bleeding	21		
Central nervous bleeding	7		
Lung hemorrhage	5		
Intestinal bleeding	3		
Gastric bleeding	3		
Miscellaneous	4		
Birth trauma and umbilical bleeding	7		

available for the continuous treatment of the whole haemophilic population of this country" [14].

Therefore, bovine antihemophilic globulin (AHG, FVIII) was produced in Oxford, UK, and first used to cover tooth extractions. The treatment was effective and the rise in FVIII was measured by the newly developed thromboplastin generation test [15]. However, the material showed some antigenic properties—an early recognition of inhibitor or antibody development. This led the Oxford scientists to develop an alternative animal source of FVIII—porcine FVIII [16]. The first patient to be treated with porcine plasma was in 1954; he had developed inhibitory antibodies following injection of bovine material needed to cover surgery for a gunshot wound [16]. The first clinical report of the use of porcine FVIII in the treatment of inhibitors was in 1984 [17].

The scientist, Ethel Bidwell, led much of the early fractionation work at Oxford, and in 1961 the first patient to be treated with human factor IX (FIX) concentrate was reported [18]. A 4-year-old boy, with severe hemophilia B, had developed a large hematoma following a difficult venepuncture and the resulting hemorrhage had become infected resulting in osteomyelitis of the radius. A through-the-elbow amputation was performed in June 1960 under cover of FIX concentrate. The patient, aged 39 in 1995, qualified as an architectural technician, drove, and played golf [19,20].

The life of people with hemophilia was revolutionized by the development of cryoprecipitate. Judith Pool, in the USA, had

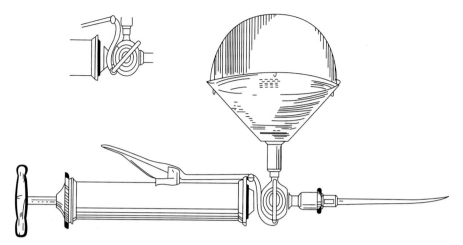

Figure 2 Blundell's syringe for the direct transfusion of blood. Reproduced from [11].

discovered that if plasma was cooled to a very low temperature in the test tube, a "cryoprecipitate" developed, which contained fibrinogen and FVIII [21]. As Kasper has recalled [22], the genius of Pool was her leap from the laboratory observation to the practical idea of using this to prepare cryoprecipitate in a closed-bag system from a single blood donation—possible in an ordinary blood bank [23]. This meant that people with hemophilia could learn to treat themselves at home for the first time. Such treatment is still used in parts of the developing world.

During the 1970s, human freeze-dried (lyophilized) FVIII and FIX became available and patients were able to treat themselves more conveniently at home. In the UK, blood donors were British for the manufacture of NHS concentrates whereas commercial products were manufactured from mostly American donor plasma. The donor pool size could be between 10 000 and 20 000 donations and the cryoprecipitate was produced from large-pool fresh frozen plasma. The FVIII was extracted using ethanol and salt (Cohn's fractionation) and the final product was freeze-dried or lyophilized. It was reconstituted by adding water and (self-)administered intravenously. Such products were not heated until 1985.

The availability of these products resulted in a dramatic increase in treatment. The lives of patients with hemophilia were improved because they could self-treat at home as soon as spontaneous bleeds occurred. However, there was no viral inactivation and this treatment resulted in the epidemics of human immunodeficiency virus (HIV) and HCV.

Human immunodeficiency virus

The epidemic of HIV in hemophilic patients occurred during the years 1978–1985, and was largely caused by USA-derived commercial concentrate. The first patient to seroconvert in the UK was treated in 1979 for abdominal bleeding and he developed non-A non-B hepatitis (HCV) followed by HIV [24].

When an HIV test became available in 1985 it was possible to retrospectively test stored samples from patients with hemophilia to establish the dates of seroconversion. In this way, a cohort of 111 patients with HIV with known dates of seroconversion was identified (Figure 3) [25]. The median age was 22 years (range 2–77) and the median date of infection was January 1983 (range December 1979 to July 1985). All these patients were coinfected with HCV either at or before the time of HIV infection. This cohort was closely monitored clinically, and serial CD4 counts were assessed regularly from 1982. It was established that there was a linear decline of CD4 count from the normal of 800/μL and on average acquired immunodeficiency syndrome (AIDS) developed when the CD4 count reached 50 [26].

The epidemic of HIV in hemophilic patients in the USA showed an increase in deaths per million from 0.50 in the 1970s to 60 by 1990 [27]. In the UK, 1246 of 7250 patients with hemophilia were infected with HIV. Observations on this well-characterized cohort resulted in a series of publications charting the course of the epidemic [28–30]. Highly active antiretroviral therapy became available in the early 1990s and as a result deaths from HIV were reduced (Figure 4) [30].

Hepatitis C virus

The epidemic of HCV was a much longer one, from 1961 to 1985. The first patients became infected from the first large-pool plasma-derived FIX concentrates, used in 1961, and the epidemic ended with the dry heating of concentrates in 1985. Thus, all patients with HIV were coinfected with HCV either at the time of HIV infection or before. The natural history of HCV in a population of 310 patients whose date of infection was known showed that 25 years after infection with HCV 19% had progressed to death from liver disease and that HIV was a significant cofactor for progression [31].

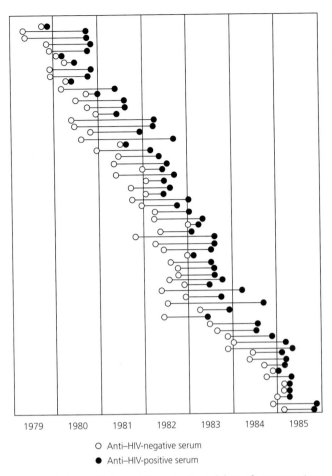

O Anti–HIV-negative serum

● Anti–HIV-positive serum

Figure 3 Patients with hemophilia and estimated dates of seroconversion in human immunodeficiency virus (HIV). Reproduced from [25]. With permission of John Wiley and Sons.

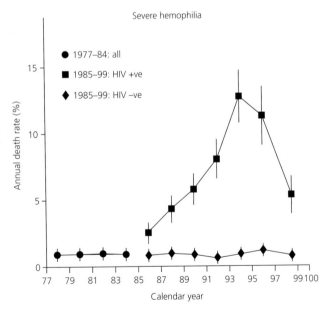

Figure 4 Impact of human immunodeficiency virus (HIV) on mortality rates in the UK hemophilia population. Reproduced from [29]. With permission of Nature Publishing Group.

However, the first recognition that hepatitis was a hazard of blood transfusion was a publication as early as 1943 [32], reporting seven cases of jaundice occurring 1–4 months after transfusion of whole blood or plasma, and a publication in 1946 [33], showing the increased risk of pooled plasma. Thus, it was not surprising that large-pool clotting factor concentrates should cause hepatitis; however, this was difficult to characterize in the absence of a test for HCV until 1991. There was also enthusiasm for the new concentrates among both patients and their treaters. In a historical interview, Dr Rosemary Biggs explained:

> "The next thing that started to crop up was that patients started to get jaundice, and we felt at that time that they were better alive and having jaundice than dead with haemophilia" [34].

In an anonymous leader written in 1981 it was also recognized that:

> "In some cases early death from liver disease may be the price paid by haemophiliacs for the improved quality of life afforded by the easy availability of clotting factor concentrates" [35].

In 1985, it was shown that following a first exposure to plasma-derived clotting factor concentrate there was a high risk, approaching 100%, of non-A non-B hepatitis irrespective of whether the donors were of NHS or USA commercial origin, although the hepatitis from commercial product was more severe, with a shorter incubation period [36]. Once testing had become available, from 1991, it was possible to characterize the HCV epidemic in hemophilic patients more clearly [31]. Approximately one-third of those infected with HCV were also infected with HIV. It was found that the relative hazard of death for those coinfected with HIV and HCV was 19 times compared with those infected with HCV alone [31].

Many patients with hemophilia have been "cured" or "cleared" of HCV with interferon-based therapies, most recently with pegylated interferon and ribavirin. In an international multi-center cohort study, 147 patients maintained a sustained viral response up to 15 years after treatment whereas in 148 unsuccessfully treated patients the cumulative incidence of endstage liver failure was 13% [37].

The ultimate cure for endstage liver failure is liver transplantation, and a small number of transplants have been performed in hemophilic patients. A report in 2002 described 11 hemophilic patients who were monoinfected with HCV and who had been successfully transplanted. Since the liver is the site of synthesis of clotting factors, on average, 36 h post-transplant the patients no longer needed treatment with clotting factor concentrate: liver transplantation is essentially "gene therapy" for hemophilia [38].

New products

The epidemics of HIV and HCV were the stimuli to achieve safe plasma-derived products using viral inactivation processes. These were effectively introduced in 1985 and no HIV or HCV transmissions following exposure to clotting factor concentrates have occurred since that time. The first-generation products were conventionally fractionated and heated in lyophilized state ("dry heated"). These have now been withdrawn. Second-generation products involve dry superheating at 80°C for 72h; solvent/detergent; pasteurization; and heating in hot vapor. Third-generation products are prepared by monoclonal immunoadsorption directed to either FVIII or von Willebrand factor, the carrier protein for FVIII [39].

In 1984, a series of landmark papers were published in *Nature* describing the structure of FVIII and the cloning of the gene [40]. This enabled the manufacture of recombinant FVIII and the investigation of such products in worldwide trials. The results of a study in 107 patients, including pharmacokinetics, treatment for home therapy, surgery, and in previously untreated patients (PUPs), who were mostly children, demonstrated that it had biologic activity similar to plasma FVIII and was safe and efficacious in the treatment of hemophilia [41]. This meticulous study showed, for the first time, the natural history of the treatment in PUPs and the development of inhibitors (antibodies to FVIII)—six of 21 children developed inhibitors. It soon emerged that the three recombinant products, two full-length FVIII, and one B-domain deleted, had similar inhibitor incidences of 25% [42,43]. Inhibitors have now emerged as the biggest challenge in the treatment of hemophilia.

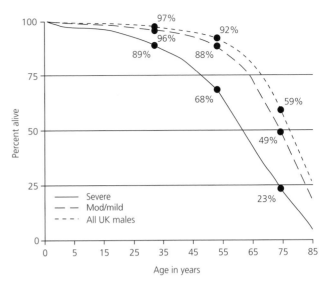

Figure 5 Survival in 6018 men with hemophilia not infected with human immunodeficiency virus (HIV) between 1977 and 1998 and in the general male UK population. Reproduced from [46]. With permission of John Wiley and Sons.

The future

The outlook for people with hemophilia is now very good. In a study of 6018 people with hemophilia in the UK between 1977 and 1998, who were not infected with HIV, the median life expectancy was 63 years for those with severe hemophilia and 75 years for those with nonsevere hemophilia. This approaches that for the normal male population (Figure 5) [47].

Variant Creutzfeldt–Jakob disease

Even though plasma-derived concentrates are very safe with respect to HIV and hepatitis transmission, and also recombinant products used predominantly in the developed world, there remains the possibility of variant Creutzfeldt–Jakob disease (vCJD), particularly in the UK.

The peak exposure of the UK population to vCJD through the food chain was in 1998 when nearly 400 000 cattle were infected with bovine spongiform encephalopathy (BSE). There has been almost no BSE since 2000. A small epidemic of vCJD in humans, as a result of ingestion of infected beef, has peaked with a total 176 cases (www.cjd.ed.ac.uk).

There have now been four cases of transmission by blood from donors incubating vCJD [44]. Thus, surveillance of the UK hemophilia population is ongoing because many patients were treated with plasma-derived concentrates manufactured from UK-derived plasma between 1980 (when the epidemic of BSE began) and 2001 (when concentrates derived from non-UK plasma were used exclusively) [45]. Abnormal prion protein has been demonstrated at postmortem in the splenic tissue of a patient with hemophilia who died from other causes [46].

Notes on this edition

This third edition of *The Textbook of Hemophilia* gives a perspective on the "state of the art" in 2013, the 50th anniversary year of the World Federation of Hemophilia. We have asked our authors to update their chapters to include new information and we have expanded the treatment section to include new treatments and those in development such as gene therapy. Within three-quarters of a century, the life expectancy for people with hemophilia has increased from less than 20 years to near 70 years in the developed parts of the world: the section *birth to old age* celebrates this. Many patients with hemophilia have been, and continue to be, enthusiastic to participate in trials of newer treatments resulting in increased life expectancy. However, effective treatment is rarely free from side-effects and these have been devastating for a generation of people with hemophilia and therefore it is important to remain vigilant. There are still many challenges, but as history has shown, hemophilia is one of the best examples in medicine where advances in basic science are rapidly translated into clinical practise. Worldwide, people with hemophilia can look forward to a bright future.

References

1 Ingram GIC. The history of haemophilia. *J Clin Pathol* 1976; **29**: 469–79.

2 Otto JC. *Review of American Publications in Medicine, Surgery and the Medical Repository*, VI(I): 1–4. New York: Auxillary Branches of Sciences, 1803.

3 Hilgartner M. Historical Annotation 'An account of an hemorrhagic disposition existing in certain families'. *Haemophilia* 1997; **3**: 154–6.

4 Dennison M. *The Last Princess*. London: Weidenfeld and Nicolson, 2007.

5 Zeepvat C. *Prince Leopold: The untold story of Queen Victoria's youngest son*. Gloucester: Sutton Publishing, 1998.

6 Massie RK. *Nicholas and Alexandra*. London: Gollanz, 1968.

7 Rogaev EI, Grigorenko AP, Faskhutdinova G, Kittler ELW, Moliaka YK. Genotype analysis identifies the cause of the "royal disease". *Science* 2009; **326**: 817.

8 Bulloch W, Fildes P. *Treasury of Human Inheritance*, Parts V and VI, Section XIVa, "Haemophilia." London: Dulan and Co., 1911.

9 Birch C La F. *Hemophilia, Clinical and Genetic Aspects*. University of Illinois, Urbana: 1937.

10 Biggs R. Thirty years of haemophilia treatment in Oxford. *Br J Haematol* 1967; **13**: 452–63.

11 Lane S. Successful transfusion of blood. *Lancet* 1840; **i**: 185–8.

12 Cohn EJ, Strong LE, Hughes WL, *et al.* Preparation and properties of serum and plasma proteins. *J Am Chem Soc* 1946; **68**: 459–75.

13 McMillan CW, Diamond LK, Surgenor DM. Treatment of classical haemophilia: the use of fibrinogen rich in FVIII for haemorrhage and surgery. *N Engl J Med* 1961; **265**: 224–30 and 277–83.

14 Macfarlane RG, Biggs R, Bidwell E. Bovine anti haemophilic globulin in the treatment of haemophilia. *Lancet* 1954; **i**: 1316–19.

15 Biggs R, Douglas AS. The thromboplastin generation test. *J Clin Pathol* 1953; **6**: 23.

16 Giangrande P. Porcine factor VIII. *Haemophilia* 2012; **18**: 305–9.

17 Kernoff PBA, Thomas ND, Lilley PA, Matthews KB, Goldman E, Tuddenham EG. Clinical experience with polyelectrolyte fractionated porcine FVIII concentrate in the treatment of haemophiliacs with antibodies to factor VIII. *Blood* 1984; **63**: 31–41.

18 Bidwell E. The purification of antihaemophilic globulin from animal plasma. *Br J Haematol* 1955; **1**: 35–45 and 386–9.

19 Biggs R, Bidwell E, Handley DA, *et al.* The preparation and assay of Christmas factor (factor IX) concentrate and its use in the treatment of two patients. *Br J Haematol* 1961; **7**: 349–64.

20 Rizza CR. Historical annotation: The first patient to receive factor IX concentrate in the UK: a recollection. *Haemophilia* 1995; **1**: 210–12.

21 Pool JG, Hershgold EJ, Pappenhagen AR. High potency antihaemophilic factor concentrate prepared from cryoglobulin precipitate. *Nature* 1964; **18**: 203–12.

22 Kasper CK. Judith Pool and the discovery of cryoprecipitate. *Haemophilia* 2012; **18**: 833–5.

23 Pool JGP, Shannon AE. Production of high-potency concentrates of anti-haemophilic globulin in a closed-bag system. *N Engl J Med* 1965; **273**: 1443–7.

24 Lee CA, Webster A, Griffiths PD, Kernoff PBA. Symptomless HIV infection after more than ten years. *Lancet* 1990; **i**: 426.

25 Lee CA, Phillips A, Elford J, *et al.* The natural history of human immunodeficiency virus infection in a haemophilic cohort. *Br J Haematol* 1989; **73**: 228–34.

26 Phillips AN, Lee CA, Elford J, *et al.* Serial CD4 lymphocyte counts and the development of AIDS. *Lancet* 1991; **337**: 389–92.

27 Chorba TL, Holman RC, Strine TW. Changes in longevity and causes of death among persons with haemophilia A. *Am J Haematol* 1991; **37**: 243–6.

28 Darby SC, Rizza CR, Doll R, Spooner RJD, Stratton IM, Thakrar B. Incidence of AIDS and excess of mortality associated with HIV in haemophiliacs in the United Kingdom: report on behalf of the Directors of Haemophilia Centres in the UK. *Br Med J* 1989; **298**: 1064–8.

29 Darby SC, Ewart W, Giangrande PLF, Dolin PJ, Spooner RJD, Rizza CR, on behalf of the UK Haemophilia Directors Organisation. Mortality before and after HIV infection in the complete UK population of haemophiliacs. *Nature* 1995; **377**: 79–82.

30 United Kingdom Haemophilia Centre Doctors' Organisation (UKHCDO). The impact of mortality rates in the complete UK haemophilia population. *AIDS* 2004; **18**: 525–33.

31 Yee TT, Griffioen A, Sabin CA, Dusheko G, Lee CA. The natural history of HCV in a cohort of haemophilic patients infected between 1961 and 1985. *Gut* 2000; **47**: 845–51.

32 Beeson PB. Jaundice occurring one to four months after transfusion of blood or plasma. *J Am Med Assoc* 1943; **121**: 1332–4.

33 Spurling N, Shone J, Vaughan J. The incidence, incubation period and symptomatology of homologous serum jaundice. *Br Med J* 1946; **2**: 409–11.

34 Historical Annotation. Witnessing medical history: an interview with Dr Rosemary Biggs. *Haemophilia* 1998; **4**: 769–77.

35 Leader. *Br Med J* 1981; **283**: 1.

36 Kernoff PBA, Lee CA, Karayiannis P, Thomas HC. High risk of non-A non-B hepatitis after a first exposure to volunteer or commercial clotting factor concentrates: effects of prophylactic immune serum globulin. *Br J Haematol* 1985; **60**: 469–79.

37 Posthouwer D, Yee TT, Makris M, *et al.* Antiviral therapy for chronic hepatitis C in patients with inherited bleeding disorders: an international, multicenter cohort study. *J Thromb Haemost* 2007; **5**: 1624–9.

38 Wilde J, Teixeira P, Bramhall SR, Gunson B, Multimer D, Mirza DF. Liver transplantation in haemophilia. *Br J Haematol* 2002; **117**: 952–6.

39 Lee CA. Coagulation factor replacement therapy. In: Hoffbrand AV, Brenner MK (eds.) *Recent Advances in Haematology*, 6th edn. Edinburgh: Churchill Livingstone, 1992: 73–88.

40 Vehar GA, Key B, Eaton D, *et al.* Structure of human FVIII. *Nature* 1984; **312**: 337–42.

41 Scharz RS, Abildgaaard CF, Aledort LM, *et al.* Human recombinant DNA-derived antihaemophilic factor (factor VIII) in the treatment of haemophilia. *N Engl J Med* 1990; **323**: 1800–5.

42 Bray GL, Gompertz ED, Courter S, *et al.* A multicenter study of recombinant FVIII (Recombinant): safety, efficacy, and inhibitor risk in previously untreated patients with haemophilia A. *Blood* 1994; **83**: 2428–35.

43 Lusher JM, Lee CA, Kessler CM, Bedrosian CL, for the Refacto Phase 3 Study Group. The safety and efficacy of B-domain deleted recombinant factor VIII concentrate in patients with severe haemophilia A. *Haemophilia* 2003; **9**: 38–49.

44 Llewelyn CA, Hewitt PE, Knight RS, *et al.* Possible transmission of variant Creutzfeldt–Jakob disease by blood transfusion. *Lancet* 2004; **363**: 417–21.

45 Zaman SM, Hill FGH, Palmer B, *et al.* The risk of variant Creutzfeldt–Jakob disease among UK patients with bleeding disorders, known to have received potentially contaminated products. *Haemophilia* 2011; **17**: 931–7.

46 Peden A, McCardle L, Head MW, *et al.* Variant CJD infection in the spleen of a neurologically asymptomatic UK adult patient with haemophilia. *Haemophilia* 2010; **16**: 296–304.

47 Darby SC, Kan SW, Spooner RJ, *et al.* Mortality rates, life expectancy, and causes of death in people with haemophilia A or B in the United Kingdom who were not infected with HIV. *Blood* 2007; **110**: 815–25.

PART I

Introduction

CHAPTER 1

Overview of hemostasis

Kathleen Brummel Ziedins and Kenneth G. Mann

University of Vermont, College of Medicine, VT, USA

Introduction

The maintenance of blood fluidity and protection from blood leakage provide major biophysical challenges for the organism. Nature has evolved a highly complex, integrated, and dynamic system which balances the presentations of procoagulant, anticoagulant, and fibrinolytic systems. These systems function collectively to maintain blood within the vasculature in a fluid state while at the same time providing potent leak attenuating activity which can be elicited upon vascular perforation to provide the rapid assembly of a thrombus principally composed of platelets and fibrin to attenuate extravascular blood loss. The dynamic control of this system is such that the coagulation response is under the synergistic control of a variety of blood and vascular inhibitors, resulting in a process that is regionally restricted to the site of vascular damage and does not propagate throughout the vascular system. The rapid coagulation response is also tightly linked to the vascular repair process during which the thrombus is removed by the fibrinolytic system which is also activated regionally to provide clot removal coincident with vascular repair.

A list of important procoagulant, anticoagulant, and fibrinolytic proteins, inhibitors, and receptors can be seen in Table 1.1.

Importance of complex assembly to coagulation

Laboratory data combined with clinical pathology lead to the conclusion that the physiologically relevant hemostatic mechanism is primarily composed of three procoagulant vitamin K-dependent enzyme complexes (which utilize the proteases factor VIIa, factor IXa, and factor Xa) and one anticoagulant vitamin K-dependent complex (which utilizes the proteases thrombin, meizo, and α-thrombin) [1,2] (Figure 1.1). These complexes—extrinsic factor Xase (tissue factor–factor VIIa complex), intrinsic factor Xase (factor VIIIa–factor IXa complex) [3], and the protein Case complex (thrombin–thrombomodulin) [4]—are each composed of a vitamin K-dependent serine protease, a cofactor protein and a phospholipid membrane; the latter provided by an activated or damaged cell. The membrane-binding properties of the vitamin K-dependent proteins are a consequence of the post-translational γ-carboxylation of these macromolecules [5]. The cofactor proteins are either membrane binding (factor Va, factor VIIIa), recruited from plasma, or intrinsic membrane proteins (tissue factor, thrombomodulin). Cofactor–protease assembly on membrane surfaces yields enhancements in the rates of substrate processing ranging from 10^5 to 10^9-fold relative to rates observed when the same reactions are limited to solution-phase biomolecular interactions between the individual proteases (factor VIIa, factor IXa, and factor Xa) and their corresponding substrates [6–8] (Figure 1.2a). Membrane binding, intrinsic to complex assembly, also localizes catalysis to the region of vascular damage. Thus, a system selective for regulated, efficient activity presentation provides for a regionally limited, vigorous arrest of hemorrhage.

Additional complexes associated with the "intrinsic" pathway are involved in the surface contact activation of blood [3]. However, the association of the contact-initiating proteins (factor XII, prekallikrein, high-molecular-weight kininogen) with hemorrhagic disease is uncertain [9].

Of equal importance to the procoagulant processes is regulation of anticoagulation by the stoichiometric and dynamic inhibitory systems. The extant effectiveness of the inhibitory functions is far in excess of the potential procoagulant responses. These inhibitory processes provide activation thresholds, which require presentation of a sufficient concentration of tissue factor prior to significant thrombin generation [10]. Antithrombin and tissue factor pathway inhibitor [11] are the primary stoichiometric inhibitors while the proteolytic thrombin–thrombomodulin–protein C system (protein Case, Figure 1.1) is dynamic in its function.

Textbook of Hemophilia, Third Edition. Edited by Christine A. Lee, Erik E. Berntorp and W. Keith Hoots.
© 2014 John Wiley & Sons, Ltd. Published 2014 by John Wiley & Sons, Ltd.

Table 1.1 Procoagulant, anticoagulant, and fibrinolytic proteins, inhibitors, and receptors.

Protein	Molecular weight (kDa)	Plasma concentration		Plasma $t_{1/2}$ (days)	Clinical manifestation[a]		Functional classification
		nmol/L	µg/mL		H	T	
Procoagulant proteins and receptors							
Factor XII	80	500	40	2–3	–		Protease zymogen
HMW kininogen	120	670	80		–		Cofactor
LMW kininogen	66	1300	90				Cofactor
Prekallikrein	85/88	486	42				Protease zymogen
Factor XI	160	30	4.8	2.5–3.3	+/–		Protease zymogen
Tissue factor	44			N/A			Cell-associated cofactor
Factor VII	50	10	0.5	0.25	+	+/–	VKD protease zymogen
Factor X	59	170	10	1.5	+		VKD protease zymogen
Factor IX	55	90	5	1	+		VKD protease zymogen
Factor V	330	20	6.6	0.5	+	+	Soluble pro-cofactor
Factor VIII	285	1.1–1.5[b]	0.3–0.4[b]	0.3–0.5	+	–	Soluble pro-cofactor
VWF	255 (monomer)	Varies	10		+		Platelet adhesion carrier for FVIII
Factor II	72	1400	100	2.5	+	–	VKD protease zymogen
Fibrinogen	340	7400	2500	3–5	+	+/–	Structural protein cell adhesion
Factor XIII	320	94	30	9–10	+	+/–	Transglutaminase zymogen
Anticoagulant proteins, inhibitors, and receptors							
Protein C	62	65	4	0.33		+	Proteinase zymogen
Protein S	69	300	20	1.75		+	Inhibitor/cofactor
Protein Z	62	47	2.9	2.5	+/–		Cofactor
Thrombomodulin	100	N/A	N/A	N/A			Cofactor/modulator
Tissue factor pathway inhibitor	40	1–4	0.1	6.4×10^{-4} to1.4×10^{-3}			Proteinase inhibitor
Antithrombin	58	2400	140	2.5–3			Proteinase inhibitor
Heparin cofactor II	66	500–1400	33–90	2.5	+	+/–	Proteinase inhibitor
Fibrinolytic proteins, inhibitors, and receptors							
Plasminogen	88	2000	200	2.2			Proteinase zymogen
t-PA	70	0.07	0.005	0.00167			Proteinase zymogen
u-PA	54	0.04	0.002	0.00347			Proteinase zymogen
TAFI	58	75	4.5	0.00694		+	Carboxypeptidase
PAI-1	52	0.2	0.01	<0.00694			Proteinase inhibitor
PAI-2	47/60	<0.070	<0.005	–			Proteinase inhibitor
α2-Antiplasmin	70	500	70	2.6	+		Proteinase inhibitor
u-PAR	55						Cell membrane receptor

H, hemorrhagic disease/hemophilia; HMW/LMW, high/low molecular weight; N/A, not applicable; PAI-1, plasminogen activator inhibitor–1; T, thrombotic disease/thrombophilia; TAFI, thrombin activatable fibrinolysis inhibitor; t-PA, tissue-type plasminogen activator; u-PA, urokinase-type plasminogen activator; uPAR, urokinase receptor; VKD; vitamin K-dependent proteins; VWF, von Willebrand factor.

+, Presence of phenotype; –, absence of phenotype; ±, some individuals present with the phenotype and others do not.

[a]Clinical phenotype; the expression of either hemorrhagic or thrombotic phenotype in deficient individuals.

[b]Modified from [36,37].

Extrinsic pathway to blood coagulation

The initiating event in the generation of thrombin involves the binding of membrane-bound tissue factor with plasma factor VIIa [12]. The latter is present in blood at ∼0.1 nM [∼1–2% of the factor VII concentration (10 nM)] [13]. Plasma factor VIIa does not express proteolytic activity unless it is bound to tissue factor; thus factor VIIa at normal blood level has no significant activity toward either factor IX or factor X prior to its binding to tissue factor. The inefficient active site of factor VIIa permits its escape from inhibition by the antithrombin present in blood. Vascular damage [14] or cytokine-related presentation of the active tissue factor triggers the process by interaction with activated factor VIIa, which increases the catalytic constant k_{cat} of the enzyme and increases the rate of factor X activation by four orders of magnitude [15]. This increase is the result of the improvement in catalytic efficiency and the membrane binding of factor IX and factor X.

The tissue factor–factor VIIa complex (extrinsic factor Xase) (Figure 1.2) catalyzes the activation of both factor IX and factor

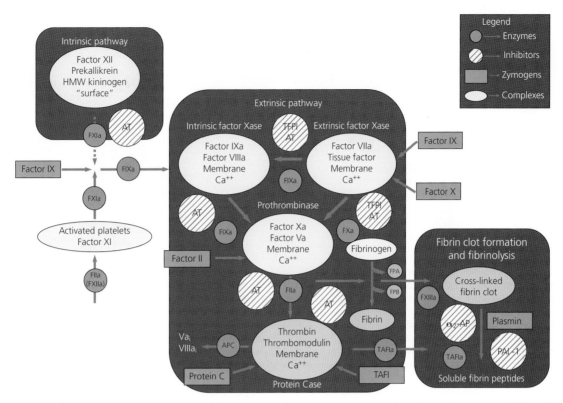

Figure 1.1 Overview of hemostasis. Coagulation is initiated through two pathways: the primary extrinsic pathway (shown on the right) and the intrinsic pathway (historically called the *contact* or *accessory pathway*, shown on the left). The components of these multistep processes are illustrated as follows: enzymes (*circles*), inhibitors (*hatched circles*), zymogens (*boxes*), or complexes (*ovals*). Fibrin formation is also shown as an oval. The intrinsic pathway has no known bleeding etiology associated with it, thus this path is considered accessory to hemostasis. Upon injury to the vessel wall, tissue factor, the cofactor for the extrinsic factor Xase complex, is exposed to circulating factor VIIa and forms the vitamin K-dependent complex, the extrinsic factor Xase. Factor IX and factor X are converted to their serine proteases factor IXa (FIXa) and factor Xa (FXa), which then form the intrinsic factor Xase and the prothrombinase complexes, respectively. The combined actions of the intrinsic and extrinsic factor Xase and the prothrombinase complexes lead to an explosive burst of the enzyme thrombin (IIa). In addition to its multiple procoagulant roles, thrombin also acts in an anticoagulant capacity when combined with the cofactor thrombomodulin in the protein Case complex. The product of the protein Case reaction, activated protein C (APC), inactivates the cofactors Va and VIIIa. The cleaved species, factors Va$_i$ and VIIIa$_i$, no longer support the respective procoagulant activities of the prothrombinase and intrinsic Xase complexes. Once thrombin is generated through procoagulant mechanisms, thrombin cleaves fibrinogen, releasing fibrinopeptide A and B (FPA and FPB) and activate factor XIII to form a cross-linked fibrin clot. Thrombin–thrombomodulin also activates thrombin activatable fibrinolysis inhibitor (TAFIa) that slows down fibrin degradation by plasmin. The procoagulant response is downregulated by the stoichiometric inhibitors tissue factor pathway inhibitor (TFPI) and antithrombin (AT). TFPI serves to attenuate the activity of the extrinsic factor Xase trigger of coagulation. Antithrombin directly inhibits thrombin, factor IXa, and factor Xa. The intrinsic pathway provides an alternative route for the generation of factor IXa. Thrombin has also been shown to activate factor XI. The fibrin clot is eventually degraded by plasmin-yielding soluble fibrin peptides. α-AP, α-antiplasmin; HMW, high molecular weight; PAI-1, plasminogen activator inhibitor-1. Modified from [32].

X, the latter being the more efficient substrate [16]. Thus, the initial product formed is factor Xa. Feedback cleavage of factor IX by membrane-bound factor Xa enhances the rate of generation of factor IXa in a cooperative process with the tissue factor–factor VII complex [17].

The initially formed, membrane-bound factor Xa activates small amounts of prothrombin to thrombin [18]. This initial prothrombin activation provides the thrombin essential to the acceleration of the hemostatic process by serving as the activator for platelets [19], factor V [20], and factor VIII [21] (Figure 1.1). Once factor VIIIa is formed, the factor IXa generated by tissue factor–factor VIIa combines with factor VIIIa on the activated platelet membrane to form the "intrinsic factor Xase"

(Figure 1.2a), which becomes the major activator of factor X. The factor VIIIa–factor IXa complex is 10^9-fold more active as a factor X activator and 50 times more efficient than tissue factor–factor VIIa in catalyzing factor X activation [22,23]; thus, the bulk of factor Xa is ultimately produced by the factor VIIIa–factor IXa complex (Figure 1.2).

As the reaction progresses, factor Xa generation by the more active "intrinsic factor Xase" complex exceeds that of the "extrinsic factor Xase" complex [24]. In addition, the "extrinsic factor Xase" complex is subject to inhibition by tissue factor pathway inhibitor (Figure 1.2b) [25]. As a consequence, most (>90%) of factor Xa is ultimately produced by the factor VIIIa–factor IXa complex in the tissue factor-initiated hemostatic

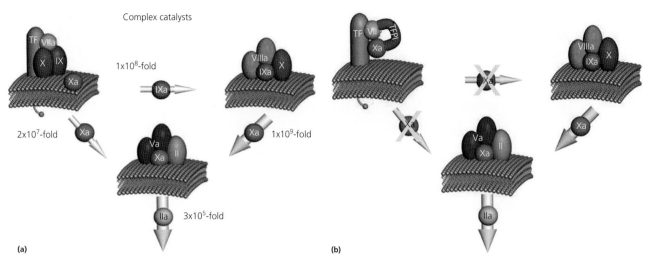

Figure 1.2 Vitamin K-dependent complex assembly. **(a)** The factor Xa generated by the tissue factor–factor VIIa complex activates a small amount of thrombin which activates factor V and factor VIII leading to the presentation of the intrinsic factor Xase (factor VIIIa–factor IXa) and prothrombinase (factor Va–factor Xa) complexes. At this point in the reaction, factor IXa generation is cooperatively catalyzed by membrane-bound factor Xa and by the tissue factor–factor VIIa complex. The thick arrow representing factor Xa generation is cooperatively catalyzed by factor VIIIa-factor IXa and by the tissue factor-factor VIIa complex. **(b)** The tissue factor pathway inhibitor (TFPI) interacts with the tissue factor–factor VIIa–factor Xa product complex to block the tissue factor-initiated activation of both factors IX and factor X. Inhibition of the extrinsic factor Xase complex results in the factor VIIIa–factor IXa complex (intrinsic factor Xase), becoming the only viable catalyst for factor X activation. These slides were modified and used with permission from the "Dynamics of Hemostasis," Haematologic Technologies, K.G. Mann, 2002 [35]. (See also Plate 1.2.)

processes. In hemophilia A and hemophilia B, the "intrinsic factor Xase" complex cannot be assembled, and amplification of factor Xa generation does not occur [26]. Factor Xa combines with factor Va on the activated platelet membrane receptors and this factor Va–factor Xa "prothrombinase" catalyst (Figure 1.2a) converts prothrombin to thrombin. Prothrombinase is 300 000-fold more active than factor Xa alone in catalyzing prothrombin activation [6].

Attenuation of the procoagulant response

The coagulation system is tightly regulated by the inhibitory systems. The tissue factor concentration threshold for reaction initiation is steep and the ultimate amount of thrombin produced is largely regulated by the concentrations of plasma procoagulants and the stoichiometric inhibitors and the constituents of the dynamic inhibition processes [24]. Tissue factor pathway inhibitor blocks the tissue factor–factor VIIa–factor Xa product complex, thus effectively neutralizing the "extrinsic factor Xase" complex (Figure 1.2b) [27]. However, tissue factor pathway inhibitor is present at low abundance ($\sim$2.5 nM) in blood and can only delay the hemostatic reaction [28]. Antithrombin, normally present in plasma at twice the concentration (3.2 μM) of any potential coagulation enzyme, neutralizes all the procoagulant serine proteases primarily in their uncomplexed states [11].

The dynamic protein C system is activated by thrombin binding to constitutive vascular thrombomodulin (protein

Case). This complex activates protein C to activated protein C (Figure 1.1) [4]. Activated protein C competes in binding with factor Xa and factor IXa and cleaves factor Va and factor VIIIa, eliminating their respective complexes [20]. The protein C system, tissue factor pathway inhibitor, and activated protein C cooperate to produce steep tissue factor concentration thresholds, acting like a digital "switch," allowing or blocking thrombin formation [10].

In humans, the zymogen factor XI which is present in plasma and platelets has been variably associated with hemorrhagic pathology [29]. Factor XI is a substrate for thrombin and has been invoked in a "revised pathway of coagulation" contributing to factor IX activation (Figure 1.1) [30]. *In-vitro* importance of the thrombin activation of factor XI is evident only at low tissue factor concentrations [26].

Factor XII, prekallikrein, and high-molecular-weight kininogen (Figure 1.1) do not appear to be fundamental to the process of hemostasis [31]. The contribution of these contact pathway elements to thrombosis remains an open question and further experimentation is required to resolve this issue [31].

Conclusion

Advances in genetics, protein chemistry, bioinformatics, physical biochemistry, and cell biology provide an array of information with respect to normal and pathologic processes leading to hemorrhagic or thrombotic disease. The challenge for the 21st century will be to merge mechanism-based, quantitative data with epidemiologic studies and subjective clinical experience associated with the tendency to bleed or thrombose and with the therapeutic management of individuals with thrombotic or hemorrhagic disease. *In-vitro* data and clinical experience with individuals with thrombotic and hemorrhagic disease will ultimately provide algorithms which can combine the art of clinical management with the quantitative science available to define the phenotypes vis-á-vis the outcome of a challenge or the efficacy of an intervention [28–34].

Acknowledgment

The authors were supported by HL46703 from the National Institutes of Health National Heart, Lung, and Blood Institute and by the Systems Biology program ARO-W911NF-10-1-0376.

References

1 Mann KG, Nesheim ME, Church WR, Haley P, Krishnaswamy S. Surface-dependent reactions of the vitamin K-dependent enzyme complexes. *Blood* 1990; **76**: 1–16.

2 Brummel-Ziedins K, Orfeo T, Jenny NS, Everse SJ, Mann KG. Blood coagulation and fibrinolysis. In: Greer JP, Foerster J, Lukens J, Rodgers GM, Paraskevas F, Glader B (eds.) *Wintrobe's Clinical Hematology*. Philadelphia: Lippincott Williams & Wilkins, 2003: 677–774.

3 Davie EW, Ratnoff OD. Waterfall sequence for intrinsic blood clotting. *Science* 1964; **145**: 1310–12.

4 Esmon CT. The protein C pathway. *Chest* 2003; **124**: 26S–32S.

5 Stenflo J. Contributions of Gla and EGF-like domains to the function of vitamin K-dependent coagulation factors. *Crit Rev Eukaryot Gene Expr* 1999; **9**: 59–88.

6 Nesheim ME, Taswell JB, Mann KG. The contribution of bovine Factor V and Factor Va to the activity of prothrombinase. *J Biol Chem* 1979; **254**: 10952–62.

7 van Dieijen G, Tans G, Rosing J, Hemker HC. The role of phospholipid and factor VIIIa in the activation of bovine factor X. *J Biol Chem* 1981; **256**: 3433–42.

8 Komiyama Y, Pedersen AH, Kisiel W. Proteolytic activation of human factors IX and X by recombinant human factor VIIa: effects of calcium, phospholipids, and tissue factor. *Biochemistry* 1990; **29**: 9418–25.

9 Davie EW. A brief historical review of the waterfall/cascade of blood coagulation. *J Biol Chem* 2003; **278**: 50819–32.

10 van't Veer C, Golden NJ, Kalafatis M, Mann KG. Inhibitory mechanism of the protein C pathway on tissue factor-induced thrombin generation. Synergistic effect in combination with tissue factor pathway inhibitor. *J Biol Chem* 1997; **272**: 7983–94.

11 Olson ST, Bjork I, Shore JD. Kinetic characterization of heparin-catalyzed and uncatalyzed inhibition of blood coagulation proteinases by antithrombin. *Methods Enzymol* 1993; **222**: 525–59.

12 Nemerson Y. Tissue factor and hemostasis. *Blood* 1988; **71**: 1–8.

13 Morrissey JH, Macik BG, Neuenschwander PF, Comp PC. Quantitation of activated factor VII levels in plasma using a tissue factor mutant selectively deficient in promoting factor VII activation. *Blood* 1993; **81**: 734–44.

14 Osterud B. The role of platelets in decrypting monocyte tissue factor. *Semin Hematol* 2001; **38**: 2–5.

15 Bom VJ, Bertina RM. The contributions of Ca^{2+}, phospholipids and tissue-factor apoprotein to the activation of human blood-coagulation factor X by activated factor VII. *Biochem J* 1990; **265**: 327–36.

16 Osterud B, Rapaport SI. Activation of factor IX by the reaction product of tissue factor and factor VII: additional pathway for initiating blood coagulation. *Proc Natl Acad Sci USA* 1977; **74**: 5260–4.

17 Lawson JH, Mann KG. Cooperative activation of human factor IX by the human extrinsic pathway of blood coagulation. *J Biol Chem* 1991; **266**: 11317–27.

18 Butenas S, DiLorenzo ME, Mann KG. Ultrasensitive fluorogenic substrates for serine proteases. *Thromb Haemost* 1997; **78**: 1193–201.

19 Brass LF. Thrombin and platelet activation. *Chest* 2003; **124**: 18S–25S.

20 Mann KG, Kalafatis M. Factor V: a combination of Dr Jekyll and Mr Hyde. *Blood* 2003; **101**: 20–30.

21 Fay PJ. Subunit structure of thrombin-activated human factor VIIIa. *Biochim Biophys Acta* 1988; **952**: 181–90.

22 Mann KG, Krishnaswamy S, Lawson JH. Surface-dependent hemostasis. *Semin Hematol* 1992; **29**: 213–26.

23 Ahmad SS, Rawala-Sheikh R, Walsh PN. Components and assembly of the factor X activating complex. *Semin Thromb Hemost* 1992; **18**: 311–23.

24 Hockin MF, Jones KC, Everse SJ, Mann KG. A model for the stoichiometric regulation of blood coagulation. *J Biol Chem* 2002; **277**: 18322–33.

25 Girard TJ, Warren LA, Novotny WF, *et al.* Functional significance of the Kunitz-type inhibitory domains of lipoprotein-associated coagulation inhibitor. *Nature* 1989; **338**: 518–20.

26 Cawthern KM, van't Veer C, Lock JB, DiLorenzo ME, Branda RF, Mann KG. Blood coagulation in hemophilia A and hemophilia C. *Blood* 1998; **91**: 4581–92.

27 Baugh RJ, Broze GJ, Jr, Krishnaswamy S. Regulation of extrinsic pathway factor Xa formation by tissue factor pathway inhibitor. *J Biol Chem* 1998; **273**: 4378–86.

28 Novotny WF, Brown SG, Miletich JP, Rader DJ, Broze GJ, Jr. Plasma antigen levels of the lipoprotein-associated coagulation inhibitor in patient samples. *Blood* 1991; **78**: 387–93.

29 Seligsohn U. Factor XI deficiency. *Thromb Haemost* 1993; **70**: 68–71.

30 Gailani D, Broze GJ, Jr. Factor XI activation in a revised model of blood coagulation. *Science* 1991; **253**: 909–12.

31 Colman RW. Contact activation pathway: Inflammatory, fibrinolytic, anticoagulant, antiadhesive and antiangiogenic activities. In: Colman RW, Hirsh J, Marder VJ, Clowes AW, George JN (eds.) *Hemostasis and Thrombosis: Basic Principles and Clinical Practice*. Philadelphia: Lippincott Williams & Wilkins, 2001: 103–21.

32 Undas A, Brummel-Ziedins KE, Mann KG. Antithrombotic properties of aspirin and resistance to aspirin: beyond strictly antiplatelet actions. *Blood* 2007; **109**: 2285–92.

33 Brummel-Ziedins K, Vossen CY, Rosendaal FR, Umezaki K, Mann KG. The plasma hemostatic proteome: thrombin

generation in healthy individuals. *J Thromb Haemost* 2005; **3**: 1472–81.

34 Mann KG, Brummel-Ziedins K, Undas A, Butenas S. Does the genotype predict the phenotype? Evaluations of the hemostatic proteome. *J Thromb Haemost* 2004; **2**: 1727–34.

35 Mann KG. *Coagulation Explosion: Tissue Factor Pathway*. Haematologic Technologies, 2002.

36 Butenas S, Parhami-Seren B, Mann, KG. The influence of von Willebrand factor on factor VIII activity measurements. *J Thromb Haemost* 2009; **7**(1): 132–7.

37 Butenas S, Parhami-Seren B, Undas A, Fass DN, Mann KG. The "normal" factor VIII concentration in plasma. *Thromb Res* 2010; **126**(2): 119–23.

CHAPTER 2
Cellular processing of factor VIII and factor IX

Michael U. Callaghan[1] and Randal J. Kaufman[2]
[1] Children's Hospital of Michigan, Michigan, USA
[2] Sanford-Burnham Medical Research Institute, California, USA

Factor VIII and hemophilia A

Hemostasis is a tightly controlled process that enables plasma and cellular blood components to perform their functions in a fluid phase. However, upon damage to the lining of a blood vessel, an insoluble clot must be formed at the site of injury to minimize loss of blood components. This process is initiated by activation of platelets and the formation of a primary platelet plug followed by the coordinated and highly regulated formation of a stable fibrin cross-linked network. Hemostasis is further facilitated by the regulated interaction of the vitamin K-dependent proteases, protease cofactors, membrane surfaces and receptors, calcium ions, and protease inhibitors. This occurs through the rapid and sequential activation of three separate vitamin K-dependent serine proteases, factors VII (VII), factor IX (IX), and factor X (FX), with their cofactors, tissue factor, factor VIII (FVIII), and factor V (FV), that make up the intrinsic, extrinsic, and common coagulation pathways, respectively. These pathways act to rapidly and efficiently cleave the vitamin K-dependent zymogen prothrombin to its active serine protease form, thrombin, at the site of injury, leading to cleavage of soluble fibrinogen to insoluble fibrin and clot formation.

Factor VIII travels in the plasma in an inactive form that is cleaved by thrombin to form FVIIIa. FVIIIa acts as an essential cofactor for FIXa in the intrinsic coagulation cascade, amplifying FIXa activity by several orders of magnitude. The physiologic significance of these pathways is evident from genetic deficiencies that result in bleeding disorders. In the absence of FVIII, clot formation is impaired leading to prolonged bleeding. Mutations in *F8*, the gene coding for coagulation FVIII, leading to deficiency of FVIII or impaired FVIII function, result in the clinical disease hemophilia A. Hemophilia was recognized for over 2000 years as an X-linked bleeding disorder characterized by spontaneous bleeding into joints and muscles and severe bleeding from trauma. Treatment of hemophilia A has steadily improved since the discovery in the 19th century that whole blood transfusion improved coagulation in patients with hemophilia. In the 1980s the gene for FVIII was cloned and this discovery led quickly to the production of recombinant FVIII in mammalian cells for replacement therapy in patients. Proteins involved in the coagulation cascade require post-translational modifications for appropriate secretion, plasma half-life, and function. Recombinant DNA technology has provided the ability to produce safe and efficacious preparations of FVIII, as well as FIX, for protein replacement therapy. Gene therapy approaches for hemophilia B have shown promise in clinical trials, and gene therapy trials for hemophilia A are approaching but will need to consider the requirement for proper post-translational modification in protein secretion and function.

Factor VIII expression

The site of *in-vivo* expression of FVIII has not been definitively determined. However, animal experiments involving transplant livers from a wild-type animal to a FVIII-deficient animal have resulted in production of FVIII in the previously deficient animal [1], and transplantation of livers from FVIII-deficient animals into wild-type animals did not result in FVIII deficiency suggesting other sites of production as well [2]. Immunohistochemical studies have detected FVIII in hepatocytes [3], and studies have identified FVIII mRNA in a variety of organs [4]. However, most definitive characterization of the site of FVIII synthesis was performed in the mouse and demonstrated it is produced in sinusoidal endothelial cells, as well as additional vascular endothelial beds in the body [5,6].

Domain structure of factor VIII

Factor VIII and FV are homologous glycoproteins that serve as cofactors for proteolytic activation of FX and prothrombin, respectively. These cofactors act to increase the V_{max} of substrate activation by four orders of magnitude. They have a conserved domain organization of A1-A2-B-A3-C1-C2 [7] (Figure 2.1). The A domains of FV and FVIII are homologous to the A domains of the plasma copper-binding protein ceruloplasmin. Copper was detected in FVIII and its presence is associated with

Textbook of Hemophilia, Third Edition. Edited by Christine A. Lee, Erik E. Berntorp and W. Keith Hoots.
© 2014 John Wiley & Sons, Ltd. Published 2014 by John Wiley & Sons, Ltd.

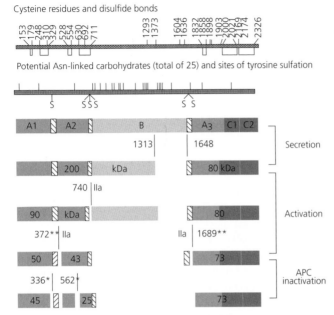

Cysteine residues and disulfide bonds

Potential Asn-linked carbohydrates (total of 25) and sites of tyrosine sulfation

Figure 2.1 Domain structure and processing of factor VIII (FVIII). The structural domains of FVIII are depicted: A1 domain (1-336), A2 domain (372-740), B domain (740-1648), A3 domain (1690-2020), and the C domains (2021-2332). On top the pairing of disulfide bonds is shown. Below are represented the potential N-linked glycosylation sites (vertical bars up). Three regions (stippled areas) rich in acidic amino acid residues lie between domains A1 and A2, A2 and B, B and A3 contain sites of tyrosine sulfation (s). Intracellularly, FVIII is cleaved within the B domain after Arg1313 and Arg1648 to generate an approximately 200 kDa peptide and the 80 kDa light chain. The two cleavages required for thrombin activation are indicated (**). The sites for activated protein C (APC) cleavage and inactivation are also shown (*).

functional FVIII activity [8]. One mole of reduced Cu(I) was detected in recombinant FVIII and likely resides within a type 1 copper ion-binding site within the A1 domain that uses Cys310 as a ligand [9]. The C domains are homologous to phospholipid-binding proteins, such as milk-fat globule protein, suggesting a role in phospholipid interaction. Whereas the amino acid sequences in the A and C domains are 40% identical between FV and FVIII, there is only limited homology between the B domains. However, the B domains of both proteins have conserved the addition of a large number of asparagine-linked oligosaccharides as well as a large number of serine/threonine-linked oligosaccharides, suggesting a role of the carbohydrate in cofactor function.

The crystal structure of a B domain-less FVIII was solved revealing a triangular heterotrimer composed of the three A domains with the A1 domain interacting with the C2 domain and the A3 domain interacting with the C1 domain [10,11]. These crystal structure and biochemical studies have yielded an in-silico model of the activated FVIII-activated FIX complex with FIXa wrapping across the side of FVIIIa and forming an

extended area of interaction including large portions of both the heavy and light chains of FVIII [11]. Interestingly these FVIII structures contain two Cu^{2+} ions and one or two Ca^{2+} ions and three asparagine-linked carbohydrate moieties which are essential to the structure [10].

Factors VIII and V have aminoterminal signal peptides of 19 and 28 amino acid residues, respectively, that are removed upon translocation into the endoplasmic reticulum (ER). FV is secreted from hepatocytes as a single-chain polypeptide of 330 kDa. In contrast, FVIII is processed within the secretory pathway in the cell to yield a heterodimer comprised primarily of a heavy chain extending up to 200 kDa (primarily two species from residues 1 to 1313 or 1648, where residue 1 is the aminoterminal amino acid after signal peptide cleavage) in a metal-ion dependent association with an 80 kDa light chain (residues 1649 to 2332) (Figure 2.1). This association is stabilized by noncovalent interactions between the aminoterminal and carboxyterminal ends of the FVIII light chain with the amino terminus of mature von Willebrand factor (VWF). VWF interaction stabilizes FVIII upon secretion from the cell, inhibits FVIII binding to phospholipids, and increases the half-life of FVIII circulating in plasma [12]. The ratio of VWF to FVIII is maintained at 50:1, where an increase or decrease in the plasma VWF level results in a corresponding change in the level of FVIII.

Factor V and FVIII circulate in plasma as inactive precursors that are activated through limited proteolysis by either thrombin or activated FX (FXa). Thrombin activation of FVIII results in cleavage initially after Arg 740 and subsequently after Arg residues 372 and 1689. Cleavage at Arg372 and 1689 are both required for activation of FVIII procoagulant activity. The cleavage at 1689 releases activated FVIII from VWF, thereby relieving the inhibitory activity of VWF on FVIII permitting the activated form of FVIII to interact with negatively charged phospholipids. Thrombin-activated FVIII consists of a heterotrimer of a 50 kDa A1-domain derived polypeptide, a 43 kDa A2-domain derived polypeptide, and a 73 kDa derived light chain fragment. Upon thrombin activation, the B domains of both FV and FVIII are released. B-domain-deleted F8 genes are now used in many gene therapy experiments and in the production of recombinant FVIII protein by many pharmaceutical companies. These deletions have employed various short modified linkers between the A3 and C1 domains [13–18]. The aminoterminal sides of the thrombin cleavage sites within FV and FVIII are rich in acidic amino acids, and contain the post-translationally modified amino acid, tyrosine sulfate. Stability and activity of FVIII depends on interactions between subunits with dissociation of the A2 domain resulting in inactivity and mutations that alter interdomain interactions affecting stability and function [19].

Disulfide bond formation

Factor VIII and FV also have a conserved disulfide bonding pattern in which two disulfide bonds occur within the A1 and

A2 domains, whereas only the small disulfide loop is present in their A3 domains. In addition, each C domain in FV and VIII contains one disulfide bond [20]. There are a number of nondisulfide bonded cysteine residues within FVIII; one cysteine residue is not oxidized in each A domain and there are four cysteine residues within the B domain that are also likely not oxidized. Disulfide bond formation occurs in the oxidizing environment of the ER and it is possible that protein thiol-disulfide isomerases such as protein disulfide isomerase are important to ensure proper disulfide bond formation and exchange occurs prior to exit from the ER. FVIII contains a total of eight disulfide bonds; interestingly, seven of these are found in FV. Replacement of cysteine residues with glycine in any of the seven conserved bonding pairs in FVIII resulted in impaired secretion while elimination of the disulfide loop pairing residues 1899 and 1903 in FVIII resulted in improved secretion [21].

Asparagine- and serine/threonine-linked glycosylation

Addition of N-linked oligosaccharides to many glycoproteins is an obligatory event for the folding and assembly of newly synthesized polypeptides. The presence of oligosaccharides is often required for the efficient transport of individual glycoproteins through the secretory pathway [22,23]. In addition, N-linked glycosylation frequently affects the plasma half-life and biologic activity of glycoproteins. The consensus site for N-linked glycosylation is Asn-Xxx-Ser/Thr where Xxx may be any amino acid except for proline. The utilization of a particular consensus site for N-linked oligosaccharide attachment is determined by the structure of the growing polypeptide. As a consequence, proteins expressed in heterologous cells most frequently exhibit occupancy of N-linked sites very similar to that of the native polypeptide.

After addition of the high mannose containing oligosaccharide core structure (composed of glucose$_3$-mannose$_9$-N-acetylglucosamine$_2$) to consensus asparagine residues, trimming begins with the removal of the three terminal glucose residues that is mediated by the action of glucosidases I and II. Glucosidase I removes the terminal α1–3 glucose and glucosidase II subsequently removes the two α1–2 glucose residues. Glucose trimming is required for binding to the protein chaperones calnexin and calreticulin within the lumen of the ER. Prolonged association with Calnexin (CNX) and/or Calreticulin (CRT) is observed when proteins are unfolded, misfolded, or unable to oligomerize. CNX and CRT bind most avidly to monoglucosylated forms of the N-linked core structure. Removal of the third glucose from the oligosaccharide core structure correlates with release from CNX and CRT and transport to the Golgi apparatus. The selectivity in binding of unfolded glycoproteins to CRT and CNX is mediated by reglucosylation of the deglucosylated N-linked oligosaccharide. This reglucosylation activity is performed by a uridine diphosphate (UDP)-glucose:glycoprotein glucosyltransferase (UGT). Only

unfolded, mutant, or unassembled proteins are subject to reglucosylation. Reglucosylated proteins rebind CNX and/or CRT and in this manner, unfolded proteins are retained in the ER through a cycle on CNX/CRT interaction, glucosidase II activity, and UGT activity. Subsequent to glucose trimming in the ER, at least one α1–2-linked mannose is removed by an ER α1–2 mannosidase prior to transport out of the ER. This system acts as a quality control mechanism allowing only properly folded FV or FVIII to be translocated out of the ER for secretion while sequestering or sending misfolded proteins to the proteasome through ER associated degradation (ERAD) pathways.

Upon transit through the Golgi apparatus, a series of additional carbohydrate modifications occur that are separated spatially and temporarily and involve the removal of mannose residues by Golgi mannosidases I and II and the addition of N-acetylglucosamine, fucose, galactose, and sialic acid residues. These reactions occur by specific glycosyltransferases that modify the high mannose carbohydrate to complex forms. Also within the Golgi apparatus, O-linked oligosaccharides are attached to the hydroxyl of serine or threonine residues through an O-glycosidic bond to N-acetylgalactosamine. Serine and threonine residues subject to glycosylation are frequently clustered together and contain an increased frequency of proline residues in the region, especially at positions −1 and +3, relative to the glycosylated residue. Galactose, fucose, and sialic acid are frequently attached to the serine/threonine-linked N-acetylgalactosamine. O-glycosylation occurs in the Golgi complex concomitant complex processing of with N-linked oligosaccharides.

Factor V and FVIII contain a large number of N-linked oligosaccharides. Comparison of the N-linked oligosaccharides present on recombinant FVIII expressed in mammalian cells to human plasma-derived FVIII indicated that both proteins display similar occupancy and complexity at the N-linked sites [12]. However, a detailed analysis demonstrated that differences in the microheterogeneity of oligosaccharides present on human plasma-derived FVIII and recombinant FVIII produced in baby hamster kidney cells do exist [24]. The light chains of FVIIIa and FVa migrate as doublets upon sodium dodecyl sulfate polyacrylamide gel electrophoresis (SDS-PAGE) due to differences in the complexity of N-linked oligosaccharides present on the light chain [25]. The difference in complexity of the N-linked sugars on the light chain does not affect FVIII activity. The majority of N-linked oligosaccharides within FVIII and FV occur within the B domain. N-linked oligosaccharides within the FV and FVIII B domains may be important to interact with the protein chaperone complex, lectin mannose-binding 1 (LMAN1)/multiple coagulation factor deficiency 2 (MCFD2) for facilitated transport from the ER to the Golgi compartment [26] (Figure 2.2). Mutations in either of the subunits of this heterodimeric complex cause combined deficiency of coagulation FV and FVIII [27]. MCFD2 appears to recruit FV and FVIII to the LMAN1 cargo complex and LMAN1 acts to recycle

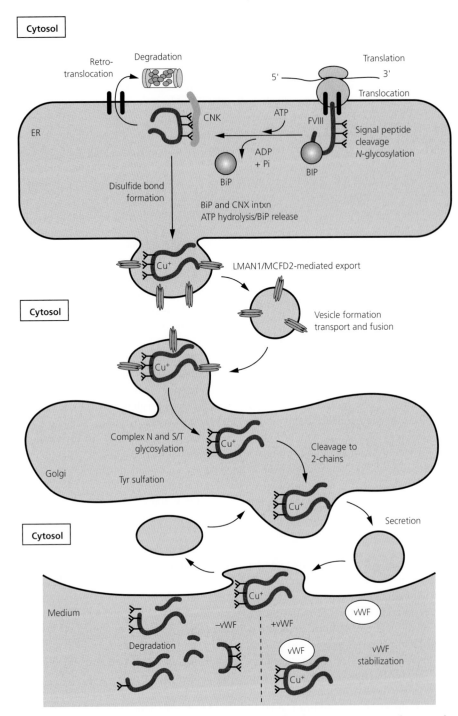

Figure 2.2 Synthesis, processing, and secretion of factor VIII (FVIII) in mammalian cells. The FVIII primary translation product is translocated into the lumen of the endoplasmic reticulum (ER) where *N*-linked glycosylation occurs. A fraction of FVIII binds tightly to the protein chaperone BiP and requires adenosine triphosphate (ATP) binding for release A portion of FVIII is retrotranslocated into the cytoplasm and is degraded by the cytosolic 26S proteasome ADP bound BiP has increased affinity for FVIII. Another fraction of the molecules interact with the lectins calnexin/calreticulin and then with the protein chaperone complex LMAN1/MCFD2 for transit to the Golgi apparatus. In the Golgi apparatus, additional processing occurs that includes complex modification of carbohydrate on *N*-linked sites, addition of carbohydrate to serine and threonine residues, sulfation of tyrosine residues, and cleavage of the protein to the mature heavy and light chains. ADP, adenosine diphosphate; CNX calnexin; vWF, von Willebrand factor.

MCFD2 back to the ER. In the absence of LMAN1, MCFD2 is secreted from the cell [28]. Patients that have MCFD2 mutations exhibit lower circulating levels of FV and FVIII compared to those with LMAN1 mutations [29].

Detailed analysis of recombinant FVIII demonstrated that 3% of the total sugar chains contain a Galα1-3Gal group on some of the outer chains of the bi-, tri-, and tetra-antennary complex-type sugar chains that is absent on FVIII derived from human plasma. This structure was present in Kogenate (prepared from baby hamster kidney cells) and not in recombinate [prepared from Chinese hamster ovary (CHO) cells] [24]. The α1-3 galactosyltransferase that produces this structure is expressed in most nonprimate mammalian cells and primates frequently develop antibodies to this structure. Approximately 1% of immunoglobulin in human plasma is directed toward this moiety, so it is expected that antibodies should be detected. A limited clinical trial did not detect any difference in the efficacy and/or half-life of FVIII that contains the Galα1-3Gal group. Therefore, there is no evidence of detrimental effects of this structure present on recombinant FVIII. However, increasingly, regulatory agencies are requiring detailed characterization of glycosylation and some pharmaceutical companies have gone to production in human cell lines to produce recombinant FVIII with glycosylation patterns most similar to native plasma FVIII [30].

Chaperone-assisted factor VIII folding

Factor VIII protein is secreted at markedly lower levels than similar proteins including FV [31]. Secretion of FV and FVIII in the proper tertiary and quaternary structure requires considerable chaperone-dependent folding assistance in the ER. FVIII folding is considerably onerous than even the homologous protein FV and this accounts for the major difference in secretion efficiency [25]. Misfolded, unfolded, or defective proteins are retained for refolding in the ER, degraded through ER-associated degradation (ERAD) by retrotranslocation into the cytosol and degradation by the 26S proteasome, or subject to macroautophagy where bulk segments of the ER are digested by autophagosomes [23,32].

Newly synthesized FVIII interacts with the ER luminal chaperone immunoglobulin-binding protein (BiP/GRP78), a member of the heat shock protein 70 (hsp70) family which exhibit a peptide-dependent adenosine triphosphatase (ATPase) activity. As FVIII is translated and translocated into the ER, BiP interacts with FVIII transiently and retains FVIII within the ER lumen. Increased expression of FVIII induces transcription of the BiP(Hsp5a) gene [33] and the level of BiP inversely correlates with FVIII secretion efficiency. Overexpressed BiP complexes with FVIII to retain it in the ER [34]. Interestingly, porcine FVIII does not exhibit strong interaction with BiP and is secreted more efficiently [35]. Site-directed mutation of Phe-309Ser in FVIII reduces interaction with BiP and improves FVIII secretion efficiency [36,37]. Disassociation of wild-type

FVIII from BiP requires more ATP than does dissociation of the Phe309Ser mutant from BiP [36,38]. Recently, chemical chaperones were shown to improve FVIII secretion [39]. In addition, accumulation of misfolded FVIII in the ER lumen was sufficient to increase production of reactive oxygen species (ROS) [40]. Significantly, treatment with antioxidant butylated hydroanisole either *in vitro* or *in vivo* upon *FVIII* gene delivery to the liver in mice prevented UPR activation, reduced ROS production and cell death, and improved FVIII folding and secretion [40].

An increase in FVIII synthesis causes it to accumulate in the ER in a misfolded and aggregated state, inducing the expression of protein chaperones, eventually leading to apoptosis [33]. These findings contributed to the discovery a tripartite signaling system, termed the unfolded protein response (UPR), that evolved to adapt the ER protein folding capacity with the ER protein folding load [32,41]. The UPR is composed of three ER transmembrane sensors, IRE1α, PERK, and ATF6α, that signal to attenuate general protein synthesis and increase transcription of genes encoding ER components for protein folding, protein trafficking, and degradation of misfolded proteins to decrease the toxic accumulation of misfolded proteins in the ER lumen.

Tyrosine sulfation

Sulfate addition to tyrosine as an O^4-sulfate ester is a common post-translational modification of secretory proteins that occurs in the *trans*-Golgi apparatus and is mediated by tyrosylprotein sulfotransferase that utilizes the activated sulfate donor 3'-phosphoadenosine 5'-phosphosulfate (PAPS). This modification occurs on many secretory proteins including a number of proteins that interact with thrombin, such as hirudin, fibrinogen, heparin cofactor II, α2-antiplasmin, vitronectin, and bovine FX. In addition, both FV and FVIII contain multiple sites of tyrosine sulfation [42,43]. Tyrosine sulfation can modulate the biologic activity, binding affinities, and secretion of specific proteins. For example, tyrosine sulfation at the carboxy terminus of hirudin increases its binding affinity to the anion binding exosite of thrombin.

Recombinant FVIII contains six sites of tyrosine sulfation at residues 346, 718, 719, 723, 1664, and 1680 [44]. All sites are sulfated to near completion, so it does not appear that this modification is inefficient in CHO cells, with 1.5–8% nonsulfation compared to complete sulfation in recombinant FVIII produced in human cell lines [30]. Site-directed mutagenesis was used to change individual or multiple tyrosine residues to the conserved residue phenylalanine in order to identify their role in FVIII function. Tyrosine sulfation at all six sites was required for full FVIII activity. In addition, mutagenesis of Tyr1680 to Phe demonstrated that sulfation at that residue was required for high-affinity interaction with VWF [42]. In the absence of tyrosine sulfation at 1680 in FVIII, the affinity for VWF was reduced by fivefold. In contrast, mutation at residue Tyr1664 did not affect VWF interaction. The significance of the Tyr1680 sulfation *in vivo* is made evident by the presence of a Tyr1680 to Phe mutation that causes a moderate hemophilia A, likely due to reduced interaction with VWF and decreased plasma half-life [45]. The other sites of tyrosine sulfation within FVIII affect the rate of cleavage by thrombin at the adjacent thrombin cleavage site. It was suggested that thrombin selectively utilizes the tyrosine sulfate residues adjacent to cleavage sites in FV and FVIII to facilitate interaction and/or cleavage.

Phosphorylation of serine and threonine residues

Phosphate has been observed in FV and FVIII, although its significance remains unknown. Exposure of FV and FVIII to activated platelets results in phosphorylation of serine residues in FV and primarily threonine residues in FVIII [46]. Phosphorylation can occur within the heavy chain of FVa and both the heavy chain and light chains of FVIII, possibly within the acidic acid rich regions. Phosphorylation of FVIII by casein kinase II is thought to occur within the acidic regions 337 through 372 and 1649 through 1689. Although the kinase responsible for the phosphorylation remains unknown, it may be related to casein kinase II [47]. Partially phosphorylated FVa was shown to be more sensitive to APC inactivation, suggesting phosphorylation of these cofactors may down regulate their activity.

Proteolytic processing

Factor VIII proteolytic processing within the B domain after arginine residues 1313 and 1648 can saturate the proteolytic machinery of the cell. Both arginine residues at 1313 and 1648 have consensus sites for *furin*/PACE cleavage (Lys-Arg-Xaa-Arg). In this case, secretion of heavy chains that extend to residue 1648 and secretion of light chains that extend to 1313 can be detected. In addition, some single chain FVIII is detected in conditioned medium from transfected mammalian cells and in heparin-treated human plasma [12,48]. Recently however, a mutation altering a furin cleavage site in canine FVIII was shown to result in increased FVIII activity that was attributed to increased stability, possibly a consequence of reducing dissociation of the heavy and light chains [49]. These observations have contributed to interest in developing single chain FVIII protein for therapeutic use in hemophilia [50].

Summary

Eukaryotic cells contain an extensive machinery to modify polypeptides that transit the secretory compartment. In the case of coagulation FVIII, a large number of post-translational modifications occur; many are required for secretion of the polypeptide and others are required for functional activity of the polypeptide. Proper synthesis and secretion of FVIII requires that the primary translation product is modified by signal peptide cleavage and core high mannose oligosaccharide addition upon translocation into the lumen of the ER. Within the ER, FVIII requires trimming of glucose residues on the core

N-linked glycans for transport to the Golgi compartment. In the Golgi compartment additional modifications occur that include: (1) tyrosine sulfation of six residues that are required for efficient activation by thrombin and for high-affinity VWF interaction; (2) extensive addition of oligosaccharides to many Ser/Thr residues within the B domain; (3) complex modification of *N*-linked glycans; and (4) cleavage of single-chain FVIII to its heavy and light chain species. To date, there do not appear to be any specific post-translational modifications that significantly limit secretion and/or functional activity of FVIII. Further studies are required to elucidate the effect of FVIII expression in different cell types in order to identify the importance that subtle differences in post-translational modifications may have on their secretion, *in vivo* half-life, and function. These considerations will be important when considering different cells and tissues as targets for gene therapy.

Factor IX and hemophilia B

Hemophilia B is caused by mutations in the *F9* gene leading to deficient or defective FIX in its role as a serine protease in the intrinsic coagulation cascade. These mutations result in slow clot formation and prolonged bleeding. Hemophilia B was recognized as a clinical entity distinct from hemophilia A when it was noted that mixing plasma from patients with one hemophilia corrected the prolonged clotting times from patients with the other hemophilia [51]. The primary structure of human FIX was determined from affinity-purified FIX from plasma and the cDNA sequence was cloned using oligonucleotides derived from the bovine FIX amino acid sequence [52–54]. This work led to the development of recombinant FIX produced in CHO cells for clinical use in patients with hemophilia B [55]. Prior to being secreted from hepatocytes, FIX undergoes γ-carboxylation, *O*- and *N*-linked glycosylation, phosphorylation, sulfation, disulfide bond formation, and β-hydroxylation as well as cleavage of the signal peptide and propeptide. Recent gene therapy trials in hemophilia B using adenovirus-associated viral vector delivery to hepatocytes have shown safety and efficacy [56]. Improved understanding of the mechanisms of FIX processing and secretion has important implications for both production of recombinant FIX and future gene therapy trials in hemophilia B as evidenced by the incorporation of the recently described gain of function Padua mutation in new gene therapy protocols [57].

Domain structure of factor IX

The domain structures of the vitamin K-dependent coagulation factors FVII, FIX, and FX, and prothrombin, protein C, and protein S deduced from their cDNA sequences demonstrate that they contain common structural features [58] (Figure 2.3). All contain a signal peptide that is required for translocation into the lumen of the ER. This is followed by a propeptide that directs vitamin K-dependent γ-carboxylation of the mature

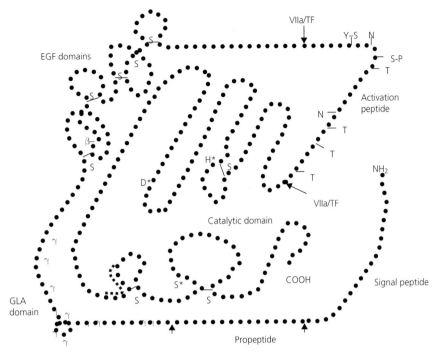

Figure 2.3 Domain structure and processing of factor IX (FIX). FIX is composed of a signal peptide, propeptide, γ-carboxyglutamic acid domain (GLA), epidermal growth factor (EGF)-like domains, activation peptide, and serine protease catalytic domain. Short arrows represent intracellular processing sites that cleave away the signal peptide and propeptide. The long arrows represent the cleavages required for activation by factor VIIa/tissue factor (VIIa/TF) or FXIa. The 35 amino acid activation peptide is indicated. γ represents γ-carboxyglutamic acid and β represents β-hydroxyaspartic acid. The 330-338 loop that interacts with factor VIII is shown by a dotted line. Also indicated are sites of addition of asparagine-linked oligosaccharides (N), serine or threonine-linked oligosaccharides (S and T, respectively), tyrosine sulfation (Y-S), and serine phosphorylation (S-P).

polypeptide. Upon transit through the *trans*-Golgi apparatus the propeptide is cleaved away by furin. The aminoterminus of the mature protein contains a γ-carboxyglutamic acid rich region (Gla) that includes a short α-helical stack of aromatic amino acids. Then there are two epidermal growth factor (EGF)-like domains. In FIX, protein C, and FX, the aminoterminal EGF domain contains ß-hydroxyaspartic acid (Hya) at homologous locations. The next region is the activation peptide (12-52 residues) that is glycosylated on asparagine residues and is released by specific proteolysis accompanying activation. The remainder of the vitamin K-dependent protease comprises the serine protease catalytic triad that is absent in protein S.

Disulfide bond formation

The vitamin K-dependent coagulation factors, exemplified by FIX, have conserved disulfide bonds. Generally, three disulfide bonds occur within each EGF domain, and several disulfide bonds occur within the serine protease catalytic domain. In addition, FIX has a disulfide bond that connects the aminoterminal half with the carboxyterminal half of the protein so that after activation, the two portions of the molecule do not dissociate. In FIX, cysteine residues at 18 and 23 within the Gla domain form a small essential disulfide loop where mutations at either cysteine residue results in severe hemophilia B [59].

Asparagine- and serine/threonine-linked glycosylation

With the development of recombinant FIX produced in CHO cells for the treatment of hemophilia B, a detailed characterization and comparison of the carbohydrate structures was performed between plasma-derived and recombinant-derived FIX [60]. In both plasma- and recombinant-derived FIX, Asn157 and Asn167 within the activation peptide are fully occupied with complex-type *N*-glycans [61]. Recombinant FIX contains tetra-antennary, tetra-sialylated, and core fucosylated glycans at both sites. Plasma-derived FIX contains bi-, tri-, and tetra-antennary, sialylated glycans, with and without fucose. Both molecules have a range of minor structures; however, the glycans present on plasma-derived FIX are considerably more heterogeneous and diverse. The diversity may be a consequence of the plasma pool. Recent work has demonstrated production of FIX in human hepatoma cells produced a glycosylation pattern more similar to plasma FIX [62] and the addition of glycosylation sites through mutagenesis increased half-life considerably [63].

Both plasma- and recombinant-derived FIX contain a number of *O*-linked oligosaccharides. In the first FIX EGF domain, serine residues 53 and 61 are uniformly *O*-glycosylated. The EGF1 domain in both recombinant- and plasma-derived

FIX contains nonclassic *O*-linked glycans at Ser53 and Ser61. Ser53 contains Xyl-Xyl-Glc-Ser and Ser61 contains the tetrasaccharide with a terminal sialic acid (NeuAc), NeuAc-Gal-GlcNac-Fuc-Ser61 [61,64]. This indicates that CHO cells (the cells used as a host to produce recombinant FIX) have the enzymatic machinery to produce the structures present on plasma-derived FIX that is synthesized in human hepatocytes and that it is not saturated at high expression levels. The carbohydrate structure at Ser61 in FIX contains fucose-linked tetrasaccharide with a terminal sialic acid. Ser61 within the first EGF domain of FIX has the consensus sequence (C-X-X-G-G-T/S-C) for fucosyl modification of *O*-linked sugars and is also found in FVII, but not in FX. However, a crystal structure of FIX demonstrated that both these *O*-linked modifications reside on the face of the EGF domain that apparently does not interact with other components of the FX-ase complex [65]. In addition to serine-linked oligosaccharide addition in the first EGF domain, both plasma-derived and recombinant-derived FIX molecules are partially occupied by *O*-linked glycans at residues Thr159, Thr169, Thr172, and Thr179 as well as at yet unidentified additional sites [61]. The function of these *O*-linked glycans remains unknown.

γ-Carboxylation of glutamic acid residues

The vitamin K-dependent coagulation factors contain the post-translationally modified amino acid γ-carboxyglutamic acid (Gla). The Gla residues are essential for these proteins to attain a calcium-dependent conformation and for their ability to bind phospholipid surfaces, an essential interaction for their function. The precursor of the vitamin K-dependent coagulation factors contain a propeptide that directs γ-carboxylation of up to 12 glutamic acid residues at the aminoterminus of the mature protein all of which is completed prior to translocation out of the ER [66,67]. The propeptides (residues −18 to −1 in FIX) of these factors share amino acid similarity by conservation of the γ-carboxylase recognition site and the site for furin cleavage of the propeptide.

The residues that are carboxylated in FIX are glutamic acid residues 7, 8, 15, 17, 20, 21, 26, 27, 30, 33, 36, and 40. Mutations at residues 6, 7, 17, 21, 27, 30, or 33 result in moderate to severe hemophilia B, indicating their functional importance. High level expression of the vitamin K-dependent plasma proteins in transfected mammalian cells is limited by the ability of the mammalian host cell to efficiently perform γ-carboxylation of aminoterminal glutamic acid residues and also to efficiently cleave the propeptide [58,68,69]. Analysis of FIX expressed in CHO cells revealed that the protein had a much lower specific activity compared to the natural human plasma-derived protein. The reduced specific activity was attributed to both the limited ability of CHO cells to cleave the propeptide of FIX as well to efficiently perform γ-carboxylation [55,69]. Generally, expression of FIX at levels greater than $1\,\mu g/10^6$ cells/day saturates the activity for most cells studied [68]. Overexpression of the γ-carboxylase did not improve γ-carboxylation of FIX when coexpressed in transfected mammalian cells [55]. These results suggest that the amount of carboxylase protein is not a limiting factor to direct vitamin K-dependent γ-carboxylation *in vivo*. Several possibilities exist for the inability of the overexpressed γ-carboxylase to improve FIX carboxylation *in vivo*. First, the overexpressed γ-carboxylase may be mislocalized within the secretory pathway. It is possible that another protein, such as a protein chaperone, may be required to utilize a more complex substrate such as FIX as opposed to a small peptide substrate. It is possible that another cofactor, possibly reduced vitamin K, is limiting for FIX carboxylation *in vivo*. Finally, as furin-mediated propeptide cleavage becomes limiting, the presence of the propeptide may interfere with gamma carboxylation [68]. Further information on the mechanism of γ-carboxylation reaction *in vivo* is required in order to elucidate the rate-limiting step for γ-carboxylation *in vivo*.

Recombinant FIX produced in CHO cells contains 11.8 Gla residues/mole of FIX, compared to plasma-derived FIX that contains 12 Gla residues/mole. The difference resides in the inefficient carboxylation of residues 36 and 40 within recombinant FIX [70]. In contrast to the first 10 Gla residues in FIX, glutamic acid residues 36 and 40 are not conserved in the other vitamin K-dependent coagulation factors. To date, no functional difference is observed between fully carboxylated FIX and FIX deficient in Gla at residues 36 and 40.

β-Hydroxylation of aspartic acid and asparagine

Blood coagulation factors FIX and FX, protein C, and protein S contain the modified amino acid erythro-ß-hydroxyaspartic acid in the first EGF domain. In addition, one molecule of β-hydroxy aspartic acid is found in each of the three carboxy-terminal EGF domains in protein S. Hydroxylation of both aspartic acid and asparagine is catalyzed by aspartyl ß-hydroxylase, requires 2-ketoglutarate and Fe^{+2}, and is inhibited by agents that inhibit 2-ketoglutarate-dependent dioxygenases. This enzyme recognizes a consensus sequence C-X-X-X-X-X-X-X-X-C in the β-sheet and C-X-D/N-X-X-X-X-Y/F-X in the antiparallel β-sheet [71]. β-Hydroxylation is unnecessary for high-affinity calcium binding to the first EGF domain [72]. In addition, inhibition of ß-hydroxylation of FIX expressed in mammalian cells did not reduce functional activity in FIX [73]. It is interesting that only 0.3 mol/mol of plasma FIX is modified by ß-hydroxylation at Asp64 and this same amount of ß-hydroxylation occurs in recombinant FIX expressed at high levels in CHO cells [73].

Tyrosine sulfation

Plasma-derived and recombinant-derived FIX are sulfated on Tyr155. Whereas plasma-derived FIX is mostly sulfated, recombinant FIX is approximately 15% sulfated [60,61]. This is one unusual example where a sulfated tyrosine occurs adjacent to an occupied *N*-linked glycosylation site (at asparagine residue 157). Plasma-derived FIX and plasma-derived FIX differ in their *in-vivo* recovery, where the absolute recovery of plasma-derived

FIX is approximately 50% and the recovery of recombinant FIX is approximately 30%. Studies suggest Tyr sulfation on FIX may be responsible for the difference in the recovery of these two sources of FIX [61]. For example, infusion of recombinant FIX enriched for full sulfation at Tyr155 demonstrated an equivalent recovery to plasma-derived FIX (approximately 50%). Similarly, removal of the sulfate as well as phosphate from plasma-derived FIX resulted in a molecule having a recovery similar to recombinant FIX. Finally, administration of recombinant FIX to hemophilia B dogs and isolation of the circulating FIX yielded species that were enriched with tyrosine sulfate compared to the starting material. The sum of these observations suggests that Tyr sulfation at 155 in FIX can influence *in-vivo* recovery.

Phosphorylation of serine and threonine residues

Phosphate has been observed in FIX, although its significance remains unknown. Plasma-derived FIX is fully phosphorylated at Ser158 whereas recombinant FIX contains no phosphate at this position [61,74]. FIX produced in myotubes had considerably less phosphorylation at Ser158 compared to plasma-derived FIX but maintained similar specific activity [75]. The presence or absence of phosphate or sulfate on FIX has no effect on the *in-vitro* clotting activity.

Factor IX Padua

Recently, a mutation R338L at an arginine residue that is highly conserved in FIX across mammalian species results in eightfold higher FIX activity and predisposition to thrombosis [76]. This site is important for interaction with FX and results in more efficient binding of FX by FIX. Recent studies have suggested that FIX Padua may be used as a transgene for gene therapy trials [57] and a recently initiated gene therapy trial is using FIX Padua.

Proteolytic processing

The requirement for propeptide processing for FIX function was first made apparent by identification mutations resulting in hemophilia B that prevent processing of the FIX propeptide. Mutations of the Arg at the P1 or P4 positions inhibit propeptide cleavage and the resultant FIX is secreted into the plasma but is nonfunctional due to the presence of the propeptide [77]. This mutant is unable to bind phospholipid vesicles and may also display reduced γ-carboxylation of glutamic acid residues [78]. It is likely that the presence of the propeptide yields a molecule that is defective in phospholipid interaction due to an inability to undergo a calcium-dependent conformation in the Gla domain.

Characterization of the amino acid requirements around the propeptide cleavage site has identified that both the P1 and P4 arginine are important for efficient processing mediated by *furin* and subtillisin-like proprotein convertase (PACE4) [79]. Overexpression of *furin* in transfected cells as well as in transgenic animals improves the processing ability to yield fully processed proteins [68]. Recombinant FIX is produced by coexpression with *furin*/PACE to ensure complete processing of the propeptide.

Summary

Factor IX undergoes a remarkable number of varied posttranslational modifications prior to secretion from the hepatocyte. Cotranslational translocation into the lumen of the ER occurs concomitantly with signal peptide cleavage and addition of core high mannose oligosaccharides to the polypeptide is followed in the ER by glucose trimming of the *N*-linked oligosaccharide core structures, γ-carboxylation of 12 aminoterminal glutamic acid residues, and β-hydroxylation of a portion of molecules on residue Asp64 occurs. Upon transit into the Golgi compartment additional modifications occur that include: (1) complex modification of *N*-linked oligosaccharides; (2) tyrosine sulfation at Tyr155; (3) Ser/Thr glycosylation at residues Ser61 and Ser53 as well as several Thr residues within the activation peptide; and (4) cleavage of the propeptide. In addition, FIX isolated from human plasma is phosphorylated at Ser158 within the activation peptide. A majority of the modifications within FIX occur within the activation peptide and may regulate activation of FIX. Appropriate γ-carboxylation and propeptide cleavage are essential for functional secretion and activity of secreted FIX. Both of these activities are easily saturated upon expression of FIX in heterologous cells. The large number of other modifications likely also affects FIX activity by mechanisms that are not understood to date. Further studies are required to elucidate the effect of FIX expression in different cell types in order to identify the importance that subtle differences in post-translational modifications may have on their secretion, *in-vivo* half-life, and function. These considerations will be important when considering different cells and tissues as targets for gene therapy.

Acknowledgments

RJK is supported by NIH grants HL057346 and HL052173.

References

1 Marchioro TL, Hougie C, Ragde H, Epstein RB, Thomas ED. Hemophilia: role of organ homografts. *Science* 1969; **163**(3863): 188–90.

2 Webster WP, Zukoski CF, Hutchin P, Reddick RL, Mandel SR, Penick GD. Plasma factor VIII synthesis and control as revealed by canine organ transplantation. *Am J Physiol* 1971; **220**(5): 1147–54.

3 Zelechowska MG, van Mourik JA, Brodniewicz-Proba T. Ultrastructural localization of factor VIII procoagulant antigen in human liver hepatocytes. *Nature* 1985; **317**(6039): 729–30.

4 Wion KL, Kelly D, Summerfield JA, Tuddenham EG, Lawn RM. Distribution of factor VIII mRNA and antigen in human liver and other tissues. *Nature* 1985; **317**(6039): 726–9.

5 Lesley Everett C, Cleuren AA, Khoriaty R, Ginsburg D. Coagulation factor VIII is synthesized in endothelial cells. *Blood* 2013; **122**(21).

6 Fahs SA, Hille MT, Montgomery RR. Transcriptional analysis of a tissue-specific factor VIII knockout model demonstrates the importance of endothelial factor viii synthesis. *Blood* 2013; **122**(21).

7 Toole JJ, Knopf JL, Wozney JM, *et al.* Molecular cloning of a cDNA encoding human antihaemophilic factor. *Nature* 1984; **312**(5992): 342–7.

8 Bihoreau N, Pin S, de Kersabiec AM, Vidot F, Fontaine-Aupart MP. Copper-atom identification in the active and inactive forms of plasma-derived FVIII and recombinant FVIII-delta II. *Eur J Biochem* 1994; **222**(1): 41–8.

9 Tagliavacca L, Moon N, Dunham WR, Kaufman RJ. Identification and functional requirement of Cu(I) and its ligands within coagulation factor VIII. *J Biol Chem* 1997; **272**(43): 27428–34.

10 Shen BW, Spiegel PC, Chang CH, *et al.* The tertiary structure and domain organization of coagulation factor VIII. *Blood* 2008; **111**(3): 1240–7.

11 Ngo JC, Huang M, Roth DA, Furie BC, Furie B. Crystal structure of human factor VIII: implications for the formation of the factor IXa–factor VIIIa complex. *Structure* 2008; **16**(4): 597–606.

12 Kaufman RJ, Wasley LC, Dorner AJ. Synthesis, processing, and secretion of recombinant human factor VIII expressed in mammalian cells. *J Biol Chem* 1988; **263**(13): 6352–62.

13 Paik SH, Kim YJ, Han SK, Kim JY, Park H, Park YI. Comparability studies of new 3rd generation recombinant human factor VIII GreenGene F after improvement of formulation and viral inactivation/removal process. *Biologicals* 2012; **40**(6): 405–14.

14 Stennicke HR, Kjalke M, Karpf DM, *et al.* A novel B-domain O-glycoPEGylated FVIII (N8-GP) demonstrates full efficacy and prolonged effect in hemophilic mice models. *Blood* 2013; **121**(11): 2108–16.

15 Thim L, Vandahl B, Karlsson J, *et al.* Purification and characterization of a new recombinant factor VIII (N8). *Haemophilia* 2010; **16**(2): 349–59.

16 Heinz S, Schuttrumpf J, Simpson JC, *et al.* Factor VIII-eGFP fusion proteins with preserved functional activity for the analysis of the early secretory pathway of factor VIII. *Thromb Haemost* 2009; **102**(5): 925–35.

17 Wiken M, Sjoberg K. Analysis of samples from patients treated with ReFacto for the presence of anti-SQ-peptide specific antibodies. *Semin Thromb Hemost* 2002; **28**(3): 297–308.

18 Kaufman RJ, Powell JS. Molecular approaches for improved clotting factors for hemophilia. Hematology/the Education Program of the American Society of Hematology. *Am Soc Hematol Educ Prog* 2013; **2013**: 30–6.

19 Pipe SW, Eickhorst AN, McKinley SH, Saenko EL, Kaufman RJ. Mild hemophilia A caused by increased rate of factor VIII A2 subunit dissociation: evidence for nonproteolytic inactivation of factor VIIIa in vivo. *Blood* 1999; **93**(1): 176–83.

20 McMullen BA, Fujikawa K, Davie EW, Hedner U, Ezban M. Locations of disulfide bonds and free cysteines in the heavy and light chains of recombinant human factor VIII (antihemophilic factor A). *Protein Sci* 1995; **4**(4): 740–6.

21 Selvaraj SR, Scheller AN, Miao HZ, Kaufman RJ, Pipe SW. Bioengineering of coagulation factor VIII for efficient expression through elimination of a dispensable disulfide loop. *J Thromb Haemost* 2012; **10**(1): 107–15.

22 Sousa M, Parodi AJ. The molecular basis for the recognition of misfolded glycoproteins by the UDP-Glc:glycoprotein glucosyltransferase. *EMBO J* 1995; **14**(17): 4196–203.

23 Ferris SP, Kodali VK. Glycoprotein folding and quality control. *Dis Models Mech* 2014 (in press).

24 Hironaka T, Furukawa K, Esmon PC, *et al.* Comparative study of the sugar chains of factor VIII purified from human plasma and from the culture media of recombinant baby hamster kidney cells. *J Biol Chem* 1992; **267**(12): 8012–20.

25 Pittman DD, Tomkinson KN, Kaufman RJ. Post-translational requirements for functional factor V and factor VIII secretion in mammalian cells. *J Biol Chem* 1994; **269**(25): 17329–37.

26 Cunningham MA, Pipe SW, Zhang B, Hauri HP, Ginsburg D, Kaufman RJ. LMAN1 is a molecular chaperone for the secretion of coagulation factor VIII. *J Thromb Haemost* 2003; **1**(11): 2360–7.

27 Zhang B, Cunningham MA, Nichols WC, *et al.* Bleeding due to disruption of a cargo-specific ER-to-Golgi transport complex. *Nat Genet* 2003; **34**(2): 220–5.

28 Nyfeler B, Zhang B, Ginsburg D, Kaufman RJ, Hauri HP. Cargo selectivity of the ERGIC-53/MCFD2 transport receptor complex. *Traffic* 2006; **7**(11): 1473–81.

29 Zhang B, Spreafico M, Zheng C, *et al.* Genotype–phenotype correlation in combined deficiency of factor V and factor VIII. *Blood* 2008; **111**(12): 5592–600.

30 Kannicht C, Ramstrom M, Kohla G, *et al.* Characterisation of the post-translational modifications of a novel, human cell line-derived recombinant human factor VIII. *Thromb Res* 2013; **131**(1): 78–88.

31 Lynch CM, Israel DI, Kaufman RJ, Miller AD. Sequences in the coding region of clotting factor VIII act as dominant inhibitors of RNA accumulation and protein production. *Hum Gene Ther* 1993; **4**(3): 259–72.

32 Kaufman RJ. Orchestrating the unfolded protein response in health and disease. *J Clin Invest* 2002; **110**(10): 1389–98.

33 Dorner AJ, Wasley LC, Kaufman RJ. Increased synthesis of secreted proteins induces expression of glucose-regulated proteins in butyrate-treated Chinese hamster ovary cells. *J Biol Chem* 1989; **264**(34): 20602–7.

34 Morris JA, Dorner AJ, Edwards CA, Hendershot LM, Kaufman RJ. Immunoglobulin binding protein (BiP) function is required to protect cells from endoplasmic reticulum stress but is not required for the secretion of selective proteins. *J Biol Chem* 1997; **272**(7): 4327–34.

35 Brown HC, Gangadharan B, Doering CB. Enhanced biosynthesis of coagulation factor VIII through diminished engagement of the unfolded protein response. *J Biol Chem* 2011; **286**(27): 24451–7.

36 Swaroop M, Moussalli M, Pipe SW, Kaufman RJ. Mutagenesis of a potential immunoglobulin-binding protein-binding site enhances secretion of coagulation factor VIII. *J Biol Chem* 1997; **272**(39): 24121–4.

37 Tagliavacca L, Wang Q, Kaufman RJ. ATP-dependent dissociation of non-disulfide-linked aggregates of coagulation factor VIII is a rate-limiting step for secretion. *Biochemistry* 2000; **39**(8): 1973–81.

38 Dorner AJ, Wasley LC, Kaufman RJ. Protein dissociation from GRP78 and secretion are blocked by depletion of cellular ATP levels. *Proc Natl Acad Sci USA* 1990; **87**(19): 7429–32.

39 Roth SD, Schuttrumpf J, Milanov P, *et al.* Chemical chaperones improve protein secretion and rescue mutant factor VIII in mice with hemophilia A. *PloS one* 2012; **7**(9): e44505.

40 Malhotra JD, Miao H, Zhang K, et al. Antioxidants reduce endoplasmic reticulum stress and improve protein secretion. *Proc Natl Acad Sci USA* 2008; **105**(47): 18525–30.

41 Cao SS, Kaufman RJ. Unfolded protein response. *Curr Biol* 2012; **22**(16): R622–6.

42 Michnick DA, Pittman DD, Wise RJ, Kaufman RJ. Identification of individual tyrosine sulfation sites within factor VIII required for optimal activity and efficient thrombin cleavage. *J Biol Chem* 1994; **269**(31): 20095–102.

43 Pittman DD, Tomkinson KN, Michnick D, Selighsohn U, Kaufman RJ. Posttranslational sulfation of factor V is required for efficient thrombin cleavage and activation and for full procoagulant activity. *Biochemistry* 1994; **33**(22): 6952–59.

44 Pittman DD, Wang JH, Kaufman RJ. Identification and functional importance of tyrosine sulfate residues within recombinant factor VIII. *Biochemistry* 1992; **31**(13): 3315–25.

45 Higuchi M, Wong C, Kochhan L, et al. Characterization of mutations in the factor VIII gene by direct sequencing of amplified genomic DNA. *Genomics* 1990; **6**(1): 65–71.

46 Rand MD, Kalafatis M, Mann KG. Platelet coagulation factor Va: the major secretory platelet phosphoprotein. *Blood* 1994; **83**(8): 2180–90.

47 Kalafatis M, Rand MD, Jenny RJ, Ehrlich YH, Mann KG. Phosphorylation of factor Va and factor VIIIa by activated platelets. *Blood* 1993; **81**(3): 704–19.

48 Ganz PR, Tackaberry ES, Palmer DS, Rock G. Human factor VIII from heparinized plasma. Purification and characterization of a single-chain form. *Eur J Biochem* 1988; **170**(3): 521–8.

49 Siner JI, Iacobelli NP, Sabatino DE, et al. Minimal modification in the factor VIII B-domain sequence ameliorates the murine hemophilia A phenotype. *Blood* 2013; **121**(21): 4396–403.

50 Schulte S. Innovative coagulation factors: albumin fusion technology and recombinant single-chain factor VIII. *Thromb Res* 2013; **131**(Suppl. 2): S2–6.

51 Schulman E, Smith CH. Hemorrhagic disease in an infant due to deficiency of a previously undescribed coagulation factor. *AMA Am J Dis Child* 1952; **84**(6): 758–60.

52 Andersson LO, Borg H, Miller-Andersson M. Purification and characterization of human factor IX. *Thromb Res* 1975; **7**(3): 451–9.

53 Choo KH, Gould KG, Rees DJ, Brownlee GG. Molecular cloning of the gene for human anti-haemophilic factor IX. *Nature* 1982; **299**(5879): 178–80.

54 Kurachi K, Davie EW. Isolation and characterization of a cDNA coding for human factor IX. *Proc Natl Acad Sci USA* 1982; **79**(21): 6461–4.

55 Kaufman RJ, Wasley LC, Furie BC, Furie B, Shoemaker CB. Expression, purification, and characterization of recombinant gamma-carboxylated factor IX synthesized in Chinese hamster ovary cells. *J Biol Chem* 1986; **261**(21): 9622–8.

56 Nathwani AC, Tuddenham EG, Rangarajan S, et al. Adenovirus-associated virus vector-mediated gene transfer in hemophilia B. *N Engl J Med* 2011; **365**(25): 2357–65.

57 Finn JD, Nichols TC, Svoronos N, et al. The efficacy and the risk of immunogenicity of FIX Padua (R338L) in hemophilia B dogs treated by AAV muscle gene therapy. *Blood* 2012; **120**(23): 4521–3.

58 Davie EW. Biochemical and molecular aspects of the coagulation cascade. *Thromb Haemost* 1995; **74**(1): 1–6.

59 Wojcik EG, van den Berg M, van der Linden IK, Poort SR, Cupers R, Bertina RM. Factor IX Zutphen: a Cys18->Arg mutation results in formation of a heterodimer with alpha 1-microglobulin and the inability to form a calcium-induced conformation. *Biochem J* 1995; **311**(Pt 3): 753–9.

60 White GC, 2nd, Beebe A, Nielsen B. Recombinant factor IX. *Thromb Haemost* 1997; **78**(1): 261–5.

61 Bond MD, Jankowski MA, Huberty MC. Structural analysis of recombinant human factor IX. *Blood* 1994; **84**: 194a.

62 Enjolras N, Dargaud Y, Perot E, Guillaume F, Becchi M, Negrier C. Human hepatoma cell line HuH-7 is an effective cellular system to produce recombinant factor IX with improved post-translational modifications. *Thromb Res* 2012; **130**(5): e266–73.

63 Brooks AR, Sim D, Gritzan U, et al. Glycoengineered Factor IX Variants with Improved Pharmacokinetics and Subcutaneous Efficacy. *J Thromb Haemost* 2013 (in press).

64 Hase S, Nishimura H, Kawabata S, Iwanaga S, Ikenaka T. The structure of (xylose)2glucose-O-serine 53 found in the first epidermal growth factor-like domain of bovine blood clotting factor IX. *J Biol Chem* 1990; **265**(4): 1858–61.

65 Brandstetter H, Bauer M, Huber R, Lollar P, Bode W. X-ray structure of clotting factor IXa: active site and module structure related to Xase activity and hemophilia B. *Proc Natl Acad Sci USA* 1995; **92**(21): 9796–800.

66 Bristol JA, Ratcliffe JV, Roth DA, Jacobs MA, Furie BC, Furie B. Biosynthesis of prothrombin: intracellular localization of the vitamin K-dependent carboxylase and the sites of gamma-carboxylation. *Blood* 1996; **88**(7): 2585–93.

67 Fryklund L, Borg H, Andersson LO. Amino-terminal sequence of human factor IX: presence of gamma-carboxyl glumatic acid residues. *FEBS Lett* 1976; **65**(2): 187–9.

68 Wasley LC, Rehemtulla A, Bristol JA, Kaufman RJ. PACE/furin can process the vitamin K-dependent pro-factor IX precursor within the secretory pathway. *J Biol Chem* 1993; **268**(12): 8458–65.

69 Rehemtulla A, Roth DA, Wasley LC, et al. In vitro and in vivo functional characterization of bovine vitamin K-dependent gamma-carboxylase expressed in Chinese hamster ovary cells. *Proc Natl Acad Sci USA* 1993; **90**(10): 4611–15.

70 Gillis S, Furie BC, Furie B, et al. gamma-Carboxyglutamic acids 36 and 40 do not contribute to human factor IX function. *Protein Sci* 1997; **6**(1): 185–96.

71 Stenflo J, Stenberg Y, Muranyi A. Calcium-binding EGF-like modules in coagulation proteinases: function of the calcium ion in module interactions. *Biochim Biophys Acta* 2000; **1477**(1–2): 51–63.

72 Sunnerhagen MS, Persson E, Dahlqvist I, et al. The effect of aspartate hydroxylation on calcium binding to epidermal growth factor-like modules in coagulation factors IX and X. *J Biol Chem* 1993; **268**(31): 23339–44.

73 Derian CK, VanDusen W, Przysiecki CT, et al. Inhibitors of 2-ketoglutarate-dependent dioxygenases block aspartyl beta-hydroxylation of recombinant human factor IX in several mammalian expression systems. *J Biol Chem* 1989; **264**(12): 6615–18.

74 Atoda H, Yokota E, Morita T. Characterization of a monoclonal antibody B1 that recognizes phosphorylated Ser-158 in the activation peptide region of human coagulation factor IX. *J Biol Chem* 2006; **281**(14): 9314–20.

75 Arruda VR, Hagstrom JN, Deitch J, *et al.* Posttranslational modifications of recombinant myotube-synthesized human factor IX. *Blood* 2001; **97**(1): 130–8.

76 Simioni P, Tormene D, Tognin G, *et al.* X-linked thrombophilia with a mutant factor IX (factor IX Padua). *N Engl J Med* 2009; **361**(17): 1671–5.

77 Bentley AK, Rees DJ, Rizza C, Brownlee GG. Defective propeptide processing of blood clotting factor IX caused by mutation of arginine to glutamine at position -4. *Cell* 1986; **45**(3): 343–8.

78 Diuguid DL, Rabiet MJ, Furie BC, Liebman HA, Furie B. Molecular basis of hemophilia B: a defective enzyme due to an unprocessed propeptide is caused by a point mutation in the factor IX precursor. *Proc Natl Acad Sci USA* 1986; **83**(16): 5803–7.

79 Rehemtulla A, Kaufman RJ. Preferred sequence requirements for cleavage of pro-von Willebrand factor by propeptide-processing enzymes. *Blood* 1992; **79**(9): 2349–55.

PART II

Hemophilia A

CHAPTER 3

Molecular basis of hemophilia A

Geoffrey Kemball-Cook[1] and Keith Gomez[2]

[1] University College London, London, UK
[2] Royal Free and University College London Medical School, London, UK

Introduction

It is now 30 years since the factor VIII (FVIII) protein was first purified [1], leading to the subsequent cloning of the gene [2]. Detection of causative mutations in the FVIII gene (*F8*) was initially slow and laborious, but recent years have seen great advances in the technology for detection of variations in *F8*. These, coupled with the recently published crystal structure of FVIII [3,4], have paved the way for a much greater understanding of the relationship between FVIII structure and the function of the cofactor in coagulation. There are still many questions to answer as to how FVIIIa (the thrombin-activated form of FVIII) interacts with phospholipid membranes and promotes the activity of activated factor IX (FIXa) so enormously in the activation of factor X (FX). Comprehensive mutation detection is often now performed by polymerase chain reaction (PCR) and direct sequencing of all exons. Because of the size and complexity of the *F8* gene this is still a considerable undertaking in many centers. FVIII function in coagulation is briefly described below.

Structure and function of the factor VIII gene (*F8*) and protein

F8 gene

The human *F8* gene was cloned between 1982 and 1984 simultaneously by two groups [2,5]. At the time, the gene was the largest described (186 kb), and is still one of the largest. Mapping positioned the *F8* gene in the most distal band (Xq28) of the long arm of the X chromosome. As shown in Figure 3.1, the gene contains 26 exons, 24 of which vary in length from 69 to 262 base pairs (bp); the remaining much larger exons, 14 and 26, contain 3106 and 1958 bp, respectively. However, the large majority of exon 26 is 3′ untranslated sequence, so that exon 14 bears by far the most coding sequence, largely that of the B domain. The spliced FVIII mRNA is approximately 9 kb in length and predicts a precursor protein of 2351 amino acids.

Production of factor VIII protein

After removal of the 19 peptide secretory leader sequence, FVIII has a mature sequence of 2332 amino acids with the domain structure A1–*a1*–A2–*a2*–B–*a3*–A3–C1–C2 [6]. Figure 3.1 shows the relationship between the domains and the cDNA exons. FVIII circulates in plasma complexed noncovalently with von Willebrand factor (VWF), which acts as a plasma carrier, apparently protecting it from proteolysis and rapid clearance.

The domain structure of FVIII is very similar to that of coagulation factor V (FV) [7], although the B domains are unrelated in sequence and FV lacks the short acidic *a1*, *a2*, and *a3* sequences. The A domains of FVIII and FV are homologous to ceruloplasmin and hephaestin (which share the domain structure A1–A2–A3), and homology of the FVIII and FV C domains has been noted with slime mold discoidin I [6], milk-fat globule membrane protein [8], and a receptor tyrosine kinase found in breast carcinoma cells [9]. There is no significant homology between the B domain of FVIII and any other protein sequence in the human genome; however, the B domains of FVIII and FV share the characteristic that they are large and very heavily *N*-glycosylated, a factor that may be crucial in their intracellular folding and processing.

Factor VIII is highly sensitive to proteolytic processing after secretion, and only a small fraction of circulating FVIII is in the single-chain form: the majority consists of heavy chains of variable length (consisting of the A1 and A2 domains together with variable lengths of B domain) linked noncovalently to light chains consisting of the A3, C1, and C2 domains. Expression of active recombinant FVIII lacking the entire length of the B domain has confirmed that this domain is unnecessary for activation of the protein or procoagulant function [10]: a cleavage after R759 (probably by thrombin) during coagulation serves to remove it. In contrast, the FV B domain is important for normal activation of the cofactor.

The function of FVIII is to accelerate the activation of FX by FIXa on a suitable phospholipid surface, thus amplifying the clotting stimulus many-fold, and specific proteolytic cleavages

Textbook of Hemophilia, Third Edition. Edited by Christine A. Lee, Erik E. Berntorp and W. Keith Hoots.

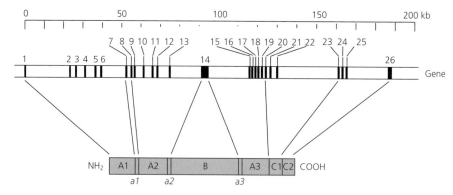

Figure 3.1 Linear representation of the *F8* gene showing (above) the 26 exons and (below) the domain organization of the protein based on amino acid homology comparisons.

between the domains both activate and inactivate the cofactor. It is clear that the active form (FVIIIa) consists of a heterotrimer of an A1–*a1* chain linked by a metal cation-dependent bond to the A3–C1–C2 chain; with the A2–*a2* chain held by electrostatic association between the A1 and A2 domains. Inactivation and loss of procoagulant function occurs through either spontaneous dissociation of A2–*a2* or proteolysis of FVIIIa by activated protein C (aPC).

Until quite recently, three-dimensional structural analysis of FVIII was based largely upon homology models using the separate structures of similar domains. In 2008, two groups independently solved the structure of B-domain-deleted FVIII by X-ray crystallography at intermediate resolution [3,4]. This demonstrated that the heterotrimer consists of the five expected globular domains with a metal ion bridge between the A1 and A3 domains. The C1, C2, and A3 domains contain phospholipid-binding regions that serve to anchor the cofactor on the negatively charged surface of activated platelets that form the platform for coagulation amplification. The crystal structure has been used to produce a putative model of the "tenase" complex in which FVIIIa and FIXa interact over an extensive surface including two high-affinity binding sites for FIXa in A2 and one in A3. The main advantage of the crystal structure is that it allows mapping of naturally occurring hemophilia A missense mutations with accurate prediction of the deleterious effects of mutating specific residues. Although this clearly represents a major advance, there are still a number of questions that remain to be answered regarding the purpose of the B domain, the mechanisms by which FVIIIa accelerates the catalytic function of FIXa and the interaction between FVIII and VWF that serves to stabilize FVIII in the circulation.

F8 gene defects found in hemophilia A

F8 gene defects associated with hemophilia A may be divided for convenience into three categories: (1) gross gene rearrangements; (2) insertions or deletions of genetic sequence of a size varying from 1 bp up to the entire gene; and (3) single DNA base substitutions resulting in either amino acid replacement ("missense"), premature peptide chain termination ("nonsense" or stop mutations), or mRNA splicing defects. These classes are described briefly below.

At its last update in late 2012, the international online hemophilia A mutation database HADB (http://hadb.org.uk) listed over 5200 individual reports of *F8* variants, including all insertion/deletions and single-base DNA replacements, whether directly submitted to the database or derived from journal reports. Updating continues actively and the database is expected to expand further during 2014/2015.

The overall incidence of hemophilia A does not vary appreciably between different ethnic groups [11]. All classes of defects can result in severe disease. However, the single most clinically important defect is a gene rearrangement (an inversion) involving *F8* intron 22 (see below), which results in approximately 50% of all severe disease cases worldwide. Inversions are omitted from the database as they are almost entirely identical both genetically and by phenotype, and therefore highly redundant. Apart from the intron 22 inversion there are few repetitive mutations, with most genetic defects caused by private mutations. This indicates a high degree of spontaneous mutations in the *F8* gene. Studies in small populations have occasionally shown a preponderance of a single mutation, suggesting a founder effect. But these are often found with mild disease and it is then unclear whether they are causative or act as a marker for a disease-associated haplotype. For full details of the other categories readers should consult the database. A summary of mutations listed in the online database is given in Table 3.1.

Gene rearrangements

As noted above, gross gene rearrangements of *F8* consist almost entirely of a unique inversion the mechanism of which was described in 1993 [12,13], and which is now known to be responsible for approximately 50% of all cases of severe hemophilia A. Prior to these studies, PCR amplification of all 26 *F8*

Table 3.1 Summary of unique mutation data available from analysis of 5243 individual reports in the online hemophilia A database at http://hadb.org.uk.

Hemophilia A unique mutations		Disease severity where reported				Inhibitor status where reported	
		Severe (%)	Moderate (%)	Mild (%)	Variable (%)	Positive (%)	Negative (%)
Total unique mutations	2107	1213 (62)	173 (9)	361 (19)	202 (10)	326 (21)	1250 (79)
Unique single-base variants	1349	565 (46)	142 (11)	349 (28)	185 (15)	153 (15)	873 (85)
Missense	983	293 (33)	118 (13)	325 (36)	164 (18)	84 (11)	670 (89)
Stop	208	183 (93)	6 (3)	0 (0)	7 (4)	54 (32)	114 (68)
Splice	158	89 (61)	18 (12)	24 (17)	14 (10)	15 (14)	89 (86)
Unique insertions	146	117 (89)	7 (5)	2 (2)	5 (4)	26 (25)	78 (75)
Unique deletions	612	531 (92)	24 (4)	10 (2)	12 (2)	147 (33)	299 (67)
Small (<50 bp)	357	291 (88)	18 (5)	10 (3)	12 (4)	64 (24)	205 (76)
Large (>50 bp)	255	240 (98)	6 (2)	0 (0)	na	83 (47)	94 (53)

The distribution of these mutations among severe, moderate, and mild disease, and relation to inhibitor status where known, are given. *F8* inversions invariably result in severe disease, but are not included in the database because of their high redundancy: inversions are responsible for about 45% of all severe disease.
na, Not applicable.

exons detected mutations in only about 50% of cases of severe hemophilia. However, reverse transcription (RT)-PCR of *F8* mRNA from most of the remaining severe cases showed that no amplification was possible between exons 22 and 23, suggesting a rearrangement within the *F8* gene in this region.

Unusually, the intron separating exons 22 and 23 (IVS22) contains a CpG island associated with two additional transcripts, originally termed *F8A* [14] and *F8B* [15]. *F8B* is a transcript of 2.5 kb and is transcribed in the same direction as the *F8* gene, using a private exon plus *F8* exons 23–26. *F8A* is transcribed in the opposite direction to the *F8* gene; furthermore, two additional copies of *F8A* were found approximately 300 and 400 kb telomeric to the *F8* gene [14]. Thus, the large majority of the "missing" cases of severe hemophilia were explained by homologous recombination between the 9.5 kb intronic sequence (now termed *int22h-1*) and one of the two extragenic homologs of this sequence (*int22h-2* and *int22h-3*). The recombination occurs during the meiotic division of gametogenesis, resulting in a large inversion and translocation of the gene sequence including exons 1–22 away from exons 23–26 (Figure 3.2a,b). Of these two common types of intron 22 inversion, the distal homolog is responsible for the majority of the severe hemophilia A inversion cases, while crossover with the proximal copy results in a further minority of cases [16].

Most laboratories now carry out initial screening for the intron 22 inversion in all cases of severe hemophilia A. Whilst Southern blotting provides a relatively laborious screening method, it is able to detect some rarer, nonstandard gene rearrangements involving intervening sequence (IVS) 22. In most centers detection is now performed more rapidly by a long-range or inverse PCR method [17].

Even with the recognition of the IVS22 rearrangements a residual 5% (approximately) of severely affected hemophiliacs

with no known defect remained. Most of these cases were found to be caused by a different inversion resulting from recombination between a 1.0 kb sequence in intron 1 (*int1h-1*) and a homologous sequence *int1h-2* approximately 140 kb upstream of *F8* [18]. Recombination of these sequences results in separation of the *F8* promoter–exon 1 sequence from the remainder of the *F8* gene (Figure 3.2a,c): this inversion may account for approximately 2–5% of severe hemophilia A cases.

Very recently, a third rearrangement involving a different homologous sequence in intron 1—*int1R-1*—has been described. In this case, the matching repeat sequence is situated 386 kb upstream of *F8* in the *IKBKG* gene. The frequency of this rearrangement as a cause for hemophilia A is unknown [19].

Anti-FVIII inhibitor development is a significant complication in hemophilia A: 21% of intron 22 inversion cases have demonstrated inhibitors [20], an identical rate to the average across all mutations but lower than that in cases caused by large deletions or nonsense mutations.

Single-base substitutions in the *F8* gene

Substitution of single bases in *F8* exons may result in amino acid substitutions ("missense" variants) or the introduction of stop codons causing premature peptide chain truncation ("nonsense" variants). In addition, single-base substitution at mRNA splicing sites (at or near the intron–exon boundaries) can result in splice variants, which may or may not also include an amino acid alteration.

As of late 2012, there were over 4000 individual reports of single-base substitutions in the hemophilia A database, with over 1300 *unique* (different) variants listed: the actual reports are far too numerous to show here (even condensed to one line per unique mutation), and readers may access the database directly for phenotypic information. This includes FVIII clotting activity (FVIII:C) and circulating protein antigen (FVIII:Ag)

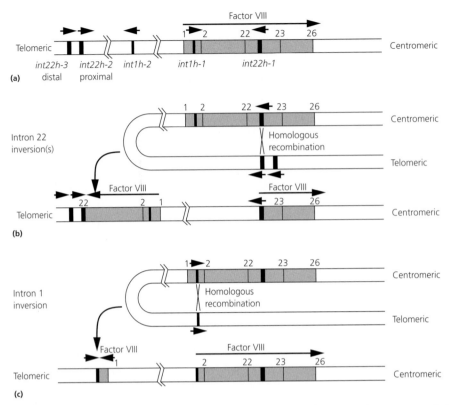

Figure 3.2 Simplified representation of the gene inversion mechanisms resulting in severe hemophilia A, involving sequences in introns 1 and 22 of the *F8* gene. Recombination between homologous sequences in intron 22 and ~400 kb telomeric to the gene leads to separation of exons 1–22 from exons 23–26, with the former sequence inverted and relocated to the site of the telomeric homologous sequence (**a and b**); alternatively, recombination between the intron 1 sequence and its telomeric homolog results in relocation and inversion of exon 1 (**a and c**).

levels, disease severity, anti-FVIII inhibitor status, and journal reference (where available) for each report. Some overall analysis, however, is presented here (Table 3.1).

The unique single-base variants are made up of 983 unique missense mutations (i.e. resulting in an amino acid substitution), 208 unique stop mutations, and 158 unique splice variants. The distribution by exon is given in Table 3.2. Exon 14 contains approximately 10 times as much coding sequence as the other exons and has a much higher burden of causative mutations generally; however, missense mutations are actually very poorly represented per kilobase of coding sequence, reflecting the dispensability of the B domain for functional activity.

Table 3.1 gives some stratification of unique single-base mutations by disease severity and anti-FVIII inhibitor status. While missense mutations and splice variants are associated with all disease severities, stop mutations (as expected) result almost exclusively in severe disease (93% of cases).

In 1026 single-base cases in which inhibitor status is known, 153 are reported as inhibitor positive (15%, broadly in accord with published studies on inhibitor incidence) with about 70% of these associated with severe disease. Stop mutations result in a much higher proportion of cases with positive inhibitor status (32%, 54 of 168) in comparison with the missense mutation group, in which only 11% (84 of 754) are inhibitor positive, or the splice variant group, in which only 15 of 104 cases had inhibitor development. Remarkably, of the 54 unique stop mutations associated with the generation of anti-FVIII antibodies *in vivo*, only six are found in the first 11 exons, and only two in exons 1–7. The reasons for this highly skewed distribution of inhibitor-positive cases relative to the position of the stop mutation in the FVIII mRNA are unknown, although various hypotheses have been formulated. The distribution of inhibitor-negative cases essentially follows the size of each coding exon.

Although nearly 60% of unique single-base mutations have been reported only once, with over 3000 individual missense reports in the database, it is to be expected that many other single-base mutations occur in multiple reports. Forty-seven unique mutations have been reported independently on 10 occasions or more, with 29 of those reported independently over 25 times: there are now two missense mutations which have been reported over 100 times. This suggests some enhanced predisposition to replication errors at the local chromatin level, whether caused by the well-known CpG dinucleotide effect, by specific sequence motifs (e.g. "runs" or repetitions of a particular base such as adenine), or by other local factors.

Table 3.2 Summary of the distribution of 2107 unique mutations in the online database by *F8* exon.

F8 exon		Point mutations			Deletions		Insertions
Number	Size (bp)	Missense	Nonsense (stop)	Splicing	Small	Large	
1	343	25	2	9	3	na	1
2	122	19	2	5	8	na	6
3	123	49	0	7	6	na	3
4	213	66	8	9	4	na	3
5	69	16	1	8	5	na	3
6	117	26	3	9	5	na	2
7	222	61	5	4	13	na	5
8	262	40	8	1	9	na	3
9	172	40	4	13	12	na	6
10	94	20	4	8	7	na	2
11	215	56	6	7	5	na	1
12	151	31	8	6	4	na	1
13	210	60	5	7	18	na	5
14	3106	79	89	7	153	na	67
15	154	39	4	9	8	na	0
16	213	53	14	6	12	na	2
17	229	47	3	3	10	na	10
18	183	49	5	3	11	na	6
19	117	24	2	9	8	na	4
20	72	10	1	0	5	na	2
21	86	13	7	3	0	na	2
22	156	30	6	6	5	na	4
23	145	47	3	6	13	na	1
24	149	18	6	7	8	na	2
25	177	26	5	6	13	na	5
26	1959	39	6	0	12	na	0
Total		983	208	158	357	255	146

Total unique single base (point) mutations: 1349. Total unique mutations of all types: 2107.
na, not applicable.

Frequently, both the disease severity and FVIII activity measurement are highly variable within the cases for a single mutation. For example, the common mutation Arg2169His (2150) has been reported 105 times, with FVIII:C activity varying from <1% to 40% of normal plasma values (matched by FVIII:Ag values ranging from <1% to 50%). The tremendous variability in these multiple reports suggests that additional factors besides the defined mutation in the *F8* gene influence circulating FVIII protein levels. It is now well known that mutations in at least two genes coding for proteins involved in glycoprotein trafficking in the endoplasmic reticulum (ER) and Golgi apparatus can result in reductions in the secreted levels of both FVIII and FV, resulting in the rare disorder of combined FVIII and FV deficiency [21]. FVIII deficiency may also be seen in von Willebrand disease, particularly the 2N subtype. However, it is likely that there are additional unknown factors, both genetic and environmental.

Now that accurate structural information about normal FVIII and its domains is available it is possible to make interpretations as to the cause of hemophilia at the level of protein structure. The large group of missense mutations in the database might be expected to provide a fertile area for analysis, correlating FVIII function with protein structure, and increasing our understanding of "molecular pathology" in hemophilic mutation cases. However, it is crucial to understand that in order to make interpretations about either FVIII function in plasma, or the ability of a variant molecule to be secreted, it is necessary to know circulating protein (FVIII:Ag) levels as well as activity (FVIII:C) levels. Comparison of these levels gives information about whether a missense mutation results in a functionally normal protein that is poorly secreted or unstable (type I defect) or a dysfunctional protein that circulates at a normal level (type II defect). In practice, type I defects are easily identified as the activity and antigen levels are similar. With type II defects, the mutation may have mixed effects, but the predominant feature will be that the protein is dysfunctional. Thus, although the antigen level might by reduced, sometimes markedly so, the activity will be significantly lower still. Arbitrarily, an activity:antigen ratio of <0.7 is considered indicative of a type II defect. The designation of missense mutations as type I or II equates with the earlier terms "CRM negative" (cross-reacting material) or "CRM positive" that were used when serum from patients with severe hemophilia and inhibitors was used to detect FVIII protein levels in test samples.

Unfortunately, data on plasma FVIII:Ag level (in addition to FVIII:C) are available for only a minority of the unique missense reports despite the availability of commercial enzyme-linked immunosorbent assay (ELISA) kits. In addition, for two-thirds of cases where antigen levels are reported, the levels are reduced broadly in parallel with activity, indicating that the hemophilic mutations result in defective secretion or instability of an otherwise functionally active cofactor. Since we understand the mechanisms of protein folding, chaperoning, secretion, and clearance so poorly, it is extremely difficult to make mechanistic explanations of why these amino acid changes result in low plasma levels in this group. Possibilities include mutations abolishing existing cysteine residues known to be involved in disulfide bridge formation, introducing new cysteine residues which may promote novel illegitimate disulfide bond formation, or mutations at, or near, site(s) of binding to VWF, which may result in defective association with the plasma carrier for FVIII.

In the remaining one-third of missense mutation cases in which plasma activity and antigen levels are both known, FVIII:Ag levels are essentially normal (or only mildly reduced) while FVIII:C levels are grossly reduced or even undetectable. This indicates that the mutation causes hemophilia by generation of a functionally inactive molecule that is secreted and circulates normally. This smaller class of missense mutations gives strong clues as to which amino acids are crucial for functional interactions in this enormous molecule, and attempts have been made to interpret type II mutations in terms of structure–function relationships (see for example [22–26]).

Rationalization of the effects of some of these missense mutations is fairly simple: for example, modifications of proteolytic sites known to be required for FVIII activation [Arg391Cys/His (372), Ser392Pro/Leu (373), Arg1708Cys (1689)] all result in normal circulating FVIII protein levels with functional activity in the range 13% or below. Other mutations would be expected to have their effect by modifying interaction with one of the ligands of FVIII (e.g. VWF, factor IXa, phospholipid membrane), resulting in reduced functional activity. For example, three mutations with very low FVIII activity and normal antigen levels are associated with N-glycosylation variants. Ile585Thr (566) leads to a new glycosylation at Asn583 (564) affecting a FIXa binding site; Met1791Thr (1772) predicts a new N-glycosylation at Asn1789 (1770), also close to a FIXa-binding region; and, unexpectedly, loss of an N-glycosylation site at Asn601 (582) resulting from the Ser603Arg (584) mutation also results in a dysfunctional protein. There are many other examples in the literature.

Mutations impacting the stability of the heterotrimeric form of activated FVIII (FVIIIa) may give rise to hemophilic consequences. A number of mutations that are widely separated in the linear sequence of FVIII cluster at the interdomain interfaces and produce discrepancies in measured FVIII activity depending on which laboratory assay is used. FVIII activity is normally measured by either a one-stage or two-stage clotting assay or a chromogenic assay. In many laboratories the chromogenic and two-stage assays are considered to measure FVIII activity by a similar methodology. In the vast majority of hemophiliacs, the FVIII activity is the same whichever assay is used, but in a small, but distinct, group of cases of mild or moderate hemophilia caused by missense mutations the results vary. This can cause problems in clinical management, with uncertainty as to which assay truly reflects the patient's phenotype. In classical "assay discrepancy" the one-stage assay produces higher activity levels than the two-stage assay. There are now some 20 unique mutations in this group with the one-stage assay producing levels that are up to fivefold higher than the two-stage assay. Among the first of this class of mutants that were described are Ala303Glu (284), Ser308Leu (289), and Arg550Cys (531). Studies of mutations in this group using thrombin generation methods suggest that the lower, chromogenic value more accurately reflects the clinical phenotype [27]. In a rarer group with "inverse assay discrepancy" the results with the one-stage assay are lower. There are at least five unique mutations in this group (personal communication, Dr Mike Makris, Sheffield Haemophilia and Thrombosis Centre, UK). In both situations, the chromogenic assay value tends to agree with the two-stage clotting assay value.

Some explanation for the mechanism behind this assay discrepancy phenomenon can be derived from mapping of the mutations in the crystal structure of FVIII (Figure 3.3). Although the structure is of nonactivated FVIII rather than FVIIIa, it does provide an indication of the position, and interaction between, adjacent domains. The majority of the "discrepant" mutations occur at the interface between the A2 domain and the A1 or A3 domains. As the A2 domain is a separate polypeptide chain that is held within the complex by electrostatic forces, mutations in these residues are likely to affect the strength of that interaction. The chromogenic and two-stage assays include a longer incubation time than the one-stage assay, leading to greater dissociation of the A2 domain in mutants with weakened attachment. Prolonging the incubation time in the one-stage assay leads to lower levels, confirming that this is the likely mechanism. However, some of the mutants are at the interface between the A3 and C1 domains (which are also covalently attached) indicating that destabilization of interactions between other domains can also affect function. It is generally felt that the two-stage or chromogenic values correlate better with the clinical phenotype and it is noteworthy that in the few cases where thrombin generation has been measured the results correlate better with these assays.

The mechanism of "inverse assay discrepancy" is likely to be more diverse. The first mutant in this group that was fully studied, Tyr365Cys (346), is close to a thrombin-cleavage site, with a resulting reduction in the rate of activation by thrombin. In this case, the assays with longer incubation times allow for

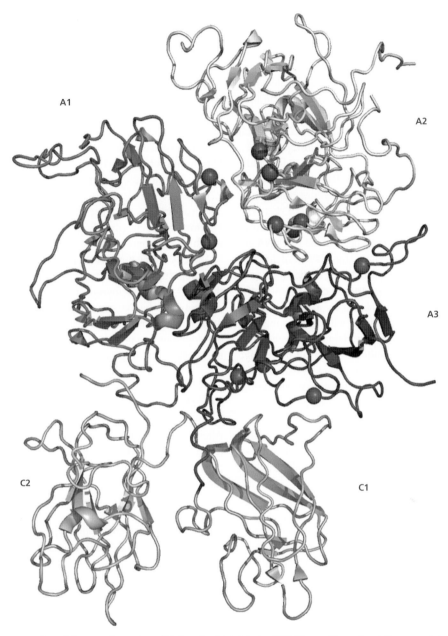

Figure 3.3 Ribbons representation of the crystal structure of B-domain-deleted factor VIII. The positions of mutations associated with classical assay discrepancy are shown by red spheres (in Plate 3.3). These cluster in two groups: at the interface between the A2 domain and the A1 and A3 domains and at the interface between the A3 and C1 domains. PDB ID: 2R7E. (See also Plate 3.3.)

more mutant protein to become activated, producing higher measured activity levels.

Although these mutants represent a small group, it is becoming clear that reliance on the one-stage FVIII:C assay as the sole functional test in the diagnosis of nonsevere hemophilia A might lead to the diagnosis being missed.

It is a reasonable assumption that approximately two-thirds of all hemophilic missense mutations will cause the phenotype by defective FVIII secretion or stability while the remaining one-third generate a dysfunctional molecule. However, only

performance of FVIII:Ag assays allows assignment of a particular mutation into the appropriate category of molecular pathology: in the absence of these data, apparently sophisticated analyses of interspecies residue conservation or structural modeling may be misleading.

Sequence insertions and deletions

The hemophilia A mutation database at http://hadb.org.uk lists both *F8* insertions and the much more numerous deletions. *F8* deletions are divided for convenience into large (>50 bp) and small (<50 bp).

Sequence insertions

There are 310 individual reports of insertions associated with hemophilia A: however, these are composed of just 146 unique insertion events, the vast majority of which are very short (less than 10 bp), with a very small number of larger insertions such as long interspersed elements (LINE) [28] or Alu repeats [29]. Many of the repetitious reports consist of insertions of an additional adenine base at the site of a run of adenines; for example, there are more than 60 separate unrelated cases of insertion of an A into a run of eight As at codons 1458–1460 (1439–1441), and a further 31 cases of insertion of A into a run of nine As at codons 1210–1213 (1191–1194). Runs of As in the *F8* cDNA are not uncommon, and these insertions (and small deletions) result from DNA polymerase slippage during replication.

Although the vast majority of insertions cause frame-shifts resulting in severe hemophilia (Table 3.1), a small number of "A-run" insertion cases are associated with low but measurable FVIII activity levels and only moderate (or even mild) disease severity. This probably results from a small percentage of normal mRNA molecules being produced by "corrective" slippage errors on the mutant template during transcription: a small number of cases with measurable plasma FVIII:Ag provides supportive evidence.

Of the 146 unique insertions, 104 have inhibitor status reported, with 25% of cases inhibitor positive (Table 3.1)—a very similar percentage to that found in the small deletions subgroup, as may be expected.

Sequence deletions

Small deletions subgroup (<50 bp)

There are 623 individual small deletion reports in the database, composed of 357 unique small deletions, of which 47% (168/357) are of single bases. As with small insertions almost all the multiple reports are of deletions of a single A in a run of As: for example, there are no less than 112 separate reports of an A deletion in a run of nine As at codons 1210–1213 (1191–1194), which is also a hotspot for single-base insertions.

Small deletions generally cause frame-shifts and are almost all associated with severe disease; however, as with small insertions, there are a small number of moderate or mild cases, often associated with "A-runs" but also with in-frame deletions of a single amino acid. Overall inhibitor development at 24% of all unique cases with known status is closely comparable with a value of 25% for all insertion frame-shifts, and somewhat lower than the overall figure for all nonsense point mutations (32%).

Large deletions subgroup (>50 bp)

There are 264 individual reports in the database, probably comprising close to that number of unique large deletions (detection methods are fairly imprecise so it is difficult to compare different reports where the deleted sequence may be simply given as "10 kb" or "exons 1–5"): the deletions range from just a few hundreds of bases up to more than 210 kb, deleting the entire gene, and are responsible for about 4% of severe hemophilia A cases.

Large deletions in the *F8* gene almost invariably give rise to severe disease with no measurable FVIII activity or antigen. Unexpectedly, however, there are several independent reports of moderate disease (quoting low but measurable FVIII activity levels), most associated with exon-skipping deletions toward the C-terminus of the FVIII protein, involving exon 22, exons 23–24, and exon 25. Remarkably, secretion of hypoactive FVIII lacking C-terminal amino acid sequences may occur in these cases, alleviating the disease severity: this is supported by *in-vitro* expression of a FVIII variant lacking the C2 domain which retains some cofactor activity [30].

There is a very high level of inhibitor development (47%) in this subgroup of cases (83/177)—far higher than that found for the small deletion subgroup (24%): clearly, there is a relationship between the size of deletion and the likelihood of inhibitor development. Grouping all deletions yields an overall inhibitor development rate of 33% (147 of 446; Table 3.1), similar to the nonsense mutation group (32%).

Conclusion

After nearly 30 years of mutation hunting in hemophilia A, the technology of detection has reached the point where, in large centers with substantial cohorts of patients, causative mutations can be found in around 95% of cases. The remaining small percentage of undetermined genetic causes may suggest that there are unknown gene rearrangements still to be found, or that there are other causes outside the *F8* gene; however, there remains an understandable impetus for afflicted families to have their mutation defined for prenatal diagnosis.

Rather surprising, considering the number of years over which mutations have been accumulating in the database, is the fact that novel mutations continue to be added at a largely undiminished pace, and there are several large centers which have not as yet submitted their own mutation lists. How many more disease-causing mutations exist within this remarkable protein is yet to be determined.

Public database

The Haemophilia A Mutation Database is available at: http://hadb.org.uk

Mutation nomenclature

Numbering of DNA bases and amino acids in this chapter follows the guidelines of the Human Genome Variation Society

(HGVS). +1 refers to the "A" of the ATG translation start codon for nucleotide numbering, and also the methionine residue that this codes for in amino acid numbering. Most earlier publications use amino acid numbering based on the mature protein: subtraction of 19 from the amino acid numbering given here generates the previous commonly used numbering. This legacy numbering is shown in parentheses thus (XXX) when specific residues are referred to in the text.

Disease severity

In this chapter "disease severity" refers to categorization by means of laboratory tests for FVIII activity (FVIII:C), while "clinical phenotype" refers to assessment by clinical criteria such as number of treatment episodes, severity of bleeding or other indicators. Generally, the disease severity of hemophilia A (in this chapter and elsewhere) is categorized into three groups based on the results of FVIII:C assays. FVIII:C values below 1% of normal are defined as severe disease; 1–5% are defined as moderate, and 5–40% as mild. The disease severity as measured by a FVIII:C assay is rarely in disagreement with severity of clinical phenotype; however, there are rare cases in which the two are not concordant.

References

1 Rotblat F, Goodall AH, O'Brien DP, Rawlings E, Middleton S, Tuddenham EG. Monoclonal antibodies to human procoagulant factor VIII. *J Lab Clin Med* 1983; **101**: 736–46.

2 Gitschier J, Wood WI, Goralka TM, *et al.* Characterization of the human factor VIII gene. *Nature* 1984; **312**: 326–30.

3 Ngo JC, Huang M, Roth DA, Furie BC, Furie B. Crystal structure of human factor VIII: Implications for the formation of the factor IXa–factor VIIIa complex. *Structure* 2008; **16**: 597–606.

4 Shen BW, Spiegel PC, Chang CH, *et al.* The tertiary structure and domain organization of coagulation factor VIII. *Blood* 2008; **111**: 1240–7.

5 Toole JJ, Knopf JL, Wozney JM, *et al.* Molecular cloning of a cDNA encoding human antihaemophilic factor. *Nature* 1984; **312**: 342–7.

6 Vehar GA, Keyt B, Eaton D, *et al.* Structure of human factor VIII. *Nature* 1984; **312**: 337–42.

7 Kane WH, Davie EW. Cloning of a cDNA coding for human factor V, a blood coagulation factor homologous to factor VIII and ceruloplasmin. *Proc Natl Acad Sci USA* 1986; **83**: 6800–4.

8 Stubbs JD, Lekutis C, Singer KL, Bui A, Yuzuki D, Srinivasan U, Parry G. cDNA cloning of a mouse mammary epithelial cell surface protein reveals the existence of epidermal growth factor-like domains linked to factor VIII-like sequences. *Proc Natl Acad Sci USA* 1990; **87**: 8417–21.

9 Johnson JD, Edman JC, Rutter WJ. A receptor tyrosine kinase found in breast carcinoma cells has an extracellular discoidin I-like domain. *Proc Natl Acad Sci USA* 1993; **90**: 5677–81.

10 Eaton D, Rodriguez H, Vehar GA. Proteolytic processing of human factor VIII. Correlation of specific cleavages by thrombin, factor Xa, and activated protein C with activation and inactivation of factor VIII coagulant activity. *Biochemistry* 1986; **25**: 505–12.

11 Stonebraker JS, Bolton-Maggs PH, Soucie JM, Walker I, Brooker M. A study of variations in the reported haemophilia A prevalence around the world. *Haemophilia* 2010; **16**: 20–32.

12 Naylor J, Brinke A, Hassock S, Green PM, Giannelli F. Characteristic mRNA abnormality found in half the patients with severe haemophilia A is due to large DNA inversions. *Hum Mol Genet* 1993; **2**: 1773–8.

13 Lakich D, Kazazian HH, Jr, Antonarakis SE, Gitschier J. Inversions disrupting the factor VIII gene are a common cause of severe haemophilia A. *Nat Genet* 1993; **5**: 236–41.

14 Levinson B, Kenwrick S, Lakich D, Hammonds G, Jr, Gitschier J. A transcribed gene in an intron of the human factor VIII gene. *Genomics* 1990; **7**: 1–11.

15 Levinson B, Kenwrick S, Gamel P, Fisher K, Gitschier J. Evidence for a third transcript from the human factor VIII gene. *Genomics* 1992; **14**: 585–9.

16 Antonarakis SE, Rossiter JP, Young M, *et al.* Factor VIII gene inversions in severe hemophilia A: Results of an international consortium study. *Blood* 1995; **86**: 2206–12.

17 Liu Q, Nozari G, Sommer SS. Single-tube polymerase chain reaction for rapid diagnosis of the inversion hotspot of mutation in hemophilia A. *Blood* 1998; **92**: 1458–9.

18 Bagnall RD, Waseem N, Green PM, Giannelli F. Recurrent inversion breaking intron 1 of the factor VIII gene is a frequent cause of severe hemophilia A. *Blood* 2002; **99**: 168–74.

19 Pezeshkpoor B, Rost S, Oldenburg J, El-Maarri O. Identification of a third rearrangement at Xq28 that causes severe haemophilia A as a result of homologous recombination between inverted repeats. *J Thromb Haemost* 2012; **10**: 1600–8.

20 Oldenburg J, El-Maarri O, Schwaab R. Inhibitor development in correlation to factor VIII genotypes. *Haemophilia* 2002; **8**(Suppl. 2): 23–9.

21 Zhang B, McGee B, Yamaoka JS, *et al.* Combined deficiency of factor V and factor VIII is due to mutations in either LMAN1 or MCFD2. *Blood* 2006; **107**: 1903–7.

22 Liu ML, Shen BW, Nakaya S, *et al.* Hemophilic factor VIII C1- and C2-domain missense mutations and their modeling to the 1.5-angstrom human C2-domain crystal structure. *Blood* 2000; **96**: 979–87.

23 David D, Ventura C, Moreira I, *et al.* The spectrum of mutations and molecular pathogenesis of hemophilia A in 181 Portuguese patients. *Haematologica* 2006; **91**: 840–3.

24 Venceslá A, Corral-Rodríguez MA, Baena M, *et al.* Identification of 31 novel mutations in the *F8* gene in Spanish hemophilia A patients: structural analysis of 20 missense mutations suggests new intermolecular binding sites. *Blood* 2008; **111**: 3468–78.

25 Sirocova N, Tsourea V, Vicol M, *et al.* Factor VIII mutations in 42 Moldovan haemophilia A families, including 12 that are novel. *Haemophilia* 2009; **15**: 942–51.

26 Trossaërt M, Boisseau P, Quemener A, *et al.* Prevalence, biological phenotype and genotype in moderate/mild hemophilia A with discrepancy between one-stage and chromogenic factor VIII activity. *J Thromb Haemost* 2011; **9**: 524–30.

27 Trossaërt M, Regnault V, Sigaud M, Boisseau P, Fressinaud E, Lecompte T. Mild hemophilia A with factor VIII assay discrepancy:

using thrombin generation assay to assess the bleeding phenotype. *J Thromb Haemost* 2008; **6**: 486–93.

28 Kazazian HH, Jr, Wong C, Youssoufian H, Scott AF, Phillips DG, Antonarakis SE. Haemophilia A resulting from de novo insertion of L1 sequences represents a novel mechanism for mutation in man. *Nature* 1988; **332**: 164–6.

29 Sukarova E, Dimovski AJ, Tchacarova P, Petkov GH, Efremov GD. An Alu insert as the cause of a severe form of hemophilia A. *Acta Haematol* 2001; **106**: 126–9.

30 Wakabayashi H, Griffiths AE, Fay PJ. Factor VIII lacking the C2 domain retains cofactor activity in vitro. *J Biol Chem* 2010; **285**: 25176–84.

CHAPTER 4

Prophylaxis

Kathelijn Fischer and H. Marijke van den Berg
University Medical Centre, Utrecht, the Netherlands

Rationale for prophylaxis

The prevention of bleeds by prophylactic clotting factor replacement therapy has now been advocated for almost half a century. It started with the observation that the clinical phenotype of patients with moderate hemophilia was very different from those with severe hemophilia [1]. Patients with moderate hemophilia and factor VIII (FVIII)/factor IX activities of 0.01–0.05 IU/mL bled only after trauma and had a fairly normal life expectancy, while patients with severe hemophilia (FVIII/IX <0.01 IU/mL) had spontaneous severe muscle and joint bleeds followed by early crippling hemophilic arthropathy, with a life expectancy of only 20 years. Because of this observation, it seemed logical to supply the missing clotting factor in patients with severe hemophilia and increase the level of clotting factor activity above 0.01 IU/mL. Besides the established effect of prophylaxis on the prevention of joint damage, there is also data that support a reduction in the occurrence of intracranial hemorrhages [2]. Although there is already decades of evidence on the effectiveness of prophylaxis for patients with severe hemophilia, there is still an ongoing debate concerning when to start, which dose to use, and the effects on joint damage. However, one should keep the clear clinical example of moderate hemophilia in mind: only a limited amount of FVIII or IX is needed to correct hemostasis and prevent bleeding. Continuous replacement therapy can prevent bleeding—no further study is needed to confirm this—similar to the observation for the need of parachutes [3].

Introduction of prophylaxis

Using her own Swedish product, Professor Inga Marie Nilsson from Malmö, was the first to start prophylactic replacement therapy in boys with severe hemophilia A [3]. The patients who first started on prophylactic therapy were those with frequent bleeds. In these first studies, it was demonstrated that the number of bleeds decreased and that these patients lost fewer days from school or work. After the discovery of cryoprecipitate [4], this Swedish initiative was repeated in the Netherlands by Professor Van Creveld, who also reported a reduction in the number and the severity of bleeds [5]. Concomitant with the increased availability of clotting factors, the use of prophylaxis was extended. Moreover, it was observed that early prophylaxis was more effective in preventing arthropathy, and that radiologic joint damage could not be reversed by prophylaxis. So, in subsequent years, prophylaxis was started earlier, before the occurrence of joint damage [6,7]. The benefit of prophylaxis for children with severe hemophilia A and B is equal; most studies described in this chapter include both hemophilia A and B patients, and the beneficial effects on the prevention of bleeding are similar.

Consequently, "primary prophylaxis," defined as the start of regular continuous treatment before the age of 2 years or after the occurrence of the first joint bleed [8], was recommended. After favorable experience, prophylaxis increasingly became the treatment of choice for boys with severe hemophilia, and was recommended by World Health Organization (WHO)/World Federation of Hemophilia (WFH) experts [9].

After publication of favorable results from two randomized controlled trials (RCTs) in children [10,11], the first version of the Cochrane review, that stated that there was insufficient evidence to support prophylaxis in children with severe hemophilia, was revised in favor of prophylaxis [12].

Prophylaxis in children

Based on observational studies and two RCTs, the benefits of prophylaxis in children are well established (Table 4.1). The first of the two RCTs was performed in the USA and published in 2007 [11]. In this trial, patients with FVIII <0.02 IU/mL, with normal joints on physical examination and imaging studies, were randomized to receive prophylaxis (25 IU/kg every other day) or enhanced episodic treatment (40 IU/kg, followed by 20 IU/kg after 24 and 72 h). Magnetic resonance imaging (MRI)

Textbook of Hemophilia, Third Edition. Edited by Christine A. Lee, Erik E. Berntorp and W. Keith Hoots.
© 2014 John Wiley & Sons, Ltd. Published 2014 by John Wiley & Sons, Ltd.

Table 4.1 Outcome and costs reported in studies comparing on-demand treatment (OD) with prophylaxis (PR).

Study	Design	Patients (n) (OD/PR)	Follow-up (years)	Age at evaluation (years)	Annual Joint bleeds (OD/PR)	Consumption (IU/kg/year) (OD/PR)
Children						
Aledort *et al.* [48].	Prospective cohort	411/66	5	13	16.5 vs 5.7	1038 vs 2772
Smith *et al.* [49].	Retrospective cohort	90/27	2	7[a]	NA	1015 vs 3323[a]
Manco-Johnson [11]	Prospective RCT	33/32	4	6	4.9 vs 0.6	1819 vs 5770[c]
ESPRIT, Gringeri [12]	Prospective RCT	23/22	4	10	5.5 vs 1[a,b]	1803 vs 4008
Adults						
Schramm *et al.* [50].	Retrospective cohort	670/335	1	35	7.7 vs 3.4	1224 vs 3208
Fischer *et al.* [35].	Retrospective complete cohort	103/49	1	22	16.9 vs 5.1	1488 vs 1612
Steen Carlsson *et al.* [51].	Retrospective complete cohort	61/95	11	Adults	NA	780 vs 3024
Liou *et al.* [52].	Retrospective complete cohort	37/13	5	38 vs 17	31.9 vs 7.8[a]	1325 vs 1824[a]
Collins *et al.* [53].	Prospective cross-over	20/19	0.5	36.9	30 vs 0[a]	1630 vs 4552
POTTER, Tagliaferri *et al.* [26].	Prospective observational	36/27	5	17–60	18.3 vs 2.9[b]	1749 vs 3733[b]

Values are given as means.

NA, not applicable; RCT, randomized controlled trial.

[a]Median values.

[b]Calculated based on published data.

[c]Data provided by author.

and radiography were primary endpoints. In total, 32 patients started prophylaxis at a mean age of 1.6 years and were followed for 4 years. As expected, outcome at the age of 6 years was significantly better in the prophylaxis group: 45% (13/29) of patients treated with the enhanced on-demand regimen had joint damage on MRI vs 7% (2/27) of patients treated with prophylaxis ($P < 0.01$). Differences in the number of bleeds experienced and FVIII consumption were even more significant.

Results of the Italian RCT (ESPRIT) comparing prophylactic (30 IU/kg three times a week) with on-demand treatment (minimum 25 IU/kg every 12–24 hours until bleed was resolved) in 40 children with FVIII <0.01 IU/mL were published in 2011 [12]. Here, patients started prophylaxis at a mean age of 4.1 years and were followed for a median of 7 years. During follow-up, 4/21 patients (19%) switched from prophylactic to on-demand treatment, and 5/19 patients (26%) switched from on-demand to prophylactic treatment. Even in the intention-to-treat analysis, the outcome was significantly worse in the on-demand group with radiologic joint abnormalities in the majority of patients in the on-demand arm (14/19: 74%), vs in 6/21 (29%) of patients in the prophylaxis arm. Again, prophylaxis was associated with significantly fewer joint bleeds and more FVIII consumption (Table 4.1).

When to start prophylaxis

The timing of the initiation of prophylaxis is important: "primary prophylaxis," i.e. prophylaxis started before the age of 2 years or after the first joint bleed, has been recommended for all boys with severe hemophilia [8].

Mostly, it is issues of venous access and parental acceptance that hamper prophylaxis in young boys. Therefore, it has been recommended to individualize the initiation of prophylaxis according to patient characteristics [13]. Such an approach takes the large variability in the onset of joint bleeding into account. The onset of joint bleeding ranges from 0.2 to 5.8 years, with a median around 1.6 years [14,15]. It has been suggested that arthropathy is best prevented if prophylaxis is started before the second [16] or third [13] joint bleed, but the benefits of starting before the first joint bleed have not been established. Strong support for an early start of prophylaxis can also be obtained from the Swedish experience [17]. In their analysis of 121 patients with severe hemophilia, it was shown that the age at start of prophylaxis was an independent predictor for the development of arthropathy, but dose and interval of prophylaxis at the start of prophylactic treatment were not. A subgroup analysis of the ESPRIT study also suggested that prophylaxis was more effective when started before the age of 3 years [11].

It has been well established that frequent infusions are most efficient at preventing bleeds [18]. A practical strategy to start prophylaxis in very young boys is to follow the example of Dr Petrini and start with once-weekly infusions. This approach is more acceptable for parents and may reduce the need for central venous catheters. After starting once-weekly infusions, the Swedish aim to increase the frequency of infusions to three times weekly or every other day as soon as possible [19]. Others advocate increasing frequency according to bleeding patterns, increasing the number of weekly infusions stepwise at the occurrence of each joint bleed or severe bleed until patients achieve a frequency of three times a week or every other day rate in both arms (Table 4.2). Dosing in the PK arm was calculated to achieve minimum trough levels of 1% FVIII with dosing every third day. Therefore, clotting factor consumption was very high in both arms.

Lindvall *et al.* performed a cross-over study comparing standard prophylaxis (on average 2000 IU every other day) to daily prophylaxis using PK driven doses to achieve similar or higher trough levels than those achieved using standard dosing [43]. Overall, a 30% reduction in treatment costs was achieved. Although this study was too small to achieve statistically significant differences, there was a clear trend towards a considerable reduction in consumption. Although overall bleeding appeared slightly increased, more follow-up is needed to determine whether this also affects joint outcome.

In conclusion, these data suggest that different prophylactic regimens are effective in preventing bleeds, but consumption is only reduced using lower dose and/or more frequent infusions.

Future issues in prophylaxis

Now that the positive effects of early prophylaxis in young boys have been confirmed by two RCTs and the body of evidence concerning prophylaxis in adults is increasing, it is expected that the use of prophylaxis will further increase in countries with available products. Intermediate-dose regimens may be effectively used in countries with limited resources.

Currently, there is increasing debate about the use of prophylaxis in patients with inhibitors to prevent the development of target joints and arthropathy, both before and during immune tolerance treatment, and in patients who failed immune tolerance. However, bypassing agents are less effective than FVIII or IX, and the results of prophylaxis with bypassing agents may not be as favorable as with normal concentrates in patients without inhibitors.

The development of clotting factor products with a prolonged half-life will be an important step forward. Their use will allow for prophylactic regimens with less frequent infusions or a lower dose. Especially less frequent infusions are expected significantly to reduce the burden of treatment for younger patients and improve adherence.

Conclusion

It has been proven that early prophylactic therapy can prevent bleeds and arthropathy. Although an increasing number of countries use primary prophylaxis, the general market prices for clotting products have not been reduced in the last 20 years. Since primary prophylaxis is most effective in preventing arthropathy, this should be the treatment of choice for young children. There is no reason to expose our next generation of hemophiliacs to the risk of bleeding, while we have a good and safe therapy available and gene therapy on our doorstep. The aim is to continue prophylaxis in adulthood; only some patients with milder bleeding patterns and normal muscles and joints may be able to reduce the intensity of their regimen.

In our discussions with authorities, it may be best to rephrase prophylaxis as replacement therapy, which better reflects the real need for this treatment.

References

1 Ahlberg A. Haemophilia in Sweden VII. Incidence, treatment and prophylaxis of arthropathy and other musculo-skeletal manifestations of haemophilia A and B. *Acta Orthop Scand* 1965; **77**(Suppl.): 5–99.

2 Witmer C, Presley R, Kulkarni R, Soucie M, Manno S, Raffini L. Associations between intracranial haemorrhage and prescribed prophylaxis in a large cohort of haemophilia patients in the United Stated. *Br J Haematol* 2010; **152**: 211–16.

3 White GC. Parachutes and prophylaxis: they both work! *J Thromb Haemost* 2006; **4**(6): 1226–7.

4 Nilsson IM, Blomback M, Ahlberg A. Our experience in Sweden with prophylaxis on haemophilia. *Bibl Haematol* 1970; **34**: 111–24.

5 Pool JG, Shannon AE. Production of high-potency concentrates of antihemophilic globulin in a closed-bag system. *N Engl J Med* 1965; **273**: 1443–7.

6 Van Creveld S. Prophylaxis of joint hemorrhages in hemophilia. *Acta Haematol* 1971; **45**: 120 –7.

7 Löfqvist T, Nilsson IM, Berntorp E, Pettersson H. Haemophilia prophylaxis in young patients—a long-term follow-up. *J Intern Med* 1997; **241**(5): 395–400.

8 Fischer K, Van der Bom JG, Mauser-Bunschoten EP, *et al.* Changes in treatment strategies for severe haemophilia over the last 3 decades: effects on clotting factor consumption and arthropathy. *Haemophilia* 2001; **7**: 446–52.

9 Ljung RCR, Aronis-Vournas S, Kurnik-Auberger K, *et al.* Treatment of children with haemophilia in Europe: a survey of 20 centres in 16 countries. *Haemophilia* 2000; **6**: 619–24.

10 Berntorp E, Astermark J, Bjorkman S, *et al.* Consensus perspectives on prophylactic therapy for haemophilia: summary statement. *Haemophilia* 2003; **9**(Suppl. 1): 1–4.

11 Manco-Johnson MJ, Abshire TC, Shapiro AD, *et al.* Prophylaxis versus episodic treatment to prevent joint disease in boys with severe hemophilia. *N Engl J Med* 2007; **357**(6): 535–44.

12 Gringeri A, Lundin B, von MS, Mantovani L, Mannucci PM. A randomized clinical trial of prophylaxis in children with hemophilia A (the ESPRIT Study). *J Thromb Haemost* 2011; **9**(4): 700–10.

13 Fischer K, Van der Bom JG, Mauser-Bunschoten EP, *et al.* Effects of postponing prophylactic treatment on long-term outcome in patients with severe haemophilia. *Blood* 2002; **99**: 2337–41.

14 Van Dijk K, Fischer K, Van der Bom JG, Grobbee DE, Van den Berg HM. Variability in clinical phenotype of severe haemophilia: the role of the first joint bleed. *Haemophilia* 2005; **11**: 438–43.

15 Pollmann H, Richter H, Ringkamp H, Jürgens H. When are children diagnosed as having severe haemophilia and when do they start to bleed? A 10-year single-centre PUP study. *Eur J Pediatr* 1999; **158** (Suppl. 3): 166–70.

16 Kreuz W, Escuriola-Ettingshausen C, Funk M, Schmidt H, Kornhuber B. When should prophylactic treatment in patients with haemophilia A and B start? The German experience. *Haemophilia* 1998; **4**: 413–17.

17 Astermark J, Petrini P, Tengborn L, Schulman S, Ljung RCR, Berntorp E. Primary prophylaxis in severe haemophilia should be started at an early age but can be individualized. *Br J Haematol* 1999; **105**: 1109–13.

18 Schimpf K, Fischer B, Rothmann P. Die ambulante dauerbehandlung der Hämophilie A. *Dtsch Med Wochenschr* 1976; **101**(5): 141–8.

19 Petrini P. What factors should influence the dosage and interval of prophylactic treatment in patients with severe haemophilia A and B? *Haemophilia* 2001; **7**: 99–102.

20 Meunier S, Trossaërt M, Berger G, et al. [French guidelines. Long term prophylaxis for severe haemophilia A and B children to proevent haemophiliac arthropathy.] *Arch Pediatr* 2009; **16**(12): 1571–8.

21 Feldman BM, Pai M, Rivard GE, et al. Tailored prophylaxis in severe hemophilia A: interim results from the first 5 years of the Canadian Hemophilia Primary Prophylaxis Study. *J Thromb Haemost* 2006; **4**(6): 1228–36.

22 Kurnik K, Bidlingmaier C, Engl W, Chehadeh H, Reipert B, Auerswald G. New early prophylaxis regimen that avoids immunological danger signals can reduce FVIII inhibitor development. *Haemophilia* 2010; **16**(2): 256–62.

23 Gouw SC, Van der Bom JG, Van den Berg HM. Treatment-related risk factors of inhibitor development in previously untreated patients with hemophilia A: the CANAL cohort study. *Blood* 2007; **109**(11): 4648–54.

24 Jansen NW, Roosendaal G, Bijlsma JW, DeGroot J, Theobald M, Lafeber FP. Degenerated and healthy cartilage are equally vulnerable to blood-induced damage. *Ann Rheum Dis* 2008; **67**(10): 1468–73.

25 Acharya SS. Exploration of the pathogenesis of haemophilic joint arthropathy: understanding implications for optimal clinical management. *Br J Haematol* 2012; **156**(1): 13–23.

26 Tagliaferri A, Rivolta GF, Coppola A, et al. Prophylaxis versus on-demand therapy through economic report (POTTER) study: Preliminary data from the final 5-year analysis. *Haemophilia* 2012; **18**(Suppl. 3): 160–1.

27 Fischer K, Hermans C. The European Principles of Haemophilia Care: a pilot investigation of adherence to the principles in Europe. *Haemophilia* 2013; **19**: 35–43.

28 Biss TT, Chan AK, Blanchette VS, Iwenofu LN, McLimont M, Carcao MD. The use of prophylaxis in 2663 children and adults with haemophilia: results of the 2006 Canadian national haemophilia prophylaxis survey. *Haemophilia* 2008; **14**(5): 923–30.

29 Zappa S, McDaniel M, Marandola J, Allen G. Treatment trends for haemophilia A and haemophilia B in the United States: results from the 2010 practice patterns survey. *Haemophilia* 2012; **18**(3): e140–e153.

30 Van Dijk K, Fischer K, Van der Bom JG, Scheibel E, Ingerslev J, Van den Berg HM. Can long-term prophylaxis for severe haemophilia be stopped in adulthood? Results from Denmark and the Netherlands. *Br J Haematol* 2005; **130**(1): 107–12.

31 Richards M, Altisent C, Batorova A, et al. Should prophylaxis be used in adolescent and adult patients with severe haemophilia? A European survey of practice and outcome data. *Haemophilia* 2007; **13**(5): 473–9.

32 Hang MX, Blanchette VS, Pullenayegum E, McLimont M, Feldman BM. Age at first joint bleed and bleeding severity in boys with severe hemophilia A: Canadian Hemophilia Primary Prophylaxis Study. *J Thromb Haemost* 2011; **9**(5): 1067–9.

33 Molho P, Rolland N, Lebrun T, et al. Epidemiological survey of the orthopedic status of severe haemophilia A and B patients in France. *Haemophilia* 2000; **6**: 23–32.

34 Steen Carlsson K, Hojgard S, Lindgren A, et al. Costs of on-demand and prophylactic treatment for severe haemophilia in Norway and Sweden. *Haemophilia* 2004; **10**: 515–26.

35 Fischer K, Van der Bom JG, Molho P, et al. Prophylactic versus on demand strategies for severe haemophilia: a comparison of costs and long-term outcome. *Haemophilia* 2002; **8**: 745–52.

36 Fischer K, Grobbee DE, Van den Berg HM. RCTs and observational studies to determine the effects of prophylaxis in severe haemophilia. *Haemophilia* 2007; **13**: 345–50.

37 Nicholson A, Berger K, Bohn R, et al. Recommendations for reporting economic evaluations of haemophilia prophylaxis: a nominal groups consensus statement on behalf of the Economics Expert Working Group of The International Prophylaxis Study Group. *Haemophilia* 2008; **14**(1): 127–32.

38 Noone D, O'Mahony B, van Dijk JP, Prihodova L. A survey of the outcome of prophylaxis, on-demand treatment or combined treatment in 18–35-year old men with severe haemophilia in six countries. *Haemophilia* 2013; **19**(1): 44–50.

39 Feldman BM, Berger K, Bohn R, et al. Haemophilia prophylaxis: how can we justify the costs? *Haemophilia* 2012; **18**: 680–4.

40 Matucci M, Messori A, Donati-Cori G, et al. Kinetic evaluation of four Factor VIII concentrates by model-independent methods. *Scand J Haematol* 1985; **34**(1): 22–8.

41 Ahnström J, Berntorp E, Lindvall K, Björkman S. A 6-year follow-up of dosing, coagulation factor levels and bleedings in relation to joint status in the prophylactic treatment of haemophilia. *Haemophilia* 2004; **10**: 689–97.

42 Collins PW, Blanchette VS, Fischer K, et al. Break-through bleeding in relation to predicted factor VIII levels in patients receiving prophylactic treatment for severe haemophilia A. *J Thromb Haemost* 2009; **7**: 413–20.

43 Lindvall K, Astermark J, Bjorkman S, et al. Daily dosing prophylaxis for haemophilia: a randomized crossover pilot study evaluating feasibility and efficacy. *Haemophilia* 2012; **18**(6): 855–9.

44 Khair K, Gibson F, Meerabeau L. The benefits of prophylaxis: views of adolescents with severe haemophilia. *Haemophilia* 2012; **18**(3): e286–9.

45 Richards M, Williams M, Chalmers E, et al. A United Kingdom Haemophilia Centre Doctors' Organization guideline approved by the British Committee for Standards in Haematology: guideline on the use of prophylactic factor VIII concentrate in children and adults with severe haemophilia A. *Br J Haematol* 2010; **149**(4): 498–507.

46 Fischer K, Steen Carlsson K, Petrini P, et al. Intermediate-dose versus high-dose prophylaxis for severe haemophilia: comparing outcome and costs since the 1970s. *Blood* 2013; **122**: 1129–36.

47 Valentino LA, Mamonov V, Hellmann A, et al. A randomized comparison of two prophylaxis regimens and a paired comparison of on-demand and prophylaxis treatments in hemophilia A management. *J Thromb Haemost* 2012; **10**(3): 359–67.

48 Aledort LM, Haschmeyer RH, Pettersson H. A longitudinal study of orthopaedic outcomes for severe factor-VIII-deficient haemophiliacs. The Orthopaedic Outcome Study Group. *J Intern Med* 1994; **236**: 391–9.

49 Smith PS, Teutsch SM, Shaffer PA, Rolka H, Evatt B. Episodic versus prophylactic infusions for hemophilia A: a cost-effectiveness analysis. *J Pediatr* 1996; **129**: 424–31.

50 Schramm W, Royal S, Kroner B, *et al.* Clinical outcomes and resource utilization associated with haemophilia care in Europe. *Haemophilia* 2002; **8**: 33–43.

51 Steen Carlsson K, Hojgard S, Glomstein A, *et al.* On-demand vs. prophylactic treatment for severe haemophilia in Norway and Sweden: differences in treatment characteristics and outcome. *Haemophilia* 2003; **9**(5): 555–66.

52 Liou WS, Tu TC, Cheng SN, *et al.* Secondary prophylaxis treatment versus on-demand treatment for patients with severe haemophilia A: comparisons of cost and outcomes in Taiwan. *Haemophilia* 2011; **17**(1): 45–54.

53 Collins P, Faradji A, Morfini M, Enriquez MM, Schwartz L. Efficacy and safety of secondary prophylactic vs. on-demand sucrose-formulated recombinant factor VIII treatment in adults with severe hemophilia A: results from a 13-month crossover study. *J Thromb Haemost* 2010; **8**(1): 83–9.

PART III

Inhibitors to factor VIII

CHAPTER 5

Inhibitors to factor VIII: immunology

Jean-Marie R. Saint-Remy and Marc G. Jacquemin
University of Leuven, Leuven, Belgium

Introduction

The immune response toward factor VIII (FVIII) presents several characteristics that make it unique. Antibodies to FVIII are made by healthy individuals, by patients suffering from hemophilia A, and by patients affected by some autoimmune diseases. FVIII is an autoantigen in the first and third of these situations. In the second instance, FVIII is administered intravenously and on a recurrent basis. The purpose of this chapter is to review our current understanding of the homeostasis of the anti-FVIII response, to summarize information recently gathered from animal models, and to update data obtained from relevant clinical observations.

Homeostasis of the antifactor VIII immune response

The production of antibodies to FVIII, analogous to the immune response to any soluble glycoprotein, depends on the interaction between specific B and T lymphocytes. The repertoire of T cells is established primarily in the thymus. The role of the latter is threefold:

1 To eliminate T cells that do not recognize major histocompatibility class (MHC) class I or class II determinants, a process through which CD4⁻CD8⁻ T cells mature into CD8⁺ or CD4⁺, respectively.
2 To eliminate T cells that recognize with high affinity the complex of self epitopes and MHC determinants.
3 To select a population of regulatory T cells expressing CD25.

Observations in mice and humans have established that in some circumstances FVIII-specific T cells can be found in the periphery, which indicates that the thymic selection does not eliminate all T cells with the capacity to react with FVIII.

By contrast, the B-cell repertoire is continuously replenished over the lifespan. Random rearrangement of the B-cell receptor

(BCR) in the bone marrow generates cells with the potential of reacting with FVIII. The majority of autoreactive B cells are eliminated before entering the periphery. However, B cells use a number of mechanisms by which they can further diversify in the periphery. This is rendered possible by somatic hypermutation, which is a property of B cells. It involves the random introduction of mutations in antibody hypervariable regions, followed by affinity-driven selection.

All conditions are therefore assembled for an immune response to FVIII to emerge: specific T and B cells are present. However, the mechanisms by which the immune response is kept under control, i.e. without emergence of inhibitor antibodies, are many: specific cells maintained in a state of anergy or unresponsiveness, the presence of anti-idiotypic antibodies, and regulatory T cells are but a few of these mechanisms. However, subtle alterations in this equilibrium can rapidly lead to the production of antibodies.

Lessons from animal models

Significant progress in our understanding of how anti-FVIII murine antibodies are elicited has been made since the mouse hemophilia A model became available. Strains with target disruption of exons 16 or 17 mimic the situation of severe hemophilia A patients and have been used to study the conditions under which antibodies are generated. Injection of physiologic quantities of human rFVIII by the intravenous route elicits a strong antibody response, with T-cell activation observed after only 3 days [1]. An additional insight gleaned from FVIII immunization in hemophilia A mice is that von Willebrand factor (VWF) may somehow affect the immunogenicity of FVIII, both by reducing the overall antibody response toward FVIII and by modifying the profile of antibody specificity [2]. These results must be interpreted with caution since the protective effect of VWF is dependent on the model and it can also be recapitulated by administration of other foreign proteins [3].

Textbook of Hemophilia, Third Edition. Edited by Christine A. Lee, Erik E. Berntorp and W. Keith Hoots.
© 2014 John Wiley & Sons, Ltd. Published 2014 by John Wiley & Sons, Ltd.

The mouse model of haemophilia A has been exploited for the testing of various approaches of immunomodulation. Thus, information on how to suppress an immune response gleaned from other fields of immunologic research has been implemented in haemophilia A mice [1,4]. Several studies highlighted the potential role of modified antigen-presenting cells expressing FVIII [5,6] and of regulatory T cells (reviewed in [7]) in controlling the anti-FVIII immune response. FVIII gene therapy also offers an opportunity to prevent an immune response to FVIII in adult mice and dogs [8]. All these studies have opened therapeutic opportunities to prevent inhibitor formation, but have fallen short for the complete suppression of an ongoing inhibitor formation. A full suppression of an established immune response to FVIII has only recently been achieved by gene therapy [9].

Immune tolerance induction (ITI) by prolonged administration of FVIII has been widely used for the last two decades to treat patients with inhibitor. The mechanism of action of ITI is still unknown. A mouse model of ITI based on an implantable venous-access device system has only recently been developed [10]. *In vitro*, concentrations of FVIII equivalent to what would be achieved in a patient under ITI results in induction of apoptosis of FVIII-specific memory B cells [11]. Animal models of hemophilia will no doubt continue to shed light on the mechanisms controlling the immune response to FVIII, in addition to providing valuable alternative therapies for inhibitors.

Clinical observations

Characterization of antifactor VIII antibodies
Physicochemical characteristics
Antibody specificity
Mapping B-cell epitopes on FVIII has been the subject of many studies [12]. The presence of antibodies to FVIII is often confused with the presence of inhibitor antibodies, which constitute only a subset of antibodies with functional properties related essentially to the epitope they recognize.

To date, clusters of B-cell epitopes have been identified primarily on the C2 and A2 domains [12,13]. However, in the case of the C2 epitopes, it is known that the three-dimensional conformation is important for full antibody recognition, as shown by the importance of the disulfide bridge within this domain.

The diversity of antibodies recognizing a given cluster have recently been outlined by the characterization of a large collection of mouse monoclonal antibodies recognizing the FVIII C2 domain. Competition experiments between such antibodies and patient polyclonal antibodies demonstrated the existence of the different types of anti-C2 antibodies among patients' anti-FVIII antibodies [14].

Additional clusters of B-cell epitopes have been described on the A3 [15] and C1 [13] domains, the frequency of which is unclear.

Antibody isotype and genetic origin
The anti-FVIII antibody response recruits all subclasses of immunoglobulin G (IgG), but the IgG4 isotype is somewhat overrepresented [16], considering that IgG4 accounts for only 3% of the total IgG concentration in plasma. IgG4 is associated with long-term exposure to antigens [17], a situation that characterizes hemophilia A patients with long-standing inhibitors. Immortalization of B lymphocytes as well as phage display has provided information on antibodies directed to the A2, A3, C1, and C2 domains, and have helped to determine the repertoire of immunoglobulin genes coding for anti-FVIII antibodies [18,19].

Functional properties
Kinetics of factor VIII inactivation
One usually distinguishes two types of inhibitor antibodies: type 1 antibodies completely inhibit FVIII procoagulant activity following second-order kinetics, while type 2 antibodies follow more complex kinetics and cannot inhibit FVIII completely [20]. The reason for such a difference is not known. It may be related to different mechanisms of FVIII inactivation and/or to differences in affinity, although it is possible that interaction with VWF plays a role. Indeed, Gawryl and Hoyer [21] reported that, for most type 2 inhibitors, FVIII inactivation was partial only when the antibody was in the presence of VWF. The later observation that antibodies to the A3 and C2 domains competed with VWF for binding to FVIII provided an explanation for the effect of VWF on inhibitor kinetics. It is noteworthy that antibodies competing with VWF and with a sufficiently high affinity for FVIII can inactivate FVIII completely (type I inhibitor), albeit following complex kinetics because binding to FVIII requires the preliminary dissociation of the FVIII–VWF complex [19]. Alternatively, VWF can be required for inhibitor activity. In such a case, it is likely that antibodies reduce the rate of dissociation of FVIIIa from VWF [22].

In contrast, rare antibodies only partially inhibit FVIII even in the absence of VWF [21,22]. The human monoclonal antibody LE2E9, which was derived from a patient with mild hemophilia A with inhibitor, recognizes the FVIII C1 domain and inhibits only 85% FVIII activity in the absence of VWF. The mechanism of action of this antibody is still under investigation, but its high affinity ($K_d = 0.5 \times 10^{-9}$ mol/L) indicates that, when it is present in excess over FVIII, all FVIII molecules must be complexed to the antibody [22]. Antibodies such as LE2E9 probably, therefore, reduce the cofactor activity of the FVIII molecule in the X–ase complex.

Whatever the precise reason for this difference, the distinction between type 1 and type 2 inhibitors remains useful. Thus, type 1 inhibitors are most often observed in severe hemophilia A patients who respond to FVIII infusions by producing high antibody titers. In contrast, type 2 inhibitors are observed preferentially in mild or moderate hemophilia A patients, in previously untreated patients (PUPs) mounting a transitory response to FVIII infusion, and in patients producing antibodies toward FVIII molecules altered by preparation procedures [23]. This distinction is also relevant for the bleeding phenotype and response to treatment. Type 2 inhibitor patients usually present with skin and soft tissue bleeding rather than the joint and intraorgan bleeding observed in patients with type 1 inhibitors. In addition, eradication of the inhibitor, either spontaneously or as the result of infusion with high doses of FVIII, is readily achieved in patients with type 2 inhibitors, whereas type 1 inhibitor patients are far less responsive [24].

Mechanisms of factor VIII inactivation

One usually distinguishes two main categories of inhibitor antibodies. In the first case, antibodies bind to or within short distance of a site of FVIII that is involved in its function. It is worth noting that almost all possibilities have been illustrated by the study of mouse or human anti-FVIII antibodies. Thus, antibodies have been observed that inhibit the binding of FVIII to phospholipids (PL), to VWF [12], to FIXa [12,15], and to thrombin or FXa [25], thereby interfering with thrombin cleavage.

In addition to this generic steric hindrance mechanism, antibodies can be formed to epitopes that are accessible only when the molecule is either bound to VWF or activated. Such antibodies are much more difficult to distinguish from polyclonal antibody populations, making it difficult to determine either their prevalence and/or their clinical relevance [26].

Recently, antibodies with catalytic activity to FVIII have been described, demonstrating a strong correlation between such an activity and the titer of inhibitor antibodies. Their presence is detectable in ∼50% of hemophilia A patients with inhibitors [27]. Highly purified preparations of polyclonal anti-FVIII antibodies exert this catalytic activity when contaminating enzymes are excluded.

Notably, the majority of anti-FVIII antibodies do not interfere with FVIII function, as evaluated by current assay systems [13]. However, it is not yet clear whether or not such "nonfunctional" antibodies have a pathophysiologic role. It has been suggested that such antibodies could increase the clearance rate of FVIII from the circulation [28], perhaps thereby increasing the uptake of FVIII–immunoglobulin complexes by phagocytic cells. The relevance and specificity of noninhibitory antibodies need to be further monitored as a recent study demonstrated that a significant proportion of patients without a history of positive inhibitor measured by the Bethesda test have anti-FVIII antibodies [29].

Factor VIII-specific T cells

Several clinical observations indicate that FVIII-specific T cells support the development of the humoral response to FVIII. In some patients with an established humoral response to FVIII, human immunodeficiency virus (HIV) infection leads to a decline in FVIII inhibitor as well as T-cell counts [30]. A large proportion of anti-FVIII antibodies belong to the IgG4 subclass

[16]. This pinpoints a role for T cells in the development of the humoral response to FVIII since isotype switching is T-cell dependent. Lastly, hypermutations have been consistently detected in the genes coding for the variable part of cloned anti-FVIII antibodies [18,19]. This indicates that B cells secreting anti-FVIII antibodies undergo affinity maturation processes that require specific T-cell help. The observation that polymorphisms in the T cell *CTLA-4* gene influence the incidence of inhibitor development [31] further supports a role of T cells in inhibitor production.

Factor VIII-specific T cells have been identified in the peripheral blood of hemophilia A patients with inhibitor using T-cell proliferation assays with native FVIII [32]. The epitope(s) recognized by such T cells have been mapped using synthetic peptides covering the entire FVIII molecule [33]. In severe hemophilia A patients with inhibitor, FVIII-specific T cells recognizing a large array of peptides scattered over the entire FVIII molecule have been detected. T cells proliferating in response to such peptides have also been identified in hemophilia A patients without an inhibitor and in healthy individuals [33]. Unexpectedly, FVIII-specific T cells have also been isolated in patients who underwent a successful immune tolerance induction with FVIII [34].

Only minor qualitative or quantitative differences have been identified between FVIII-specific T cells isolated from healthy individuals and T cells isolated from hemophilia A patients with or without inhibitor. However, more clear-cut differences between normal individuals and hemophilia A patients with an inhibitor have been observed when FVIII- specific T cells were examined at the clonal level. The epitope specificity of the T-cell lines characterized so far is also more restricted than that observed when peptides are used to stimulate CD4$^+$ T cells isolated from blood of hemophilia A patients or from normal individuals [35,36].

The phenotype of the FVIII-specific T cells may be different in patients with or without inhibitor. FVIII-specific clones responding to the same epitope have been isolated from two *repeatedly* infused brothers, of whom only one has not developed a clinically significant inhibitor. In the initial phase of the immune response against FVIII, clones were T helper (TH) 17/TH1- or TH1/TH2-polarized, whereas all clones isolated later were TH2-polarized cells. In contrast, all clones from the brother who did not develop an inhibitor were TH1-polarized, indicating that tolerance to FVIII can be maintained even with circulating TH1-polarized cells that respond vigorously to *in-vitro* FVIII stimulation [37]. Two populations of FVIII-specific T cells may therefore coexist in the periphery. One population is detectable in normal individuals and in hemophilia A patients irrespective of inhibitor status and is demonstrable only when the entire FVIII-specific T-cell repertoire is screened through the use of peptides. A second population of bona fide pathogenic T cells is present only in patients with inhibitor antibodies and may produce a different set of interleukins.

Factor VIII is present in relatively low concentration in plasma (0.2 μg/mL, 1 nM), which raises the question of how FVIII can be presented by professional antigen presenting cells to T cells. Capture of FVIII by human dendritic cells is mediated at least in part by macrophage mannose receptor (CD206) expressed on dendritic cells and by mannose-terminating glycans on FVIII. However, the interaction between FVIII and CD206 is blocked by VWF [38] so that *in vivo* it cannot be excluded that other mechanisms could be exploited by antigen-presenting cells to present FVIII to T cells. The C1 domain is also involved in capture of FVIII by DC as an antibody to C1 inhibits FVIII binding to *C1* [39]. It has therefore been speculated that modulation of FVIII uptake by antigen-presenting cells may provide novel therapeutic approaches for treatment of inhibitor formation in patients with hemophilia A.

Infection and/or inflammation give signals to antigen-presenting cells, which increase the ability of the immune system to recognize a foreign antigen. This may explain why surgical intervention is associated with a higher risk of inhibitor development than treatment with similar doses of FVIII for other conditions, such as bleeding [40].

Future perspectives

Many questions remain concerning the immune response to FVIII. However, it is clearly worth pursuing these types of investigations. Beyond the primary goal, which is to provide new methods to prevent and/or suppress the production of inhibitors in patients, more broadly applicable information will undoubtedly be gathered.

The anti-FVIII immune response represents the only known situation in which allo- and autoimmune responses are observed concurrently and in which patients at risk can be followed longitudinally. This offers the possibility of studying the way in which tolerance is established in central and peripheral organs. With the help of suitable animal models and experiments carried out at the clonal level (including transgenic animals), there is little doubt that mechanisms leading to anti-FVIII immune responses will be progressively unraveled.

References

1 Qian J, Collins M, Sharpe AH, Hoyer LW. Prevention and treatment of factor VIII inhibitors in murine hemophilia A. *Blood* 2000; **95**: 1324–9.

2 Behrmann M, Fasold H, Pasi J, *et al.* Von Willebrand factor modulates factor VIII immunogenicity: comparative study of different plasma-derived and recombinant factor VIII concentrates in a hemophilia A mouse model. *Thromb Haemost* 2002; **88**: 2221–9.

3 Qadura M, Waters B, Burnett E, *et al.* Recombinant and plasma-derived factor VIII products induce distinct splenic cytokine microenvironments in hemophilia A mice. *Blood* 2009; **114**: 871–80.

4 Wroblewska A, Reipert BM, Pratt KP, Voorberg J. Dangerous liaisons: how the immune system deals with factor VIII. *J Thromb Haemost* 2012; **11**: 47–55.

5 Lei TC, Scott DW. Induction of tolerance to factor VIII inhibitors by gene therapy with immunodominant A2 and C2 domains presented by B cells as Ig fusion proteins. *Blood* 2005; **105**: 4865–70.

6 Su RJ, Epp A, Feng J, *et al.* Suppression of the immune response to FVIII in hemophilia A mice by transgene modified tolerogenic dendritic cells. *Mol Ther* 2011; **19**: 1896–904.

7 Cao O, Loduca PA, Herzog RW. Role of regulatory T cells in tolerance to coagulation factors. *J Thromb Haemost* 2009; **7**(Suppl. 1): 88–91.

8 Sabatino DE, Lange AM, Altynova ES, *et al.* Efficacy and safety of long-term prophylaxis in severe hemophilia A dogs following liver gene therapy using AAV vectors. *Mol Ther* 2011; **19**: 442–9.

9 Finn JD, Ozelo MC, Sabatino DE, *et al.* Eradication of neutralizing antibodies to factor VIII in canine hemophilia A after liver gene therapy. *Blood* 2010; **116**: 5842–8.

10 Madoiwa S, Kobayashi E, Kashiwakura Y, *et al.* Immune response against serial infusion of factor VIII antigen through an implantable venous-access device system in haemophilia A mice. *Haemophilia* 2012; **18**: e323–30.

11 Hausl C, Ahmad RU, Sasgary M, *et al.* High-dose factor VIII inhibits factor VIII-specific memory B cells in hemophilia A with factor VIII inhibitors. *Blood* 2005; **106**: 3415–22.

12 Scandella DH. Properties of anti-factor VIII antibodies in haemophilia A patients. *Semin Thromb Haemost* 2000; **26**: 137–42.

13 Gilles JGG, Arnout J, Vermylen J, *et al.* Anti-Factor VIII antibodies of haemophiliac patients are directed primarily towards nonfunctional determinants and do not exhibit isotypic restriction. *Blood* 1993; **82**: 2452–61.

14 Meeks SL, Healey JF, Parker ET, *et al.* Nonclassical anti-C2 domain antibodies are present in patients with factor VIII inhibitors. *Blood* 2008; **112**: 1151–3.

15 Fijnvandraat K, Celie PHN, Turenhout EAM, *et al.* A human alloantibody interferes with binding of factor IXa to the factor VIII light chain. *Blood* 1998; **91**: 2347–52.

16 Andersen BR, Terry WD. Gamma G4-globulin antibody causing inhibition of clotting Factor VIII. *Nature* 1968; **217**: 174–5.

17 Aalberse RC, Schuurman J. IgG4 breaking the rules. *Immunology* 2002; **105**: 9–19.

18 van den Brink EN, Bril WS, Turenhout EA, *et al.* Two classes of germline genes both derived from the V(H)1 family direct the formation of human antibodies that recognize distinct antigenic sites in the C2 domain of factor VIII. *Blood* 2002; **99**: 2828–34.

19 Jacquemin MG, Desqueper BG, Benhida A, *et al.* Mechanism and kinetics of factor VIII inactivation: study with an IgG4 monoclonal antibody derived from a hemophilia A patient with inhibitor. *Blood* 1998; **92**: 496–506.

20 Biggs R, Austen DE, Denson KW, *et al.* The mode of action of antibodies which destroy factor VIII. II. Antibodies which give complex concentration graphs. *Br J Haematol* 1972; **23**: 137–55.

21 Gawryl M, Hoyer L. Inactivation of factor VIII coagulant activity by two different types of human antibodies. *Blood* 1982; **60**: 1103–8.

22 Jacquemin MG, Benhida A, Peerlinck K, *et al.* A human antibody directed to the factor VIII C1 domain inhibits factor VIII cofactor activity and binding to von Willebrand factor. *Blood* 2000; **95**: 156–65.

Table 7.1 (a) Prevalence of inhibitors in hemophilia A. The table presents the prevalence estimate (as the upper boundary of the confidence interval) for inhibitors in hemophilia A as reported by relevant publications. The prevalence estimate has been recalculated from the number of events and number of exposed or (*) the reported rate and number of exposed.

Study	Sample	Rate (upper 95% confidence limit)
Strauss, *N Engl J Med*, 1969	143	0.18
Ikkala, *Scand J Haematol*, 1969	90	0.21
Brinkhouse, *Thromb Diath Haem*, 1972	1486*	0.08
Kasper, *Thromb Diath Haem*, 1973	325	0.13
Biggs, *Br J Haematol*, 1974	1625*	0.07
Rizza, *Br Med J*, 1983	4321	0.07
Gill, *Prog Clin Biol Res*, 1984	1522*	0.16
Schwarzinger, *Am J Hematol*, 1987	57	0.30
Izquierdo-Ramirez, *Bol Med H Inf Mexico*, 1988	298	0.11
Rasi, *Br J Haematol*, 1990	110	0.26
Sultan, *Thromb Haemost*, 1992	2870	0.08
Mahasanda,S, *Asian J Trop Med Pub Health*, 1993	101	0.14
Rosendaal, *Blood*, 1993	447	0.09
Aronis, *Haemophilia*, 1995	82	0.37
Yee, *Br J Haematol*, 1999	419	0.06
Oren, *Acta Haematol*, 1999	58	0.40
Rieger, *Thromb Haemost*, 1999	1345*	0.22
UKHCDO, Internal Report, 2000	4979	0.06
Rizza, *Haemophilia*, 2001	4826	0.06
Ghosh, *Haemophilia*, 2001	352	0.11
Wang, *Haemophilia*, 2010	1435	0.05
Serban, *Hämostaseologie*, 2011	494	0.19
Company, *Behbood Journal*, 2011	104	0.28
Webert, *Haemophilia*, 2011	2435	0.04

Table 7.1 (b) Incidence of inhibitors in previously untreated severe hemophilia A patients. The table presents the estimate of the incidence (as the upper boundary of the confidence interval) for inhibitors in hemophilia A as reported by relevant publications. The incidence estimate has been recalculated from the number of events and number of subject at risk or (*) the reported rate and number of subjects at risk. Due to inconsistency in the reporting of follow-up, the approximate cumulative incidence has been reported.

Study	Sample	Rate (upper 95% confidence limit)
Lusher, *Ann Haematol*, 1991	82	0.12
Addiego, *Lancet*, 1993	89	0.38
Lusher, *N Engl J Med*, 1993	93	0.25
Peerlink, *Blood*, 1993	76	0.13
Bray, *Blood*, 1994	79	0.32
Schimpf, *Thromb Haemost*, 1995	22	0.27
Yee, *Br J Haematol*, 1997	37	0.17
Rokicka-Milewska, *Ann Hematol* (Abstr), 1999	28	0.21
El Alfy, *Haemophilia*, 2000	25	0.31
Courter, *Semin Haematol*, 2001	101	0.41
Mauser-Bunschoten, *Haemophilia*, 2001	59	0.36
Yoshioka, *Int J Hematol*, 2003	47	0.40
Escuriola-Ettinghausen, *Haemophilia*, 2006	57	0.34
Kreuz, *Thromb Haemost* (Abstr), 2005	37	0.29
Morado, *Haemophilia*, 2005	48	0.43
Goudemand, Blood, 2006	148	0.21
Gringeri, *Haemophilia*, 2006	31	0.26
Gouw, *Blood*, 2007	263	0.32
Pollman, *Haemophilia*, 2007	16	0.45
Chalmers, *Haemophilia*, 2008	304	0.26
Delumeau, *Thromb Haemost*, 2008	30	0.20
Musso, *Haemophilia*, 2008	13	0.39
Bidlingmaier, *Haemophilia*, 2009	52	0.54
Strauss, *Haemophilia*, 2011	292	0.15
Shirahata, *Haemophilia*, 2011	141	0.34
Klukowska, *Thromb Research*, 2011	39	0.18
Awerswald, *Haemophilia*, 2012	55	0.42
Mancuso, *J Thromb Haemost*, 2012	318	0.31
Gouw, *N Engl J Med*, 2013	517*	0.36

two large European studies is around 13%, and it is 16.4% in the white population of a US study [13] who also showed an increased prevalence in black (26.8%) and Hispanic (24.5%) patients. A recent critical appraisal of the variability of estimates of prevalence of hemophilia A worldwide [14], investigating variation due to source of information, census, and time convincingly showed that the reported prevalence of hemophilia has a strong positive correlation with the wealth of the reporting country and steadily increases over time. The prevalence and epidemiology of inhibitors was not directly investigated, but it is likely that the same factors affect the reported prevalence of inhibitors. Noticeably, a recent appraisal of the prevalence of inhibitors in the Canadian Hemophilia Registry, performed with a stringent epidemiologic method [15], showed a low prevalence both in the overall (3.3%) and in severe patient (8.9%) populations. Analysis of the trend over time showed fairly stable estimates from 2003 to 2009 for all categories with the exception of severe hemophilia A, where the prevalence fell from 13.8% to 9.2%. Epidemiology of inhibitors in moderate and mild hemophilia patients is discussed elsewhere in this book.

Hemophilia B

Much less data are available to estimate the prevalence of inhibitors in hemophilia B [15–20]. Overall the prevalence spans from 1.5% to 3.6%, with the upper limit of the 95% confidence interval for the bigger study at 2% [18]. As for hemophilia A, the prevalence was lower in the analysis of the Canadian Hemophilia Registry with prevalence in the overall population of 0.6% and in severe patients of 2.1%.

Inhibitor incidence in previously untreated patients

Hemophilia A

Several reports have been published about the cumulative incidence of inhibitors in PUPs (Table 7.1b). The best estimate of the risk of inhibitors in PUPs is around 25%, with the mean time to inhibitor development around 14 to 20 ED, which for patients on standard prophylaxis is 1–2 months from the beginning of treatment. The determinants of inhibitor risks in PUPs will be reviewed elsewhere in this book; in this paragraph, we will focus on briefly appraising the nature and quality of the existing evidence, particularly looking at the issue of comparative immunogenicity. Every attempt to provide an interpretation of the causes of inhibitor occurrence, even in the framework of the most inclusive and extensive systematic review [1], has been immediately criticized for the component relative to the comparative immunogenicity of different factor VIII molecules [12]. As demonstrated in a subsequent systematic review [2], the relative strength of factor VIII brand or class is significantly lower than that of other risk factors (i.e. family history, reason for or intensity of treatment) and significantly confounded by study characteristics (i.e. study design and time, testing frequency). The two largest cohorts of PUPs ever studied, the Research of Determinants of Inhibitor Development (RODIN) study cohort [21] and the EUHASS cohort [9], though not yet published in a peer-reviewed form, confirmed both the overall cumulative incidence of inhibitors in PUPs and the nonsignificant difference among different concentrates or plasma-derived and recombinant products. The overall cumulative incidence of inhibitor development within the first 50 ED in the last interim analysis of EUHASS was 25% (95% confidence interval 20.1–30.5%). Time to inhibitor was 14 ED [interquartile range (IQR) 9–23]. The overall inhibitor incidence in the RODIN study was 32% (95% CI 28.4–35.8%) and the cumulative incidence of high responding inhibitors was 22.2% (19.1–25.7%). A randomized controlled study addressing the differential immunogenicity of plasma-derived and recombinant factor concentrates in PUPs is underway (the Survey of Inhibitors in Plasma-Product Exposed Toddlers or SIPPET study, http://www.sippet.org).

Hemophilia B

The incidence of factor IX (FIX) inhibitors reported in the literature is between 1.5 and 3% of all patients with hemophilia B and between 9 and 23% of severely affected FIX-deficient patients [18,22–25]. In the EUHASS data collection, the overall cumulative incidence of inhibitor development within the first 50 ED was 7.7% (95% CI 1.6–20.9) and time to inhibitor was 7 ED.

Inhibitor incidence in previously treated patients

The risk of inhibitor development in previously treated patients (PTPs) is low but not null, and can be considered as the "baseline risk for inhibitor development" after a patient had become tolerant to factor VIII [26]. The estimate of the baseline risk of inhibitors in PTPs is critical information in any assessment of treatment-related inhibitors, which is what PTPs have been proposed for as the ideal hemophilic subset [27], and which is what

is required by regulatory authorities [28]. Unfortunately, investigators and regulators were and are keen to accept uncontrolled PTP series for the scope, without contextually measuring the baseline risk of inhibitor in patients not exposed (i.e. switched) to the drug under evaluation. Historically, on proposing the use of uncontrolled case series of PTP for the assessment of the immunogenicity of factor concentrates [27], it was implicitly assumed that the inhibitor rate from historical controls was an economic way of accounting for the baseline risk of inhibitors. The concept of baseline risk was soon lost, leading to the assumption that any inhibitor observed in PTP studies was related to the molecule the patient was receiving, which completely ignores the multicausality mechanism of inhibitor development. Though not critical when roughly assessing the suitability of a new molecule for use as substitution therapy [29], the multicausality principle has to be taken into account when comparing for safety (i.e. in terms of adverse event rates, like inhibitors) or effectiveness (i.e. in terms of bleeding rate) two different regimens or two different formulations.

The incidence of inhibitors in large and well-characterized populations of PTPs (Table 7.1c) is estimated at 0.2% patient

Table 7.1 (c) Cumulative incidence of inhibitors in previously treated severe hemophilia A patients. The table presents the estimate of the incidence (as the upper boundary of the confidence interval) for inhibitors in hemophilia A as reported by relevant publications. The incidence estimate has been recalculated from the number of events and number of person-years (PY) at risk or the reported rate and number of subjects at risk. Only studies allowing the calculation of the cumulative incidence has been plotted. (*) Recalculated incidence rate was 0.0037.

Study	PY	Rate (upper 95% confidence limit)
Aygoren-Pursun, *Thromb Haemost*, 1997	39	0.05
White II, *Thromb Haemost*, 1997	328	0.01
Aznar, *Haemophilia*, 1998	48	0.04
Abshire, *Thromb Haemost*, 2000	121	0.02
Courter, *Semin Haematol*, 2001	565	0.01
Vossebeld, *Haemophilia*, 2003	280	0.01
Gringeri, *Br J Haematol*, 2004	13	0.24
Smith, *Haemophilia*, 2005	29	0.10
Kempton, *Haemophilia*, 2006	3268	0.00(*)
Yoshioka, *Int J Haematol*, 2006	206	0.06
Nemes, *Haemophilia*, 2007	28	0.07
Singleton, *Thromb Haemost*, 2007	157	0.04
Pollmann, *Haemophilia*, 2007	331	0.01
Delumeau, *Thromb Haemost*, 2008	447	0.01
Blanchette, *J Thromb Haemost*, 2008	27	0.07
Musso, *Haemophilia*, 2008	300	0.01
Recht, *Haemophilia*, 2009	47	0.10
Recht, *Haemophilia*, 2009	55	0.12
Young, *Haemophilia*, 2009	70	0.03
Den Uijl, *Haemophilia*, 2009	85	0.02
Oldenburg, *Haemophilia*, 2010	457	0.02
Windyga, *Haemophilia*, 2010	8	0.39
Vidovic, *Haemophilia*, 2010	77	0.02
Bacon, *Haemophilia*, 2011	283	0.01

year, with an upper 95 CI at 0.4% patient year [1,2,30]. The best source to estimate the baseline risk of clinically relevant inhibitors is constituted by large registry data [5,31–34]. The reports from studies provide a measure of the risk of inhibitors in PTPs that is reliable, consistent, and reproducible. Interestingly, the incidence and cumulative rates have progressively increased by a factor of 3 over time, from 0.15 to 0.53% person-years [32–34]. This might be a spurious effect due to increased awareness and more accurate and frequent inhibitor testing; it might, alternatively, reflect more widespread use of prophylaxis, higher factor consumption, or more frequent switching; it might finally parallel the temporal trends toward more frequent allergic and autoimmune disorders observed in the general population. Ten times more inhibitors are usually detected in registration trials testing new drugs, which might again be the consequence of closer testing or suboptimal screening at baseline. All the registration trial in PTPs are by definition switching trials. A few non-registration studies [35–40] explored the rate of inhibitors after switching. While ruling out any major effect of switching (lying well within the 0.2–0.3% patient-years risk of inhibitors measured in PTPs), some of the studies [37,38] showed how critically pre-existing, locally undiagnosed inhibitors may confound the assessment (7.9% on centrally retested samples). It must be also appreciated that the vast majority of the inhibitors detected after switching are transient, even after exposure to highly immunogenic products [35,36]. In view of the scanty knowledge about risk factors for inhibitor development in PTPs, uncontrolled cohorts or their univariate metaanalysis [8] cannot provide trustable comparative assessments; baseline risk and attributable risk fraction need to be accounted for, ideally incorporating control groups as unconfounded as possible. Hierarchical Bayesian appraisal and multivariable analysis will then shed much brighter light on our knowledge about inhibitor rates [41]. The EUHASS project is for the first time providing a prospective parallel observation of inhibitor rates in PTPs, which was 0.29/100 patient-years (95% CI 0.19–0.44) for hemophilia A and 0.06/100 patient-years (95% CI 0.00–0.35) for hemophilia B. The inhibitor rate in severe hemophilia A PTPs was 0.20/100 patient-years of treatment (95% CI 0.12–0.28) and for severe hemophilia B PTPs 0.05/100 patient-years (95% CI 0.00–0.25). As mentioned above, several reports have focused during the last few years on the rate of inhibitor development in mild hemophilia A patients, who seem to follow a completely different pattern and will be discussed in a separate section of this book.

Natural history of inhibitors in hemophilia A

After adjusting for the increased mortality rate in inhibitor patients, the observation that prevalence is lower than incidence clearly indicates that not all patients who develop inhibitors will continue to have them for their entire lives. Some of these inhibitors will spontaneously disappear, other will be cleared with immunotolerance (ITI) treatment. The epidemiology of the natural history of inhibitors is extremely fascinating, but very little is actually known about the long-term history of inhibitors in the absence of ITI. A seminal observation of spontaneous resolution of inhibitors in patients who continued to be exposed to standard doses of factor VIII was reported by Rizza and Matthews [42], and recently confirmed by a report that nontolerized inhibitors may present different patterns over time including not only "stable positivity" or "stable negativity," but also a third category of "unstable" inhibitors [43]. Similarly, spontaneous clearance of inhibitors in up to 2/3 of cases was reported in absence of ITI in a large Italian cohort [44].

References

1 Wight J, Paisley S. The epidemiology of inhibitors in haemophilia A: a systematic review. *Haemophilia* 2003; **9**(4): 418–35.

2 Iorio A, Halimeh S, Holzhauer S, et al. Rate of inhibitor development in previously untreated hemophilia A patients treated with plasma-derived or recombinant factor VIII concentrates: a systematic review. *J Thromb Haemost* 2010; **8**(6): 1256–65.

3 Ragni MV, Ojeifo O, Feng J, et al. Risk factors for inhibitor formation in haemophilia: a prevalent case-control study. *Haemophilia* 2009; **15**(5): 1074–82.

4 Gouw SC, Van den Berg HM, Oldenburg J, et al. F8 gene mutation type and inhibitor development in patients with severe hemophilia A: systematic review and meta-analysis. *Blood* 2012; **119**(12): 2922–34.

5 Kempton CL, Soucie JM, Abshire TC. Incidence of inhibitors in a cohort of 838 males with hemophilia A previously treated with factor VIII concentrates. *J Thromb Haemost* 2006; **4**(12): 2576–81.

6 Calvez T, Laurian Y, Goudemand J. Inhibitor incidence with recombinant vs. plasma-derived FVIII in previously untreated patients with severe hemophilia A: homogeneous results from four published observational studies. *J Thromb Haemost* 2008; **6**(2): 390–2.

7 Aledort LM, Navickis RJ, Wilkes MM. Can B-domain deletion alter the immunogenicity of recombinant factor VIII? *J Thromb Haemost* 2011; **9**(11): 2180–92.

8 Iorio A, Marcucci M, Makris M. Concentrate related inhibitor risk: is a difference always real? *J Thromb Haemost* 2011; **9**(11): 2176–9.

9 Makris M, Calizzani G, Fischer K, et al. EUHASS: The European Haemophilia Safety Surveillance System. *Thromb Res* 2011; **127**(Suppl. 2): S22–5.

10 Iorio A, Marcucci M. Clinical trials and haemophilia: does the Bayesian approach make the ideal and desirable good friends? *Haemophilia* 2009; **15**(4): 900–3.

11 Lee ML, Roth DA. A Bayesian approach to the assessment of inhibitor risk in studies of factor VIII concentrates. *Haemophilia* 2005; **11**(1): 5–12.

12 Scharrer I, Ehrlich HJ. Reported inhibitor incidence in FVIII PUP studies: comparing apples with oranges? *Haemophilia* 2004; **10**(2): 197–8.

13 Carpenter SL, Michael Soucie J, Sterner S, Presley R. Increased prevalence of inhibitors in Hispanic patients with severe haemophilia A enrolled in the Universal Data Collection database. *Haemophilia* 2012; **18**(3): e260–5.

14 Stonebraker JS, Bolton-Maggs PHB, Soucie JM, Walker I, Brooker M. A study of variations in the reported haemophilia A prevalence around the world. *Haemophilia* 2010; **16**(1): 20–32.

15 Webert KE, Rivard GE, Teitel J, *et al.* Low prevalence of inhibitor antibodies in the Canadian haemophilia population. *Haemophilia* 2011; **14**: 1–6.

16 Biggs R. Jaundice and Antibodies directed against factors viii and ix in patients treated for haemophilia or Christmas disease in the United Kingdom. *Br J Haematol* 1974; **26**(3): 313–29.

17 Ehrenforth S, Kreuz W, Scharrer I, *et al.* Incidence of development of factor VIII and factor IX inhibitors in haemophiliacs. *Lancet* 1992; **339**(8793): 594–8.

18 Katz J. Prevalence of factor IX inhibitors among patients with haemophilia B: results of a large scale North American survey. *Haemophilia* 1996; **2**: 28–31.

19 Serban M, Mihailov D, Pop L, *et al.* Development of inhibitors in haemophilia. Ongoing epidemiological study. *Hämostaseologie* 2011; **31**(Suppl. 1): S20–3.

20 Sultan Y. Prevalence of inhibitors in a population of 3435 hemophilia patients in France. French Hemophilia Study Group. *Thromb Haemost* 1992; **67**(6): 600–2.

21 Gouw S, Van den Berg M, Van der Bom JG. Factor VIII prophylaxis and inhibitor development in previously untreated patients with severe hemophilia A: The RODIN study. *Haemophilia* 2012; **18**(3): 1–208.

22 Briet E. Factor IX inhibitor in hemophilia B patients: their incidence and prospects for development with high purity factor IX products. *Blood Coag Fibrinol* 1991; **2**: 47–50.

23 Ljung RCR. Gene mutations and inhibitor formation in patients with hemophilia B. *Acta Haematol* 1995; **94**(1): 49–52.

24 Warrier I, Ewenstein BM, Koerper MA, *et al.* Factor IX inhibitors and anaphylaxis in hemophilia B. *J Pediatr Hematol/Oncol* 1997; **19**(1): 23–7.

25 Ljung R, Petrini P, Tengborn L, Sjörin E. Haemophilia B mutations in Sweden: a population-based study of mutational heterogeneity. *Br J Haematol* 2001; **113**(1): 81–6.

26 Manuel DG, Rosella LC. Commentary: assessing population (baseline) risk is a cornerstone of population health planning—looking forward to address new challenges. *Int J Epidemiol* 2010; **39**(2): 380–2.

27 White GC, DiMichele D, Mertens K, *et al.* Utilization of previously treated patients (PTPs), noninfected patients (NIPs), and previously untreated patients (PUPs) in the evaluation of new factor VIII and factor IX concentrates. Recommendation of the Scientific Subcommittee on Factor VIII and Fact. *Thromb Haemost* 1999; **81**(3): 462.

28 European Medicines Agency (EMA). Guideline on the clinical investigation of recombinant and human plasma-derived factor VIII products. 2011; p. EMA/CHMP/BPWP/144533/2009.

29 Glasziou P, Chalmers I, Rawlins M, McCulloch P. When are randomised trials unnecessary? Picking signal from noise. *Br Med J Clin Res* 2007; **334**(7589): 349–51.

30 Kempton CL. Inhibitors in previously treated patients: a review of the literature. *Haemophilia* 2010; **16**(102): 61–5.

31 Mcmillan CW, Shapiro SS, Whitehurst D, Hoyer LW, Rao AV, Lazerson J. The natural history of factor VIII:C inhibitors in patients with hemophilia A: a national cooperative study. II . Observations on the initial development of factor VIII:C inhibitors. *Blood* 1988; **71**: 344–8.

32 Colvin BT, Hay CR, Hill FG, Preston FE. The incidence of factor VIII inhibitors in the United Kingdom, 1990–93. Inhibitor Working Party. United Kingdom Haemophilia Centre Directors Organization. *Br J Haematol* 1995; **89**(4): 908–10.

33 Darby SC, Keeling DM, Spooner RJD, *et al.* The incidence of factor VIII and factor IX inhibitors in the hemophilia population of the UK and their effect on subsequent mortality, 1977–99. *J Thromb Haemost* 2004; **2**(7): 1047–54.

34 Hay CRM, Palmer B, Chalmers E, *et al.* Incidence of factor VIII inhibitors throughout life in severe hemophilia A in the United Kingdom. *Blood* 2011; **117**(23): 6367–70.

35 Mauser-Bunschoten EP, Rosendaal FR, Nieuwenhuis HK, Roosendaal G, Briët E, Van den Berg HM. Clinical course of factor VIII inhibitors developed after exposure to a pasteurised Dutch concentrate compared to classic inhibitors in hemophilia A. *Thromb Haemost* 1994; **71**(6): 703–6.

36 Peerlink K, Arnout J, Di Giambattista M, *et al.* Factor VIII inhibitors in previously treated haemophilia A patients with a double virus-inactivated plasma derived factor VIII concentrate. *Thromb Haemost* 1997; **77**(1): 80–6.

37 Giles A, Rivard G, Teitel J, Walker I. Surveillance for factor VIII inhibitor development in the Canadian Hemophilia A population following the widespread introduction of recombinant factor VIII replacement therapy. *Transfusion Sci* 1998; **19**(2): 139–48.

38 Rubinger M, Lillicrap D, Rivard GE, *et al.* A prospective surveillance study of factor VIII inhibitor development in the Canadian haemophilia A population following the switch to a recombinant factor VIII product formulated with sucrose. *Haemophilia* 2008; **14**(2): 281–6.

39 Bacon CL, Singleton E, Brady B, *et al.* Low risk of inhibitor formation in haemophilia A patients following en masse switch in treatment to a third generation full length plasma and albumin-free recombinant factor VIII product (ADVATE®). *Haemophilia* 2011; **17**(3): 407–11.

40 Singleton E, Smith J, Kavanagh M, Nolan B, White B. Low risk of inhibitor formation in haemophilia patients after a change in treatment from Chinese hamster ovary cell-produced to baby hamster kidney cell-produced recombinant factor VIII. *Thromb Haemost* 2007; **98**(6): 1188–92.

41 European Medicines Agency (EMA). Guideline on clinical trials in small populations. 2006; p. CHMP/EWP/83561/2005.

42 Rizza C, Matthews M. Effect of frequent factor VIII replacement on the level of factor VIII antibodies in haemophiliacs. *Br J Haematol* 1982; **52**: 13–24.

43 Caram C, De Souza RG, De Sousa JC, *et al.* The long-term course of factor VIII inhibitors in patients with congenital haemophilia A without immune tolerance induction. *Thromb Haemost* 2011; **105**(1): 59–65.

44 Tagariello G, Iorio A, Matino D, *et al.* High rate of spontaneous inhibitor clearance during the long term observation study of a single cohort of 524 haemophilia A patients not undergoing immunotolerance. *J Hematol Oncol Pharm* 2013; **6**: 63–70.

CHAPTER 8

Inhibitors to factor VIII: mild and moderate hemophilia

Kathelijne Peerlinck and Marc Jacquemin
KULeuven and University Hospitals, Leuven, Belgium

Introduction

Until the late 1990s, inhibitors in mild/moderate hemophilia A were considered to be very rare. However, since the publication of Hay *et al.* [1] in 1998 on behalf of the UK Haemophilia Centre Directors Organisation, it has been appreciated that inhibitors in mild/moderate hemophilia are more frequent than previously thought. Clinical problems associated with inhibitors in mild/moderate hemophilia are often considerable, since in the majority of cases adult patients are confronted with a change in phenotype from mild/moderate to severe and they suddenly experience spontaneous severe bleeding. Although some of the risk factors for inhibitor development are similar to those in severe hemophilia, others are specific for mild/moderate hemophilia. The study of the immune response in mild/moderate hemophilia A can help to elucidate some of the mechanisms underlying inhibitor formation and disruption of tolerance. Treatment of bleeding episodes and eradication of inhibitors in mild/moderate hemophilia require specific management and special attention should be paid to the prevention of this complication.

Incidence and prevalence

Patients with mild/moderate hemophilia are at lower risk of inhibitor development than severely affected patients. The prevalence of these inhibitors has been estimated to be between 3 and 13% [2–4]. In a prospective study of inhibitor incidence among 1306 hemophilia A patients, only 6% of the inhibitors were found in patients with factor VIII (FVIII) >0.03 IU/mL [5]. Sixteen (28%) of 57 new inhibitors reported between January 1990 and January 1997 in the UK Haemophilia Centre Doctors' Organisation (UKHCDO) inhibitor register, arose in patients with mild or moderate hemophilia [1]. The annual incidence of inhibitors in the UK was 3.5/1000

registered with severe hemophilia and 0.84/1000 patients registered with mild/moderate hemophilia [6]. Preliminary analysis of the INSIGHT study, including >2500 unselected patients with nonsevere hemophilia, all of them having received treatment with FVIII between 1980 and 2010, showed development of inhibitors in 4.3% [95% confidence interval (CI) 3.6–5.2] at a median age of 37 [interquartile range (IQR) 15–60] years and after a median of 25 (IQR 15–57) exposure days to FVIII concentrates [7].

In a prospective study in the Netherlands, the incidence of inhibitor development following intensive treatment with FVIII for surgery was 4% in 56 unselected patients with mild/moderate hemophilia [8].

Clinical presentation

Usually the presence of an inhibitor in patients with mild/moderate hemophilia is suggested by a change in bleeding pattern: patients start to experience severe spontaneous bleeding whereas they used to bleed only after trauma or surgery. This change in bleeding pattern is explained by cross-reactivity of the inhibitor with the mutated FVIII of the patient resulting in a residual FVIII:c level of <0.01 IU/mL [9–11]. The bleedings occur often in muscles and joints as in severe congenital hemophilia but sometimes the bleeding pattern is more reminiscent of acquired hemophilia with the occurrence of large cutaneous bruising, and gastrointestinal and urogenital bleeding [1]. Occasionally, there is no change in residual FVIII level but an inhibitor is detected in the Bethesda assay and/or there is lack of efficiency of FVIII transfusions [11–13]. In some cases, the specificity of the immune response reverts over time from neutralisation of both mutated self and transfused normal FVIII to tolerance to self, resulting in a recovery of the original basal FVIII level and response to desmopressin, despite the persistence of antibodies to exogenous FVIII [1,7,11,12].

Textbook of Hemophilia, Third Edition. Edited by Christine A. Lee, Erik E. Berntorp and W. Keith Hoots.
© 2014 John Wiley & Sons, Ltd. Published 2014 by John Wiley & Sons, Ltd.

Risk factors

Intensive exposure to factor VIII

Inhibitors in mild/moderate hemophilia occur more commonly later in life and an episode of intensive treatment with FVIII concentrate (e.g. for bleeding, trauma or surgery) seems to precede detection of the inhibitor in most reported cases. In the series reported by Hay et al. [1], 16 out of 26 inhibitors were detected after such intensive replacement therapy and in this series no particular concentrate was implicated.

In a case–control study including 36 subjects with nonsevere hemophilia and an inhibitor, intensive treatment (≥6 days) in the preceding year was strongly associated with inhibitor development [odds ratio (OR) 4.64]. The association between intensive treatment and inhibitor development was greater in those ≥30 years of age (OR 13.54) than in those <30 years (OR 1.55). In those >30 years of age, surgery (orthopedic surgery in 11/14), was more likely the indication for intensive FVIII treatment compared with those <30 years ($P = 0.01$). The inhibitor occurred within 12 weeks of the intensive FVIII treatment in 17/18 patients [14].

In a Dutch retrospective study [15], 10 out of 138 patients with nonsevere hemophilia developed an inhibitor after treatment with FVIII. Seven of these 10 inhibitors occurred after intensive treatment for surgery and, in five of the 10 inhibitor patients, FVIII was administered by continuous infusion.

The risk of inhibitor development in nonsevere hemophilia associated with intensive treatment is clearly multifactorial and may be influenced by the indication for intensive treatment (surgery/type of surgery), the age of the patient, and the way of administration (i.e. continuous infusion vs bolus).

Genetic background

In severe hemophilia the risk of inhibitor formation is associated with the type of mutation. More disruptive mutations in the *FVIII* gene such as intron 22 inversions, large gene deletions, and stop codons are associated with about a 35% risk of inhibitor formation, compared to only about 5% in those with missense mutations and small deletions [16]. Missense mutations in the light chain are more often (12%) associated with inhibitors than are missense mutations in other parts of the *FVIII* gene (3.9%) [16]. In patients with mild/moderate hemophilia and inhibitors, certain missense mutations seem to predispose to inhibitor formation. In the series of Hay et al. [1] seven out of nine mutations were clustered in a region at the junction between the C1 and C2 domain. The two remaining mutations affected the A2 domain. Clustering of the mutations in these regions has been confirmed in most other reported cases of mild/moderate hemophilia with inhibitor and some particular mutations such as Arg2150His and Arg593Cys seem to be overrepresented [1,8,9,11,12,17–20]. Some point mutations associated with an increased incidence of inhibitor in patients with mild/moderate hemophilia A are illustrated in Figure 8.1.

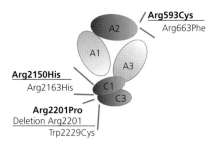

Figure 8.1 *FVIII* mutations responsible for mild/moderate hemophilia A and associated with a high incidence of inhibitor development.

In the Haemophilia A Mutation, Structure, Test and Resource Site (HAMSTeRS) database (http://hadb.org.uk), about 50 point mutations responsible for mild/moderate hemophilia A have been identified in patients with inhibitor. However, further studies are still required to determine the impact of each of these mutations on the incidence of inhibitor development. Further information is also required on the influence of polymorphisms of genes involved in the regulation of the immune response to FVIII in patients with mild/moderate hemophilia A [21,22].

Analysis of the immune response to factor VIII in mild/moderate hemophilia A

To determine why some mutations located in the A2, C1, or C2 domains of the FVIII molecule are more frequently associated with the presence of inhibitor, the humoral and cellular responses to FVIII were analysed at the polyclonal and clonal level.

Analysis of FVIII produced by patients with mild/moderate hemophilia A demonstrated that mutations at residues Arg593, Arg2150, Arg2159, or Ala2201 eliminates FVIII epitopes (antigenic determinants) recognized by inhibitor antibodies [7,12,23–26].

The T-cell response to FVIII was studied in a mild hemophilia A patient carrying an Arg2150His substitution in the C1 domain and who presented with a high titer inhibitor toward normal but not self FVIII. The FVIII-specific T cells of this patient recognized a peptide encompassing residue Arg2150, the residue mutated in the patients' *FVIII* gene and did not recognize recombinant FVIII carrying the substitution Arg2150His. Thus, the C1 domain of wild-type FVIII contains T-cell epitopes that are absent in FVIII carrying the mutation Arg2150His [27] (Figure 8.1).

These observations demonstrate that Arg2150His FVIII and normal FVIII can be distinguished by the immune system not only at the B-cell level but also at the T-cell level. Recently, similar observations have been made with patients carrying the mutation at residues Ala2201 [28] and Arg593 [29], suggesting that this type of phenomenon may occur in patients carrying mutations responsible for mild/moderate hemophilia A and predispose to inhibitor formation to normal FVIII administered as substitution therapy. It is hypothesized that in some patients, activated T cells recognizing exogenous FVIII will also support the activation of B cells producing antibodies directed against both exogenous and self FVIII. In such cases, the phenotype of the patient becomes that of severe hemophilia A.

Interestingly, some T cells recognize antigenic peptides corresponding to the wild-type normal FVIII sequence and to the mutated one. However, in such cases, quantitative differences have been seen in the stimulation of the T cells or in the affinity of the major histocompatibility complex (MHC) class II/peptide complex with the T-cell receptor, suggesting that the immune response is elicited by wild type rather than by self FVIII [27,29]. Sometimes, the presence of T cell recognizing self FVIII is only transient [28]. In such cases, the importance of the interaction of T cells with self FVIII is unclear.

Surprisingly, successful immune tolerance induction by FVIII in hemophilia A patients with inhibitor may occur without deletion of FVIII-specific T cells. FVIII-specific T cells recognizing allogeneic normal FVIII were detected and expanded *in vitro* 1 year after complete elimination of the inhibitor by prolonged administration of FVIII and transient administration of corticosteroids in one patient with mild hemophilia A [30]. It is presently unknown whether the persistence of such FVIII-specific T cells may influence the long-term tolerance to FVIII in successfully desensitized patients.

The FVIII A and C domains are schematically represented in Figure 8.1. The B domain is not shown. Some of the mutations in the A2 domain and at the junction of the C1/C2 domains responsible for mild/moderate hemophilia A and associated with an increased incidence of inhibitor development [1] are indicated. The mutations preventing the binding of some inhibitor antibodies recognizing wild-type normal FVIII are underlined [7,23,25]. Mutations of residues modifying T-cell epitopes are highlighted in bold [27–29].

Treatment

Bleeding episodes

Bleeding episodes in patients with mild/moderate hemophilia who developed an inhibitor are often particularly severe and sometimes life threatening. Bypass therapy with activated prothrombin complex concentrates or recombinant activated factor VII can be used to control bleeding and has the advantage of avoiding anamnesis. Some patients can be treated successfully with deamino-D-arginine vasopressin (DDAVP), especially those patients whose basal FVIII level did not significantly decrease and whose inhibitor does not seem to cross-react with their endogenous FVIII [1,11,12] or once adequate circulating FVIII levels have returned. DDAVP does not cause anamnesis in those patients despite the presence of high-responding inhibitors [1].

Inhibitor eradication

Published data on immune tolerance induction in patients with mild/moderate hemophilia and inhibitors are very scarce. In the series reported by Hay *et al.* [1], immune tolerance induction was attempted in eight patients using different regimens. The Malmo regime [high-dose FVIII combined with cyclophosphamide and intravenous immunoglobulin G (IgG)] was used successfully in two patients and with a partial response in a further two patients, the Van Creveld regime (low-dose FVIII every other day) was used unsuccessfully in one patient and with partial success in a further patient; and the Bonn regime was used unsuccessfully in one patient and with partial success in another patient. The overall success rate of immune tolerance of two out of eight patients seems lower than the reported success rate in severe hemophilia.

Other reported treatments have included immunomodulatory drugs such as corticosteroids, cyclophosphamide, anti-CD20 monoclonal antibody rituximab [8,31–34], and avoidance of re-exposure to FVIII using desmopressin and bypassing agents to treat bleeding episodes [35]. Currently available data are not sufficient to offer evidence-based advice on the optimal treatment of inhibitors in patients with mild/moderate hemophilia A and the management of these patients remains controversial at this point. Preliminary data from a retrospective and prospective data collection in France and Belgium [36,37] suggest that immune tolerance induction could be more effective than no specific treatment or immunomodulating drugs in preventing risk of anamnesis of the inhibitor after re-exposure to FVIII.

Prevention

Maximal use of desmopressin for the treatment of patients with mild/moderate hemophilia A is certainly useful to prevent the development of inhibitors in these patients. Avoidance of intensive courses of treatment with FVIII concentrates has to be considered especially in those patients known to harbor one of the high-risk mutations or having a relative who developed an inhibitor. It is not clear at this moment whether administration of FVIII as bolus injections or as continuous infusion infers different risks. Identification of the underlying mutation in patients with mild/moderate hemophilia A is useful to have an indication of their risk of inhibitor formation.

Conclusion

The occurrence of an inhibitor in a patient with mild/moderate hemophilia A is often a dramatic event. Bleeding episodes can be particularly severe, force patients to change their lifestyle completely, and may be life threatening. Avoidance of treatment with FVIII concentrates by using desmopressin where possible is the single most effective way to prevent this complication in mild/moderate hemophilia A patients. It is not clear at this moment whether immune tolerance induction, immunosuppression, or a combination of both should be used to eradicate the inhibitor. Again, avoidance of exposure to FVIII by using bypassing agents [FVIII inhibitor bypass activity (FEIBA) or activated recombinant FVII (rFVIIa)] and desmopressin to treat bleeding episodes, might be an interesting option.

References

1 Hay CR, Ludlam CA, Colvin BT, et al. Factor VIII inhibitors in mild and moderate-severity haemophilia A. Thromb Haemost 1998; **79**: 762–6.

2 Lusher JM, Arkin S, Abildgaard CF, et al. Recombinant factor VIII for the treatment of previously untreated patients with haemophilia A. N Engl J Med 1993; **328**: 453–9.

3 Sultan Y, and the French Haemophilia Study Group. Prevalence of inhibitors in a population of 3435 haemophilia patients in France. Thromb Haemost 1992; **67**: 600–2.

4 Rizza CR, Spooner RGD. Treatment of haemophilia and related disorders in Britain and Northern Ireland during 1976–80: report on behalf of the directors of haemophilia centres in the United Kingdom. Br Med J 1983; **286**: 929–32.

5 McMillan CW, Shapiro SS, Whitehurst D, et al. The natural history of factor VIII:c inhibitors in patients with haemophilia A: A national cooperative study. II; Observations on the initial development of factor VIII:c inhibitors. Blood 1988; **71**: 344–8.

6 Rizza CR, Spooner RJD Giangrande PLF, on behalf of the UK Haemophilia Centre Doctors' Organisation (UKHCDO). Treatment of haemophilia in the UK 1981–96. Haemophilia 2001; **7**: 349–59.

7 Eckhardt C, van Velzen AS, Peters M, et al. Factor VIII gene (F8) mutation and risk of inhibitor development in nonsevere haemophilia A. Blood 2013; **122**: 1954–62.

8 Eckhardt CL, Mauser-Bunschoten EP, Peters M, Leebeek FW, van der Meer FJ, Fijnvandraat K. Inhibitor incidence after intensive FVIII replacement for surgery in mild and moderate haemophilia A: a prospective national study in the Netherlands. Br J Haematol 2012; **157**: 747–52.

9 Fijnvandraat K, Turenhout EAM, van den Brink EN, et al. The missense mutation Arg593 -> Cys is related to antibody formation in a patient with mild haemophilia A. Blood 1997; **89**: 4371–7.

10 Vlot AJ, Wittebol S, Strengers PFW, et al. Factor VIII inhibitor in a patient with mild haemophilia A and an Asn618-Ser mutation responsive to immune tolerance induction and cyclophosphamide. Br J Haematol 2002; **117**: 136–40.

11 Santagostino E, Gringeri A, Tagliavacca L, et al. Inhibitors to factor VIII in a family with mild haemophilia: Molecular characterization and response to factor VIII and desmopressin. Thromb Haemost 1995; **74**: 619–21.

12 Peerlinck K, Jacquemin M, Arnout J, et al. Antifactor VIII antibody inhibiting allogeneic but not autologous factor VIII in patients with mild haemophilia A. Blood 1999; **93**: 2267–73.

13 Kesteven PJ, Holland LJ, Lawrie AS, et al. Inhibitor to factor VIII in mild haemophilia. Thromb Haemost 1984; **52**: 50–2.

14 Kempton CL, Soucie JM, Miller CH, et al. In non-severe hemophilia A the risk of inhibitor after intensive factor treatment is greater in older patients: a case–control study. J Thromb Haemost 2010; **8**: 2224–31.

15 Eckhardt CL, Menke LA, van Ommen CH, et al. Intensive perioperative use of factor VIII and the Arg593->Cys mutation are risk factors for inhibitor development in mild/moderate hemophilia A. J Thromb Haemost 2009; **7**: 930–7.

16 Goodeve AC, Peake IR, et al. The molecular basis of haemophilia A: genotype–phenotype relationships and inhibitor development. Semin Thromb Haemost 2003; **29**: 23–30.

17 Thompson AR, Murphy MEP, Liu M, et al. Loss of tolerance to exogenous and endogenous factor VIII in a mild haemophilia A patient with an Arg593 to Cys mutation. Blood 1997; **90**: 1902–10.

18 Fernandez-Lopez O, Garcia-Lozano JR, Nunez-Vasquez R, et al. The spectrum of mutations in Southern Spanish patients with hemophilia A and identification of 28 novel mutations. Haematologica 2005; **90**: 707–10.

19 Knobe KE, Villoutreix BO, Tengborn LI, et al. Factor VIII inhibitors in two families with mild haemophilia A: structural analysis of the mutations. Haemostasis 2000; **30**: 268–79.

20 Franchini M, Girelli D, Olivieri O, et al. Tyr2105Cys mutation in exon 22 of FVIII gene is a risk factor for the development of inhibitors in patients with mild/moderate haemophilia A. Haemophilia 2006; **12**: 448–51.

21 Astermark J, Wang X, Oldenburg J, et al. Polymorphisms in the CTLA-4 gene and inhibitor development in patients with severe hemophilia A. J Thromb Haemost 2007; **5**: 263–5.

22 Astermark J, Oldenburg J, Carlson J, et al. Polymorphisms in the TNFA gene and the risk of inhibitor development in patients with hemophilia A. Blood 2006; **108**: 3739–45.

23 Jacquemin M, Benhida A, Peerlinck K, et al. A human antibody directed to the factor VIII C1 domain inhibits factor VIII cofactor activity and binding to von Willebrand factor. Blood 2000; **95**: 156–63.

24 Suzuki H, Shima M, Arai M, et al. Factor VIII Ise (R2159C) in a patient with mild haemophilia A, an abnormal Factor VIII with retention of function but modification of C2 epitopes. Thromb Haemost 1997; **77**: 862–7.

25 d'Oiron R, Lavergne JM, Lavend'homme R, et al. Deletion of Alanine 2201 in the FVIII C2 domain results in mild haemophilia A by impairing FVIII binding to vWF and phospholipids and destroys a major FVIII antigenic determinant involved in inhibitor development. Blood 2004; **103**: 155–7.

26 Gilles JG, Lavend'homme R, Peerlinck K, et al. Some factor VIII (FVIII) inhibitors recognise a FVIII epitope(s) that is present only on FVIII–vWF complexes. Thromb Haemost 1999; **82**: 40–5.

27 Jacquemin M, Vantomme V, Buhot C, et al. CD4+ T-cell clones specific for wild-type factor VIII: a molecular mechanism responsible for a higher incidence of inhibitor formation in mild/moderate haemophilia A. Blood 2003; **101**: 1351–8.

28 James EA, Kwok WW, Ettinger RA, et al. T-cell responses over time in a mild hemophilia A inhibitor subject: epitope identification and transient immunogenicity of the corresponding self-peptide. J Thromb Haemost 2007; **5**: 2399–407.

29 James EA, van Haren SD, Ettinger RA, et al. T-cell responses in two unrelated hemophilia A inhibitor subjects include an epitope at the factor VIII R593C missense site. J Thromb Haemost 2011; **9**: 689–99.

30 Pautard B, D'Oiron R, Li Thiao Te V, *et al.* Successful immune tolerance induction by FVIII in hemophilia A patients with inhibitor may occur without deletion of FVIII-specific T cells. *J Thromb Haemost* 2011; **9**: 1163–70.

31 Capel P, Toppet M, Van Remoor E, *et al.* Factor VIII inhibitor in mild haemophilia. *Br J Haematol* 1986; **62**: 786–7.

32 White B, Cotter M, Byrne M, *et al.* High responding factor VIII inhibitors in mild haemophilia—is there a link with recent changes in clinical practice? *Haemophilia* 2000; **6**: 113–15.

33 Carcao M, St Louis J, Poon MC, *et al.* Inhibitor Subcommittee of Association of Hemophilia Clinic Directors of Canada. Rituximab for congenital haemophiliacs with inhibitors: a Canadian experience. *Haemophilia* 2006; **12**: 7–18.

34 Dunkley S, Kershaw G, Young G, *et al.* Rituximab treatment of mild haemophilia A with inhibitors: a proposed treatment protocol. *Haemophilia* 2006; **12**: 663–7.

35 Robbins D, Kulkarni R, Gera R, *et al.* Successful treatment of high titer inhibitors in mild haemophilia A with avoidance of factor VIII and immunosuppressive therapy. *Am J Hematol* 2001; **68**: 184–8.

36 d'Oiron R, Volot F, Reynaud J, *et al.* Impact of choice of treatment for bleeding episodes on inhibitor outcome in patients with mild/moderate hemophilia A and inhibitors. *Semin Hematol* 2006; **43**(1 Suppl. 1): S3–9.

37 d'Oiron R, Pipe SW, Jacquemin M. Mild/moderate haemophilia A: new insights into molecular mechanisms and inhibitor development. *Haemophilia* 2008; **14**(Suppl. 3): 138–46.

CHAPTER 9

Inhibitors to factor VIII/IX: immune tolerance

Donna M. DiMichele

National Institutes of Health, Maryland, USA

Introduction

Antibody eradication is the ultimate goal of inhibitor management. The sole clinically proven strategy for achieving antigen-specific tolerance to factor VIII (FVIII) or factor IX (FIX) is immune tolerance induction (ITI). As recently reviewed, our current knowledge about ITI in hemophilia A (HA) and hemophilia B (HB) has historically been derived from small cohort studies and retrospective registries [1]. ITI practise in severe HA has been further impacted by prospective cohort data [2,3], and the results of a prospective randomized ITI (I-ITI) trial [4]. Due to the lower FIX inhibitor incidence (1.5–3%), and despite the significant morbidity associated with allergic reactions that often herald FIX antibody development and complicate attempts at eradication, there are no comparable data to inform an evidence-based approach to the prevention and eradication of FIX inhibitors [5]. Ultimately, successful inhibitor prevention and eradication strategies for both HA and HB will emerge from the clinical translation of the evolving knowledge of the immune mechanisms involved in antibody development and immune tolerance.

This chapter discusses current understanding of immune tolerance outcome and outcome predictors for severe HA and for HB from the published literature, and will review the current consensus practise recommendations for ITI. It will also summarize how the current understanding of the immunology of FVIII and FIX antibody formation and tolerance might inform current investigative priorities that could impact future therapeutic and preventative tolerance strategies.

Immune tolerance for factor VIII inhibitors

Role of host factors in immune tolerance induction outcome

Historical ITI success rates of >50% in HA ITI have been defined by variably stringent clinical and laboratory endpoints [6]. Although undergoing additional refinement based on emerging population-based pharmacokinetic data [7], successful ITI has most recently been defined by both an undetectable inhibitor titer [≤0.6 Bethesda units (BU) by Bethesda or Nijmegen assays], and a normal FVIII recovery (≥66% of expected) and half-life (≥6h) [4].

Among host-related variables known to influence inhibitor development, only race and *F8* genotype have been studied in relation to ITI outcome. With respect to impact of race and/or ethnicity, data from several investigative cohorts have suggested but not proven a lower ITI success rate among black people [4,8,9].The impact of *F8* genotype on ITI outcome has so far been retrospectively examined in a single study of 156 high responder (HR) (historical titer ≥5 BU) subjects [3]. *F8* mutations associated with a lower risk of inhibitor development also predicted a statistically higher rate of ITI success in a multivariate analysis.

Role of treatment factors in immune tolerance induction outcome

The International Immune Tolerance Registry (IITR), the German registry, and the North American Immune Tolerance Registry (NAITR) all retrospectively identified parameters that influence both success rate and time to successful ITI in severe HA high-titer inhibitor patients [8,10,11]. Lower pre-ITI, historical peak and, in the NAITR, ITI peak titers, have uniformly and statistically correlated with ITI success [8,10,11]. The role of inhibitor titer, including pre-ITI titer, is being prospectively examined in two observational studies [2,3].

In the I-ITI study, pre-ITI titer <10 BU was a primary determinant of the "good risk" cohort that defined subject eligibility and therefore not evaluable as an outcome variable. However, historical peak titer ($P = 0.02$) and peak titer on ITI ($P = 0.002$) did inversely correlate with outcome in a univariate logistical regression analysis [4]. In a multivariate analysis of these data, ITI peak titer alone remained a significant predictor of outcome ($P = 0.002$), prospectively validating the observation made in the NAITR [8].

Textbook of Hemophilia, Third Edition. Edited by Christine A. Lee, Erik E. Berntorp and W. Keith Hoots.
© 2014 John Wiley & Sons, Ltd. Published 2014 by John Wiley & Sons, Ltd.

Other treatment variables with variable significance that were examined in at least one registry include older age at ITI initiation [8,10]; interval of >5 years between inhibitor diagnosis and start of ITI [8,10]; and ITI interruption of more than 2 weeks [11]. The I-ITI study also used these variables to define the "good risk" cohort for this trial, and, therefore, could not evaluate their predictive role in ITI outcome [4].

Factor VIII dose and dosing regimen

The role of FVIII dosing regimen in the eradication of HR inhibitors has been controversial due to conflicting data generated by the registries [8,10]. While the IITR observed better ITI outcomes with daily FVIII doses of ≥200 IU/kg/day, the NAITR reported a more significant impact of FVIII dose (≥50 IU/kg/day) on time to successful tolerance. Ultimately, a metaanalysis of both registries determined that for patients with historical inhibitor titers <200 BU and immediate pre-ITI titers <10 BU, FVIII dose did not impact ITI outcome [12].

Understanding the comparative cost-effectiveness and morbidity associated with nondaily lower dose regimens may be critical to the broader global access to ITI. In an attempt to prospectively study the effect of FVIII dose on both the overall rate of ITI success and time to success, the I-ITI trial randomized 134 good risk severe HA HR inhibitor subjects from 55 participating centers to receive either 200 IU/kg/day or 50 IU/kg thrice weekly FVIII for up to 33 months (Figure 9.1) [4]. At the time of early study termination, 70% of the 66 subjects who reached an evaluable study endpoint achieved ITI success with either regimen. However, sample size was inadequate to demonstrate statistical equivalence in dose effectiveness [4]. Although the study did not observe an FVIII dose effect on the overall time to tolerance, dose was noted to impact the time from the start of ITI to achievement of both a negative titer and a normal FVIII recovery (Table 9.1) [4].

The I-ITI study observed a significant impact of dose on inhibitor-related hemorrhage. The rate of all intercurrent bleeding (hemorrhages/ month) was notably higher with low-dose FVIII throughout all phases of ITI, but over twofold higher ($P = 0.00024$) between start of ITI and achievement of a negative inhibitor titer (Table 9.2) [4]. Since one major objective of timely tolerance induction is the reduction of hemorrhage-related morbidity, these data add another important dimension to the future evaluation of ITI cost-effectiveness. Additional analyses of both the epidemiology of bleeding during ITI and the impact of hemorrhage on ITI pharmacoeconomics are ongoing.

Factor VIII product type

Subsequent to the first observation of greater ITI success with a von Willebrand factor (VWF) containing FVIII product [13], similarly successful rates of tolerance have been achieved in good and poor risk inhibitor patients using both recombinant and plasma-derived FVIII [1,14]. International prospective studies, controlled for other variables known to impact ITI outcome, will be required to delineate the role of product type in successful tolerance. Two observational studies are prospectively examining ITI outcome predictors, including FVIII product type [2,3]. The Rescue Immune Tolerance Study (RES.I.ST) planned to study this question directly by randomizing ITI-naïve poor risk hemophilia inhibitor patients to receive 200 IU/kg/day of either recombinant or plasma-derived VWF-containing FVIII, but was terminated early for futility [15].

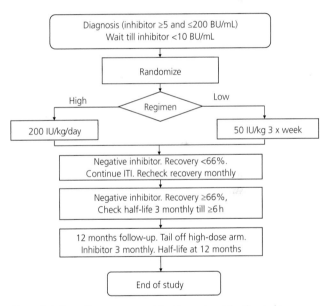

Figure 9.1 Flow-diagram summarizing the protocol for the study, randomization, and monitoring of ITI and prophylaxis. BU: Bethesda unit. Reproduced from [4].

Table 9.1 Time to achieve immune tolerance induction (ITI) milestones by treatment arm in the International Immune Tolerance study reported as median (IQ range) months [4].

	n	Low dose	*n*	High dose	*P*
Phase 1 (Start of ITI to negative titer)	29	9.2 (4.9–17.0)	31	4.6 (2.8–13.8)	0.017
Phase 2 (Negative titer to 1st normal recovery)	27	13.6 (8.7–19.0)	23	6.9 (3.5–12.0)	0.001
Phase 3 (Normal recovery to tolerance)	24	15.5 (10.8–22.0)	22	10.6 (6.3–20.5)	0.096

Table 9.2 All bleed rates (bleeds/month) by treatment arm and phase of immune tolerance induction (ITI) in the International Immune Tolerance Study [4].

	Dose (n)	Mean	Median	(IQ range)	P value
Phase 1	Low (58)	0.623	0.564	(0.093– 0.886)	0.00024
	High (57)	0.282	0.000	(0.000– 0.440)	
Phase 2	Low (27)	0.127	0.000	(0.000– 0.073)	0.283
	High (22)	0.087	0.000	(0.000– 0.000)	
Phase 3	Low (24)	0.150	0.000	(0.000– 0.148)	0.552
	High (22)	0.033	0.000	(0.000– 0.000)	
Phase 4	Low (24)	0.175	0.150	(0.000– 0.290)	0.112
	High (22)	0.102	0.000	(0.000– 0.231)	

Phase 1: start of ITI to negative titer; Phase 2: negative titer to first normal recovery; Phase 3: normal recovery to tolerance; Phase 4: prophylaxis following successful tolerance.
IQ, interquartile.

Past, current, and future role of immune modulation in immune tolerance induction

Cyclophosphamide and immunoglobulin, historically part of the Malmö ITI regimen [16], were subsequently demonstrated to confer no outcome advantage relative to standard ITI [17,18]. Furthermore, concern about cyclophosphamide-related complications and the technical difficulty of performing extracorporeal immunoadsorption limit the current use of this strategy in young children.

Renewed interest in immune modulation has focused on selective B-cell depletion using rituximab (IDEC Pharmaceuticals, San Diego, CA, USA), a humanized monoclonal antibody to B-cell CD20 antigen. The largest retrospective study of inhibitor eradication with rituximab in congenital HA reported an initial complete response (CR) rate (defined by negative inhibitor titer) of 40% and partial response (PR) rate (defined by titer <5 BU with effective FVIII bleeding prophylaxis) of 27% among 15 patients treated with 4–12 infusions administered as 4 consecutive weekly doses of 375 mg m^{-2} [19]. A sustained CR or PR was ultimately achieved in seven (47%) patients over an observational period of >108 weeks. Of note, 10/12 patients receiving concomitant FVIII ITI at doses of 100–200 IU/kg/day achieved an initial CR (six patients) or PR (four patients). Of these, seven (58%) had sustained clinical benefit, while none of the three patients treated in the absence of concomitant FVIII achieved any response to rituximab therapy [19].

The frequency of immediate and long-term complications of anti-CD20 therapy in children is still unclear, but continues to be progressively informed by therapeutic intervention studies in disorders other than hemophilia. Infusion reactions including nausea and headache, as well as serum sickness and opportunistic infections have so far occurred infrequently among children [19]. Progressive multifocal leukoencephalopathy, previously described in persons with autoimmune and lymphoproliferative disorders [20], has not been reported in persons with hemophilia. Nonetheless, caution and careful surveillance are recommended as more aggressive immunosuppressive therapeutic approaches are applied to antibody eradication in congenital hemophilia, particularly in children.

The considerable progress made in our understanding of the immunology of FVIII antibody development and eradication may eventually enable a safe and more uniformly successful approach to treatment [21,22]. The mechanisms of central and peripheral tolerance; the antigen-presenting roles of dendritic (with or without cytokine costimulation) and memory B cells in primary and secondary anti-FVIII immune responses, respectively; the immune regulatory effect of CD4+, CD8+, CD4+/CD25+ T-regulatory cells, specific T–B cell costimulatory interactions and apoptotic fibroblasts on these responses; as well as the respective roles of memory B and plasma cells and anti-idiotype antibodies in ongoing anti-FVIII antibody production are all now better understood [21,22]. However, all potentially important immunologic mechanisms of tolerance have been studied in animals. Several such observations were or are being corroborated through the *in-vitro* study of hemophilic inhibitor plasma. Further progress requires both *in-vivo* corroborative studies and the prospective mechanistic study of immunologic tolerance in association with clinical ITI studies.

Finally, animal data continues to suggest that the use of gene transfer technology to modulate immune responses with the goal of FVIII inhibitor prevention and treatment remains an intriguing future therapeutic possibility [23]. Additional proof of principle has emerged from successful long-term inhibitor eradication of high-titer FVIII inhibitors in three of four hemophilic dogs who underwent liver-directed gene transfer with a canine FVIII–adeno-associated virus (AAV) plasmid constructs [24], suggesting that gene therapy could provide the future therapeutic key to the effective maintenance and re-establishment of FVIII tolerance.

Translation into clinical practise: recommendations for immune tolerance induction in severe hemophilia A patients with high-titer inhibitors

Three independent groups simultaneously developed carefully graded consensus recommendations for the current practise of ITI in patients with severe HA and high-titer (>5 BU) inhibitors, based on critical reviews of the existing literature [25–27]. The schema developed by the International Consensus Panel (ICP) is represented in Figure 9.2 [27].

22 Waters B, Lillicrap D. The molecular mechanisms of immunomodulation and tolerance induction to factor VIII. *J Thromb Haemost* 2009; **7**(9): 1446–56.

23 Scott DW, Lozier JN. Gene therapy for haemophilia: prospects and challenges to prevent or reverse inhibitor formation. *Br J Haematol* 2012; **156**(3): 295–302.

24 Finn JD, Ozelo MC, Sabatino DE, *et al.* Eradication of neutralizing antibodies to factor VIII in canine hemophilia A after liver gene therapy. *Blood* 2010; **116**(26): 5842–8.

25 Astermark J, Morado M, Rocino A, *et al.* Current European practice in immune tolerance induction therapy in patients with haemophilia and inhibitors. *Haemophilia* 2006; **12**(4): 363–71.

26 Hay CR, Brown S, Collins PW, Keeling DM, Liesner R. The diagnosis and management of factor VIII and IX inhibitors: a guideline from the United Kingdom Haemophilia Centre Doctors Organisation. *Br J Haematol* 2006; **133**(6): 591–605.

27 DiMichele DM, Hoots WK, Pipe SW, Rivard GE, Santagostino E. International workshop on immune tolerance induction: consensus recommendations. *Haemophilia* 2007; **13**(Suppl. 1): 1–22.

28 Benson G, Auerswald G, Elezovic I, *et al.* Immune tolerance induction in patients with severe hemophilia with inhibitors: expert panel views and recommendations for clinical practice. *Eur J Haematol* 2012; **88**(5): 371–9.

29 Coppola A, Di Minno MN, Santagostino E. Optimizing management of immune tolerance induction in patients with severe haemophilia A and inhibitors: towards evidence-based approaches. *Br J Haematol* 2010; **150**(5): 515–28.

30 Mancuso ME, Berardinelli L. Arteriovenous fistula as stable venous access in children with severe haemophilia. *Haemophilia* 2010; **16**(Suppl. 1): 25–8.

31 Lozier JN, Tayebi N, Zhang P. Mapping of genes that control the antibody response to human factor IX in mice. *Blood* 2005; **105**(3): 1029–35.

32 Sawamoto Y, Shima M, Yamamoto M, *et al.* Measurement of anti-factor IX IgG subclasses in haemophilia B patients who developed inhibitors with episodes of allergic reactions to factor IX concentrates. *Thromb Res* 1996; **83**(4): 279–86.

33 Christophe OD, Lenting PJ, Cherel G, *et al.* Functional mapping of anti-factor IX inhibitors developed in patients with severe hemophilia B. *Blood* 2001; **98**(5): 1416–23.

34 Nayak S, Cao O, Hoffman BE, *et al.* Prophylactic immune tolerance induced by changing the ratio of antigen-specific effector to regulatory T cells. *J Thromb Haemost* 2009; **7**(9): 1523–32.

35 Cao O, Loduca PA, Herzog RW. Role of regulatory T cells in tolerance to coagulation factors. *J Thromb Haemost* 2009; **7**(Suppl. 1): 88–91.

36 Brackmann HH. Induced immunotolerance in factor VIII inhibitor patients. *Prog Clin Biol Res* 1984; **150**: 181–95.

37 Nilsson IM, Berntorp E, Zettervall O. Induction of split tolerance and clinical cure in high-responding hemophiliacs with factor IX antibodies. *Proc Natl Acad Sci USA* 1986; **83**(23): 9169–73.

38 Chitlur M, Warrier I, Rajpurkar M, Lusher JM. Inhibitors in factor IX deficiency a report of the ISTH–SSC international FIX inhibitor registry (1997–2006). *Haemophilia* 2009; **15**(5): 1027–31.

39 Ewenstein BM, Takemoto C, Warrier I, *et al.* Nephrotic syndrome as a complication of immune tolerance in hemophilia B. *Blood* 1997; **89**(3): 1115–16.

40 Cross DC, Van Der Berg HM. Cyclosporin A can achieve immune tolerance in a patient with severe haemophilia B and refractory inhibitors. *Haemophilia* 2007; **13**(1): 111–14.

41 Klarmann D, Martinez Saguer I, Funk MB, *et al.* Immune tolerance induction with mycophenolate–mofetil in two children with haemophilia B and inhibitor. *Haemophilia* 2008; **14**(1): 44–9.

42 Mingozzi F, Liu YL, Dobrzynski E, *et al.* Induction of immune tolerance to coagulation factor IX antigen by in vivo hepatic gene transfer. *J Clin Invest* 2003; **111**(9): 1347–56.

43 Dobrzynski E, Fitzgerald JC, Cao O, Mingozzi F, Wang L, Herzog RW. Prevention of cytotoxic T lymphocyte responses to factor IX-expressing hepatocytes by gene transfer-induced regulatory T cells. *Proc Natl Acad Sci USA* 2006; **103**(12): 4592–7.

44 Cooper M, Nayak S, Hoffman BE, Terhorst C, Cao O, Herzog RW. Improved induction of immune tolerance to factor IX by hepatic AAV-8 gene transfer. *Hum Gene Ther* 2009; **20**(7): 767–76.

45 Kelly ME, Zhuo J, Bharadwaj AS, Chao H. Induction of immune tolerance to FIX following muscular AAV gene transfer is AAV-dose/FIX-level dependent. *Mol Ther* 2009; **17**(5): 857–63.

CHAPTER 10

Prophylaxis in inhibitor patients

Alessandro Gringeri

Baxter Innovations GmbH, Vienna, Austria

Introduction

In patients with high-titer inhibitors, therapy with factor VIII (FVIII) or factor IX (FIX) concentrates is ineffective, requiring the use of inhibitor bypassing agents, such as activated prothrombin complex concentrate (aPCC; anti-inhibitor coagulant complex; factor eight inhibitor bypassing activity, FEIBA VH; Baxter AG, Vienna, Austria) or recombinant activated factor VII (rFVIIa or eptacog alfa; NvoSeven, Novo Nordisk A/S, Bagsvaerd, Denmark). Both bypassing agents have been shown to control at least 80–90% of bleeding episodes, including perioperative bleeding, in patients with high titer inhibitors [1–3]. However, their hemostatic effect is variable and does not equal that of FVIII replacement [1]. Consequently, compared with hemophilia patients without inhibitors, individuals with inhibitors are at increased risk for severe hemorrhage [4]. In inhibitor patients, severe joint disease may more likely develop after only a few bleeding episodes, due to protracted, chronic hemarthrosis, and it may result in more significant functional limitations [5,6]. Compared with inhibitor-free patients, those with inhibitors miss more time from school or work, require hospitalization with a higher frequency, and suffer greater pain, arthropathy, and loss of mobility [6]. Yet surgical interventions are less likely to be used in inhibitor patients with joint damage due to the greater potential for bleeding complications [7]. As a result, inhibitor patients often experience significantly impaired mobility and a lower quality of life (QOL) [8]. In addition to this enormous personal toll, inhibitory antibodies also disproportionately absorb health-care resources. According to a 2003 study conducted in Italy, the average annual cost of care for inhibitor patients was €220 000, with replacement therapy accounting for 99% of these costs [9] and mainly attributable to treatment for target joints and orthopedic surgery. Hence, the need for prophylaxis may be even more compelling for patients with severe hemophilia A and inhibitors.

While the benefit of prophylaxis in patients without inhibitors is now well recognized [10,11], prophylaxis in inhibitor patients does not represent the standard of care yet. Prophylaxis with bypassing agents may substantially improve their QOL, especially for those who are ineligible for immune tolerance induction (ITI) or have failed ITI.

Evidence on primary prophylaxis with bypassing agents

The main goal of hemophilia care is the prevention of life-threatening hemorrhages and joint bleeding, the latter being crucial to maintain pristine joints and prevent development of crippling arthropathy [12]. Primary prophylaxis means regular long-term treatment started before the age of 2 years and/or after no more than one joint bleed, whereas secondary prophylaxis includes all long-term regular treatments started after a second joint bleed and or at an older age [12]. This approach is valid also for patients with inhibitors, who equally deserve to have preserved joint health. Nevertheless, prophylaxis with bypassing agents is infrequently introduced in small children as soon as the inhibitor develops and before the occurrence of bleeding episodes, prior to the start of or during ITI treatment.

Very limited experience on bypassing agent prophylaxis in children after inhibitor development and before ITI has been published so far [13]. Jiménez-Yuste et al. reported their experience in three children aged 1–2 years when they started prophylaxis with rFVIIa after inhibitors developed. Prophylaxis was carried out for a median of 9 months (minimum to maximum: 8–22 months) with 90–100 μg/kg daily: in this time period, patients showed no bleeding in joints and muscles [13]. Even more limited is the experience published on prophylaxis with aPCC in these patients, due to its more infrequent use before ITI. In fact, some treating physicians are concerned about the potential anamnestic response provoked by traces of FVIII contained in the aPCC, which can be an issue while awaiting a decline in inhibitor levels before initiating ITI. Today, rFVIIa at a dose of 90–270 μg/kg daily is more frequently for

Textbook of Hemophilia, Third Edition. Edited by Christine A. Lee, Erik E. Berntorp and W. Keith Hoots.

prophylaxis when ITI is delayed to allow the inhibitor level to decline to <10 BU [14].

Evidence on prophylaxis with bypassing agent during immune tolerance induction

The largest and longest experience of bypassing therapy during ITI aPCC was a component of the original Bonn ITI protocol [15], and it has continued to be used in patients at high risk for bleeding [16]. The use of aPCC in prophylaxis was reported in 22 patients at the dose of 50 U/kg twice a day during high-dose ITI treatment with FVIII 100–150 IU/kg bid. In ITI, 50% of patients showed pristine joints at the physical and radiologic examination; only three patients showed a deterioration of joint health, the remaining patients having remained stable or improved [16]. Brackmann et al. [17] described the unfavorable use of rFVIIa in association with ITI in four patients aged from 0.5 to 26 years and with a dosage ranging from 90 μg/kg twice a day to 2–3 times a week. The duration of prophylaxis ranged from 2 to 27 months. No adverse events were reported. Nevertheless, rFVIIa prophylaxis at a dose of 90 μg/kg daily was administered to a 4-year-old boy with a high-titer FVIII inhibitor. During rFVIIa prophylaxis, the joint bleeding rate halved from about 3.8 bleeds a month when the patient was treated on demand at 1.6/month [18]. Moreover, rFVIIa was administered prophylactically initially at a dose of 160 μg/kg daily and afterward reduced to 90 μg/kg daily to a boy undergoing ITI who was frequently bleeding. During rFVIIa prophylaxis, no spontaneous bleeding episodes occurred [19].

FEIBA prophylaxis was prescribed at a dose of 50–100 U/kg daily (increased up to 100 U/kg twice daily for breakthrough bleeding) to 22 children aged 0.1–6 years undergoing ITI [20]. During FEIBA prophylaxis, the median annual joint bleeding rate was 1 (minimum to maximum: 0–6), without evidence of arthropathy was seen in 6/8 patients evaluated radiographically. Cheng et al. [21] reported five patients who had received ITI treatment and FEIBA prophylaxis at 50–75 U/kg/day

administered 1–3 times weekly. The frequency of bleeding episodes decrease in all patients to 0.98 joint bleeds/100 days total of bleeds with a 90% reduction as compared to the baseline joint bleeds (14.8 bleeds/100 days). More recently, Valentino [22] carried out a metaanalysis of six studies where data on bleeding rate was available before and during prophylaxis in a total of 34 inhibitor patients: among the four patients in this group who received ITI concomitantly, annual joint bleeding episodes decreased by an average of 79%.

Evidence from retrospective and prospective cohorts on secondary prophylaxis with bypassing agents after immune tolerance induction failure

Whether or not prophylaxis had been prescribed before or during ITI, children and adults who failed ITI treatment or who have never undergone ITI require prophylactic treatment in order to prevent life-threatening hemorrhages, reduce joint bleeding, slow down the progression of existing joint damage, and maintain or improve health-related QOL.

There is a substantial amount of published evidence on the efficacy of prophylaxis in children and adults with bypassing agents, provided by retrospective and prospective cohorts [13,22–32]. Tables 10.1 and 10.2 summarize the main studies where bleeding rate in patients on aPCC or rFVIIa prophylaxis was compared to previous on-demand treatment. The overall bleeding reduction rate was greater than 60% with both bypassing agents. No thromboembolic events were reported. Moreover, seven pediatric patients aged 1.5–11.8 years (median age: 6.0 years) were reported to be treated immediately after having failed ITI with FEIBA at 60–100 IU/kg dosages once or twice daily, every other day, or 3 times weekly, for a median duration of 6.9 years (minimum to maximum: 0.8–17.1 years) [30]. The mean annual joint bleeding rate was 1.5 [95% confidence intervals (CI), 0.7–3.0], muscle bleeding rate being 0.9 (95% CI, 0.6–1.2 episodes/year). No patient experienced major joint damage during prophylaxis.

Table 10.1 Bleeding rate reduction evidence in patients who underwent activated prothrombin complex concentrate (aPCC) prophylaxis.

References	Year	Total patients	Patients on ITI	Reduction of bleeding % (mean)
Ewenstein et al. [23]	2004	16	–	53
Ewing et al. [24]	2007	7	–	69
Schino et al. [25]	2006	4	–	75
DiMichele & Negrier [26]	2006	14	–	53 (10–85)
Leissinger et al. [27]	2007	5	–	78
Jimenez-Yuste et al. [13]	2009	5	–	43
Valentino [22]	2010	6	3	84
Lambert et al. [28]	2009	13	5	78
Antunes et al. [29]	2009	2	–	53 (38–83)
Total		**72**	**8**	**65**

Table 10.2 Bleeding rate reduction evidence in patients who underwent prophylaxis with rFVIIa.

References	Year	Total patients	Patients on immune tolerance induction	Reduction of bleeding % (mean)
Young *et al.* [31]	2005	2	–	64–74
Morfini *et al.* [32]	2007	13	–	68
Young *et al.* [33]	2012	86	–	46 (52[a])
Total		**101**	–	**61**

[a]Bleeding reduction in patients with one bleeding or more a month.

Long-term secondary prophylaxis (12 and 25 months) with rFVIIa was described [31] in two hemophilia patients aged 3 and 15 years, prophylactic regimens being 200 μg/kg every 6 and 12 h, respectively. Bleeding rate decreased during rFVIIa prophylaxis from 2.3 to 0.6 bleeds/ month, and from 2.2 to 0.8 bleeds/month, respectively. A retrospective survey [32] reported 13 inhibitor patients treated prophylactically with rFVIIa in different European centers using various regimens that ranged from 200 to 1540 μg/kg weekly administered in one to seven injections for between 4 months and 4 years. A mean reduction of 68% in bleeding frequency during prophylaxis was observed (minimum to maximum, 0–100%).

The most numerous collections of retrospective cases have been recently published [33]: data on 86 patients from 14 countries who were prescribed secondary prophylaxis with rFVIIa were collected by professional medical record abstractors. Median age at rFVIIa prophylaxis initiation was 6 years (minimum to maximum, 0.1–52.0 years). The median duration was 288 days (interquartile range, 128–615 days). The reduction of bleeding rate was 46% (95% CI, 38–54%) in patients with at least one bleeding episodes prior to starting prophylaxis and 52% (95% CI, 43–61%) in patients with at least one bleeding episode per month prior to starting prophylaxis. Surprisingly, bleeding rate reduction in the bleeding and frequently bleeding population was higher for traumatic bleeds [51% (95% CI, 36–67%) and 58% (95% CI, 40–75%), respectively] than spontaneous bleeds [27% (95% CI, 11–43%) and 30% (95% CI, 12–47%], respectively).

Evidence from randomized clinical trials on secondary prophylaxis with bypassing agents

A prospective randomized double-blind parallel group trial of secondary prophylaxis evaluated the efficacy of two different doses of rFVIIa to reduce bleeding frequency in patients with high bleeding frequency [34]. Following a 3-month preprophylaxis period when patients were treated on demand, 22 patients with at least 12 bleeds were randomized to receive rFVIIa prophylaxis either at the dose of 90 or 270 μg/kg daily for 3 months. This study showed that bleeding frequency was significantly reduced by 45% and 59% during prophylaxis with 90 or 270 μg/kg, respectively, but no significant difference was observed between the two prophylactic doses. In the 3-month postprophylaxis period when patients were again treated on demand with rFVIIa, the bleeding frequency increased again, but not at the preprophylaxis levels (27% and 50% lower, respectively) with a difference statistically significant. Prophylaxis with rFVIIa showed to improve health-related quality of life (HRQOL) for inhibitor patients and decrease the number of school/work days lost and of hospitalization days [35]. No thromboembolic events were reported during the prophylaxis treatment period [34].

Recently, a randomized clinical trial [36] compared the efficacy and safety of aPCC prophylaxis with on-demand therapy with a cross-over design: 33 patients with at least six bleeding episodes in the previous 6 months were randomly assigned to either 6 months of on-demand therapy or 6 months prophylaxis. After the initial 6-month treatment period and a 3-month washout period when all patients were treated on demand, patients crossed over to the alternative treatment period. During the prophylaxis period, a 62% reduction in total bleeding events was observed in 26 patients who completed the two study periods, from a mean (±SD) number of bleeding events of 13.1 ± 7.1 during the on-demand treatment period to 5.0 ± 5.0 bleeding events (P < 0.001). Similar bleeding reduction was observed for joint bleeding events (61%, from 10.8 ± 7.6 to 4.2 ± 4.3). Target joint bleeding events were reduced by 72% during the prophylaxis period as compared with the on-demand period (P < 0.001). The study showed a subgroup of patients (62%) with a good response to aPCC prophylaxis, defined as a reduction of 50% or more in overall bleeding, with a reduction rate of 84% and six patients with no bleeding during the prophylaxis period. Patients with a good response also showed a statistically significant improvement in HRQOL, less days lost to school and work [37], and stabilization of or improvement in joint range of motion [38]. Among the 34 enrolled patients, there were no thromboembolic events reported, but two patients had intracranial hemorrhages (one died) during on-demand treatment and another patient died from bleeding, when on prophylaxis, underscoring the substantial health risks associated with persistent factor VIII inhibitors [36].

Very recently, a prospective, randomized, parallel trial compared annualized bleed rate (ABR) in patients using aPCC prophylactically to those treated on demand over the 12-month study period [39]. Thirty-six hemophilia A or B subjects, with median ages of 23.5 years, were enrolled: 17 were randomized to aPCC prophylaxis at a dose of 85 ± 15 U/kg every other day and 19 were randomized to the on-demand arm with aPCC at dosages per their treating physician. This study confirmed what was already shown by the previous randomized cross-trial; in fact, the median ABR for subjects in the prophylaxis arm (7.9) was significantly lower (−72.5%) than subjects in the on-demand arm (28.7) ($P = 0.0003$). Four serious adverse events were deemed related to FEIBA: the occurrence of HBs antibody in four patients, determined to be due to antibody passive transfer. No thromboembolic events or laboratory signals of thrombogenicity were reported. Moreover HRQOL showed to be negatively associated with ABR, proving that HRQOL can be improved by lowering bleeding frequency [40].

Discussion

Patients with severe hemophilia A and B and high-level inhibitors are at increased risk for severe bleeding episodes compared with patients without inhibitors. On-demand therapy with bypassing agents is not always effective in rapidly resolving bleeding and cannot prevent recurrent bleeding that inevitably leads to hemophilic arthropathy. Bypassing agent prophylaxis may therefore represent a valuable approach for narrowing the gap between inhibitor and noninhibitor patients.

Findings from long-term experience with the prophylactic use of bypassing agents, a numerous series of case histories published, and, more importantly, results from prospective randomized clinical trials indicate that bypassing agents can effectively prevent bleeding. Still, robust evidence is missing to show its efficacy in preserving joint function or at least in slowing down the development of crippling arthropathy, which can limit the adoption of this treatment approach.

There are other important barriers to bypassing agent prophylaxis (Table 10.3). One of these is represented by cost of bypassing agent prophylaxis. The randomized cross-over clinical trial on aPCC prophylaxis previously described [36] has shown that prophylaxis cost was 2.5-fold that of on-demand treatment. This calculation does not take into account health-related direct medium- and long-term costs associated with the development of target joints, arthropathy, and the need for

orthopedic surgery and mobility-assistance devices, without mentioning indirect costs and HRQOL. Conversely, Jiménez-Yuste et al. switched five well-selected patients from on-demand to aPCC prophylaxis, and monthly treatment costs decreased by a median of 62.1% (range: 8.6–69.2%) [13]. This reduction in costs was likely related to the significant reduction in bleeding rate during aPCC prophylaxis [41].

Another important limitation is represented by the presence of patients relatively unresponsive to bypassing agent prophylaxis at the dosing regimens used and such low responsiveness is so far unpredictable. To overcome unresponsiveness some treating physicians have increased dose and frequency of bypassing agents or even used them in combination [42].

Endogenous thrombin potential (ETP) measured by thrombin generation assay (TGA) has been used to monitor bypassing agents prophylaxis particularly during surgery [43]. Escuriola and Kreuz [30] reported their experience with ETP, which exceeded 80% of normal after aPCC infusion in the majority of the patients. Interestingly, mean trough ETP levels between regular prophylactic infusions tested 2.6-fold higher than the inhibitor plasma control mean.

Finally, a barrier is possibly represented by the relative low convenience of bypassing agent prophylaxis, requiring frequent dosing. This can be particularly demanding with rFVIIa that showed lower efficacy with less frequent dosing as compared to daily dosing [33,34], which is necessitated by the shorter half-life of rFVIIa compared with that of aPCC, and might diminish the appeal of rFVIIa as a prophylactic modality. Conversely, dosing and/or time-consuming preparation and infusion might diminish the appeal of aPCC. These causes of inconvenience might in turn decrease patient adherence and jeopardize treatment effectiveness.

In conclusion, bypassing agents have been shown to be capable of significantly reducing bleeding rate in most patients and improving HRQOL. Long-term real-life prospective cohort studies are needed in order to provide a better picture of the impact of this approach on the health of patients with high-responding inhibitors.

Disclosure

The author was appointed to write this chapter when he was employed at the Department of Clinical Sciences and Community Health, Università degli Studi di Milano, Milan, Italy, as Associate Professor of Internal Medicine. Presently, he is employed at Baxter Innovations GmbH, Vienna, Austria as Medical Director, Global Medical Affairs Hemophilia.

Table 10.3 Barriers to bypassing agent prophylaxis in inhibitor patients.

Low evidence of long-term impact on joint health
High short-term costs
Unresponsiveness of a minority of patients
Unpredictability of response
Low convenience due to frequent dosing and/or long preparation and infusion time

References

1 Astermark J, Donfield SM, DiMichele DM, et al. A randomized comparison of bypassing agents in hemophilia complicated by an

inhibitor: the FEIBA NovoSeven Comparative (FENOC) Study. *Blood* 2007; **109**: 546–51.

2 Key NS, Aledort LM, Beardsley D, *et al*. Home treatment of mild to moderate bleeding episodes using recombinant factor VIIa (Novoseven) in haemophiliacs with inhibitors. *Thromb Haemost* 1998; **80**: 912–18.

3 Négrier C, Lienhart A, Numerof R, *et al*. SURgical interventions with FEIBA (SURF): international registry of surgery in haemophilia patients with inhibitory antibodies. *Haemophilia* 2013; **19**: e143–50.

4 Leissinger CA. Use of prothrombin complex concentrates and activated prothrombin complex concentrates as prophylactic therapy in haemophilia patients with inhibitors. *Haemophilia* 1999; **5**: 25–32.

5 Soucie JM, Cianfrini C, Janco RL, *et al*. Joint range-of-motion limitations among young males with hemophilia: prevalence and risk factors. *Blood* 2004; **103**: 2467–73.

6 Morfini M, Haya S, Tagariello G, *et al*. European study on orthopaedic status of haemophilia patients with inhibitors. *Haemophilia* 2007; **13**: 606–12.

7 Teitel JM, Carcao M, Lillicrap D, *et al*. Orthopaedic surgery in haemophilia patients with inhibitors: a practical guide to haemostatic, surgical and rehabilitative care. *Haemophilia* 2009; **15**: 227–39.

8 Scalone L, Mantovani LG, Mannucci PM, Gringeri A. Quality of life is associated to the orthopaedic status in haemophilic patients with inhibitors. *Haemophilia* 2006; **12**: 154–62.

9 Gringeri A, Mantovani LG, Scalone L, Mannucci PM, for the COCIS Study Group. Cost of care and quality of life for patients with hemophilia complicated by inhibitors: the COCIS Study Group. *Blood* 2003; **102**: 2358–63.

10 Manco-Johnson MJ, Abshire TC, Shapiro AD, *et al*. Prophylaxis versus episodic treatment to prevent joint disease in boys with severe hemophilia. *N Engl J Med* 2007; **357**: 535–44.

11 Gringeri A, Lundin B, von Mackensen S, *et al*. A randomized clinical trial of prophylaxis in children with haemophilia A (the ESPRIT study). *J Thromb Haemost* 2011; **9**: 700–10.

12 Berntorp E, Astermark J, Bjorkman S, *et al*. Consensus perspectives on prophylactic therapy for haemophilia: summary statement. *Haemophilia* 2003; **9**(Suppl. 1): 1–4.

13 Jiménez-Yuste V, Alvarez MT, Martín-Salces M, *et al*. Prophylaxis in 10 patients with severe haemophilia A and inhibitor: different approaches for different clinical situations. *Haemophilia* 2009; **15**: 203–9.

14 DiMichele DM, Hoots WK, Pipe SW, *et al*. International workshop on immune tolerance induction: consensus recommendations. *Haemophilia* 2007; **13**: 1–22.

15 Brackmann HH, Gormsen J. Massive factor-VIII infusion in haemophiliac with factor-VIII inhibitor, high responder. *Lancet* 1977; **2**: 933.

16 Brackmann HH, Oldenburg J, Schwaab R. Immune tolerance for the treatment of factor VIII inhibitors—twenty years' "Bonn protocol". *Vox Sang* 1996; **70**(Suppl. 1): 30–5.

17 Brackmann HH, Effenberger E, Hess L, *et al*. NovoSeven in immune tolerance therapy. *Blood Coag Fibrinoly* 2000; **11**(Suppl. 1): S39–44.

18 Saxon BR, Shanks D, Jory CB, Williams V. Effective prophylaxis with daily recombinant factor VIIa (rFVIIa-Novoseven) in a child with high titre inhibitors and a target joint. *Thromb Haemost* 2001; **86**: 1126–7.

19 Blatny J, Kohlerova S, Zapletal O, *et al*. Prophylaxis with recombinant factor VIIa for the management of bleeding episodes during immune tolerance treatment in a boy with severe haemophilia A and high-response inhibitors. *Haemophilia* 2008; **14**: 1140–2.

20 Kreuz W, Escuriola-Ettingshausen C, Mentzer D. Factor VIII inhibitor bypass activity (FEIBA) for prophylaxis during immune tolerance induction (ITI) in patients with high-responding inhibitors. *Blood* 2000; **96**: 266a Abstract: 1141.

21 Cheng SN, Chen YC, Chiang JL. FEIBA prophylaxis in hemophilia A patient with inhibitors decreases bleeding episodes, improves joint function and enhance quality of life. *Haemophilia* 2006; **12**(Suppl. 2): PO 371.

22 Valentino LA. Assessing the benefits of FEIBA prophylaxis in haemophilia patients with inhibitors. *Haemophilia* 2010; **16**: 263–71.

23 Ewenstein B, Giangrande PLF, Morfini M, Tjonnfjord G, Kraut E, Luu H. Evaluation of FEBIA for prophylaxis in patients with inhibitors. *Haemophilia* 2004; **10**(Suppl. 3): 22 PO 10. Abstract.

24 Ewing NP, Pullens L, De Guzman C. Anamnesis in patients with hemophilia and inhibitors who receive activated prothrombin complex concentrates for prophylaxis. *J Thromb Haemost* 2007; **5**(Suppl. 2): P-T-158 Abstract.

25 Schino M, Mancuso G, Morfini M, *et al*. aPCC (FEIBA) home therapy retrospective survey in long-term secondary prophylaxis on hemophilia A patients with factor VIII inhibitor. *Haemophilia* 2006; **12**(Suppl. 2):14 PO 424.

26 DiMichele D, Négrier C. A retrospective postlicensure survey of FEIBA efficacy and safety. *Haemophilia* 2006; **12**: 352–62.

27 Leissinger CA, Becton DL, Ewing NP, Valentino LA. Prophylactic treatment with activated prothrombin complex concentrate (FEIBA) reduces the frequency of bleeding episodes in paediatric patients with haemophilia A and inhibitors. *Haemophilia* 2007; **13**: 249–55.

28 Lambert T, Rothschild C, Goudemand J, *et al*. Secondary prophylaxis with activated prothrombin complex concentrates (APCC) reduces bleeding frequency in haemophilia A patients with inhibitors. *J Thromb Haemost* 2009; **7**(Suppl. 2): 1131.

29 Antunes M, Santos A, Diniz MJ. Prophylatic treatment of hemophilia A patients with inhibitors. *J Thromb Haemost* 2009; **7**(Suppl 2): 825.

30 Ettingshausen CE, Kreuz W. Early long-term FEIBA prophylaxis in haemophilia A patients with inhibitor after failing immune tolerance induction: A prospective clinical case series. *Haemophilia* 2010; **16**: 90–100.

31 Young G, McDaniel M, Nugent DJ. Prophylactic recombinant factor VIIa in haemophilia patients with inhibitors. *Haemophilia* 2005; **11**: 203–7.

32 Morfini M, Auerswald G, Kobelt RA *et al*. Prophylactic treatment of haemophilia patients with inhibitors: clinical experience with recombinant factor VIIa in European Haemophilia Centres. *Haemophilia* 2007; **13**: 502–7.

33 Young G, Auerswald G, Jimenez-Yuste V, *et al*. PRO-PACT: retrospective observational study on the prophylactic use of recombinant factor VIIa in hemophilia patients with inhibitors. *Thromb Res* 2012; **130**(6): 864–70.

34 Konkle BA, Ebbesen LS, Erhardtsen E *et al*. Randomized, prospective clinical trial of recombinant factor VIIa for secondary prophylaxis in hemophilia patients with inhibitors. *J Thromb Haemost* 2007; **5**: 1904–13.

35 Hoots WK, Ebbesen LS, Konkle B, *et al.* Secondary prophylaxis with recombinant activated factor VII improves health-related quality of life of haemophilia patients with inhibitors. *Haemophilia* 2008; **14**: 466–75.

36 Leissinger C, Gringeri A, Antmen B, *et al.* Anti-inhibitor coagulant complex prophylaxis in hemophilia with inhibitors. *N Engl J Med* 2011; **365**: 1684–92.

37 Gringeri A, Leissinger C, Cortesi PA, *et al.* Health-related quality of life in patients with haemophilia and inhibitors on prophylaxis with anti-inhibitor complex concentrate: results from the Pro-FEIBA study. *Haemophilia* 2013 doi: 10.1111/hae.12178 [Epub ahead of print].

38 Leissinger CA, Gringeri A, Valentino L, Cortesi PA. Joint disease and the potential for improved joint health in inhibitor patients who have a good response to aPCC prophylaxis: data from the PRO-FEIBA Study [abstract]. *Blood* 2012; **120**: 3374.

39 Antunes S, Tangada S, Stasyshyn O, *et al.* A prospective, open-label, randomized, parallel study with AICC to evaluate the efficacy and safety of prophylactic versus on-demand treatment in hemophilia A or B subjects with inhibitors [abstract]. *J Thromb Haemost* 2013; **11**(Suppl. 2): PB 4.58–6.

40 Stasyshyn O, Antunes S, Mamanov V, *et al.* Health-related quality of life in hemophilia patients with inhibitors receiving prophylaxis with antiinhibitor coagulant complex (AICC): results from AICC prophylaxis study. *J Thromb Haemost* 2013; **11**(Suppl. 2): PB 2.58–5.

41 Gringeri A. Bypassing agent regimens and costs for prophylaxis in patients with inhibitors. *Haemophilia* 2009; **15**: 1336–7.

42 Auerswald G. [Long-term prophylaxis in congenital haemophilia with inhibitors—experiences with rFVIIa.] *Hamostaseologie* 2007; **27**: 123–8.

43 Dargaud Y, Lienhart A, Meunier S, *et al.* Major surgery in a severe haemophilia A patient with high titre inhibitor: use of the thrombin generation test in the therapeutic decision. *Haemophilia* 2005; **11**: 552–8.

CHAPTER 11

Inhibitors to factor VIII: treatment of acute bleeds

Claude Negrier

Edouard Herriot Hospital, University of Lyon, France

Introduction

The treatment of acute bleeds in patients who have developed inhibitors to factor VIII (FVIII) has benefited in the last decades from the development of new drugs, which has dramatically improved the prognosis of patients who experience such events. Several therapeutic agents are available to treat bleeds in hemophiliacs with inhibitors, but no single agent is efficacious in all patients or all circumstances. Although the management of patients with high-responding inhibitors is still complex and remains a medical challenge in some clinical situations, these products may not only ameliorate the pain, but also reduce the risk of muscular and skeletal damage. They also improve the educational and work prospects for these patients as well as enhancing their social participation and quality of life. However, an increased morbidity is associated with these acute bleeds that require early treatment with the most adapted concentrate.

Clinical context

Acute bleeds may occur in various clinical contexts, but two characteristics influence product choice to achieve hemostasis. Patients with low- or high-titer inhibitors are considered to exhibit the bleeding profile of a patient with severe hemophilia. This means that they suffer two to four bleeding episodes per month, although some patients demonstrate a decrease in the frequency of bleeding with aging. Most of these bleeds occur spontaneously (in everyday life) and will be successfully treated with home treatment. In contrast, some acute bleeds may be life threatening or may arise in critical situations such as perioperative periods. Although both types of clinical settings represent acute conditions, the nature of treatment to be administered may be different, depending on the titer of the inhibitor at that moment (Figure 11.1).

Classification between high and low responders

Inhibitors have been classified according to peak historical antibody titer and the presence or absence of immunologic anamnesis. A recent consensus of the FVIII and factor IX (FIX) Standardization Subcommittee of the International Society on Thrombosis and Hemostasis defined high-responding antibodies as those exhibiting a peak historical titer of >5 Bethesda units (BU) accompanied by brisk anamnesis and the consequent inability to treat hemorrhages routinely with specific factor replacement [1]. Accordingly, a low responder was defined by both a low historical peak titer (<5 BU) and a lack of anamnesis upon factor re-exposure. As a consequence, these latter patients can usually be treated with higher than usual doses of specific clotting factor concentrate to override the inhibitory effect of the antibody.

Products

The available therapeutic agents for treatment of acute hemorrhage in hemophiliacs with an inhibitor include high-dose human FVIII concentrate, porcine FVIII concentrate, activated prothrombin complex concentrates (aPCCs), and recombinant FVIIa (rFVIIa). In addition, antifibrinolytics and external removal of the inhibitory antibodies may be used as an adjunct therapy.

Human factor VIII concentrates

For low-titer inhibitors (<5 BU), high doses of FVIII concentrates may be used to achieve hemostasis [2]. Both plasma-derived and rFVIII can be administered with no objective difference in terms of *in-vivo* efficacy between these types of products. The dose is targeted to saturate the inhibitor (number of units to be infused = plasma volume in mL

Textbook of Hemophilia, Third Edition. Edited by Christine A. Lee, Erik E. Berntorp and W. Keith Hoots.
© 2014 John Wiley & Sons, Ltd. Published 2014 by John Wiley & Sons, Ltd.

PART IV

Acquired hemophilia

CHAPTER 12

Acquired inhibitors to factor VIII

Craig M. Kessler

Georgetown University Medical Center, Washington, DC, USA

Epidemiology

Recognition of the patient with acquired hemophilia (AH) and confirmation of the diagnosis have proven to be very challenging [1]. The demographics of AH have been established primarily through data collected from small clinical studies or from national surveillance registries, which are both encumbered by possible referral bias. Thus, the published prevalence (the proportion of the population found to have AH) for the disease likely represents a significant underestimate. Overall, AH has an estimated prevalence of 1.48 cases per million per year, and a reported mortality between 9% and 22% [2,3]. Recent data generated within the UK and Wales national health systems affirm the prevalence to be 1.3–1.5 per million per year [4,5]. Despite its low prevalence, the condition imposes significant clinical, medical, and economic challenges because its dramatic complications are frequently life threatening and management of bleeding events is expensive.

Age of onset for AH is distributed in a biphasic pattern, with a small peak in young individuals, primarily postpartum women and those with autoimmune diseases, and the major peak in those aged 60–80 years of either sex. AH is uncommon in children under the age of 16 years (estimated at 0.045/million/year), and may be underdiagnosed in the very elderly older than age 85 years (estimated at 14.7/million/year) [3]. Of the 172 patients in the United Kingdom Haemophilia Centre Doctors' Organisation (UKHCDO) dataset, 63% were aged 65 years to less than 85 years, and an additional 22% were aged 85 years and older [3]. The European Acquired Haemophilia Registry (EACH2), which includes 501 patients with AH from 13 European countries, has also reported a bimodal age distribution, with a small peak occurring in younger women, mainly those with peripartum AH (median age 33.9 years) [6]. In the largest published population series, 50–60% of diagnosed individuals who developed AH were previously healthy with no identified underlying disease state [2,3,7]. The clinical conditions most consistently associated with AH have included pregnancy; evolving or pre-existing autoimmune diseases; hematologic and solid tumor malignancies; and administration of certain medications (e.g. penicillin, sulfonamides, interferon-α, etc.) [8].

Pathophysiology and characteristics of autoantibodies to factor VIII

Human factor VIII (FVIII) circulates in the plasma, noncovalently bound to von Willebrand factor (VWF) protein, which chaperones it through the circulation. The sequence of the FVIII protein is composed of amino acids grouped into six domains. It has been well established that the most common epitopes for autoantibody (as well as alloantibody) binding appear to lie between amino acids 454–509 and 593 in the A2 domain, between 1804 and 1819 in the A3 domain, and between 2181 and 2243 in the C2 domain [9]. Anti-C2 antibodies inhibit the binding of FVIII to phospholipid and may also interfere with the binding of FVIII to VWF protein, whereas anti-A2 and anti-A3 antibodies impede the binding of FVIII to factor X (FX) and factor IXa (FIXa), respectively, in the intrinsic pathway FX activation complex. Congenital hemophilia patients typically have a polyclonal response consisting of antibodies to both the A2 and C2 domain, whereas AH patients typically have anti-A2 or anti-C2 antibodies but not both [10]. Autoantibodies binding to epitope sites other than those mentioned above may be clinically silent, or may be involved in other methods of FVIII inactivation, including mediating FVIII hydrolysis [11]. FVIII antibodies directed against areas in the B domain may influence clearance of FVIII from the circulation.

Most antibodies are mixtures of polyclonal immunoglobulin G1 (IgG1) and IgG4, with the IgG4 molecules mainly responsible for inhibiting clotting activity. Kappa light chains predominate. The IgG4 antibodies do not form immunoprecipitates or fix complement; thus, end-organ damage does not occur as it may with alloantibodies against FIX.

Textbook of Hemophilia, Third Edition. Edited by Christine A. Lee, Erik E. Berntorp and W. Keith Hoots.
© 2014 John Wiley & Sons, Ltd. Published 2014 by John Wiley & Sons, Ltd.

The mechanisms and kinetics by which FVIII activity is inhibited as a result of interacting with autoantibodies versus alloantibodies are quite dissimilar and not completely understood. Alloantibodies typically neutralize FVIII activity completely, following a so-called linear type I kinetics pattern. In contrast, most autoantibodies do not completely neutralize or inhibit FVIII activity and interact with FVIII via a nonlinear, nonsaturable, complex pattern of type II kinetics. The implications of this latter nonsaturable reaction process are profound: in patients with AH, residual low levels of FVIII activity may be detectable in laboratory assays; however, individuals with AH may bleed as profusely as if they had no FVIII activity [12]. The level of residual FVIII activity in the context of the presence of autoantibody inhibitors does not predict for the severity or frequency of their bleeding complications. Furthermore, these inhibitors, which follow complex kinetics, may only be quantified inexactly since the standard Bethesda assay is based on linear kinetics. This phenomenon results in routine underestimation of the potency of the autoantibody inhibitor. Thus, patients may be classified as having low titers of the autoantibody inhibitor, expressed as Bethesda units (BU), but manifest with severe bleeding [13].

It is apparent also that the contrasting interactions of auto- versus alloantibody inhibitors with FVIII result in very different clinical bleeding phenotypes. The explanations for this are not obvious; however, in contrast to the hemorrhagic arthropathy, which predominates in individuals with alloantibody inhibitors, AH is associated with more profound visceral, intramuscular, and soft-tissue bleeding. Small angle X-ray scattering (SAXS) techniques have recently suggested that "antibody cooperativity" may contribute to the different kinetic and thus perhaps clinical patterns observed between type I "classical" FVIII alloantibody inhibition and type II "nonclassical" FVIII autoantibody inhibition [14]. Other studies have indicated that the "classical" anti-C2 inhibitor antibodies interfere with the ability of FVIII to bind to phospholipid (essential for tenase complex assembly) and VWF protein while the "nonclassical" inhibitor antibodies block proteolytic activation of FVIII by thrombin or FXa in both the presence and absence of VWF protein [15]. Just as provocative are the laboratory observations that thrombin generation in patients with AH were significantly depressed compared to patients with severe hemophilia A [16]. Certainly, more examination is necessary to understand completely how the presence of autoantibodies versus alloantibodies influence the laboratory kinetics, the steric interactions with coagulation proteases and phospholipid, and the bleeding phenotypes of FVIII function in AH.

Another important but poorly elucidated aspect of AH is why the anti-FVIII autoantibody develops in the first place. The fact that AH is associated with many other autoimmune disease processes, that it occurs frequently in individuals with lymphoproliferative disorders, that it occurs predominantly in elderly persons, and that effective therapies are based on immunosuppressive regimens all suggest that an altered or compromised immune system must in some way predispose to the development of this autoimmune coagulation disease. The data generated from the Hemophilia Inhibitor Genetics Study (HIGS) demonstrate that FVIII alloantibody formation in patients with severe hemophilia A is a complex polygenic process involving polymorphisms in immune response genes, including those coding for histocompatibility locus antigen (HLA) class II alleles, interleukin 10 (IL-10), and cytotoxic T-lymphocyte antigen-4 (CTLA-4) [17]. Recently, Oldenburg *et al.* observed that the HLA class II *DRB*16* and *DQB1*0502* alleles and the *CTLA-4 + 49G* allele were present more frequently in patients with AH compared with controls [18]. If and how these immune response genes contribute to the onset of AH remains to be elucidated.

Associated disease states

Auto-FVIII antibody inhibitors frequently are associated with disease states thought to arise from a dysregulated immune system. In the largest retrospective series, an autoimmune association was found in 17–25% of cases [3,19]. Primary among such are collagen vascular disorders, including systemic lupus erythematosus (SLE) and rheumatoid arthritis (RA). Less commonly, AH is associated with more organ-specific autoimmune diseases such as myasthenia gravis, multiple sclerosis, Graves' disease, and autoimmune hemolytic anemia (HA). Associations with asthma, chronic inflammatory bowel disease, and graft-versus-host disease following allogeneic bone marrow transplant have also been reported anecdotally. The prospective EACH2 registry noted that 11.6% of AH cases were associated with autoimmune disease and most individuals had high-titer inhibitors [6]. The literature contains an ever-expanding list of autoimmune illnesses, which have been complicated by the development of AH, and compels the clinician to suspect AH in the differential diagnosis of new-onset bruising and/or bleeding in patients with these disorders.

Development of an autoanti-FVIII inhibitor is rare but a well-recognized complication of pregnancy. The UK national surveillance study estimated that AH developed in 1/350 000 of otherwise normal pregnancies [3]. The EACH2 registry reported that 8.4% of their 501 cases of AH were associated with pregnancy, primarily diagnosed in the postpartum period (range 21–120 days; median 89 days) [20]. The development of AH has been described up to a year postpartum, but these cases may be more likely associated with evolving or occult autoimmune disorders [21]. Bleeding and excessive bruising are the most common clinical manifestations but some AH in the context of pregnancy are clinically insignificant except for abnormal coagulation laboratory tests. The prognosis is overall good and mortality rates are low (0–6%) [8]. The EACH2 registry observed no mortality in this cohort [20]. Compared to AH associated with autoimmune disease, the titers of pregnancy-associated auto-FVIII antibodies run considerably lower (median 7.4 BU/mL, range 0.7–348, in the EACH2 study [20]). If the inhibitor is low titer (≤5 BU), it generally disappears spontaneously over a median of 30 months postpartum. Approximately 74% of women achieve complete remission with first-line immunosuppressive treatment [20]. Although conflicting data exist, it appears that <15% of individuals with anti-FVIII autoantibodies will experience a recurrence in subsequent pregnancies. The pathogenesis of these pregnancy-related autoantibody inhibitors directed against FVIII remains unclear.

Theoretically and anecdotally, the anti-FVIII IgG autoantibodies circulating in pregnant mothers with AH can increase the risk of severe hemorrhagic complications in the neonate at delivery due to the transplacental transfer of the antibody. Because these bleeds often involve the central nervous system, C-section delivery should be seriously considered in these patients. EACH2 reported two infants born with postnatal bleeding complications [20].

Associated malignancies, most commonly lymphoproliferative in nature, have been identified in up to 10% of patients with AH, and may be associated with a worse prognosis [8,22]. The incidence of cancer associated AH in the prospective French Surveillance des Auto antiCorps au cours de l'Hemophilie Acquise (SACHA) study was 19.5% [23] and occurred predominantly in elderly men; and, especially when observed in conjunction with lymphoproliferative disorders, is consistent with the broad range of autoimmune phenomena that frequently complicate these conditions. The etiologic role of solid tumor malignancies in AH is not so apparent. In fact, some authors consider that the appearance of FVIII autoantibodies in patients with solid tumors such as prostate cancer may well be an epiphenomenon as these neoplasms occur so commonly in the same elderly cohort as AH. In some cases, the FVIII autoantibodies have been observed to arise after treatment for cancer has been initiated; it is possible that the use of corticosteroids, cytotoxic agents, and biologic response modifiers, such as interferon-α, could have altered host immunity and predisposed the patient to the development of autoimmune phenomena. Alternatively, FVIII autoantibody inhibitors could represent a host immune response to the tumor-derived antigens, although no tumor antigen has yet been described to have homology to FVIII. The development of AH does not appear to correlate with the stage or grade of the malignancy [24]. The presence of an underlying malignancy is not a contraindication to the use of immunotherapy to suppress the production of the antibody even in cases that fail to respond to primary antitumor therapy [24]. The auto-FVIII antibody inhibitor may not remit following successful eradication of the malignancy; however, 70% of AH cases, particularly associated with low-stage/grade tumors, went into complete remission for their AH after systemic chemotherapy and/or steroids [24]. Conversely, the re-emergence of inhibitors is not always a reliable indication of tumor recurrence in patients [25].

Drug reactions to certain medications, including antibiotics such as pencillin and its derivatives, sulfonamides and chloramphenicol; anticonvulsants such as diphenylhydantoin; and BCG (bacille Calmette–Guérin) vaccination have all been associated with the development of antibodies to FVIII [2,26]. The list of putative medications has expanded rapidly over recent years as anecdotal reports in the literature increase. This may represent an increased awareness of AH and the ability to diagnose it since the cause–effect of antibody elaboration and medication exposure is not obvious. Frequently, drug-induced anti-FVIII antibodies arise after hypersensitivity reactions and remit shortly after withdrawing the offending drug. The pathophysiology remains unknown in most cases; however, the significant alterations of immune function which are induced by the administration of such medications as interferon-α and fludarabine may facilitate the appearance of autoantibodies against FVIII, as they do for other immune phenomena reported with their use, e.g. immune thrombocytopenic purpura or autoimmune HA.

Clinical manifestations of acquired hemophilia

The clinical picture of AH is characterized by acute onset of severe bleeding in individuals who previously had no history of bleeding diatheses. It is notable that the bleeding pattern is distinctly more severe and anatomically varied than that observed in congenital severe hemophilia A complicated by alloimmune inhibitors against FVIII. Patients generally present with mucocutaneous bleeding such as epistaxis and gastrointestinal bleeding, as well as soft-tissue bleeding including extensive ecchymoses and hematomas. Joint and muscle bleeding, commonly experienced by patients with congenital hemophilia A and alloinhibitors, is comparatively rare. The bleeding is usually spontaneous, although minimal trauma or surgical procedures may predispose to disproportionately extensive ecchymoses and bleeding. Over 70% of AH patients present with severe bleeding or anemia severe enough to require transfusion therapy while only about 6% remain asymptomatic except for laboratory abnormalities [6]. The bleeding is accompanied by considerable morbidity; however, mortality, ranging between 9 and 22% [2,3] frequently is due to the infectious complications of immunosuppression rather than to fatal hemorrhage. The EACH2 registry noted a mortality rate of over 26% in AH patients, in whom fatal or bleeding complications occurred in 4.5%. No deaths occurred in pregnancy-related AH.

Laboratory diagnosis

The activated partial thromboplastin time (aPTT) is prolonged as FVIII (or FIX, FXI, and FXII), for which it screens, is decreased in undiluted patient plasma. The prothrombin time (PT) and platelet function are usually normal. To determine if the elevated aPTT is due to a specific clotting factor deficiency or a pathologic circulating anticoagulant, performance of mixing studies is critical. For FVIII inhibitory antibodies of the allo or auto variety, the neutralizing expression of the inhibitor is time and temperature dependent and may require 2 h at 37°C, especially in the case of weak autoantibodies, before an accurate assessment of the inhibitor can be ascertained. A difference of 10 s or greater is indicative of a positive inhibitor screen.

To confirm the neutralization of a specific coagulation factor by auto- or alloantibody inhibitors, assays for each of the coagulation factors in the involved pathway must be performed. Lupus-like anticoagulants can be distinguished from clotting factor autoantibody inhibitors by the finding of a positive platelet neutralization assay and/or a prolonged dilute Russell's viper venom test (dRVVT), tissue thromboplastin inhibition assay, or kaolin clotting time. In addition, clinical presentation is essential to distinguishing among these possibilities, as lupus-like anticoagulants are typically found in either asymptomatic or hypercoagulable patients, and patients with AH tend to bleed.

When the presence of a specific factor inhibitor is suspected, it is imperative that the target is identified and the degree of inhibitory activity quantified. This is accomplished by incubating a source of the specific clotting factor (typically, pooled normal plasma) with increasing dilutions of the patient's plasma at 37°C for 2 h. As the antibody-containing plasma is diluted, the clotting factor concentration will appear to increase although the baseline mixture may yield a normal aPTT or FVIII activity level. The inhibitor potency is expressed most commonly worldwide in terms of BU, where 1.0 BU is the reciprocal dilution of patient test plasma permitting detection of 50% residual FVIII activity in a mixture with normal pooled plasma [27]. The Nijmegen modification of the Bethesda assay employs buffered normal plasma throughout each step of the assay, thereby minimizing shifts in pH and allowing for increased sensitivity of the inhibitor assay to detect low-titer inhibitors, e.g. ≤0.6 BU [28]. While this assay is widely accepted for research trials, particularly those in which the detection of low-titer alloantibody inhibitors is critical, it is labor intensive and is rarely needed or used in the typical clinical scenario for AH.

Other assays for detecting specific inhibitors which target clotting factor proteins rely on immunologic rather than functional methodologies. These assays, such as enzyme-linked immunoadsorbent assays (ELISAs), are extremely sensitive and may detect antibodies that do not inhibit FVIII activity *in vitro* or *in vivo*. They have thus far generally been confined to a research setting.

From the clinical perspective, the severity of bleeding cannot be predicted from the BU titer of the autoantibody inhibitor or to the level of residual FVIII activity.

Treatment

There are two major goals for the treatment of AH: the immediate control of acute and chronic bleeding and the long-term suppression/eradication of the autoantibody inhibitor. The first objective is necessary because bleeding episodes are often relentless without reversal of the coagulation deficit, and can be life threatening. The second objective is required to restore normal hemostasis and can usually be accomplished using some type of immunotherapy. An important caveat is that the level of inhibitor potency is not directly proportional to or predictive of the severity or frequency of bleeding events.

The choice of therapeutic agent to reverse bleeding depends on the severity of the bleeding, the clinical setting, and the initial and historical peak titers of antihuman FVIII inhibitors. There are no randomized controlled "head to head" studies in AH patients comparing the efficacy of the available replacement products. Several strategies, such as administration of desmopressin and concentrates of human rFVIII may raise the FVIII activity levels adequately in plasma of individuals with low-titer auto-FVIII antibody inhibitors (≤5 BU). If the inhibitor titer is high (>5 BU), or if bleeding persists despite infusions of FVIII concentrates, then FVIII bypassing agents, such as activated prothrombin complex concentrates (aPCCs) or rFVIIa, are indicated. Local measures for treatment of mucosal hemorrhage, such as antifibrinolytic agents or topical fibrin glues, may also be helpful. The use of plasma-derived or recombinant topical thrombin preparations may also spare the need for the more expensive parenteral replacement products.

The target level of FVIII activity needed to control most bleeding events is 30–50% of normal. This is generally more feasible to achieve if the inhibitor titer is <5 BU. The recommended initial dose of FVIII concentrate is 20 IU/kg for each BU of inhibitor plus 40 additional IU/kg intravenously as a bolus. The plasma FVIII activity level should be determined 10–15 min after the initial bolus and, if the incremental recovery is not adequate, another bolus dose should be administered [29]. An alternative approach is to administer an initial intravenous bolus of 200–300 IU/kg followed by continuous infusion of about 4–14 IU/kg/h [30]. These doses are estimations, and FVIII levels and clinical response should be monitored carefully throughout treatment. FVIII concentrates are generally not useful if the patient has a high-titer (>5 BU) or high-responding inhibitor. The latter may not be known until after the first dose of FVIII is administered since patients with low-titer inhibitors may be high responders, with the capacity to mount an anamnestic response after exposure to the offending antigen, e.g. FVIII.

The FVIII present in intermediate purity concentrates is associated with a large amount of VWF protein, which theoretically protects the FVIII from proteolytic inactivation and neutralization by the autoantibodies in the patient's plasma, particularly by antibodies directed against C2 domain. Thus far, this has been more of an *in-vitro* consideration than an *in-vivo* one, but it is provocative and awaits testing in a clinical setting. A similar argument has been posited for the benefits of 1-deamino-8-D-arginine vasopressin (DDAVP) for the treatment of autoantibody FVIII inhibitors, albeit low-titer ones. In this situation, DDAVP would be expected to increase both VWF protein and FVIII release into the plasma.

Porcine plasma-derived FVIII (pFVIII) concentrate was formerly considered a vital first-line therapy to achieve hemostasis in patients with AH due both to its excellent efficacy and the opportunity for close laboratory montoring (unlike for the bypassing agents, aPCCs and rFVIIa, postinfusion FVIII activity levels may be followed in the laboratory while using the porcine plasma-derived product). Unfortunately, pFVIII was removed from the market in 2004 due to its contamination with porcine parvovirus. In contrast to allo-FVIII antibody inhibitors, the cross-reactivity between antihuman FVIII autoantibodies and pFVIII is usually minimal and rarely neutralizing enough to obviate the use of pFVIII concentrate [7]. A new recombinant porcine B-domain-deleted FVIII product (OBI-1, Baxter) has recently completed phase I and II clinical trials in congenital hemophilia and alloinhibitors [31]; trials in AH are pending.

For patients with high-titer inhibitors (>5 BU), the "bypassing" agents, aPCCs and rFVIIa, are the most commonly used first-line therapies. factor eight bypassing activity (FEIBA, Baxter) is currently the only commercially available aPCC in the USA. Its main active components include activated FX and prothrombin, but the precise mechanism for its hemostatic action in AH remains poorly understood. aPCCs have been used extensively in the treatment of bleeding episodes in patients with both allo- and auto-FVIII antibody inhibitors.

Retrospective studies in subjects with AH report excellent or good hemostatic response in 86–100% of cases [32,33]. The EACH2 registry reported greater than 90% success in controlling bleeding complications with FEIBA in AH [6]. For treatment of acute bleeds, the recommended dose of FEIBA is 50–100 IU/kg infused intravenously every 8–12 h. If bleeding persists after 24–48 h, a switch to an alternative bypassing agent should be considered. Minor reactions such as headache, nausea, pruritus, skin rashes, and diarrhea have been noted. FEIBA administration may also produce an anamnestic increase in titer of autoantibody as it does in alloantibody inhibitors. Rare cases of disseminated intravascular coagulation (DIC), venous thromboembolism, and myocardial infarction have also been reported in AH [34] and a manufacturer-initiated assessment of FEIBA safety over 10 years described three cases of thrombotic complications in individuals with AH, which they attributed to patient risk factors (e.g. obesity, atherosclerosis, etc.) rather than to FEIBA [35]. In the prospective Factor Eight Inhibitor Bypassing Activity in Acquired Hemophilia (FEIBHAC) study [36], FEIBA administration was associated with two separate episodes of deep venous thromboembolism (both in the same patient) and one case of DIC out of 23 patient with AH.

There is also a small, but theoretical risk of viral and perhaps prion transmission as FEIBA is a plasma-derived product. This necessitates a careful risk to benefit analysis prior to the administration of this human plasma-derived product. It must be noted that there has never been a reported case of human immunodeficiency virus (HIV), hepatitis C virus (HCV), or variant Creutzfeldt–Jakob disease (CJD) transmission associated with the use of FEIBA.

The other widely used bypassing agent is rFVIIa (NovoNordisk). While its mechanism of action is also not fully understood, it has been demonstrated to directly activate FX and increase thrombin production on the surface of activated platelets even in the absence of FVIII and FIX. The activated platelet-specific generation of thrombin is postulated to localize its action to sites of active bleeding and tissue injury. Retrospective data collected from compassionate use programs [37] and the Hemophilia and Thrombosis Research Society (HTRS) database suggest that rFVIIa is effective or partially effective in 88% of evaluable bleeding episodes in AH. When rFVIIa concentrate was used as first-line therapy, there was 95% efficacy; when used as salvage treatment, rFVIIa yielded 83% efficacy in AH [38]. The EACH2 registry noted 91% efficacy for rFVIIa therapy versus 94% efficacy for FEIBA [6]. The major adverse effect anticipated with rFVIIa administration in AH, as with FEIBA, is the occurrence of arterial and venous thrombosis, which generally occurs at very low rates in AH, and has been noted predominantly in individuals with pre-existing atherosclerotic disease [39,40]. The retrospective HTRS registry observed one thrombotic event in 87 patients treated with rFVIIa for their AH [41] while the EACH2 registry reported 2.9% thrombotic events with rFVIIa versus 4.8% for FEIBA [42]. Thrombotic events were correlated with increased age and included 1.4% myocardial infarctions, 0.2% cerebrovascular accidents, and 1% venous thromboembolic events [42]. There is some concern that combining antifibrinolytic agents with administration of either FEIBA or rFVIIa concentrate will increase the risk for thrombotic complications. Similarly, there is concern that combining rFVIIa and FEIBA in very refractory bleeding episodes will lead to hypercoagulability.

Rapid intravenous bolus administration of 90–120 μg/kg rFVIIa, repeated every 2–3 h, depending on clinical response, is the recommended treatment regimen to reverse or prevent bleeding episodes in AH. Continuous infusion of rFVIIa is being explored as a means of simplifying the demands of frequent dosing and of reducing cost of product. The superpharmacologic dosing regimen of intravenous bolus 270 μg rFVIIa/kg, which has been popularized for treatment of bleeds associated with allo-FVIII antibody inhibitors, has not been evaluated in AH and should be used with extreme caution, if at all, due to the potentially increased thrombogenicity induced by such dosing regimens in those without congenital hemophilia A [39].

Although no randomized trials have been performed comparing FEIBA to rFVIIa in patients with AH, there appear to be more data associated with rFVIIa than FEIBA. In the EACH2 trial, 56.7% of AH patients received rFVIIa as first-line therapy for bleeding complications compared to 20.5% who received FEIBA [42]. Nevertheless, the efficacy rates in AH for both products are similar (93%) [42]. If first-line therapy fails with either product, switching to the alternative bypassing agent may prove successful. Secondary prophylaxis to diminish bleeding has been used in patients with congenital hemophilia and inhibitors, but has not yet been explored in AH. An important drawback to the use of both products is the lack of a validated laboratory technique to monitor or predict hemostatic efficacy and safety. The use of thrombin generation assays and thromboelastography is currently being explored in research settings [43,44]. Currently, when administering bypassing agents in AH, efficacy is a clinical endpoint and dosing is empirical.

Autoantibody inhibitor eradication in acquired hemophilia

The primary aim in long-term management of AH is to eradicate the FVIII autoantibodies so that further bleeding can be averted. Although in some clinical situations (e.g. postpartum women and drug-related AH) FVIII autoantibodies may remit spontaneously, most published guidelines and algorithms recommend early initiation of eradication therapy. This is usually achieved through immunosuppressive medications or immunomodulation. Delgado *et al.* reported that mortality in untreated patients with AH was significantly increased compared to those who received immunosuppressive therapy (41% vs 20%), irrespective of active bleeding, titer of autoantibody, level of residual FVIII activity, or underlying associated disease state [8]. Successful immunosuppression regimens in AH have most frequently used corticosteroids as the cornerstone, either as a single agent or in combination with cyclophosphamide. In a prospective randomized trial, Green *et al.* treated 31 subjects with prednisone 1 mg/kg/day for 3 weeks, with a 32% complete remission rate. After 3 weeks, in subjects with persistence of antibody, switching to oral cyclophosphamide 2 mg/kg/day as second-line therapy appeared more effective than continuing prednisone alone (complete remission rate 50% vs 42%) [45]. While some investigators have advocated using combination therapy first line, a metaanalysis of 20 reports and a UK surveillance study showed that although addition of cyclophosphamide improved initial complete remission rates, there was no change in overall survival [3,8]. This may be related to the high rates of adverse effects from immunosuppressive agents, including neutropenia-related infections, in this predominantly elderly population. Patients who respond to steroids fall into a good prognostic category. Median time to remission is 5–7 weeks, with overall complete remission rates ranging between 60 and 80% [46]. Single agent cyclophosphamide was significantly more effective than corticosteroids in its ability to eradicate FVIII autoantibody inhibitors; however, there was no survival advantage [8]. The EACH2 prospective registry noted higher complete remissions in inhibitor eradication with combined corticosteroids and cyclophosphamide (77% vs 58%) but this significant difference did not translate to improved survival [47].

Other immunosuppressive medications have been employed for particularly refractory autoantibody inhibitor eradication, including azathioprine, cyclosporine, FK506 (tacrolimus), mycophenolate mofetil (Cellcept), sirolimus (rapamycin), and 2-chlorodeoxyadensine. Controlled studies have not been performed to confirm their comparative safety and efficacy in sufficiently large populations.

Introduction of rituximab, a chimeric monoclonal antibody that targets the CD20 antigen, has opened new horizons in the treatment of benign hematologic diseases, and has been used to treat inhibitors in patients with both congenital and AH. Anecdotal case reports and series including over 65 patients have reported complete remission rates > 80%, which must be interpreted with some caution due to the likely bias of publishing only positive results. While this justifies a randomized prospective trial to define the exact role of rituximab in the management of AH, it cannot currently be recommended as first-line therapy [48,49]. This stance was also affirmed by the prospective EACH2 registry in which first-line rituximab therapy alone or with concurrent corticosteroids resulted in an inferior response to autoantibody inhibitor eradication versus the combination of corticosteroids and cyclophosphamide [50]. Studies in the lymphoproliferative disorders indicate that rituximab use may be associated with long-term consequences, including persistent neutropenia, reactivation of hepatitis B and C, and immunosuppression. These could be pertinent to the use of rituximab in AH therapy. Thus, in view of its long-term side-effects, its decreased effectiveness compared to other first-line therapies in eradicating the autoantibody inhibitor, its cost, and its inability to improve survival, rituximab should be relegated to second-line therapy.

Care should be exercised when considering any of these eradication strategies in pregnancy-related AH.

Other less used treatment options include administration of intravenous immunoglobulin in large doses, which often mediate a rapid but short-lived decline in autoantibody titers, perhaps due to anti-idiotypic antibodies derived from the pooled plasmas of thousands of normal donors. The usual administered dose is 2 g/kg divided in either two or five daily infusions. Intravenous immunoglobulin is rarely able to induce a complete remission when used alone (25–37% response rates, effective probably only in low-titer inhibitors) [51], but may be useful adjunctive therapy along with immunosuppressants, as part of an immune tolerance induction regimen (ITI), or with extracorporeal plasmapheresis. Combination treatment with FVIII concentrate, cyclophosphamide, and methylprednisolone, or other similar immunomodulation protocols, has reported high success rates (complete remission rate 93%) of inhibitor eradication with low recurrence rates [52,53]. The Budapest protocol employs a low-dose FVIII concentrate taper regimen (30 IU/kg/day for week 1, 20 IU/kg/day for week 2, and 15 IU/kg/day for week 3) in concert with cyclophosphamide (200 mg/day) and methylprednisolone (100 mg/day IV for week 1 and tapering over the next 2 weeks) and has reported over

90% success in autoantibody eradication [53]. In contrast, the Bonn–Malmo protocol employs a high-dose FVIII approach (100 IU/kg/day) in combination with oral cyclophosphamide (1–2 mg/kg/day), methylprednisolone (1 mg/kg/day po), plasmapheresis with exchange 5% albumin, immunoabsorption, and high-dose intravenous gammaglobulin (0.3 g/kg twice weekly). There was an 88% inhibitor eradication rate [52]. These reported excellent results were generated from small studies and remain to be tested in a randomized manner. They do appear to be a promising albeit costly treatment strategy.

In patients with AH, relapse rates of up to 20% have been reported, at a median of 7.5 months (range 1 week to 14 months) [3]. In over 50% of patients, a second complete remission could be induced, although some patients required longer term immunosuppression. Patients should be carefully followed after remission and advised to promptly report new hemorrhagic symptoms so that relapses may be detected and treated as rapidly as possible.

Additional new treatment modalities for AH await development and clinical research application. Theoretically, they could include the manufacture via recombinant technology of a preparation of combined rFII–rFX, which could provide an alternative to rFVIIa concentrate for refractory auto-FVIII inhibitors; the marketing of recombinant pFVIII concentrate (not yet in clinical trials for AH); and the development of aptimers and antibodies to activate coagulation factors to bypass the FVIII autoantibody; or development of ribonucleic acid interference therapies targeting antithrombin III. Finally, modulation of the immune system may be possible to eradicate the autoantibody. This approach remains to be tested for auto-FVIII antibodies. All of these strategies are provocative and suggest that the future for treatment of the auto-FVIII antibody inhibitors in AH is promising.

References

1 Reding MT, Cooper DL. Barriers to effective diagnosis and management of a bleeding patient with undiagnosed bleeding disorder across multiple specialties: results of a quantitative case-based survey. *J Multidiscip Health* 2012; **5**: 277–87.

2 Green D, Lechner K. A survey of 215 non-hemophilic patients with inhibitors to Factor VIII. *Thromb Haemost* 1981; **45**(3): 200–3.

3 Collins PW, Hirsch S, Baglin TP, et al. Acquired hemophilia A in the United Kingdom: a 2-year national surveillance study by the United Kingdom Haemophilia Centre Doctors' Organisation. *Blood* 2007; **109**(5): 1870–7.

4 Collins P, Macartney N, Davies R, Lees S, Giddings J, Majer R. A population based, unselected, consecutive cohort of patients with acquired haemophilia A. *Br J Haematol* 2004; **124**(1): 86–90.

5 Collins P, Budde U, Rand JH, Federici AB, Kessler CM. Epidemiology and general guidelines of the management of acquired haemophilia and von Willebrand syndrome. *Haemophilia* 2008; **14**(Suppl.) 3: 49–55.

6 Knoebl P, Marco P, Baudo F, et al. Demographic and clinical data in acquired hemophilia A: results from the European Acquired Haemophilia Registry (EACH2). *J Thromb Haemost* 2012; **10**: 622–31.

7 Kessler CM, Ludlam CA. The treatment of acquired factor VIII inhibitors: worldwide experience with porcine factor VIII concentrate. International Acquired Hemophilia Study Group. *Semin Hematol* 1993; **30**(2 Suppl. 1): 22–7.

8 Delgado J, Jimenez-Yuste V, Hernandez-Navarro F, Villar A. Acquired haemophilia: review and meta-analysis focused on therapy and prognostic factors. *Br J Haematol* 2003; **121**(1): 21–35.

9 Lollar P. Pathogenic antibodies to coagulation factors. Part one: factor VIII and factor IX. *J Thromb Haemost* 2004; **2**(7): 1082–95.

10 Prescott R, Nakai H, Saenko EL, et al. The inhibitor antibody response is more complex in hemophilia A patients than in most nonhemophiliacs with factor VIII autoantibodies. Recombinate and Kogenate Study Groups. *Blood* 1997; **89**(10): 3663–71.

11 Lacroix-Desmazes S, Moreau A, Bonnemain C, et al. Catalytic activity of antibodies against factor VIII in patients with hemophilia A. *Nat Med* 1999; **5**(9): 1044–7.

12 Gawryl MS, Hoyer LW. Inactivation of factor VIII coagulant activity by two different types of human antibodies. *Blood* 1982; **60**(5): 1103–9.

13 Boggio LN, Green D. Acquired hemophilia. *Rev Clin Exp Hematol* 2001; **5**(4): 389–404.

14 Walter JD, Werther RA, Polozova MS, et al. Characterization and solution structure of the factor VIII C2 domain in a ternary complex with classical and non-classical inhibitor antibodies. *J Biol Chem* 2013; **288**(14): 9905–14.

15 Meeks SL, Healey JF, Parker ET, Barrow RT, Pollar P. Non-classical anti-factor VIII C2 domain antibodies are pathogenic in a murine in vivo bleeding model. *J Thromb Haemost* 2009; **7**(4): 658–74.

16 Matsumoto T, Nogami K, Ogiwara K, Shima M. A putative inhibitory mechanism in the tenase complex responsible for loss of coagulation function in acquired haemophilia A patients with antic-C2 autoantibodies. *Thromb Haemost* 2012; **107**(2): 288–301.

17 Astermark J, Donfield SM, Gomperts ED, et al. The polygenic nature of inhibitors in hemophilia A: results from the Hemophilia Inhibitor Genetics Study (HIGS) Combined Cohort. *Blood* 2013; **121**(8): 1446–54.

18 Oldenburg J, Zeitler H, Pavlova A. Genetic markers in acquired haemophilia. *Haemophilia* 2010; **16**(Suppl. s3): 41–5.

19 Morrison AE, Ludlam CA, Kessler C. Use of porcine factor VIII in the treatment of patients with acquired hemophilia. *Blood* 1993; **81**(6): 1513–20.

20 Tengborn L, Baudo F, Huth-Kuhne A, et al. Pregnancy-associated acquired haemophilia A: results from the European Acquired Haemophilia (EACH2) registry. *Br J Obstet Gynaecol* 2012; **119**(12): 1529–37.

21 Solymoss S. Postpartum acquired factor VIII inhibitors: results of a survey. *Am J Hematol* 1998; **59**(1): 1–4.

22 Hauser I, Lechner K. Solid tumors and factor VIII antibodies. *Thromb Haemost* 1999; **82**(3): 1005–7.

23 Borg JY, Guillet B, LeCam-Duchez V, Goudemand J, Levesque H. Outcome of acquired haemophilia in France: the prospective SACHA (Surveillance des Auto antiCorps au cours de l'Hemophilie Acquise) registry. *Haemophilia* 2013; **19**(4): 564–70.

24 Sallah S, Wan JY. Inhibitors against factor VIII in patients with cancer. Analysis of 41 patients. *Cancer* 2001; **91**(6): 1067–74.

25 White KT, Aggarwal A, Napolitano M, Kessler CM. Autoantibody Inhibitor Eradication In Acquired Hemophilia Associated with

Cancer: a Retrospective Analysis. *Blood (ASH Annual Meeting Abstracts)* 2010; **116**(21): 1418.

26 Franchini M, Capra F, Nicolini N, *et al*. Drug-induced anti-factor VIII antibodies: a systematic review. *Med Sci Monit* 2007; **13**(4): RA55–61.

27 Kasper CK, Aledort L, Aronson D, *et al*. Proceedings: A more uniform measurement of factor VIII inhibitors. *Thromb Diath Haemorrh* 1975; **34**(2): 612.

28 Verbruggen B, Novakova I, Wessels H, Boezeman J, van den Berg M, Mauser-Bunschoten E. The Nijmegen modification of the Bethesda assay for factor VIII:C inhibitors: improved specificity and reliability. *Thromb Haemost* 1995; **73**(2): 247–51.

29 Kasper CK. Human factor VIII for bleeding in patients with inhibitors. *Vox Sang* 1999; **77**(Suppl. 1): 47–8.

30 Blatt PM, White GC, II, McMillan CW, Roberts HR. Treatment of anti-factor VIII antibodies. *Thromb Haemost* 1977; **38**(2): 514–23.

31 Kempton C, Abshire T, Deveras R, *et al*. Pharmacokinetics and safety of OBI-1, a recombinant B domain-deleted porcine factor VIII, in subjects with haemophilia A. *Haemophilia* 2012; **18**(5): 798–804.

32 Sallah S. Treatment of acquired haemophilia with factor eight inhibitor bypassing activity. *Haemophilia* 2004; **10**(2): 169–73.

33 Holme PA, Brosstad F, Tjonnfjord GE. Acquired haemophilia: management of bleeds and immune therapy to eradicate autoantibodies. *Haemophilia* 2005; **11**(5): 510–15.

34 Mehta R, Parameswaran R, Shapiro AD. An overview of the history, clinical practice concerns, comparative studies and strategies to optimize therapy of bypassing agents. *Haemophilia* 2006; **12**(Suppl. 6): 54–61.

35 Ehrlich HJ, Henzl MJ, Gomperts ED. Safety of factor VIII inhibitor bypass activity (FEIBA): 10-year compilation of thrombotic adverse events. *Haemophilia* 2002; **8**(2): 83–90.

36 Borg I-Y, Negrier C, Durieu I , *et al*. Prospective clinical and biological evaluation of antihemorrhagic treatment with factor eight inhibitor bypassing activity in acquired hemophilia, FEIBHAC Study. *J Thromb Haemost* 2011; **9**(Suppl. 02) 938–939 (abstract P-TH-545).

37 Hay CR, Negrier C, Ludlam CA. The treatment of bleeding in acquired haemophilia with recombinant factor VIIa: a multicentre study. *Thromb Haemost* 1997; **78**(6): 1463–7.

38 Sumner MJ, Geldziler BD, Pedersen M, Seremetis S. Treatment of acquired haemophilia with recombinant activated FVII: a critical appraisal. *Haemophilia* 2007; **13**(5): 451–61.

39 O'Connell KA, Wood JJ, Wise RP, Lozier JN, Braun MM. Thromboembolic adverse events after use of recombinant human coagulation factor VIIa. *J Am Med Assoc* 2006; **295**(3): 293–8.

40 Abshire T, Kenet G. Safety update on the use of recombinant factor VIIa and the treatment of congenital and acquired deficiency of factor VIII or IX with inhibitors. *Haemophilia* 2008; **14**(5): 898–902.

41 Ma A, Kessler CM, Gut RZ, Cooper DL. Treatment of acquired haemophilia with recombinant factor VIIa (rFVIIa): an updated analysis from the hemophilia and thrombosis research society (HTRS) registry. *J Thromb Haemost* 2011; **9**(Suppl. 02): 476 (abstract P-TU-532).

42 Baudo F, Collins P, Huth-Kuhne A, *et al*. Management of bleeding in acquired haemophilia A: results from the European Acquired Haemophilia (EACH2) Registry. *Blood* 2012; **120**(1): 39–46.

43 Barrowcliffe TW. Monitoring inhibitor patients with the right assays. *Semin Hematol* 2008; **45**(2 Suppl. 1): S25–30.

44 Dehmel H, Werwitzke S, Trummer A, Ganser A, Tiede A. Thrombelastographic monitoring of recombinant factor VIIa in acquired haemophilia. *Haemophilia* 2008; **14**(4): 736–42.

45 Green D, Rademaker AW, Briet E. A prospective, randomized trial of prednisone and cyclophosphamide in the treatment of patients with factor VIII autoantibodies. *Thromb Haemost* 1993; **70**(5): 753–7.

46 Collins PW. Treatment of acquired hemophilia A. *J Thromb Haemost* 2007; **5**(5): 893–900.

47 Collins PW. Therapeutic challenges in acquired factor VIII deficiency. *Hematol Am Soc Hematol Educ Prog* 2012; **Dec**: 369–74.

48 Stasi R, Brunetti M, Stipa E, Amadori S. Selective B-cell depletion with rituximab for the treatment of patients with acquired hemophilia. *Blood* 2004; **103**(12): 4424–8.

49 Franchini M. Rituximab in the treatment of adult acquired hemophilia A: a systematic review. *Crit Rev Oncol Hematol* 2007; **63**(1): 47–52.

50 Coppola A, Favaloro EJ, Tufano A, Di Minno MND, Cerbone AM, Franchini M. Acquired Inhibitors of Coagulation Factors: Part I—Acquired Hemophilia A. *Semin Thromb Hemost* 2012; **38**(05): 433–46.

51 Schwartz RS, Gabriel DA, Aledort LM, Green D, Kessler CM. A prospective study of treatment of acquired (autoimmune) factor VIII inhibitors with high-dose intravenous gammaglobulin. *Blood* 1995; **86**(2): 797–804.

52 Zeitler H, Ulrich-Merzenich G, Hess L, *et al*. Treatment of acquired hemophilia by the Bonn–Malmo Protocol: documentation of an in vivo immunomodulating concept. *Blood* 2005; **105**(6): 2287–93.

53 Nemes L, Pitlik E. New protocol for immune tolerance induction in acquired hemophilia. *Haematologica* 2000; **85**(10 Suppl.): 64–8.

PART V

Hemophilia B

CHAPTER 13

Hemophilia B: molecular basis

Keith Gomez and Pratima Chowdary

Royal Free Hospital, London, UK

Mutation nomenclature

Numbering in this chapter follows the guidelines of the Human Genome Variation (HGV) society. +1 refers to the "A" of the ATG translation start codon for nucleotide numbering and the methionine residue that this codes for in peptide numbering. Most earlier publications use a numbering based on the transcription start site or the mature protein.

Introduction

Classic hemophilia B (HB) is caused by mutations in the *F9* gene that lead to quantitative and/or qualitative deficiencies in circulating factor IX (FIX) protein. Genetic analysis is now a standard part of the diagnostic process in many hemophilia centers and has resulted in a much greater understanding of the etiology of this disorder. This facilitates screening of relatives and in the future may influence therapeutic options for individual patients. From a scientific perspective, it has led to a greater appreciation of the relationship between the structure of the FIX protein and its function. This is of fundamental importance for research and has been vital for breakthroughs such as the production of recombinant FIX. It is a cornerstone for current and future research streams such as the development of better recombinant proteins or effective gene therapy.

The process of understanding the molecular basis of HB began with characterization of *F9* in the early 1980s. Several groups described parts of the *F9* coding sequence between 1982 and 1984, and the full sequence of the entire gene was published in 1985 [1]. *F9* is located at Xq27.1 and spans 33 kbp. There are eight exons which are transcribed into a 2802-bp mRNA. This, in turn, is translated into a 461-amino acid (aa) polypeptide, from which removal of a 28-aa signal peptide and 18-aa propeptide leaves a 415-aa mature protein. The primary translation product has an estimated molecular mass of 52 kDa.

The mature protein belonging to the serine protease family is synthesized in the liver as a single-chain vitamin K-dependent glycoprotein, and is present in the blood as zymogen at a concentration of 3–5 mg/L. The two principal activators of this zymogen are activated factor XI (FXIa) and the tissue factor (TF)–FVIIa complex. Activation occurs following a double cleavage after Arg192 and Arg226, which removes a 35-aa activation peptide. The active enzyme is a two-chain serine protease with a light chain of 145 aa containing the N-terminal Gla domain, EGF1 (epidermal growth factor-like), and EGF2 domains and a heavy chain of 235 aa containing the C-terminal SP (serine protease or catalytic) domain. The released activation peptide lies between the EGF2 and SP domains. The relationship between the nucleotide sequence and the translated polypeptide is shown in Figure 13.1.

Post-translational modifications seen in FIX include disulfide bonds and the one between Cys178–Cys335 holds the two chains together after activation. The Gla domain contains 12 glutamic acid residues that are post-translationally modified to 4-carboxyglutamate. These are essential for binding the calcium ions that give the Gla domain the positive charge that is required for efficient interaction with a negatively charged phospholipid membrane. Furthermore, it has two N-linked glycosylations, four O-linked glycosylations, one hydroxylation, two phosphorylations, and one sulfation. The catalytic triad, characteristic of all members of the serine protease family, is located in the heavy chain and is made up of His267, Asp315, and Ser411. On its own, FIXa is a relatively inefficient enzyme in the activation of its preferred substrate, FX. This activity is enhanced when the enzyme is noncovalently bound to its cofactor, FVIIIa, to form the macromolecular intrinsic tenase complex. The maximum catalytic activity of this complex is achieved after docking on a negatively charged phospholipid membrane. The effect of FVIIIa is to increase the specific activity by some 50 000-fold over that of the enzyme in isolation [2].

Textbook of Hemophilia, Third Edition. Edited by Christine A. Lee, Erik E. Berntorp and W. Keith Hoots.
© 2014 John Wiley & Sons, Ltd. Published 2014 by John Wiley & Sons, Ltd.

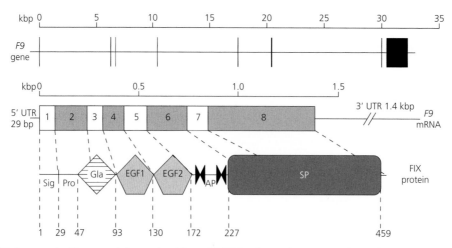

Figure 13.1 Relationship between the *F9* gene and the translated factor IX (FIX) polypeptide. Exons are depicted as vertical bars in *F9* with thickness approximating to size. In the primary mRNA, the parts of the coding sequence transcribed from each exon are shown by numbered blocks. The regions of the protein encoded by different exons are shown by dashed lines and below the protein residue numbering indicates the domain boundaries. AP, activation peptide; Gla, γ-carboxyglutamic domain; UTR, untranslated region; AP: activation peptide; EGF: epidermal growth factor; Pro: propeptide; Sig: signal peptide; SP: serine protease. The signal and propeptides are removed to form the mature protein.

The structure of the macromolecular intrinsic tenase complex has yet to be elucidated but can be inferred from the published crystal structures of porcine FIXa [3], individual domains of human FIXa [4–6], and human FVIII [7,8]. A predicted model of full-length human FIXa derived from these structures is available on the FIX mutation database on the internet (factorix. org) [9]. In the active enzyme, the light chain forms a stalk with the N-terminal Gla domain anchoring it to the phospholipid membrane. The catalytic domain is a globular structure sitting at the top of the stalk (Figure 13.2) and the neo N-terminus of the heavy chain is inserted into the catalytic domain during activation. The interface with FVIIIa is formed by one side of the protein and includes critical groups of residues in the EGF1, EGF2, and catalytic domains [8,10].

Techniques for mutation detection

Early methods of mutation detection generally relied upon distinguishing abnormal alleles by virtue of change in size of DNA fragments generated by restriction endonucleases. This is the basis of methods such as Southern blot, which can readily detect large deletions but are generally not suitable for direct detection of missense mutations. As discussed below, most cases of HB are associated with missense mutations. In this situation, the disease-associated allele could sometimes be tracked in a pedigree by linkage with known polymorphisms that modified restriction sites (restriction fragment length polymorphisms or RFLPs). There are several well-described polymorphisms that can be used for this purpose [11]. One of these is a single-nucleotide polymorphism (SNP), G/A g.20393 that codes for alanine or threonine at position 194. This has been termed the Malmö polymorphism and although it has no effect on protein

function, it does alter the epitope profile which produces variability in the results of antigen assays from different kits. The importance of these polymorphisms is that they can be used as indirect markers of mutation if the sequence at these positions in a pedigree varies between the normal and abnormal allele. Indirect methods require carriers to be heterozygous at the polymorphic marker, and there is always the possibility that recombination might lead to loss of the linkage with the mutated residue across generations. Therefore, these techniques have been superseded by DNA amplification using polymerase chain reaction (PCR) followed by direct sequencing. The primers and reaction conditions for amplification of the *F9* gene are now well standardized, making this a rapid and robust technique. The amplicons cover the coding sequence and known regulatory regions of *F9*. As PCR of the gene requires a number of amplification reactions, the possibility of simplifying the process by using mRNA as the target has been explored. Unfortunately, aberrant *F9* transcripts are found in peripheral blood, so this approach has largely been abandoned as a routine screening technique [12].

Polymerase chain reaction is generally not able to detect large deletions or other gross abnormalities in carriers because of the presence of the other (normal) allele. Although gross abnormalities represent a small group, they are nearly always associated with severe disease, making the detection of carrier status important. In the last few years, the development of new techniques has helped to tackle this problem. Of these multiplex ligation-dependent probe amplification (MLPA) and multiplex amplification and probe hybridization (MAPH) seem to be the most promising [13]. In both techniques, probes to specific sequences within the gene are amplified. The products from different probes vary by size, and are separated and quantified by electrophoresis. As the amount of amplified product is

CHAPTER 14

Factor IX inhibitors in hemophilia B

Meera B. Chitlur and Jeanne M. Lusher
Wayne State University School of Medicine, Detroit, USA

Introduction

Hemophilia B is an X-linked recessive, inherited bleeding disorder characterized by specific coagulation factor IX deficiency. While factor VIII (FVIII) deficiency (hemophilia A) is seen in approximately 80% of patients with hemophilia, factor IX (FIX) deficiency (hemophilia B) occurs in approximately 20% of patients. Hemophilia may be classified as mild (>5%), moderate (1–5%), or severe (<1%) based on the residual activity of the coagulation factor detectable in the patient's plasma. Severe hemophilia B occurs in approximately 30–45%, while 60% of those with hemophilia A have severe disease. Bleeding complications are similar for both hemophilia A and B. The availability of highly purified, virally attenuated, plasma-derived coagulation factor products and recombinant FIX concentrates has significantly diminished the complications from severe bleeding such as hemophilic arthropathy, and transmission of infectious agents have almost been obscured. The development of inhibitory antibodies is therefore the most serious and important complication seen in patients with hemophilia.

Frequency of inhibitors in hemophilia B

Factor IX inhibitors are relatively uncommon, being seen in 1–3% of persons with hemophilia B. In fact, the long-term directors of some large hemophilia centers note that they have seen no FIX inhibitors in their centers (Box 14.1). This is in striking contrast to the situation in hemophilia A, where approximately 30% of individuals with severe and moderately severe hemophilia develop inhibitors to FVIII [1,2]. Among persons with hemophilia, approximately 80% have hemophilia A, while only 20% have hemophilia B. Hemophilia B, an X-linked recessive disorder, occurs in approximately one of 30 000 male births, in all populations. Mutations causing this bleeding disorder have been found all over the FIX gene, which is located at Xq27.1; these mutations are reported and updated in the *F9* Mutation Database (www.factorIX.org) [3]. In most reports, approximately 30–45% of affected individuals have severe hemophilia B [4]. The majority of persons with hemophilia B who develop inhibitors have severe hemophilia B.

Risk factors for development of factor IX inhibitors

Genetic factors play a major role. Certain mutations in the FIX gene are associated with an increased incidence of inhibitor development. Large deletions and frame-shift mutations leading to the loss of coding information are much more likely to be associated with inhibitor development. High has reported that large deletions account for only 1–3% of all hemophilia B patients, but account for 50% of inhibitor patients [5]. In an analysis of hemophilia B patients who had anaphylactic reactions to FIX-containing products, as well as an inhibitor, Thorland *et al.* genotyped eight unrelated patients and compared their gene mutations with those found in 550 hemophilia B patients in the hemophilia B database at the time. Individuals with complete gene deletions were found to be at greatest risk for anaphylaxis. Anaphylaxis occurred more frequently in families with null mutations (large deletions, frame-shift, or nonsense mutations) than in those with missense mutations [6].

In addition to the particular FIX defect causing a patient's hemophilia B, Astermark has recently reviewed the potential role of immune response genes (noting a microsatellite polymorphism in the promoter region of the *interleukin-10* (*IL-10*) gene, which was highly associated with inhibitor formation in hemophilia A patients), environmental factors, and other concurrent immune system challenges, among others [7,8].

Textbook of Hemophilia, Third Edition. Edited by Christine A. Lee, Erik E. Berntorp and W. Keith Hoots.
© 2014 John Wiley & Sons, Ltd. Published 2014 by John Wiley & Sons, Ltd.

While race has been shown to play a definite role in the development of FVIII inhibitors, with approximately 40–50% of black individuals with hemophilia A developing a FVIII inhibitor, no such association has been found in hemophilia B.

Age and number of exposure days to factor IX at detection of factor IX inhibitors

As is the case in hemophilia A, most (but not all) individuals who develop an inhibitor to FIX do so relatively early in life (within the first 4–5 years), after a median of 9–11 exposure days (EDs) to any FIX-containing product (Box 14.2).

Anaphylaxis and other allergic reactions developing in close association with factor IX inhibitor development

With the development of plasma-derived FIX products of higher purity (e.g. monoclonal antibody purified FIX concentrates) in the 1990s, prelicensure clinical trials revealed an occasional study subject who developed anaphylaxis while being infused with the higher purity product [2]. This raised

concern that such high-purity products, which perhaps had been altered in their production, were resulting in both anaphylaxis and FIX inhibitors. As a result, an international registry of such complications was organized by Warrier *et al.* on behalf of the FVIII/FIX Subcommittee of the International Society on Thrombosis and Hemostasis (ISTH)'s Scientific and Standardization Committee (SSC) [4,9,10]. Additionally, all subsequent prelicensure clinical trials with new products included FIX inhibitors assays done at more frequent (specified) time intervals, and over a longer period of time.

Interestingly, the ISTH registry data submitted from 1997 to 2006 provided data concerning 94 individuals with inhibitors and anaphylaxis or severe reactions to FIX-containing products of various types. Some were receiving intermediate-purity plasma-derived products, while others were receiving high-purity FIX products (either recombinant or plasma derived) when the reaction occurred. Thus, there was no evidence to implicate a particular type of product [4]. This was again reconfirmed in a recent study by Recht *et al.* who conducted a retrospective, multicenter study of patients with fIX deficiency in North America and Europe. The study determined the frequency of moderate to severe allergic reactions to fIX and the frequency of inhibitor formation in those with moderate to severe allergic reactions. The results were similar to previously reported incidence and no differences were noted between patients receiving plasma-derived products and recombinant factor products [11].

However, in view of the severity of such complications occurring early in life, after very few exposures to FIX, Warrier *et al.* recommended that all infants and small children with severe hemophilia B be closely followed over their first 20 (or more) infusions (with any FIX-containing product) in a facility equipped to treat anaphylactic shock [9,10,12]. It was also recommended that genotyping be done on infants (or an affected sibling) with severe hemophilia B before such complications occurred, to know if they had a defect in the *FIX* gene (e.g. a large gene deletion) putting them at particular risk for anaphylaxis and inhibitor development [10]. Although the ISTH SSC's registry has been closed since 2006, the authors are still being contacted about new cases of anaphylactic reactions in children with severe haemophilia B.

In general, patients with an inhibitor to FIX and a history of anaphylaxis to FIX should be treated with rFVIIa—a safe, readily available recombinant product which does not contain FIX.

Management of patients with hemophilia B complicated by a factor IX inhibitor

As mentioned above, infants and young children with severe hemophilia B are at particular risk for the sudden development of anaphylactic shock (or other severe allergic reaction) and inhibitor development. While these two events are often closely related temporally, one may precede the other. Thus, a child who has developed a FIX inhibitor after relatively few EDs to FIX should be regarded as being at greater risk for anaphylactic shock with one of his next several doses of FIX. While such children are often being treated at a hemophilia treatment center (i.e. not yet on home infusion), the center should be equipped with a readily accessible "crash cart" for treating patients in shock.

Once stabilized, and with the situation being discussed with the patient's parents, they and members of the hemophilia center team can *consider* attempting desensitization with gradually increased doses of FIX. If this is successful, one can then *consider* an immune tolerance induction (ITI) regimen, using daily (or every other day) larger doses of FIX. However, while ITI regimens are often (approximately 85% of the time) successful in persons with hemophilia A complicated by a FVIII inhibitor, the success rate is much lower in hemophilia B. An average success rate here would be 40%, and ITI is fraught with complications. If success is achieved, it takes longer. More importantly, many hemophilia B patients undergoing ITI develop nephrotic syndrome approximately 7–8 months into ITI [9,12–14]. Should this occur, ITI should be stopped. Stopping FIX has resulted in improvement or cessation of edema and proteinuria in some reported patients [4]. In two patients who had developed nephrotic syndrome while on ITI, renal biopsy demonstrated membranous glomerulonephritis [13–15]. Anecdotal reports describe the efficacy of rituximab and immunosuppressive agents such as mycophenolate mofetil and cyclosporine in small numbers of difficult-to-manage FIX inhibitor patients [16–19].

Management of bleeding episodes in patients with factor IX inhibitors

The mainstays of treatment (or prevention) of bleeding episodes in individuals with hemophilia B complicated by an inhibitor to FIX are rFVIIa (Novo Nordisk's NovoSeven), and Baxter's factor VIII inhibitor bypass activity (FEIBA)-VH. Each has advantages and disadvantages [20–23]. rFVIIa is a recombinant product, and thus safe from transmission of bloodborne infections. It has been licensed for use in European countries and in North American for over a decade, and has generally proven to be safe and effective [22,23]. It can be safely used at home. However, there is no simple, readily available laboratory test for evaluating or predicting its efficacy, and the product is quite expensive [20,22,24]. While the package insert in the USA indicates a dosage range of 90–120 μg/kg/ dose, to be given every three hours if repeat doses are necessary, many hemophilia treaters are now using higher doses (e.g. 270 μg/kg/ dose), especially in children and young adults with hemophilia A complicated by an inhibitor. Anecdotal reports indicate success with a single dose in certain situations, with no adverse effects [18,25].

FEIBA-VH has also proven effective in many (but not all) bleeding situations. It is generally less expensive than rFVIIa, and if additional doses are needed, they are generally given at 12-h intervals. However, it is a plasma-derived product, and thus there is some worry about its viral safety, despite its track record of safety over many years of use. Some patients develop hives and pruritis with its use, and thus have been switched to rFVIIa.

The FEIBA NovoSeven Comparative (FENOC) study is the first head-to-head comparision of FEIBA-VH and rFVIIa in the management of bleeding episodes in patients with severe hemophilia A with inhibitors. The major conclusion from this study was that the two bypassing agents were similar but the efficacy of the products was rated differently by patients, especially during the first 12 h. The major drawbacks of the study were the lack of treatment blinding and the loss of 20% of the cohort prior to completion of the study [26]. There have been no similar studies in the hemophilia B patients with inhibitor.

References

1 Lusher J. Natural history of inhibitors in severe hemophilia A and B. In: Rodriguez-Marchan, LC (ed.) *Inhibitors in Patients with Hemophilia*. Oxford: Blackwell Science, 2002.

2 Lusher JM. Inhibitors in young boys with haemophilia. *Baillieres Best Pract Res Clin Haematol* 2000; **13**(3): 457–68.

3 Bicocchi MP, Pasino M, Rosano C, *et al*. Insight into molecular changes of the FIX protein in a series of Italian patients with haemophilia B. *Haemophilia* 2006; **12**(3): 263–70.

4 Chitlur M, Warrier I, Rajpurkar M, *et al*. Inhibitors in factor IX deficiency a report of the ISTH-SSC international FIX inhibitor registry (1997-2006). *Haemophilia* 2009; **15**(5): 1027–31.

5 High KA. Factor IX: molecular structure, epitopes, and mutations associated with inhibitor formation. *Adv Exp Med Biol* 1995; **386**: 79–86.

6 Thorland EC, Warrier I, Rajpurkar M, *et al*. Anaphylactic response to factor IX replacement therapy in haemophilia B patients: complete gene deletions confer the highest risk. *Haemophilia* 1999; **5**(2): 101–5.

7 Astermark J. Basic aspects of inhibitors to factors VIII and IX and the influence of non-genetic risk factors. *Haemophilia* 2006; **12**(Suppl. 6): 8–13; discussion 13–14.

8 Astermark J. Why do inhibitors develop? Principles of and factors influencing the risk for inhibitor development in haemophilia. *Haemophilia* 2006; **12**(Suppl. 3): 52–60.

9 Warrier I. ITI in Hemophilia B: Possibilities and problems. *Int Mon Hemophil* 2003 (10 year anniversary issue): 20–3.

10 Warrier I, Ewenstein BM, Koerper MA, *et al*. Factor IX inhibitors and anaphylaxis in hemophilia B. *J Pediatr Hematol Oncol* 1997; **19**(1): 23–7.

11 Recht M. Pollmann H, Taqliaferri A, *et al*. A retrospective study to describe the incidence of moderate to severe allergic reactions to factor IX in subjects with haemophilia B. *Haemophilia* 2011; **17**(3): 494–9.

12 Warrier I. Management of haemophilia B patients with inhibitors and anaphylaxis. *Haemophilia* 1998; **4**(4): 574–6.

13 Dharnidharka VR, Takemoto C, Ewenstein BM, *et al.* Membranous glomerulonephritis and nephrosis post factor IX infusions in hemophilia B. *Pediatr Nephrol* 1998; **12**(8): 654–7.

14 Ewenstein BM, Takemoto C, Warrier I, *et al.* Nephrotic syndrome as a complication of immune tolerance in hemophilia B. *Blood* 1997; **89**(3): 1115–16.

15 Warrier I. Factor Ix inhibitors and anaphylaxis. In: L.C. Rodriguez-Marchan (ed.) *Inhibitors in Patients with Hemophilia.* Oxford: Blackwell Science, 2002.

16 Fox RA, Neufeld EJ, Bennett CM. Rituximab for adolescents with haemophilia and high titre inhibitors. *Haemophilia* 2006; **12**(3): 218–22.

17 Lusher J. Rituximab and desensitization for a patient with factor IX deficiency. *Int Mon Hemophil* 2008; **2**: 38–40.

18 Parameswaran R, Shapiro AD, Gill JC, *et al.* Dose effect and efficacy of rFVIIa in the treatment of haemophilia patients with inhibitors: analysis from the Hemophilia and Thrombosis Research Society Registry. *Haemophilia* 2005; **11**(2): 100–6.

19 Klarmann D, Martinez Saquer I, Funk MB, *et al.* Immune tolerance induction with mycophenolate-mofetil in two children with haemophilia B and inhibitor. *Haemophilia* 2008; **14**(1): 44–9.

20 Astermark J, Rocino A, Von Depka M, *et al.* Current use of by-passing agents in Europe in the management of acute bleeds in patients with haemophilia and inhibitors. *Haemophilia* 2007; **13**(1): 38–45.

21 Brown S. Treatment of inhibitors in hemophilia B. In: Lee CA, Hoots WK (eds.) *Textbook of Hemophilia*, Vol. 1. Oxford: Blackwell Publishing, 2007.

22 Sumner MJ, Geldziler BD, Pedersen M, *et al.* Treatment of acquired haemophilia with recombinant activated FVII: a critical appraisal. *Haemophilia* 2007; **13**(5): 451–61.

23 Hedner U. Products used to treat hemophilia: Recombinant factor VIIa. In: Lee CA, Hoots WK (eds.) *Textbook of Hemophilia*, Vol. 2. Oxford: Blackwell Publishing, 2007.

24 Lacy L. Economic impact of treating inhibitor patients. *Pathophysiol Haemost Thromb* 2002; **32**(Suppl. 1): 29–32.

25 Kenet G, Lubetsky A, Luboshitz J, *et al.* A new approach to treatment of bleeding episodes in young hemophilia patients: a single bolus megadose of recombinant activated factor VII (NovoSeven). *J Thromb Haemost* 2003; **1**(3): 450–5.

26 Astermark J, Donfield SM, DeMichele DM, *et al.* A randomized comparison of bypassing agents in hemophilia complicated by an inhibitor: the FEIBA NovoSeven Comparative (FENOC) Study. *Blood* 2007; **109**(2): 546–51.

basic one is the noncompartmental method, in which the terminal $t_{1/2}$ is estimated by curve-fitting while CL, V_{ss}, MRT, and IVR are calculated directly from the data points. These parameter values are, however, not adequate to predict plasma levels as a function of time during multiple-dose treatment. This requires that the data are described by a pharmacokinetic model. If the entire curve can be described by a monoexponential function the disposition corresponds to a one-compartment model (every molecule stays in this compartment until eliminated from the body). A biexponential function corresponds to a two-compartment model depicting reversible distribution of the substance from the "central" compartment (where measurements were made) to a "peripheral" compartment. A triexponential function implies one central and two peripheral compartments, and so on.

In addition, a pharmacokinetic model can be defined from data on drug concentration (coagulation factor level) versus time by different methods. Conventional modeling entails fitting an exponential function to the data from each individual subject (as in Figures 16.1 and 16.2) and consequently requires intensive blood sampling ("rich sampling") over an adequate period of time. The number of subjects in the study is of necessity limited and studies in children can be particularly problematic. Conversely, if only a few samples are taken ("sparse sampling") from each of a large number of subjects (normally patients), the design is that of a population pharmacokinetic study. A population pharmacokinetic model is then fitted to all data from all subjects simultaneously, but not simply by pooling them. All concentration/level versus time data remain linked to the identity and characteristics of the individual patient. The core of the population pharmacokinetic model is the structural (conventional compartmental) model. However, concomitantly a covariate model describes relationships between pharmacokinetic parameters and patient characteristics, and a statistical model the variance between individuals as well as residual, or random, variance. The successful application of population pharmacokinetics to FVIII and FIX has been described [10,16,17].

Pharmacokinetics of factor VIII

In healthy persons, FVIII is presumably produced mainly in the liver and circulates in the plasma bound to the von Willebrand factor (VWF). In patients with hemophilia A, this complex is rapidly formed between infused FVIII and endogenous VWF. The binding of FVIII to VWF protects FVIII from degradation and receptor-mediated clearance [18–20]. Thus, FVIII infused as a highly purified or recombinant concentrate is cleared much faster in patients with severe von Willebrand's disease, who lack functional VWF, than in patients with hemophilia A [21,22]. Due to the very high molecular weight of the FVIII–VWF complex, it is practically confined to the plasma space. Receptor-mediated cellular uptake of the complex is probably the most

important mechanism of FVIII clearance [19,20]. Unfortunately for the engineering of FVIII analogs with prolonged activity, this suggests that blocking the clearance pathways of free FVIII cannot prolong the $t_{1/2}$ of the analog beyond that of the VWF itself [23].

When FVIII is given to adult patients as short-term infusions (typically of 5–15 min duration), plasma FVIII:C levels, on average, rise by 0.020–0.025 U/mL for every U/kg administered. Thus an infusion of 50 U/kg will normally give a peak plasma level of 1.0–1.3 U/mL. This corresponds to an initial volume of distribution (V) of 0.04–0.05 L/kg. The plasma disposition versus time curve of FVIII:C is then often approximately monophasic (Figure 16.1). Even if an irregular early phase can often be discerned it seldom contributes much to the total AUC. In addition, the peak plasma FVIII:C is often found 10–15 min after the end of the FVIII infusion, or sometimes even 1–2 h later [1,2,7,8]. The reason for this postinfusion rise in activity is not well known.

The pharmacokinetics of FVIII:C in adult patients with hemophilia A can then be summarized as a CL of 3 mL/h/kg of body weight (varying between 1.5 and 6 mL/h/kg), a V_{ss} similar to or slightly exceeding the plasma volume (0.04–0.06 L/kg), and an elimination $t_{1/2}$ ranging between 8 and 23 h [1,2,4,8–12,15,24–29]. The parameter values apply under normal physiologic conditions and in the absence of inhibitors (antibodies) to FVIII. The presence of inhibitors may give a low IVR and/or a rapid clearance of FVIII:C [30]. Other sources of interindividual variation in the pharmacokinetics of FVIII can be type of preparation, physiologic/biochemical factors, and such variation that can be related to observable characteristics of the patients (chiefly age and weight).

The differences between plasma-derived and the presently available types of recombinant FVIII are minor (except for analogs engineered to decrease CL and prolong $t_{1/2}$), even though some of them were statistically significant in comparative crossover studies. The issue of differences between FVIII products is discussed elsewhere.

Variability in the CL of endogenous VWF, as reflected by the baseline VWF level in the individual, appears to be an important source of variability in the CL and $t_{1/2}$ of FVIII. This is expected considering the co-clearance of VWF and FVIII. The CL, and level, of VWF is in turn related to blood group (group O individuals on average having lower levels of VWF [19,20,31]). It was accordingly found that the CL of B-domain-deleted recombinant FVIII correlates negatively, and the $t_{1/2}$ positively, with VWF levels in patients with hemophilia A [24]. This has been observed also with plasma-derived and full-length recombinant FVIII [25,26]. The influence of blood group has been more difficult to establish. In one study, FVIII:C had a significantly shorter mean elimination $t_{1/2}$ in patients with group O than in patients with group A [27]. Other studies [16,26] failed to confirm this finding, possibly due to lack of statistical power.

The relationship of age of the patient with the pharmacokinetics of FVIII has been studied in subjects aged 1 year and upwards [9,10,12,16,25,26]. It has also been observed that baseline VWF level increases with age [25,31], possibly reflecting a decrease in CL. Summarizing the various studies, the weight-adjusted CL of FVIII has been found to decrease with age, from on average 5 mL/h/kg at 1 year to 2.5 mL/h/kg at around 65 years of age. There appears to be no important change in distribution in patients with normal body weight. As a consequence of the change in CL, terminal $t_{1/2}$ on average increases from 8 to 15 h. There is pronounced interindividual variation around these average values.

Cross-over studies on different FVIII concentrates [9,28,29], as well as population pharmacokinetic analyses [10,16] indicate that the disposition of FVIII:C remains fairly constant within an individual, i.e. intraindividual variation in pharmacokinetics is lower than the interindividual variation. This is a prerequisite for individual dose tailoring of FVIII.

Pharmacokinetics of factor IX

Factor IX is produced by the liver and circulates in the plasma as a free molecule. Owing to its low molecular weight (55 kDa) it readily diffuses into the interstitial fluid [32]. FIX also binds rapidly and reversibly to the vascular endothelial cell surface [33]. There are conflicting data in the literature on the pharmacokinetics of plasma-derived FIX. One important reason for this is that many studies have been performed with inadequate blood sampling protocols, yielding biased or imprecise results [1,6]. The pharmacokinetics of recombinant FIX has on the other hand been characterized with generally consistent findings [5].

When plasma-derived FIX is given to adult patients as short-term infusions (typically of 5–15 min duration), plasma FIX:C levels on average rise by 0.010–0.014 U/mL for every U/kg administered. Thus an infusion of 50 U/kg will normally give a peak plasma level of 0.5–0.7 U/mL. This corresponds to an initial volume of distribution of 0.07–0.10 L/kg, which exceeds the plasma volume. This probably reflects immediate disappearance of some of the infused FIX from the plasma by binding to the endothelium. FIX:C then declines in a clearly multiexponential fashion (Figure 16.2), in which the distribution phase of the curve represents diffusion of FIX into interstitial fluid (by recent population pharmacokinetic analysis [17] the distribution phase could be subdivided into two phases with different half-lives, possibly reflecting diffusion of FIX into more and less, respectively, accessible extravascular spaces). Due to this extravascular distribution the V_{ss} of FIX is 3–4-fold greater than the plasma volume.

Table 16.1 summarizes methodologically adequate single-dose pharmacokinetic studies on FIX:C in patients with hemophilia B. The presently available recombinant FIX differs both in biochemistry and pharmacokinetics from plasma-derived FIX, with in particular a higher CL and a shorter terminal $t_{1/2}$. Its IVR is approximately two-thirds that of

Table 16.1 Reported typical mean pharmacokinetic parameter values of factor IX (FIX), compiled from studies with plasma-derived FIX (pdFIX) or recombinant FIX (rFIX). The data are condensed from a published review [5].

	CL (mL/h/kg)	IVR ([U/dL] / [U/kg])	MRT (h)	Terminal $t_{1/2}$ (h)
pdFIX	3.8–5.4	1.0–1.7	32–45	29–43
rFIX	7.5–9.1	0.75–0.96	25–30	18–23

CL, clearance; IVR in-vivo recovery; MRT, mean residence time.

plasma-derived FIX [5]. V_{ss} is on average 0.15 L/kg for plasma-derived and 0.20 L/kg for recombinant FIX.

Interindividual variation in the pharmacokinetics of plasma-derived FIX:C is difficult to estimate since the applicable studies included few patients, and only adults. No correlates or causes of interindividual variation in the standard pharmacokinetic parameters have as yet been identified. In a large study on recombinant FIX administered to 55 patients aged 4–56 years [14], both CL (in mL/h) and V_{ss} (in L) were linearly correlated (but not directly proportional) to body weight, consequently increasing during childhood and adolescence but remaining fairly constant during adulthood. Owing to the similar rises in CL and V_{ss}, neither MRT (=V_{ss}/CL) nor $t_{1/2}$ showed any significant regression with either body weight or age.

Recombinant FIX analogs with prolonged $t_{1/2}$ have been successfully designed [34–36]. Different strategies of molecular engineering gave markedly different results. GlycoPEGylation, i.e. attaching a 40-kDa polyethylene glycol (PEG) molecule to the FIX activation peptide, decreased CL to on average 0.70 mL/h/kg and increased the terminal $t_{1/2}$ to 93 h [34] in adult patients. Fusing recombinant FIX with the human immunoglobulin G$_1$ Fc domain gave an average CL of 3.1 mL/h/kg and a terminal $t_{1/2}$ of 57 h [35], while fusion with albumin decreased CL to 0.75 mL/h/kg and prolonged the $t_{1/2}$ to 92 h [36]. Attaching either the bulky 40-kDa PEG molecule or albumin to recombinant FIX impeded extravascular distribution and decreased the V_{ss} by one-half, while no corresponding change could be observed on fusion with the Fc fragment.

Application of pharmacokinetics to treatment of hemophilia

Clinical pharmacokinetics is the application of pharmacokinetic principles to the therapeutic management of patients. Adjusting the dosage of a drug according to the requirement of the individual patient is often referred to as "tailoring" the dose. Only some aspects on the methodology of pharmacokinetic dose tailoring will be described in this chapter, assuming repeated short infusions.

Targeting a FVIII:C trough level during prophylactic treatment is illustrated in Figure 16.3. A 0.01 U/mL trough level was

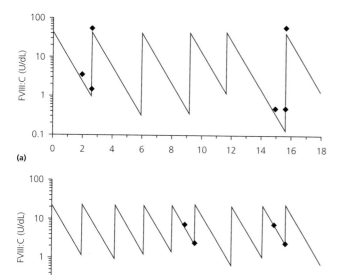

Figure 16.3 Predicted plasma factor VIII (FVIII:C, i.e. coagulant activity) levels in a patient on prophylactic therapy with FVIII [11]. The single-dose curve C(t) = 56 × e^{−1.48 × t} (where time, t, is in days) was obtained after a dose of 2300 U [8]. Multiple-dose curves were consequently plotted from the equations C(t) = (given dose/2300) × 56 × e^{−1.48 × t} which were added over time, each new curve starting when a new dose was given. **(a)** Originally prescribed dosing of 2000 U twice weekly. **(b)** Dose tailored to give a trough level of 1 U/dL (0.01 U/mL); 1000 U every 2 days. Closed diamonds represent measured control values. The two values at 0.5 U/dL are essentially "blank", or baseline, readings in the assay.

aimed for and attained. Concomitantly, the consumption of FVIII was lowered from 4000 to 3500 U/week. The pharmacokinetics of FVIII:C in this patient had been determined in a conventional intense blood sampling study on a new factor concentrate and was described by a monoexponential function. A similar study [13] was performed on FIX, with the only difference that biexponential functions had to be used.

According to guidelines for pharmacokinetic studies on new FVIII concentrates [37], 10–11 blood samples should be taken over 32–48 h. For dose tailoring during ongoing treatment, useful pharmacokinetic parameters can, however, be estimated from only a few (well-timed) determinations of coagulation factor levels, by means of Bayesian analysis [38]. This analysis is based on pharmacokinetic information in the relevant population of patients, as described by a population model which thus needs to be available beforehand. No treatment interruption (washout) is needed. The Bayesian analysis can be performed on data from practically any dosing schedule. Doses and times of preceding infusions must be known for at least five half-lives (after which <3% of a dose remains in the body) before the study infusion. The ideal use of the method is by repeated measurements during the clinical follow-up of the patient, thus accumulating and validating information over time.

Conclusion

The pharmacokinetics of FVIII and FIX have been extensively investigated and their therapeutic plasma levels are well defined in most situations. Applied pharmacokinetics has therefore become an established tool to aid dosing in the treatment of hemophilia.

References

1 Björkman S, Carlsson M. The pharmacokinetics of factor VIII and factor IX: methodology, pitfalls and applications. *Haemophilia* 1997; **3**: 1–8.

2 Björkman S, Berntorp E. Pharmacokinetics of coagulation factors. Clinical relevance for patients with haemophilia. *Clin Pharmacokinet* 2001; **40**: 815–32.

3 Björkman S. Prophylactic dosing of factor VIII and factor IX from a clinical pharmacokinetic perspective. *Haemophilia* 2003; **9** (Suppl. 1): 101–10.

4 Collins PW, Fischer K, Morfini M, Blanchette VS, Björkman S. Implications of coagulation factor VIII and IX pharmacokinetics in the prophylactic treatment of haemophilia. *Haemophilia* 2011; **17**: 2–10.

5 Björkman S. A commentary on the differences in pharmacokinetics between recombinant and plasma-derived factor IX and their implications for dosing. *Haemophilia* 2011; **17**: 179–84.

6 Björkman S, Carlsson M, Berntorp E. Pharmacokinetics of factor IX in patients with haemophilia B: methodological aspects and physiological interpretation. *Eur J Clin Pharmacol* 1994; **46**: 325–32.

7 Allain JP. Principles of in vivo recovery and survival studies. *Scand J Haematol* 1984; **33**(Suppl. 41): 123–30.

8 Björkman S, Carlsson M, Berntorp E, Stenberg P. Pharmacokinetics of factor VIII in humans: obtaining clinically relevant data from comparative studies. *Clin Pharmacokin* 1992; **22**: 385–95.

9 Björkman S, Blanchette VS, Fischer K, *et al.* Comparative pharmacokinetics of plasma-albumin-free recombinant factor VIII in children and adults: the influence of blood sampling schedule on observed age-related differences and implications for dose tailoring. *J Thromb Haemost* 2010; **8**: 730–6.

10 Björkman S, Oh M, Spotts G, *et al.* Population pharmacokinetics of recombinant factor VIII: the relationships of pharmacokinetics to age and body weight. *Blood* 2012; **119**: 612–8.

11 Carlsson M, Berntorp E, Björkman S, Lindvall K. Pharmacokinetic dosing in prophylactic treatment of hemophilia A. *Eur J Haematol* 1993; **51**: 247–52.

12 Carlsson M, Berntorp E, Björkman S, Lethagen S, Ljung R. Improved cost-effectiveness by pharmacokinetic dosing of factor VIII in prophylactic treatment of haemophilia A. *Haemophilia* 1997; **3**: 96–101.

13 Carlsson M, Björkman S, Berntorp E. Multidose pharmacokinetics of factor IX: implications for dosing in prophylaxis. *Haemophilia* 1998; **4**: 83–8.

14 Björkman S, Shapiro AD, Berntorp E. Pharmacokinetics of recombinant factor IX in relation to age of the patient: Implications for dosing in prophylaxis. *Haemophilia* 2001; **7**: 133–9.

15 Collins PW, Björkman S, Fischer K, *et al.* Factor VIII requirement to maintain a target plasma level in the prophylactic treatment of

severe hemophilia A: influences of variance in pharmacokinetics and treatment regimens. *J Thromb Haemost* 2010; **8**: 269–75.

16 Björkman S, Folkesson A, Jönsson S. Pharmacokinetics and dose requirements of factor VIII over the age range 3–74 years. *Eur J Clin Pharmacol* 2009; **65**: 989–98.

17 Björkman S, Åhlén V. Population pharmacokinetics of plasma-derived factor IX in adult patients with haemophilia B: implications for dosing in prophylaxis. *Eur J Clin Pharmacol* 2012; **68**: 969–77.

18 Weiss HJ, Sussman II, Hoyer LW. Stabilization of factor VIII in plasma by the von Willebrand factor. *J Clin Invest* 1977; **60**: 390–404.

19 Lenting PJ, van Schooten CJM, Denis CV. Clearance mechanisms of von Willebrand factor and factor VIII. *J Thromb Haemost* 2007; **5**: 1353–60.

20 Terraube V, O'Donnell JS, Jenkins PV. Factor VIII and von Willebrand factor interaction: biological, clinical and therapeutic importance. *Haemophilia* 2010; **16**: 3–13.

21 Tuddenham EGD, Lane RS, Rotblat F, et al. Response to infusions of polyelectrolyte fractionated human factor VIII concentrate in human haemophilia A and von Willebrand's disease. *Br J Haematol* 1982; **52**: 259–67.

22 Lethagen S, Berntorp E, Nilsson IM. Pharmacokinetics and hemostatic effect of different factor VIII/von Willebrand factor concentrates in von Willebrand's disease type III. *Ann Hematol* 1992; **65**: 253–9.

23 Powell JS, Josephson NC, Quon D, et al. Safety and prolonged activity of recombinant factor VIII Fc fusion protein in hemophilia A patients. *Blood* 2012; **119**: 3031–7.

24 Fijnvandraat K, Peters M, Ten Cate JW. Inter-individual variation in half-life of infused recombinant factor VIII is related to pre-infusion von Willebrand factor antigen levels. *Br J Haematol* 1995; **91**: 474–6.

25 Van Dijk K, van der Bom JG, Lenting PJ, et al. Factor VIII half-life and clinical phenotype of severe hemophilia A. *Haematologica* 2005; **90**: 494–8.

26 Barnes C, Lillicrap D, Pazmino-Canizares J, et al. Pharmacokinetics of recombinant factor VIII (Kogenate-FS) in children and causes of inter-patient pharmacokinetic variability. *Haemophilia* 2006; **12**(Suppl. 4): 40–9.

27 Vlot AJ, Mauser-Bunschoten EP, Zarkova AG, et al. The half-life of infused factor VIII is shorter in hemophiliac patients with blood group 0 than in those with blood group A. *Thromb Haemost* 2000; **83**: 65–9.

28 Fijnvandraat K, Berntorp E, ten Cate JW, et al. Recombinant, B-domain deleted factor VIII (r-VIII SQ): pharmacokinetics and initial safety aspects in hemophilia A patients. *Thromb Haemost* 1997; **77**: 298–302.

29 Tarantino MD, Collins PW, Hay CRM, et al. Clinical evaluation of an advanced category antihaemophilic factor prepared using a plasma/albumin-free method: pharmacokinetics, efficacy and safety in previously treated patients with haemophilia A. *Haemophilia* 2004; **10**: 428–37.

30 Allain JP, Frommel D. Antibodies to factor VIII. V. Patterns of immune response to factor VIII in hemophilia A. *Blood* 1976; **47**: 973–82.

31 O'Donnell J, Laffan MA. The relationship between ABO histo-blood group, factor VIII and von Willebrand factor. *Transfus Med* 2001; **11**: 343–51.

32 Thompson AR. Factor IX concentrates for clinical use. *Semin Thrombos Hemostas* 1993; **19**: 25–36.

33 Heimark RL, Schwartz SM. Binding of coagulation factors IX and X to the endothelial cell surface. *Biochem Biophys Res Commun* 1983; **111**: 723–31.

34 Negrier C, Knobe K, Tiede A, Giangrande P, Moss J. Enhanced pharmacokinetic properties of a glycoPEGylated recombinant factor IX: a first human dose trial in patients with hemophilia B. *Blood* 2011; **118**: 2695–701.

35 Shapiro AD, Ragni MV, Valentino LA, et al. Recombinant factor IX-Fc fusion protein (rFIXFx) demonstrates safety and prolonged activity in a phase 1/2a study in hemophilia B patients. *Blood* 2012; **119**: 666–72.

36 Santagostino E, Negrier C, Klamroth R, et al. Safety and pharmacokinetics of a novel recombinant fusion protein linking coagulation factor IX with albumin (rIX-FP) in hemophilia B patients. *Blood* 2012; **120**: 2405–11.

37 Lee M, Morfini M, Negrier C, Chamouard V. The pharmacokinetics of coagulation factors. *Haemophilia* 2006; **12**(Suppl. 3): 1–7.

38 Björkman S, Collins P. Measurement of factor VIII pharmacokinetics in routine clinical practice. *J Thromb Haemost* 2013; **11**: 180–2.

39 Berntorp E, Björkman S, Carlsson M, Lethagen S, Nilsson IM. Biochemical and in vivo properties of high purity factor IX concentrates. *Thromb Haemost* 1993; **70**: 768–73.

40 White G, Shapiro A, Ragni M, et al. Clinical evaluation of recombinant factor IX. *Semin Hematol* 1998; **35**(Suppl. 2): 33–8.

CHAPTER 17
Individualized dosing

Peter W. Collins

Arthur Bloom Haemophilia Centre, Cardiff, UK

Introduction

Replacement therapy can be broadly categorized into the treatment of bleeds and prevention of bleeding through prophylaxis or at the time of invasive procedures. It is well recognized that the level of factor VIII (FVIII) or IX (FIX) is useful in the management of hemophilia and it is routine practise to combine clinical observation with measurement of factor levels. Often peak and trough levels are measured and these give some information about the patient's pharmacokinetics and allow dose adjustments to be made. A more detailed estimation of a patient's factor levels after an infusion, and a better understanding of the effect of various doses and dose frequencies, is possible if an individual's pharmacokinetics are measured and used to tailor treatment. This chapter discusses the potential use of pharmacokinetic information, always combined with clinical observation, in the management of hemophilia.

Treatment of bleeding episodes

To treat acute bleeds it is common practise to aim for a predetermined peak level. The dose required to achieve the desired level is often estimated based on the patient's weight and the expected recovery of the product. There is wide variation in *in-vivo* recovery (IVR) between patients, and the finding that IVR does not correlate well with weight results in a wide inter-patient variation in the peak level achieved. There is also a wide variation within the same patients and this means that attempts to optimize therapy based on IVR are unlikely to be useful [1]. This potentially leads to variable hemostatic responses, with some patients being undertreated and others having higher levels than intended. Given the lack of reproducibility of IVR, if the clinical situation requires a specific peak level then this will need to be measured and adjusted on each occasion. Depending on the type of bleed and response to the initial infusion, the factor level will need to be maintained for a period of time and knowledge of a patient's half-life will be useful for

planning the need for further infusions and their timing and dose. For example, it is likely that a young child will need a follow-up infusion sooner than an adult to maintain the same factor levels. Although it is not common practise to base decisions about the treatment on detailed pharmacokinetic studies, peak and trough levels are commonly used to help guide therapy.

Prophylaxis

This chapter is limited to a discussion about individualisation of dose. The original concept of prophylaxis was to increase the trough level of FVIII/IX above 1 IU/dL with the aim of converting the bleeding phenotype from severe to mild [2–4], and this is a highly successful treatment strategy. Prophylaxis is usually delivered using a weight-based regimen of 20–40 IU/kg 3–4 (FVIII) or 2–3 (FIX) times a week, although good outcomes are also reported with lower dose regimens tailored on the basis of observed bleed pattern [4–7].

Studies support the hypothesis that increased time spent with a low factor level is associated with more frequent breakthrough bleeding but do not support the concept that a trough level of 1 IU/dL is applicable to all cases [8,9]. In addition to factor level, the risk factors for breakthrough bleeding on prophylaxis include physical activity, the presence of target joints and synovial hypertrophy, the degree of arthropathy, and adherence to the regimen.

The appropriate target trough level during prophylaxis varies and it is recognized that some patients bleed despite having a trough above 1 IU/dL while others do not bleed despite having an unmeasurable level. A possible explanation is that FVIII replacement affects patients' global blood clotting systems differently [10] and studies that investigate whether tailoring prophylaxis based on thrombin generation or thromboelastography, rather than factor level, will be of interest. A recent study showed that protection from joint bleeds is highly dependent on factor levels between 1 and 4 IU/dL but that joint bleeds

Textbook of Hemophilia, Third Edition. Edited by Christine A. Lee, Erik E. Berntorp and W. Keith Hoots.
© 2014 John Wiley & Sons, Ltd. Published 2014 by John Wiley & Sons, Ltd.

still occur, although more rarely, until the baseline is above 10–15 IU/dL [11]. The concept of raising the trough to just above 1 IU/dL may have been more appropriate at a time when people with hemophilia were excluded from many physical activities.

Based on these observations, if FVIII/IX is infused to maintaining levels above 15 IU/dL at all times, good outcomes could be expected but this strategy is not financially feasible. It is important to recognize that any debate around appropriate trough levels and individualized dosing of prophylaxis is essentially a discussion about cost-effectiveness.

The keys to successful individualized dosing are an accurate record of bleed pattern, a willingness to try alternative regimens (potentially for short periods of time), and regular review of bleed pattern and dosing regimen, especially soon after a change. To aid this process, the ability to easily determine an individual's FVIII/FIX pharmacokinetics and the use of this information to target a desired level, associated with knowledge of the bleed pattern, would be very useful [12]. Techniques that allow this to be done in routine clinical practise are described in Bjorkman and Collins [13].

Prophylactic regimens

There are two ways to adjust prophylaxis, by dose and/or frequency/timing; the relative importance of these depends on the individual's circumstances. Standard prophylaxis is prescribed on the basis of weight [14]; however, because neither the IVR nor the half-life of FVIII is directly proportional to weight and both vary widely between patients, this dosing strategy will result in a wide variation of trough levels. For example, in an adult who has received an infusion of 50 IU/kg, the FVIII level at 48 h may vary between 2 and 12 IU/dL and the time to reach 1 IU/dL can vary between 51 and 110 h [12,15] (Figure 17.1). The standard regimen of 20–40 IU/kg on alternate days is predicted to maintain a trough of above 1 IU/dL in almost all young children [15] but in adults, who have substantially longer half-lives [16,17], the median trough at 48 h has been shown to be >6 IU/dL [18]. These findings suggest that weight may not be the best way to prescribe prophylaxis, especially in adults, and good long-term outcomes have been reported using lower dose regimens adjusted on the basis of bleed pattern [7].

Prophylaxis should be tailored to minimize joint and significant soft-tissue bleeds with the assumption that this will translate into good long-term orthopedic outcomes [5,6,19]. This adjustment is best done collaboratively between the person with hemophilia (or their family) and their hemophilia center and relies on an accurate record of bleeds. Prophylaxis should be adjusted based on the observed pattern of bleeds, times of expected physical activity, the status of the individual's musculoskeletal system, and take into account venous access. These adjustments can be informed, and potentially made more cost-effective, by pharmacokinetic measurements.

Dose adjustment may be done very simply, for example, if a person on prophylaxis has had no breakthrough bleeds and

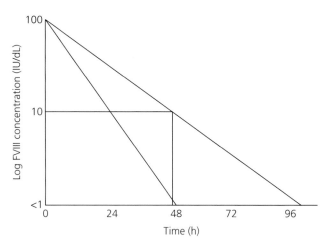

Figure 17.1 Variability in the effect of weight-based prophylaxis on factor VIII (FVIII) levels. The time for FVIII to reach 1 IU/dL after an infusion of 50 IU/kg dependent on half-life is shown. The lines depict the 5th and 95th percentile of the normal half-life in a 70-kg man. The difference in the time taken to reach 1 IU/dL when comparing the shortest half-life with the longest is 59 h suggesting that some patients need alternate-day treatment while other could be treated every 3 or 4 days. Alternatively, the data can be interpreted in terms of trough level at 48 h which varies between 2 and 12 IU/dL. This means that if a patient with a long half-life, who is taking 50 IU/kg on alternate days, had his dose reduced to 5 IU/kg, his trough may still be adequate at 1.5 IU/dL. Adapted from [32]. Reproduced with permission of John Wiley and Sons.

their trough level is measured at 6 IU/dL then their dose of FVIII/FIX could be halved and their trough would still be about 3 IU/dL, if the dose is cut by 66% the trough would be 2 IU/dL. While this may not need to be considered in a country with an unlimited supply of concentrate, in countries with limited healthcare resources the saved concentrate could allow one or two other people to be started on prophylaxis.

The principle of pharmacokinetic tailoring to a trough level of 1 IU/dL has been supported in a prospective study of patients receiving standard prophylaxis (about 30 IU/kg on alternate days) compared to patients treated every third day to achieve a trough of 1 IU/dL based on their individual pharmacokinetics. The two groups had similar numbers of bleeds and used similar amounts of FVIII; however, the standard treatment arm had trough FVIII levels of 3 IU/dL [20]. This implies that a similar outcome could have been achieved with a third of the dose using alternate-day infusions. The study suggests that through the use of pharmacokinetic dosing, a target trough level can be achieved on average, but with a great deal of variation. Although the study showed that the convenience of every third day dosing could be achieved, from a cost-effectiveness point of view, this comes at a substantially higher price compared to alternate-day dosing.

Increasing the frequency of FVIII/FIX infusions can be used to maintain a desired trough level while using substantially less FVIII/FIX or to allow a much higher trough to be achieved with the same amount of concentrate (Figure 17.2). In hemophilia B,

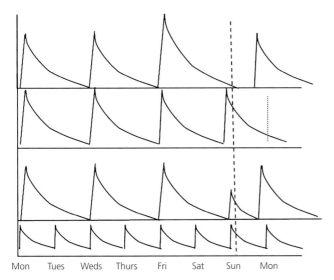

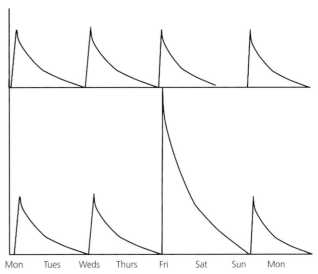

Mon   Tues   Weds   Thurs   Fri   Sat   Sun   Mon

Figure 17.2 Potential prophylactic regimens for active patients. The panels depict a hypothetical patient treated with various prophylactic regimens. The dashed line indicates a time of high physical activity on a Sunday morning, for example playing sport. The upper panel depicts 1000 IU on Monday and Wednesday and 1500 IU on Friday. This results in limited cover for activity on Sunday. An alternate-day regimen (second panel) could be used and would provide good cover on the first Sunday but on alternate weeks a lower level would be achieved (dotted line) and the patient may be vulnerable to breakthrough bleeds. The same amount of factor VIII (FVIII) as used in panel 1 will give much better cover if an extra dose of 500 IU is given on Sunday (panel 3). Alternatively, by using 500 IU daily a much higher trough level can be achieved throughout the week (panel 4). The FVIII scale is arbitrary. Adapted from [32]. Reproduced with permission of John Wiley and Sons.

Mon   Tues   Weds   Thurs   Fri   Sat   Sun   Mon

Figure 17.3 Implications of Monday, Wednesday, and Friday dosing. Upper panel depicts the factor VIII (FVIII) level of a patient on three times a week prophylaxis whose FVIII reaches 1 IU/dL after 48 h. This means that the FVIII is below 1 IU/dL throughout Sunday. The lower panel shows that to sustain FVIII above 1 IU/dL throughout Sunday, a four-fold increase is required on Friday, assuming a half-life of 12 h. The FVIII scale is arbitrary. Adapted from [32]. Reproduced with permission of John Wiley and Sons.

for example, maintaining a trough FIX level above 1 IU/dL treating 1–3 times a week, every third day or on alternate days requires an average of 240 000, 137 000, and 108 000 IU/year, respectively [21]. Similar effects are seen by increasing the frequency of FVIII infusions [22]. An important potential advantage of more frequent dosing is that, by using less concentrate, more people with hemophilia may have access to prophylaxis. For example, in a 70-kg adult with an average FVIII half-life, the baseline FVIII can be maintained above 1 IU with 100 IU/day (36 500 IU/year) compared to standard weight-based dosing (30 IU/kg alternate day) which uses about 380 000 IU/year [12].

The frequency of prophylaxis can be tailored to an individual's circumstances. For example, a very active teenager who wants to play contact sports on a daily basis might decide to take daily prophylaxis at a dose of half his alternate-day regimen during the sports season. This regimen has the advantages of a peak level each day and a much higher trough level, while not consuming more concentrate (Figure 17.2). Short-term daily prophylactic regimens may also be useful for people with target joints or those undergoing intensive physiotherapy. A study that randomized patients to their usual prophylaxis or daily prophylaxis tailored to achieve a similar trough level had

a surprisingly disappointing outcome, showing that this approach resulted in more bleeds and was more stressful for patients [23]. Daily prophylaxis is an onerous undertaking and in my anecdotal experience is successful only when patients are highly motivated to use this regimen, for example, to achieve a higher trough while using the same amount of concentrate and this situation differs from a study that involves reduction of total dose.

While people who started prophylaxis at a young age usually have well-preserved joints, those who have received on-demand treatment or started prophylaxis later in life often have significant arthropathy and this may be very severe [5,6,24]. The appropriate trough level in these circumstances is not known and must be established empirically for each patient.

It is common practise to infuse prophylaxis on a Monday, Wednesday and Friday and FIX twice a week. This has the disadvantage of allowing periods with low levels and potentially increases the risk of breakthrough bleeds. Giving an increased dose of FVIII on a Friday is a common practise but to cover the extra day for a patient with a half-life of 12 h requires a four-fold dose increase (Figure 17.3). A more cost-effective strategy which also results in substantially better levels is to give an extra infusion on Saturday (usual dose) or Sunday (half usual dose), depending on when most activity is anticipated (Figure 17.2). Infusing on alternate days avoids this problem and some families find this an easy regimen to follow. The choice of which regimen to use is individual and often depends on what the patient is used to; if alternate prophylaxis is started at a young

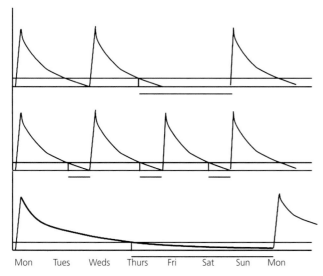

Mon   Tues   Weds   Thurs   Fri   Sat   Sun   Mon

Figure 17.4 Effect of nonadherence and hypothetical effect of a long half-life coagulation factor. Panel 1 shows that missing a dose has a very significant effect on the time spent below a hypothetical target level and this is known to be associated with an increased risk of breakthrough bleeding. The middle panel shows a standard alternate-day regimen with the same hypothetical target level. The patient spends a short period of time every second day below this level but this occurs at night. Panel 3 is a hypothetical long half-life agent. The patient achieves the same trough level but spends more time below the target level and this occurs both during the day and at night. The clinical implications of this are unknown. Adapted from [32]. Reproduced with permission of John Wiley and Sons.

age there are very few problems with adherence. In this context, it should be noted that the gold standard study in the field used alternate-day dosing [14].

Good adherence to a prophylactic regimen is key to success and any discussion about trough levels is irrelevant if doses are regularly missed because breakthrough bleeds will increase [8] (Figure 17.4). Reasons for lack of adherence need to be discussed openly between the patient and the center and any problems addressed. A better understanding of how prophylaxis works or changing the regimen to better fit the individual's lifestyle may help.

An individual's prophylactic regimen is often considered to be fixed. However, by definition, this prevents an individualized approach because a patient's circumstances and pharmacokinetics will inevitably change with age. Young children need cover throughout the week because their activity is unpredictable and often constant. Also this age group is probably the most vulnerable to the effects of hemarthroses [25]. Very active teenagers may opt for daily treatment, possible for a short period of time, for example during the part of the year when their sport is played. Young adults may need to continue intensive prophylaxis but some find that they can stop prophylaxis or use targeted prophylaxis as they gain experience of what causes their bleeds and how to avoid bleeds [5,6,26]. Older adults who undertake very limited activity, either because of work or the effect of

musculoskeletal problems, may need only a very low dose or infrequent regimen.

Our practise is to individualise prophylaxis based on all the available information and to regularly suggest that the patient tries a new regimen. If a regimen is changed, it is very important that a review takes place after 6–8 weeks, to establish whether any undesired events have occurred and also to give the patient confidence that the regimen can be adjusted again if necessary. This review can often be done by a hemophilia specialist nurse by telephone or email supported by electronic web-based bleed reporting systems [27,28].

Prophylaxis is the treatment of choice for people with severe hemophilia and the use of personalized regimens is a logical extension to weight-based dosing. Introducing cost-effective lower dose more frequent regimens may help to make prophylaxis available to more people in areas with lower healthcare budgets.

Surgery

Pharmacokinetic studies may be useful at the time of surgery but relatively few data are available to guide clinical practise. It is likely that a patient's pharmacokinetics measured in the non-bleeding state will not reflect their pharmacokinetics at the time of surgery. This is because FVIII/FIX clearance is often increased on the day of surgery due to consumption into forming clots, dilution, changes in blood volume, and, in some cases, consumptive coagulopathies. The change in perioperative clearance is likely to vary markedly dependent on the type of operation and surgical and anesthetic practise. Clearance will be difficult to predict in an individual case and will need to be measured. Increased clearance is particularly most important when planning the timing of the second perioperative infusion. In situations where clearance is high, this will need to be relatively early and, in some circumstances, may even need to be while the operation is ongoing.

These observations mean that FVIII/FIX pharmacokinetics would need to be measured regularly peri- and postoperatively to be clinically useful. To some degree this is already done in routine practise. On the day of surgery, pre- and postinfusion levels are usually performed around the preoperative infusion stage to ensure adequate levels at the time of surgery. It is also common practise to perform a fall off level in the recovery room to give some estimate of the perioperative clearance and guide the timing and amount of the next dose. The use of three or more infusions on the day of surgery, guided by measured levels, may be required.

In contrast to the increased perioperative clearance, in the postoperative period von Willebrand factor (VWF) levels are often increased and this may prolong the half-life of infused FVIII during the recovery period. FIX clearance also appears to decrease in the postoperative period although the mechanism for this is unclear [29]. Regular measurement of trough FVIII/

where exclusion of hemophilia should be part of the routine investigation. This emphasizes the importance of appropriate investigation of all cases presenting with ICH.

Failure to initiate appropriate investigations has also been highlighted in a survey from the USA published in 1999 in which neonatologists and hematologists were questioned regarding how they would investigate neonates presenting with ICH. Among neonatologists only 23% reported that they would specifically request FVIII and FIX assays in a term neonate presenting with ICH and the figure dropped to 3% in preterm infants. The figures were higher when the same questions were asked of haematologists (64% and 39%, respectively) but in many centers hematologists may not be actively involved in initiating these investigations. In light of this, it is now advised by the Medical and Scientific Advisory Council (MASAC) of the National Hemophilia Foundation in the USA that all neonates with ICH should be specifically investigated for the presence of an underlying bleeding disorder.

Treatment of hemophilia during the neonatal period

Choice of product

In the presence of acute bleeding or where prophylactic management is deemed necessary, treatment should be initiated with an appropriate factor concentrate. This applies regardless of severity, as desmopressin (DDAVP) is contraindicated during the neonatal period and up until the age of 2 years because of the risk of hyponatremia [32]. The choice of product should be governed by issues of safety and availability. In the developed world, recombinant FVIII and FIX concentrates are now widely available and neonates should have the highest priority to receive these products [31]. This is based on the likelihood that recombinant technology will be associated with the lowest risk of transmitting viral infections or prions [33]. In those parts of the world where recombinant products are not available, high-purity, virucidally inactivated, plasma-derived products remain the preferred treatment. Where prothrombin complex concentrates (PCCs) are used for the treatment of hemophilia B it should be noted that an increased risk of disseminated intravascular coagulation has been reported in neonates treated with these products.

As FVIII and FIX concentrates, particularly recombinant products, are not widely available outside hemophilia treatment centers, it is important that arrangements are made to secure a supply of an appropriate product prior to the delivery of a potentially affected neonate. Although fresh frozen plasma (FFP) is not recommended for the treatment of neonatal hemophilia, it may have a role in the presence of major hemorrhage where hemophilia is suspected but confirmatory investigations are not yet available or where other products are unavailable. FFP in this situation may be beneficial, although it will only result in a rise in factor level of a few percent at best; factor

concentrate once the diagnosis is made is the treatment of choice.

Dosing regimens

Dosing regimens for neonates are largely based on those used for older children and adults [34], as there is little published information available regarding the pharmacokinetics of replacement therapy in this age group. In view of this, careful monitoring of factor levels is likely to be particularly important. Some case reports in preterm infants with hemophilia A have shown that recovery of FVIII is similar to adults and older children but that the half-life is shorter, at 6–8 h [34–37]. In a single case report describing replacement therapy in a preterm neonate with hemophilia B, FIX recovery was similar to that seen in older children, whereas the half-life was shorter at 6 h [35].

Prophylactic treatment

Given that the incidence of ICH in neonates with severe or moderate hemophilia is 1–4% and the outcome of such bleeds can be fatal or severely disabling, some have advocated prophylactic factor replacement for all known neonates with hemophilia and for those in whom the diagnosis is highly likely [38,39]. Prophylactic use of factor concentrate is well established in the older hemophiliac both for preventing spontaneous bleeds, particularly joint bleeds, and after injury before bleeding has taken place, especially when that injury could result in ICH. In the neonate, the head and brain have been subjected to significant stress but unlike traumatic head injuries the stress is physiologic. Nevertheless, ICH occurs and the risk is increased in deliveries requiring instrumentation or cesarean section during labor [5,8]. Although early studies suggested an association between early treatment and inhibitor development [40,41], this has not been confirmed in subsequent larger studies [42,43]. Current data indicate that the genetic mutation in the *FVIII* gene is the most predictive parameter for inhibitor development. In those with a traumatic delivery, immediate treatment should be considered and in addition a high index of suspicion of ICH should be maintained. In a UK survey of hemophilia centers, only 19% of responders said they would consider prophylaxis in all severe cases but up to 62% following instrumental delivery [30]. In a survey in the USA, 89% of pediatric hematologists favored early prophylaxis with factor concentrates [44].

Conclusion

Hemophilia A and B are rare disorders but can present in the neonatal period with catastrophic bleeding. If the diagnosis is missed, not only is appropriate treatment not instituted at the time, but further bleeds may occur with attendant morbidity or even mortality before the diagnosis is eventually made. Although there has been a significant improvement in making an early diagnosis, cases continue to be missed despite a positive family history or unusual bleeding in a well neonate. It is important to encourage liaison between obstetricians, neonatologists, and hematologists in the management of the known hemophilia carrier and between hematologists and neonatologists when abnormal bleeding in a neonate occurs so that correct interpretation of the test results in the light of the clinical situation occurs. The importance of family history can be emphasized during genetic counseling of the mother so that appropriate information is given and help sought. Medical staff in attendance also need to be aware of the importance of a family history of bleeding. Written protocols for the management of the hemophilia carrier should be available in institutions where such mothers are delivered and protocols for the investigation of a bleeding neonate available in all neonatal units. Prospective studies collecting data on neonatal bleeding episodes, the contribution of routine cranial imaging, and analysis of early exposure to FVIII concentrate and inhibitor development may help determine best management in the future.

References

1 Baehner RL, Strauss H. Hemophilia in the first year of life. *N Engl J Med* 1966; **275**: 524–8.

2 Chambost H, Gaboulaud V, Coatmelec B, Rafowicz A, Schneider P, Calvez T. What factors influence the age at diagnosis of hemophilia? Results of a French cohort study. *J Paediatr* 2002; **141**: 548–52.

3 Conway JH, Hilgartner MW. Initial presentation of paediatric hemophiliacs. *Arch Pediatr Adolesc Med* 1994; **148**: 589–94.

4 Ljung R, Petrini P, Nilsson IM. Diagnostic symptoms of severe and moderate haemophilia A and B. *Acta Paediatr Scand* 1990; **79**: 196–200.

5 Klinge J, Auberger K, Auerswald G, Brackmann HH, Mauz-Körholz Ch, Kreuz W. Prevalence and outcome of intracranial haemorrhage in haemophiliacs—A survey of the paediatric group of the German Society of Thrombosis and Haemostasis (GTH). *Eur J Pediatr* 1999; **158**: S162–5.

6 Pollmann H, Richter H, Ringkamp H, Jurgens H. When are children diagnosed as having severe haemophilia and when do they start to bleed? A 10-year single centre PUP study *Eur J Pediatr* 1999; **158**: S166–70.

7 Ljung RC, Sjörin E. Origin of mutation in sporadic cases of hemophilia A. *Br J Haematol* 1999; **106**(4): 870–4.

8 Ljung R. The optimal mode of delivery for the haemophilia carrier expecting an affected infant is vaginal delivery. *Haemophilia* 2010; **16**: 415–19.

9 Towner D, Castro MA, Eby-Wilkens E, Gilbert WM. Effect of mode of delivery in nulliparous women on neonatal intracranial injury. *N Engl J Med* 1999; **341**: 1709–14.

10 Whitby EH, Griffiths PD, Rutter S, *et al.* Frequency and natural history of subdural haemorrhages in babies and relation to obstetric factors. *Lancet* 2004; **363**: 846–51.

11 Tarantino MD, Gupta SL, Brusky RM. The incidence and outcome of intracranial haemorrhage in newborns with haemophilia: Analysis of the Nationwide Inpatient Sample database. *Haemophilia* 2007; **13**: 380–2.

12 Kulkarni R, Lusher JM. Intracranial and extracranial hemorrhages in newborns with hemophilia. *J Pediatr Hematol Oncol* 1999; **21**: 289–95.

13 Kulkarni R, Lusher J. Perinatal management of newborns with haemophilia. *Br J Haematol* 2001; **112**: 264–74.

14 Kulkarni R, Soucie JM, Lusher J, *et al.* Sites of initial bleeding episodes, mode of delivery and age of diagnosis in babies with haemophilia diagnosed before the age of 2 years: report from the disease control and prevention's (CDC) universal data collection project. *Haemophilia* 2009; **15**: 1281–90.

15 Richards M, Lavigne Lissalde G, Combescure C, *et al.*, on behalf of the European Haemophilia Treatment and Standardization Board. Neonatal bleeding in haemophilia: a European cohort study. *Br J Haematol* 2011; **156**: 374–82.

16 Khair K, Baxter B, Fields P, Hann I, Leisner R. Intracranial haemorrhage in a tertiary pediatric centre: A survey of 100 children with severe haemophilia. *Haemophilia* 2002; **8**: 522–6.

17 Kletzel M, Miller CH, Becton D, Chadduck WM, Elser JM. Postdelivery head bleeding in hemophilic neonates. *Arch J Dis Child* 1989; **143**: 1107–10.

18 Plauche WC. Subgaleal haematoma. A complication of instrumental delivery. *J Am Med Assoc* 1980; **244**: 597–8.

19 Efrat Z, Akinfenwa OO, Nicolaides KH. First-trimester determination of fetal gender by ultrasound. *Ultrasound Obstet Gynecol* 1999; **13**: 305–7.

20 Whitlow BJ, Lazanakis MS, Economides DL. The sonographic identification of fetal gender from 11 to 14 weeks of gestation. *Ultrasound Obstet Gynecol* 1999; **13**: 301–4.

21 Bustamante-Aragones A, Rodriguez de Alba M, Gonzalez-Gonzalez C, *et al.* Foetal sex determination in maternal blood from seventh week of gestation and its role in diagnosing haemophilia in the foetuses of female carriers. *Haemophilia* 2008; **14**: 593–8.

22 Lavery S. Preimplantation genetic diagnosis of haemophilia. *Br J Haematol* 2009; **144**: 303–7.

23 Medical and Scientific Advisory Council (MASAC) of the National Haemophilia Foundation. MASAC guidelines for perinatal management of women with bleeding disorders and carriers of haemophilia A and B, 2009. Available at http://www.hemophilia .org/NHFWeb/MainPgs/MainNHF.aspx?menuid=57&contentid =1436

24 James AH, Hoots K. The optimal mode of delivery for the haemophilia carrier expecting an affected infant is caesarean delivery. *Haemophilia* 2010; **16**: 420–4.

25 Kadir RA, Economides DL. Obstetric management of carriers of haemophilia. *Haemophilia* 1997; **3**: 81–6.

26 Michaud JL, Rivard GE, Chessex P. Intracranial hemorrhage in a newborn with hemophilia following elective caesarean section. *Am J Pediatr Hematol Oncol* 1991; **13**: 473–5.

27 Andrew M, Paes B, Milner R, *et al.* Development of the coagulation system in the full-term infant. *Blood* 1987; **70**: 165–72.

28 Andrew M, Paes B, Milner R, *et al.* Development of the human coagulation system in the healthy premature infant. *Blood* 1988; **72**: 1998–2005.

29 Rooks VJ, Eaton JP, Ruess L, *et al.* Prevalence and evolution of intracranial hemorrhage in asymptomatic term infants. *Am J Neuroradiol* 2008; **29**: 1082–9.

30 Chalmers EA. On behalf of the UKHCDO Paediatric Working Party. Management of neonates with inherited coagulation disorders. A survey of current practice. *Haemophilia* 2002; **8**: 488.

31 Myles LM, Massicotte P, Drake J. Intracranial hemorrhage in neonates with unrecognised hemophilia A: A persisting problem. *Pediatr Neurosurg* 2001; **34**: 94–7.

32 Williams MD, Chalmers, EA, Gibson BES. Guideline: The investigation and management of neonatal haemostasis and thrombosis. *Br J Haematol* 2002; **119**: 295–309.

33 Keeling D, Tait C, Makris M, Guideline on the selection and use of therapeutic products to treat haemophilia and other hereditary bleeding disorders. A United Kingdom Haemophilia Center Doctors' Organisation (UKHCDO) guideline approved by the British Committee for Standards in Haematology. *Haemophilia* 2008; **14**: 671–84.

34 Rickard KA. Guidelines for therapy and optimal dosages of coagulation factors for treatment of bleeding and surgery in haemophilia. *Haemophilia* 1995; **1**(Suppl. 1): 8–13.

35 Kraft KE, Verlaak R, Van Heijst AFJ, *et al.* Management of haemophilia in three premature infants. *Haemophilia* 2008; **14**: 378–80.

36 Bidlingmaier C, Bergmann F, Kurnik K. Haemophilia A in two premature infants. *Eur J Pediatr* 2005; **164**: 70–2.

37 Gale RF, Hird MF, Colvin BT. Management of a premature infant with moderate haemophilia A using recombinant factor VIII. *Haemophilia* 1998; **4**: 850–3.

38 Berry E. Intracranial haemorrhage in the haemophiliac neonate—the case for prophylaxis. Available at: http://www.haemophilia-forum.org/lock/Discussion/990426.htm

39 Buchanan GR. Factor concentrate prophylaxis for neonates with haemophilia. *J Pediatr Hematol Oncol* 1999; **21**: 254–9.

40 Lorenzo JI, López A, Altisent C, Aznar JA. Incidence of factor VIII inhibitors in severe haemophilia: The importance of patient age. *Br J Haematol* 2001; **113**: 600–3.

41 Van der Bom JG, Mauser-Bunschoten EP, Fischer K, van den Berg HM. Age at first treatment and immune tolerance to factor VIII in severe haemophilia. *Thromb Haemost* 2003; **89**: 475–9.

42 Chalmers EA, Brown SA, Keeling D, *et al.* Paediatric Working Party of UKHCDO. Early factor VIII exposure and subsequent inhibitor development in children with severe haemophilia A. *Haemophilia* 2007; **13**: 149–55.

43 Gouw SC, van der Bom JG, Marijke van den Berg H. Treatment-related risk factors of inhibitor development in previously untreated patients with hemophilia A: The CANAL cohort study. *Blood* 2007; **109**: 4648–54.

44 Kulkarni R, Lusher JM, Henry RC, Kallens DJ. Current practices regarding new-born intracranial haemorrhage and obstetrical care and mode of delivery of pregnant haemophilia carriers: A survey of obstetricians, neonatologists and haematologists in the United States, on behalf of the National Hemophilia Foundation's Medical and Scientific Advisory Council. *Haemophilia* 1999; **5**: 410–15.

CHAPTER 19

Work-up of a bleeding child

Manuel D. Carcao and Victor S. Blanchette
Hospital for Sick Children, University of Toronto, Toronto, Canada

Introduction

It is important that children with bleeding symptoms are evaluated to assess if the bleeding symptoms are clinically significant and, if they are, to determine, if possible, the underlying cause(s) for the abnormal bleeding symptoms. The evaluation of a child with a suspected bleeding disorder should include:

1 A comprehensive medical history focusing on the child's history of bleeding.
2 A detailed family history with emphasis on abnormal bleeding in close relatives, and any history of parental consanguinity.
3 A detailed physical examination.
4 Initial "screening" laboratory tests followed by specific diagnostic tests.

Comprehensive medical history focusing on the child's bleeding history

Evaluation of a child who is bleeding excessively, or has a history of unusual/excessive bleeding should be approached in a structured manner, beginning with a detailed bleeding history. It is important to take into consideration the child's age as severe congenital bleeding disorders, for example severe deficiencies of factors (F) VII, VIII, IX, X, or XIII or fibrinogen, or Glanzmann thrombasthenia, are more likely to present in the neonatal period with intracranial hemorrhage (ICH), persistent bleeding from heel-stick punctures, delayed umbilical stump bleeding, or, in male infants, with bleeding following circumcision. A detailed history of the child's prior bleeds (location, severity, frequency), and of previous surgical (circumcision, dental extractions, etc.) and bleeding challenges (child birth, trauma) needs to be obtained. A child who, in the past, experienced significant bleeding challenges and did not bleed is unlikely to have a severe congenital bleeding disorder but might still have an acquired disorder. The pattern of bleeding (mucosal, deep tissue, delayed surgical) may suggest certain disorders (Table 19.1).

A great clinical challenge is the assessment of mucocutaneous bleeding symptoms (e.g. easy bruising, epistaxis, menorrhagia) that are commonly reported in healthy children without an underlying bleeding disorder. Even significant bleeding does not necessarily imply that a child has an inherited/acquired bleeding disorder since children can bleed because of other causes, e.g. gastrointestinal bleeding associated with portal hypertension and esophageal varices; bleeding associated with medications such as anticoagulants; oozing from the gums from gum disease; unexplained bruising from nonaccidental injury (child abuse); or epistaxis from local factors such as drying of the nasal mucosa, nosepicking, allergic rhinitis, and/or trauma [1]. Consequently, only a minority (10–30%) of children referred for specific bleeding symptoms (e.g. epistaxis [2] or menorrhagia [3,4]) are ultimately confirmed to have an underlying inherited/acquired bleeding disorder.

Bleeding histories are often poorly taken by healthcare professionals. Increasingly, it is recommended that a general [5] and/or organ-specific [6,7] standardized bleeding questionnaire be used when taking a bleeding history in a child to better classify a child as a "bleeder" versus a "nonbleeder" and to quantitate the bleeding severity. Over the last decade, there have been attempts to develop standardized bleeding assessment questionnaires. These questionnaires consist of a series of questions pertaining to bleeding symptoms and bleeding challenges which are then scored according to the frequency and severity of the events and the need for medical intervention. An overall bleeding score is determined. Much of the initial work to develop these bleeding questionnaires came from a group of Italian investigators working with a primarily adult population [8,9]. Since then, there have been several additions to the "palate" of available bleeding questionnaires, including a questionnaire with pediatric-specific bleeding symptoms (the Pediatric Bleeding Questionnaire or PBQ)

Textbook of Hemophilia, Third Edition. Edited by Christine A. Lee, Erik E. Berntorp and W. Keith Hoots.
© 2014 John Wiley & Sons, Ltd. Published 2014 by John Wiley & Sons, Ltd.

Table 19.1 Pattern of bleeding and representative diseases.

Type of bleeding pattern	Representative bleeding disorders
Mucosal bleeding • Epistaxis • Bruising • Gum bleeding • Menorrhagia	• Von Willebrand disease • Thrombocytopenias • Platelet function disorders • Connective tissue disorders (e.g. Ehlers–Danlos syndrome)
Deep tissue bleeding • Deep tissue hematomas • Joint bleeding • Muscle bleeding • Surgical bleeding	• Hemophilia A or B • Other factor deficiencies (e.g. factor XI, factor VII, and factor X)
Delayed surgical bleeding	Factor XIII deficiency Afibrinogenemia Disorders of fibrinolysis • Plasminogen activator inhibitor (PAI-1) deficiency [37] • α2-antiplasmin deficiency [38] • Quebec platelet disorder: disorder of increased release of platelet urokinase plasminogen activator

Table 19.2 Differential diagnosis of a low FVIII:C.

Potential diagnosis	Useful tests to confirm diagnosis
Congenital hemophilia A	Genetic testing Testing child's mother for carrier status
Type 3 VWD	VWF:Ag, VWF:RCo, factor VIII:C; VWF multimer pattern
Type 2N VWD	Factor VIII binding assays Genetic testing for type 2N VWD
Combined deficiency of factors V and VIII	PT/INR: normal in hemophilia but abnormal in combined deficiency of factors V and VIII

VWF/D, von Willebrand factor/disease.

developed by Canadian investigators [10–12]. The PBQ consists of a series of questions evaluating 13 bleeding symptoms and quantifying each on a scale of 0 (or −1) to 4. For three bleeding symptoms (bleeding after dental extractions, surgeries, and postpartum bleeding), negative scores are possible if a patient is exposed at least twice and does not bleed excessively. Using the PBQ, Canadian investigators established a PBQ score ≥2 as positive or abnormal and showed that a PBQ score of ≥2 had a very strong negative predictive value (99%) although a poor positive predictive value (14%) in predicting von Willebrand disease (VWD) in children being investigated for VWD [10]. A new single definitive bleeding assessment tool (the International Society of Thrombosis and Haemostasis/Scientific and Standardization Committee bleeding assessment tool or ISTH/SSC BAT) requires validation [13].

In addition to the bleeding history, it is also important to obtain a thorough medical history. This includes documenting all medications and herbal supplements that the child is taking as many of these are known to impair hemostatic function [14]. Renal, liver, cardiac, and endocrine disorders (e.g. hypothyroidism) should be excluded as these can result in impairment of platelet function or in acquired coagulation factor deficiencies [15]. In a child with macrothrombocytopenia, it is important to inquire about, and test for, hearing loss, cataracts, and renal failure as these can be associated with an *MYH9*-related macrothrombocytopenia (*MYH9*-RD; formerly termed May–Hegglin anomaly, or Epstein, Fechtner, and Sebastian syndromes). Oculocutaneous albinism may indicate Hermansky–Pudlak syndrome (HPS), while eczema and recurrent infections might suggest Wiskott–Aldrich syndrome (WAS).

Family history

A detailed family history in a child with a suspected bleeding disorder may provide clues to the diagnosis. An X-linked inheritance pattern is classically seen in boys with hemophilia and some congenital platelet disorders (e.g. WAS). In 50–60% of children with hemophilia A or B, the family history will be positive with affected brothers, maternal cousins, uncles, or a grandfather. An autosomal dominant pattern is seen in VWD (types 1 or 2), some platelet function disorders, and familial thrombocytopenias. Most other severe coagulation deficiencies, many platelet function disorders as well as type 3 and type 2N VWD are inherited in an autosomal recessive manner. A clue to such disorders is the presence of parental consanguinity. The finding of consanguinity in a family is particularly important in the work-up a child with a low FVIII (coagulant) level (FVIII:C) (Table 19.2).

Inherited bleeding disorders are mostly not ethnically associated, but there are notable exceptions: FXI deficiency is much more common in the Ashkenazi (European) Jewish and Basque populations [16]. FXII deficiency appears to be more common in the Oriental population [17,18].

Physical examination

The physical examination may provide certain useful clues in establishing the diagnosis of an inherited/acquired bleeding disorder. Petechiae are usually associated with quantitative [e.g. immune thrombocytopenia (ITP)] platelet disorders where the circulating platelet count is generally below 20×10^9/L. In contrast, superficial bruising without petechiae is common in patients with VWD. Deep hematomas or joint abnormalities (e.g. swelling, pain) are suggestive of hemophilia. Other physical findings may point to rare diagnoses. Oculocutaneous albinism is seen in HPS; skin hyperelasticity and joint hypermobility are

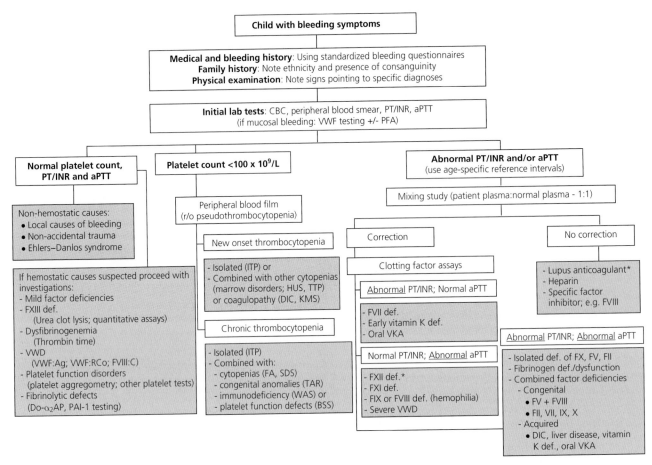

Figure 19.1 Work-up of a bleeding child: an algorithm. α2AP, α2-antiplasmin; aPTT, activated partial thromboplastin time; BSS, Bernard–Soulier syndrome; CBC, complete blood count; def, deficiency; DIC, disseminated intravascular coagulation; FA, Fanconi's anemia; HUS, hemolytic uremic syndrome; INR, international normalized ratio; ITP, immune thrombocytopenia purpura; KMS, Kasabach–Merritt syndrome; PAI-1, plasminogen activator inhibitor-1; PT, prothrombin time; SDS, Schwachman–Diamond syndrome; TAR, thrombocytopenia with absent radii; TTP, thrombotic thrombocytopenic purpura; VKA, vitamin K antagonists; VWD, von Willebrand disease; VWF:Ag, von Willebrand factor antigen level; VWF:RCo, von Willebrand factor ristocetin cofactor activity level; WAS, Wiskott–Aldrich syndrome. *Not associated with bleeding.

seen in Ehlers–Danlos syndrome (EDS); cataracts or hearing loss may be found in *MYH9*-RD; and telangiectasias can be found in hereditary hemorrhagic telangiectasia.

When examining bruises on a child, any pattern to the bruising (e.g. hand, stick, or belt injuries) needs to be noted as potentially indicative of nonaccidental injury (child abuse). The location of the bruises is also important as those associated with bleeding disorders tend to be located over sites of typical childhood trauma (e.g. the lower extremities) whereas those from nonaccidental injury are seen in unusual locations (e.g. face or chest).

Laboratory evaluation

Laboratory evaluation of a child with bleeding symptoms should begin with screening tests unless the history or family history is strongly suggestive of a particular bleeding disorder.

Screening tests, if abnormal, should then be followed by specific tests (e.g. factor assays, platelet function tests) as judged appropriate based on the history, physical examination, and results of initial testing. It is useful to have a standardized algorithmic approach to investigating children for bleeding disorders. See Figure 19.1 for one such algorithm.

Initial coagulation tests should include: a complete blood count, examination of a peripheral blood film by an experienced heathcare professional, a prothrombin time (PT) or international normalized ratio (INR), and an activated partial thromboplastin time (aPTT). Also, in patients who present with mucocutaneous bleeding, there should be specific testing for VWD and for an underlying platelet function disorder. Until about a decade ago, the traditional screening test for a platelet function disorder was the skin bleeding time (BT) but because of its drawbacks (see below) the Platelet Function Analyzer (PFA-100) test has largely replaced the BT as an initial test of platelet function in some clinics.

Complete blood count and peripheral blood film

The complete blood count (CBC) provides valuable information in the work-up of a child with a suspected bleeding disorder. The finding of anemia or of features suggestive of iron deficiency (e.g. microcytosis, hypochromasia) may be indicative of chronic bleeding. A low platelet count may indicate underlying congenital [e.g. Bernard–Soulier syndrome (BSS), type 2B VWD] or acquired thrombocytopenias [e.g. ITP, hemolytic uremic syndrome (HUS), and thrombotic thrombocytopenic purpura (TTP)]. The presence of red blood cell schistocytes provides an important clue to HUS and TTP.

Examination of a peripheral blood film is vital in diagnosing a bleeding disorder. Platelet clumping might signify type 2B VWD or might alternatively be pseudothrombocytopenia which is an artifact associated with ethylenediaminetetra-acetic acid (EDTA)-dependent antibodies against platelet surface glycoproteins. Alternative blood collection tubes (e.g. sodium citrate, hirudin) or direct collection of blood onto a microscope slide (via a pinprick) can avoid this artifact. Uniformly large platelets (mean platelet volume >12.4 femtoliters or fL) [19] may signify BSS or *MYH9*-RD while small platelets (mean platelet volume <5 fL) may indicate WAS. The finding of pale gray, almost ghost-like, platelets is suggestive of the gray platelet syndrome, or if associated with arthrogryposis, renal dysfunction, and cholestasis, of arthrogryposis–renal dysfunction–cholestasis (ARC) syndrome. The presence of Döhle-like inclusions in leukocytes accompanied by macrothrombocytopenia is suggestive of *MYH9*-RD.

Prothrombin time and the international normalized ratio

The PT is a measure of the extrinsic (FVII) and common coagulation pathway [FX, FV, FII (prothrombin), and fibrinogen], and hence is prolonged in deficiencies of these factors. Normal PT ranges vary according to the reagents used by individual laboratories. To adjust for these differences, the PT is commonly reported as the INR (the ratio of the patient's PT to a control PT raised to the power of the international sensitivity index value for the analytical system used). An abnormal INR in the presence of a normal aPTT is suggestive of FVII deficiency. Although a partial deficiency of FVII (heterozygosity for FVII) is quite common in the general population (estimated to affect 1 in 400 individuals), severe deficiency (homozygosity or compound heterozygosity for FVII mutations) is rare. Alternatively, a prolonged INR may point towards acquired bleeding disorders such as disseminated intravascular coagulation (DIC), liver disease, vitamin K deficiency, or medications, e.g. warfarin.

Activated partial thromboplastin time

The aPTT measures the intrinsic (contact factors: FXII, prekallikrein, and high-molecular-weight kininogen as well as FXI, FIX, and FVIII) and common coagulation pathways. Depending on the equipment and commercial reagents used, the aPTT may show very different sensitivities to different coagulation factors, and mild factor deficiencies may not be detected by the aPTT. The aPTT can be prolonged in isolation from the INR in any disorder that only involves clotting factors of the intrinsic pathway. The aPTT may also be affected by antiphospholipid antibodies and by heparin. In hospitalized children, particularly those in intensive or neonatal intensive care units, contamination by heparin is the most frequent cause of a prolonged aPTT. The aPTT may also be prolonged in DIC, liver disease, vitamin K deficiency, and warfarin use, but usually to a lesser extent than the PT.

A prolonged aPTT should not be interpreted as indicating that the patient is at increased risk of bleeding. The two most common situations in which the aPTT is prolonged but the child is not at increased risk of bleeding are antiphospholipid antibodies and FXII deficiency. Antiphospholipid antibodies in children tend to be postinfectious and are mostly transient with no associated increased risk of either bleeding or clotting. The exception is when there is associated acquired FII deficiency; in this rare scenario the bleeding risk is increased. Distinguishing an antiphospholipid antibody causing prolongation of the aPTT from other causes involves performing a mixing study [mixing the patient's plasma with healthy (normal) donor plasma in a ratio of 1 : 1]. In severe coagulation factor deficiencies, mixing replenishes the level of the missing factor to about 50% which is sufficient to normalize the aPTT, whereas in the presence of an antiphospholipid antibody, the aPTT remains prolonged after mixing due to the ongoing presence of the antibody.

Autoantibodies to FVIII causing acquired hemophilia A can also prolong the aPTT. In this condition, bleeding can be severe; fortunately, this condition is extremely rare in children.

It is useful to confirm a diagnosis of FXII deficiency in order to prevent the child undergoing unnecessary repeat investigations, experiencing delays in necessary procedures (e.g. surgery) or receiving blood products to correct their aPTT. Families of such children should be provided with a letter explaining their underlying disorder and emphasizing that medical intervention is not required even in the face of invasive procedures.

Combined abnormalities of the prothrombin time and activated partial thromboplastin time

Combined prolongation of the PT/INR and the aPTT can be seen in rare combined congenital factor deficiencies (combined FV and FVIII deficiency [20] and combined deficiency of vitamin K-dependent coagulation factors [21]).

More commonly, combined prolongation of the PT/INR and the aPTT is seen in acquired conditions with multiple factor deficiencies, e.g. liver disease, vitamin K deficiency, and DIC. The key laboratory tests to distinguish these entities are measurements of FV, FVII, FVIII, and FIX. In DIC, all coagulation factors, including FVIII, are reduced whereas in the other disorders, FVIII levels are normal or elevated. Liver disease and vitamin K deficiency are distinguished by the FV level, which is reduced in liver disease but normal in vitamin K deficiency.

Absent (afibrinogenemia) or very low fibrinogen levels (hypofibrinogenemias) will usually cause the PT/INR and the aPTT to be prolonged. However, mild reductions of fibrinogen may not be detected by the INR or the aPTT. For detection of such disorders, functional testing of fibrinogen using a thrombin time (TT) is useful. The TT is also useful to check for evidence of dysfibrinogenemias, which are characterized by a prolonged TT in the context of a normal fibrinogen antigen level.

Bleeding time

Traditionally, the skin BT was included as a screening test for VWD and inherited platelet function disorders. Unfortunately, the BT is invasive, time consuming, operator dependent, and not suitable for multiple repeat testing. In addition, the BT is poorly reproducible and it is a poor predictor of surgical bleeding [22]. Consequently, the PFA-100 was developed as an *ex-vivo* substitute for the BT when evaluating primary hemostasis.

Platelet function analyzer

The PFA-100 system (developed by Dade-Behring, Illinois; now owned by Siemens AG, Healthcare Sector, Henkestrasse 127, D-91052 Erlangen, Germany) provides a rapid and automated method of assessing primary hemostasis *in vitro* by measuring the time (closure time; CT) taken for platelets in a sample of anticoagulated blood under high shear to form a plug that occludes a microscopic aperture cut into a membrane coated with collagen (Col) and either epinephrine (Epi) or adenosine diphosphate (ADP) [23]. In 1998, Carcao *et al.* established the normal ranges for PFA-100 CTs in 56 normal healthy children [23]. The same group subsequently reported that both the BT and the PFA-100 were consistently abnormal in patients with type 2 and type 3 VWD. The BT, however, missed most patients with type 1 VWD whereas the PFA-100 using the Col/ADP cartridge missed far fewer cases [24]. Other recent reviews have similarly concluded that the PFA-100 has a higher sensitivity to VWD than the BT [25]. The PFA-100 has been shown to be very sensitive to acquired VWD secondary to high-flow cardiac lesions (e.g. patent ductus arteriosus, aortic stenosis, and ventricular septal defects) [26]. Several studies have shown that whereas the PFA-100 and the BT are sensitive to severe platelet function disorders both are relatively insensitive to mild platelet function disorders, particularly storage pool release defects [27]. Consequently, to detect mild platelet function disorders specific testing is required.

There are many pitfalls with using the PFA-100. PFA-100 CTs are sensitive to patient hematocrit [28], are affected by low platelet counts ($<100 \times 10^9$/L) and are sensitive to cyclooxygenase (COX) inhibitors such as aspirin and other nonsteroidal anti-inflammatory drugs.

Von Willebrand factor testing

Von Willebrand disease is the most common congenital bleeding disorder. Given that mild forms of VWD will not be detected by the aPTT and that the BT or PFA-100 CTs are not sensitive enough to rule out mild VWD, it is important to specifically test for VWD in individuals presenting with mucocutaneous bleeding. Specific tests include measurement of von Willebrand factor (VWF) antigen (VWF:Ag) using an immunologic assay, measurement of VWF function using the ristocetin cofactor assay (VWF:RCo), and FVIII:C. Depending on the results of these tests, multimer analysis and the ristocetin-induced platelet agglutination (RIPA) test may be necessary to differentiate between different types of VWD. In type 1 VWD, there is a proportional reduction in VWF:Ag and VWF:RCo levels; FVIII:C levels tend to be either normal or slightly reduced and there is a proportional reduction in all VWF multimers. In type 3 VWD, there is an absence or extremely low levels of both VWF:Ag and VWF:RCo (generally both are <5%); the FVIII:C may be as low as 1% and VWF multimers are absent.

The type 2 VWD variants are characterized by some disturbance of VWF function. In type 2A and type 2M VWD, there is minimal or no reduction in VWF:Ag while the VWF:RCo is significantly reduced causing the VWF:RCo/VWF:Ag ratio to be <0.6. The two conditions are mainly distinguished through multimer analysis: in type 2A, high-molecular-weight VWF multimers are reduced, whereas in type 2M, they are normal. Type 2B VWD also shows a low VWF:RCo/VWF:Ag ratio but is distinguished by an increase in RIPA reflecting increased binding of the abnormal VWF to platelets. This typically, but not invariably, results in moderate thrombocytopenia, most evident when such patients are stressed (e.g. surgery). Type 2N VWD is characterized by discordantly low FVIII:C levels (usually between 5 and 20%) with normal or only slightly reduced VWF:Ag and VWF:RCo levels [29]. Diagnosing type 2N requires either FVIII binding assays or genetic testing for mutations associated with type 2N VWD.

Issues in coagulation testing

For all coagulation blood tests, and in particular for VWF:Ag and VWF:RCo testing, there are many pitfalls in testing. Pre-analytical variables (i.e. variables that occur before testing) are extremely important. The correct volume of blood needs to be taken into the correct citrate tube with the correct blood to anticoagulant ratio. The blood draw should not be traumatic and the blood should not be shaken or stirred, as this may initiate clotting and result in platelet activation and consumption of both VWF and FVIII:C. Blood once taken needs to be tested within 4–6 h as many coagulation factors (e.g. VWF and FXII) are quite labile; if testing is not performed immediately, the blood needs to be centrifuged and the plasma needs to be quickly frozen at, or below −40°C. Platelet function testing becomes unreliable if not undertaken within 4 h of blood collection.

Many physiologic processes may affect coagulation testing: patient age, blood group, intercurrent illnesses, and so on. The effect of age is most notable in very young children, where the aPTT is prolonged due to physiologic reductions in some factors [e.g. vitamin K-dependent factors (FII, FVII, FIX, FX, protein C, and protein S) and contact factors such as FXII]. The interpretation of coagulation tests needs to take patient age into consideration to avoid mislabeling young children as having deficiencies in vitamin K-dependent factors (e.g. FIX).

The following increase VWF and FVIII:C levels and consequently lower aPTT values: states of high estrogen (e.g. pregnancy, oral contraceptive pills), stress (e.g. struggling or crying in children), exercise, or acute illnesses (e.g. infections, malignancies). In contrast, hypothyroidism decreases VWF levels. In postpubertal girls, VWF levels also vary with the menstrual cycle, being at their lowest levels during the menstrual and early follicular phases [30]. These variables contribute to considerable intrapatient variability in coagulation testing causing difficulties in interpreting borderline test results [31]. ABO blood group affects VWF levels. Individuals who are blood group O will have VWF levels that are 20–25% lower than non-O blood group individuals [32]. In blood group O individuals, the normal range for VWF levels can be as low as 40% [24]. It therefore becomes difficult to distinguish a blood group O individual with a VWF level of around 40% as either having VWD or as being normal.

Specific coagulation testing

The majority of bleeding disorders will be suspected following initial coagulation "screening" tests. However, certain bleeding disorders, in particular FXIII deficiency and mild platelet function disorders are not detected by these initial tests. To assess for FXIII deficiency, specific testing needs to be done. The traditional test is the urea clot solubility test but this test is limited to detecting only the most severe cases (FXIII <5% of normal) [33]. More sensitive tests are available in a few specialized laboratories [34].

Light transmission aggregometry (LTA) measures *in-vitro* platelet activation and aggregation to various strong and weak agonists in citrated platelet-rich plasma by recording changes in light transmission [35]. LTA is required for detection of mild platelet function disorders (e.g. storage pool disorders, platelet secretion defects). Additionally, a test that reflects platelet ATP release (e.g. lumi-aggregometry) is also useful. Platelet aggregation testing requires a standardized methodology, avoidance of pre-analytical variables known to affect test results (e.g. ingestion of aspirin), trained personnel, and generally must be scheduled during daytime hours [36]. Platelet aggregation testing can reveal certain classical patterns of aggregation which may suggest certain disorders (Table 19.3). Based on the results of platelet aggregation testing, more specialized testing may be appropriate (e.g. platelet GPIb/IX/V and/or GPIIb/IIIa receptor quantitation by flow cytometry), platelet morphology by transmission electron microscopy (e.g. to evaluate for disorders of

Table 19.3 Typical aggregation findings with various platelet function disorders.

Disorder	Aggregation pattern
Glanzmann thrombasthenia	Lack of aggregation to all agonists; agglutination to ristocetin is present
Bernard–Soulier syndrome	Lack of agglutination to ristocetin
Secretion defect or dense granule deficiency	Decreased aggregation with collagen and decreased secondary wave of aggregation with ADP and epinephrine
Aspirin-like defect	Lack of aggregation to arachidonic acid, decreased aggregation to collagen, and lack of secondary wave of aggregation with ADP and epinephrine
ADP receptor defect	Decreased/absent aggregation to ADP or enhanced deaggregation

ADP, adenosine diphosphate.

platelet α-granules), platelet dense granule quantitation, and immunofluorescence microscopy for myosin IIA inclusions in leukocytes (in *MYH9*-RD).

Conclusion

The work-up of a child who is bleeding involves a thorough awareness of abnormalities that can impair normal hemostasis, including abnormalities of coagulation factors, platelet disorders, and blood vessel disorders (e.g. EDS). The most important tool in establishing a correct diagnosis is a properly taken bleeding and family history which can provide clues to the diagnosis. These also guide the subsequent laboratory work-up. Most severe disorders will be quickly identified on the basis of abnormal screening tests leading to definitive diagnostic testing. The story is less clear for mild bleeding disorders (e.g. type 1 VWD and mild platelet function disorders) that tend to be associated with borderline test results. It also needs to be recognized that not all bleeding disorders will be detected by means of laboratory testing (e.g. EDS).

Acknowledgments

We would like to thank Drs Margaret Rand and Walter Kahr for their assistance in reviewing this chapter.

References

1 Gifford TO, Orlandi RR. Epistaxis. *Otolaryngol Clin N Am* 2008; **41**(3): 525–36.

2 Sandoval C, Dong S, Visintainer P, Ozkaynak MF, Jayabose S. Clinical and laboratory features of 178 children with recurrent epistaxis. *J Pediatr Hematol Oncol* 2002; **24**(1): 47–9.

3 Ahuja SP, Hertweck SP. Overview of bleeding disorders in adolescent females with menorrhagia. *J Pediatr Adolesc Gynecol* 2010; **23**(6 Suppl.): S15–21.

4 Kouides PA. Bleeding symptom assessment and hemostasis evaluation of menorrhagia. *Curr Opin Hematol* 2008; **15**(5): 465–72.

5 Rydz N, James PD. The evolution and value of bleeding assessment tools. *J Thromb Haemost* 2012; **10**(11): 2223–9.

6 Higham JM, O'Brien PM, Shaw RW. Assessment of menstrual blood loss using a pictorial chart. *Br J Obstet Gynaecol* 1990; **97**(8): 734–9.

7 Katsanis E, Luke KH, Hsu E, Li M, Lillicrap D. Prevalence and significance of mild bleeding disorders in children with recurrent epistaxis. *J Pediatr* 1988; **113**(1 Pt 1): 73–6.

8 Rodeghiero F, Castaman G, Tosetto A, *et al*. The discriminant power of bleeding history for the diagnosis of type 1 von Willebrand disease: an international, multicenter study. *J Thromb Haemost* 2005; **3**(12): 2619–26.

9 Tosetto A, Castaman G, Rodeghiero F. Bleeding scores in inherited bleeding disorders: clinical or research tools? *Haemophilia* 2008; **14**(3): 415–22.

10 Bowman M, Riddel J, Rand ML, Tosetto A, Silva M, James PD. Evaluation of the diagnostic utility for von Willebrand disease of a pediatric bleeding questionnaire. *J Thromb Haemost* 2009; **7**(8): 1418–21.

11 Biss TT, Blanchette VS, Clark DS, Wakefield CD, James PD, Rand ML. Use of a quantitative pediatric bleeding questionnaire to assess mucocutaneous bleeding symptoms in children with a platelet function disorder. *J Thromb Haemost* 2010; **8**(6): 1416–19.

12 Biss TT, Blanchette VS, Clark DS, *et al*. Quantitation of bleeding symptoms in children with von Willebrand disease: use of a standardized pediatric bleeding questionnaire. *J Thromb Haemost* 2010; **8**(5): 950–6.

13 Rodeghiero F, Tosetto A, Abshire T, *et al*. ISTH/SSC bleeding assessment tool: a standardized questionnaire and a proposal for a new bleeding score for inherited bleeding disorders. *J Thromb Haemost* 2010; **8**(9): 2063–5.

14 Ang-Lee MK, Moss J, Yuan CS. Herbal medicines and perioperative care. *J Am Med Assoc* 2001; **286**(2): 208–16.

15 Shetty S, Kasatkar P, Ghosh K. Pathophysiology of acquired von Willebrand disease: a concise review. *Eur J Haematol* 2011; **87**(2): 99–106.

16 Seligsohn U. Factor XI deficiency in humans. *J Thromb Haemost* 2009; **7**(Suppl. 1): 84–7.

17 Song KS. High incidence of plasma factor XII deficiency in normal Korean subjects. *Thromb Res* 2006; **117**(6): 732–3.

18 Gordon EM, Donaldson VH, Saito H, Su E, Ratnoff OD. Reduced titers of Hageman factor (factor XII) in Orientals. *Ann Intern Med* 1981; **95**(6): 697–700.

19 Noris P, Klersy C, Zecca M, *et al*. Platelet size distinguishes between inherited macrothrombocytopenias and immune thrombocytopenia. *J Thromb Haemost* 2009; **7**(12): 2131–6.

20 Spreafico M, Peyvandi F. Combined FV and FVIII deficiency. *Haemophilia* 2008; **14**(6): 1201–8.

21 Weston BW, Monahan PE. Familial deficiency of vitamin K-dependent clotting factors. *Haemophilia* 2008; **14**(6): 1209–13.

22 Watson HG, Greaves M. Can we predict bleeding? *Semin Thromb Hemost* 2008; **34**(1): 97–103.

23 Carcao MD, Blanchette VS, Dean JA, *et al*. The Platelet Function Analyzer (PFA-100): a novel in-vitro system for evaluation of primary haemostasis in children. *Br J Haematol* 1998; **101**(1): 70–3.

24 Dean JA, Blanchette VS, Carcao MD, *et al*. von Willebrand disease in a pediatric-based population–comparison of type 1 diagnostic criteria and use of the PFA-100 and a von Willebrand factor/collagen-binding assay. *Thromb Haemost* 2000; **84**(3): 401–9.

25 Favaloro EJ. The utility of the PFA-100 in the identification of von Willebrand disease: a concise review. *Semin Thromb Hemost* 2006; **32**(5): 537–45.

26 Vincentelli A, Susen S, Le Tourneau T, *et al*. Acquired von Willebrand syndrome in aortic stenosis. *N Engl J Med* 2003; **349**(4): 343–9.

27 Sladky JL, Klima J, Grooms L, Kerlin BA, O'Brien SH. The PFA-100 (R) does not predict delta-granule platelet storage pool deficiencies. *Haemophilia* 2012; **18**(4): 626–9.

28 Eugster M, Reinhart WH. The influence of the haematocrit on primary haemostasis in vitro. *Thromb Haemost* 2005; **94**(6): 1213–18.

29 Schneppenheim R, Budde U, Krey S, *et al*. Results of a screening for von Willebrand disease type 2N in patients with suspected haemophilia A or von Willebrand disease type 1. *Thromb Haemost* 1996; **76**(4): 598–602.

30 Knol HM, Kemperman RF, Kluin-Nelemans HC, Mulder AB, Meijer K. Haemostatic variables during normal menstrual cycle. A systematic review. *Thromb Haemost* 2012; **107**(1): 22–9.

31 Abildgaard CF, Suzuki Z, Harrison J, Jefcoat K, Zimmerman TS. Serial studies in von Willebrand's disease: variability versus "variants". *Blood* 1980; **56**(4): 712–16.

32 Jenkins PV, O'Donnell JS. ABO blood group determines plasma von Willebrand factor levels: a biologic function after all? *Transfusion* 2006; **46**(10): 1836–44.

33 Kohler HP, Ichinose A, Seitz R, Ariens RA, Muszbek L. Diagnosis and classification of factor XIII deficiencies. *J Thromb Haemost* 2011; **9**(7): 1404–6.

34 Hsieh L, Nugent D. Factor XIII deficiency. *Haemophilia* 2008; **14**(6): 1190–200.

35 Rand ML, Leung R, Packham MA. Platelet function assays. *Transfus Apher Sci* 2003; **28**(3): 307–17.

36 Hayward CP, Moffat KA, Raby A, *et al*. Development of North American consensus guidelines for medical laboratories that perform and interpret platelet function testing using light transmission aggregometry. *Am J Clin Pathol* 2010; **134**(6): 955–63.

37 Mehta R, Shapiro AD. Plasminogen activator inhibitor type 1 deficiency. *Haemophilia* 2008; **14**(6): 1255–60.

38 Carpenter SL, Mathew P. Alpha2-antiplasmin and its deficiency: fibrinolysis out of balance. *Haemophilia* 2008; **14**(6): 1250–4.

CHAPTER 20

Care of the child with hemophilia

Rolf C.R. Ljung

Skåne University Hospital, Malmö, Sweden

Introduction

The goal of the treatment of a child with hemophilia should be to ensure that both the family and the affected child perceive themselves as healthy, despite the diagnosis of hemophilia. The World Health Organization (WHO) defines health as a state of complete physical, psychological, and social well-being. The aim of this chapter is to consider various aspects of the medical and psychosocial care of children with hemophilia.

Medical care

Diagnosis and risk of inhibitor development

Healthcare professionals are highly aware that hemophilia is a hereditary disorder. However, in many countries, it is not as well recognized that the majority of babies born with hemophilia actually represent sporadic cases, i.e. the families in question have no known history of hemophilia. This lack of knowledge is a major cause of delay in the diagnosis of the disorder, since physicians simply overlook the risk of hemophilia in previously unaffected families.

Once a definite diagnosis has been made based on the results of clotting assays, it is recommended that the mutation in a family be characterized. Knowledge of the type of mutation enables carrier detection and prenatal diagnosis in the family as well as the estimation of the risk of developing inhibitors directed against factor VIII (FVIII) or factor IX (FIX) [1–3]. The development of inhibitors is the most serious complication of treatment. Other host-related factors important for inhibitor development, besides the type of mutation and thus the severity of the disease, are family history of inhibitors, ethnicity, histocompatibility locus antigen (HLA) type, and alleles of immune response modifier genes [4–6]. The age at first treatment does not seem to be a risk factor for inhibitor development by itself [7]. However, children who were treated at an early age are usually treated because of specific circumstances and those circumstances rather than age accounted for the development of

inhibitors at an early age [8]. Surgical procedures, treatment during concomitant inflammatory states, and peak treatment moments, i.e. frequent and extensive administration of high doses of factor concentrate at the start of treatment, have been suggested to increase the risk of inhibitor development and should thus be avoided [8–10].

Another aspect of early treatment currently discussed is whether the mode of administration, regular prophylactic treatment or on demand, has an impact on inhibitor development [7,9]. Starting treatment as prophylactic treatment, without bleeds or "immunological danger signals," seem to lower the risk of inhibitor development. A recent study suggests that a subgroup of patients with a high genetic risk will develop inhibitors despite protective measures while a subgroup with a lower genetic risk may be influenced by the mode of administration [10]. The impact of the type of concentrate has also been debated [11,12]. Recent studies do not show any difference in the risk for the development of inhibitors between plasma-derived and recombinant concentrates [13]. Nevertheless, administration of FVIII/FIX concentrates as treatment for a bleed should not be avoided, even if a patient is at risk of developing inhibitors. A child with hemophilia B as a result of a complete gene deletion runs a substantial risk of an anaphylactoid reaction to FIX infusions [14]. Such a response usually occurs after one of the first 10–20 infusions, therefore it is recommended that healthcare professionals who give this type of treatment are also prepared to deal with an allergic reaction.

Treatment

The most important aspect of the care of children with hemophilia is the treatment regimen that is used, which varies considerably between countries owing to differences in the level of health care that is generally available. The quality of FVIII or FIX replacement therapy in a country usually evolves from sporadic or on-demand treatment of bleeding episodes to secondary prophylaxis for those with frequent bleeds, and finally to individually tailored primary prophylaxis for all children with severe or moderate hemophilia [15]. According to a joint

---

Textbook of Hemophilia, Third Edition. Edited by Christine A. Lee, Erik E. Berntorp and W. Keith Hoots.
© 2014 John Wiley & Sons, Ltd. Published 2014 by John Wiley & Sons, Ltd.

statement made by the WHO and the World Federation of Hemophilia (WFH), initiating prophylactic treatment at an early age is considered to be the optimal form of therapy for a child with hemophilia [16]. The most refined regimens currently involve primary prophylaxis, in which treatment is begun at 12–18 months of age, before the onset of bleeding into joints or other serious bleeds [17]. The rationale behind an early start is that even a small number of joint bleeds can result in irreversible damage, as well as damage that progresses despite prophylactic therapy [18].

It has also been shown that the time point at which prophylaxis is begun is an independent factor in the evaluation of joint outcome [19]. However, it must not be forgotten that the aim of prophylactic treatment is to avoid not only arthropathy but also other serious bleedings such as intracranial hemorrhage [20]. In most cases, an early therapeutic approach is initiated by giving a dose of approximately 25 IU/kg once or twice a week via a peripheral vein, with the aim of increasing the frequency of administration as soon as possible. The ultimate goal is to reach full-scale primary prophylaxis, which usually involves the following:

- In hemophilia A, FVIII is administered at a dose of 20–40 IU/ kg/day every second day or three times weekly.
- In hemophilia B, factor IX is given at a dose of 20–40 IU/kg/ day every third day or twice weekly [15].

However, both the dose and the dose interval have to be individually tailored for each child owing to pharmacokinetic differences between patients. In older children with hemophilia A, it is possible to optimize the cost–benefit ratio of treatment by daily injections of FVIII (10–20 IU/kg) [21]. The level of the lowest concentration is more important than the peak level after injection [22]. However, it is the clinical outcome, not the achieved trough levels, that determines whether the given dose is adequate [23]. The size of the vials available is also a factor that in practise influences the dose given, especially in small children. From both a medical and a social perspective, it is best if the children can be treated at home by their parents, and that particular objective has already been accomplished for most of those patients in countries that have a well-developed system of care for people with hemophilia.

Monitoring treatment

To ensure high quality of care, children with severe hemophilia should be examined once or twice a year by a pediatrician at a comprehensive hemophilia care center. The same applies to children with mild hemophilia, although the check-ups can be done less frequently in such cases. The basic items that are recommended to be included in a biannual or annual check-up are listed in Box 20.1 [24]. Joint evaluation should be done once a year by use of a sensitive score such as the Hemophilia Joint Health Score (HJHS) 2.0 [25]. Scoring of bone changes on plain X-ray is still a valuable method; and magnetic resonance imaging (MRI) can reveal the early changes in synovia and cartilage as an aid in monitoring treatment and reveal signs of

***

Box 20.1 Important items in the biannual/annual check-up of children with hemophilia [24].

Physical examination, including physical joint score
Feedback on "daily log-book" or similar registration of bleeds and treatments
Education of the child and/or parents in venous access
Surveillance of central venous lines (e.g. position of catheter, recombinant tissue plasminogen activator/urokinase installation in catheter, blood culture, education of the child and/or parents in aseptic techniques)
Laboratory surveillance including pharmacokinetic evaluation at certain intervals [40]
Sociomedical aspects (e.g. quality of life, leisure activities, absence from school)

***

subclinical joint hemorrhage [26–30]. Ultrasound is another, more easily available, imaging technique that is increasingly used in hemophilia [31]. Quality of life can be evaluated by "Hemoqol," a disease-specific instrument validated for use in children [32]. In countries with less advanced therapy, functional tests may be a valuable tool [33,34].

Venous access

Easy venous access is a prerequisite of administering blood factor concentrates to young children with hemophilia A or B, regardless of whether this is done at the time of a bleed or as a prophylactic measure. For a child receiving on-demand treatment at home, it is preferable that the FVIII/FIX concentrate be given by the parents as soon as a bleed occurs. In such a situation, safe and easy access to a vein is essential, and the same is true for children on a prophylactic regimen. The first choice of access should be a peripheral vein and in most cases this will be successful. However, venous access can be very difficult or even impossible to accomplish in young children, thus it may be necessary to consider a central venous line (Figure 20.1). Introduction of a central venous catheter entails risks that must be weighed against the potential benefits for individual patients. Medical indications may include poor access to a peripheral vein for a planned therapy, especially the daily injections that are required for immune tolerance induction (ITI) in patients with inhibitors. An example of a combined medical and social indication is when a central venous line would enable parents to treat a young child at home. Implantation of a central venous catheter solely on psychological grounds should be discouraged— a child who is merely afraid of venepuncture needs to be helped in some other way.

Several reports have described various adverse effects associated with the use of central venous catheters in patients with hemophilia, and infections were the most frequently mentioned complications in those subjects [35]. Patients with inhibitors are at considerably higher risk for infections. Notwithstanding, easy

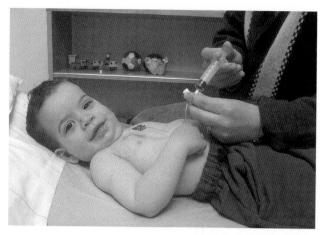

Figure 20.1 An implantable central venous line facilitates injections in children with difficult venous access in peripheral veins.

venous access is imperative for these patients, both for the treatment of acute bleeds and for ITI.

The rates of clinically manifest thrombosis have been low in the larger series of patients that have been documented, but it should be noted that routine venography was not done in most of those series. Recent reports suggest that thrombosis, although in most instances "clinically silent," is a more frequent side-effect than previously assumed [35,36]. The experiences so far suggest that the risk of catheter-related thrombosis increases after many years of use. Development of thrombosis may be related to the site of the catheter (jugular or subclavian vein), the type of concentrate used, or some genetic thrombophilic factor [37,38].

The final decision to use a central venous catheter must be a compromise between the following: the medical goal, the bleeding tendency, the social situation of the patient, and the familiarity with the devices at the particular hemophilia center. The number of complications may be reduced by taking adequate measures to maintain asepsis, both at the time of implantation and during subsequent use, and also by adopting explicit basic routines for surveillance of the systems and repeatedly educating the users. In many cases, a central venous line is indispensable for appropriate treatment, and several series on record have clearly demonstrated the benefits of these devices for hemophilic children and their families. Some centers have successfully used arteriovenous fistulae in children as an alternative to a central venous line [36].

Medication

In developed countries, most children with hemophilia are treated with recombinant FVIII/IX concentrates [37]. Drugs containing acetylsalicylic acid should not be used to relieve pain, because they inhibit platelet function and therefore have an adverse effect on coagulation. Consequently, preparations containing acetaminophen (paracetamol), alone or in combination with codeine, are recommended as analgesics. Anti-inflammatory drugs, such as celecoxib and rofecoxib, can in certain cases be useful in reducing joint pain and synovial inflammation.

Psychological care

In countries with limited resources for medical care, it is natural to focus on hemophilia itself and literally on how to help patients survive from day to day. In most countries with well-developed healthcare provisions, the ability to treat this disease has improved dramatically during the last decades owing to the introduction of FVIII and FIX concentrates. Therefore, in those nations, the focus should be switched from the disorder per se to the healthy aspects of the child with hemophilia. The connotation of the word "hemophilia" and the description of the condition have a markedly negative influence on how it is perceived by the parents and later on by the child. This disease has a dramatic history, and the attitudes of healthcare professionals and older people with hemophilia are still affected by the way the disorder used to be managed, even in industrialized countries.

The initial information given to a family with a child who has been diagnosed with hemophilia will have a pronounced effect on how this family, and in time the child himself, will cope with the disease and how it will influence daily life. Ideally, this information should be given to both parents, if possible together with older siblings. If advanced hemophilia care is available, the most important message to convey in the first discussion is that a person with hemophilia can lead a practically normal life and have a normal life expectancy.

For an optimal outcome of the crisis reaction, it is important to try to discover whether the parents think that they are to blame or that they have done something wrong in the past that might have given rise to the disease. The mother might be a genetic carrier, and thus it is obvious that she may feel responsible for her child's hemophilia.

The initial counseling should be repeated at subsequent meetings with the parents to ensure that they have received all the relevant information. Positive facts about prophylactic treatment strategies and the prospect of being able to use gene therapy to cure the disease in the future should be given together with straightforward information about possible complications, such as the development of inhibitors. Furthermore, it is important that the same doctor and nurse communicate with the family during this sensitive period in order to avoid the uncertainty and frustration that can result from slight differences in the way that individual care providers present the same information.

The child suffering from hemophilia is not the only person who is influenced by the disease; there is also a profound psychosocial effect on all the members of the family. Overprotection may become a serious problem, and the strong natural urge to safeguard the child can instead cause difficulties for the entire family. Indeed, in extreme cases, the misguided love of the parents may be more harmful to a son with hemophilia than the disorder itself. Therefore, it is essential that the pediatric hemophilia team work together with the families to support and promote normal behavior.

Social care

Hemophilia identification cards

In conjunction with the diagnosis, a patient with hemophilia should be issued with a card that states the type of the disease that the bearer has, and that also provides information about how to contact the hemophilia treatment center. It is important that the patient always carries the card and shows it when consulting a physician or undergoing dental work.

Vaccinations

Children with hemophilia can be vaccinated like any other children, but the vaccines must be given subcutaneously, not intramuscularly. It is recommended not to give concentrate at the same time as a vaccination as a measure to avoid inhibitor development. Moreover, in countries with low-purity concentrates or cryoprecipitates used for treatment, vaccination against hepatitis A and B is recommended.

Day-care center attendance and school

Attending a day-care center is no problem for a child with hemophilia, although it is recommended that the staff of the facility have access to some extra resources. The family has to avoid overprotection, and day care or other activity groups can provide just the social training and stimulation that the child needs. The school staff and students should be informed that a child has hemophilia, preferably by the parents and the child, if necessary together with the staff of the hemophilia center. If adequate prophylaxis is given, no other resources are required for medical reasons, although it is important to coordinate prophylactic treatment with the scheduling of physical education. Also, the study and vocational counselor should be told about any limitations that the disease imposes on the child's choice of profession [39].

Leisure activities

A child with hemophilia who is on adequate prophylaxis can enjoy virtually normal free-time activities, but it is best to steer clear of contact sports that involve a high risk of traumatic events. Regardless of the mode of therapy, parents should be encouraged to stimulate the child's interest in certain suitable sports (such as swimming) at an early age. A baby with haemophilia can wear a protective cap or helmet from the time he begins to stand up and until he has learned to walk steadily. However, as the child grows older, a helmet may be a social stigma that should be avoided. Parents and other people who take care of a young boy with hemophilia should be continually encouraged to observe and focus on the healthy side of the child.

References

1 Schwaab R, Brackmann HH, Meyer C, *et al.* Haemophilia A: Mutation type determines risk of inhibitor formation. *Thromb Haemost* 1995; **74**: 1402–6.

2 Giannelli F, Choo KH, Rees DJ, Boyd Y, Rizza CR, Brownlee GG. Gene deletions in patients with haemophilia B and anti-factor IX antibodies. *Nature* 1983; **303**: 181–2.

3 Gouw SC, van den Berg HM, Oldenburg J, *et al.* F8 gene mutation type and inhibitor development in patients with severe hemophilia A: systematic review and meta-analysis. *Blood* 2012; **119**: 2922–34.

4 Astermark J, Oldenburg J, Pavlova A, Berntorp E, Lefvert AK. Polymorphisms in the IL10 but not in the IL1beta and IL4 genes are associated with inhibitor development in patients with hemophilia A. *Blood* 2006; **107**: 3167–72.

5 Astermark J, Oldenburg J, Carlson J, *et al.* Polymorphisms in the TNFA gene and the risk of inhibitor development in patients with hemophilia A. *Blood* 2006; **108**: 3739–45.

6 Astermark J, Oldenburg J, Escobar M, White GC, II, Berntorp E. The Malmo International Brother Study (MIBS). Genetic defects and inhibitor development in siblings with severe hemophilia A. *Haematologica* 2005; **90**: 924–31.

7 Santagostino E, Mancuso ME, Rocino A, *et al.* Environmental risk factors for inhibitor development in children with haemophilia A: A case–control study. *Br J Haematol* 2005; **130**: 422–7.

8 Gouw SC, van den Berg HM, le Cessie S, van der Bom JG. Treatment characteristics and the risk of inhibitor development: A multicenter cohort study among previously untreated patients with severe hemophilia A. *J Thromb Haemost* 2007; **5**: 1383–90.

9 Gouw SC, van der Bom JG, Marijke van den Berg H. Treatment-related risk factors of inhibitor development in previously untreated patients with hemophilia A: The CANAL cohort study. *Blood* 2007; **109**: 4648–54.

10 Gouw SC, van den Berg HM, Fischer K, *et al.*, and the PedNet and Research of Determinants of INhibitor development (RODIN) Study Group. Intensity of factor VIII treatment and inhibitor development in children with severe hemophilia A: the RODIN study. *Blood* 2013; **121**(20): 4046–55.

11 Goudemand J, Laurian Y, Calvez T. Risk of inhibitors in haemophilia and the type of factor replacement. *Curr Opin Hematol* 2006; **13**: 316–22.

12 Gouw SC, van der Bom JG, Auerswald G, Ettinghausen CE, Tedgard U, van den Berg HM. Recombinant versus plasma-derived factor VIII products and the development of inhibitors in previously untreated patients with severe hemophilia A: The CANAL cohort study. *Blood* 2007; **109**: 4693–7.

13 Gouw SC, van der Bom JG, Ljung R, *et al.*, and the PedNet and RODIN Study Group. Factor VIII products and inhibitor development in severe hemophilia A. *N Engl J Med* 2013; **368**(3): 231–9.

14 Warrier I, Ewenstein BM, Koerper MA, *et al.* Factor IX inhibitors and anaphylaxis in hemophilia B. *J Pediatr Hematol Oncol* 1997; **19**: 23–7.

15 Nilsson IM, Berntorp E, Lofqvist T, Pettersson H. Twenty-five years' experience of prophylactic treatment in severe haemophilia A and B [see comments]. *J Intern Med* 1992; **232**: 25–32.

16 Berntorp E, Boulyjenkov V, Brettler D, *et al.* Modern treatment of haemophilia. *Bull World Health Organ* 1995; **73**: 691–701.

17 Manco-Johnson MJ, Abshire TC, Shapiro AD, *et al.* Prophylaxis versus episodic treatment to prevent joint disease in boys with severe hemophilia. *N Engl J Med* 2007; **357**(6): 535–44.

18 Kreuz W, Escuriola Ettingshausen C, Funk M, Schmidt H, Kornhuber B. When should prophylactic treatment in patients with haemophilia A and B start? The German experience. *Haemophilia* 1998; **4**: 413–17.

19 Astermark J, Petrini P, Tengborn L, Schulman S, Ljung R, Berntorp E. Primary prophylaxis in severe hemophilia should be started early but can be individualized. *Br J Haematol* 1999; **105**: 1109–13.

20 Ljung RC. Intracranial haemorrhage in haemophilia A and B. *Br J Haematol* 2008; **140**: 378–84.

21 Lindvall K, Astermark J, Björkman S, *et al.* Daily dosing prophylaxis for haemophilia: a randomized crossover pilot study evaluating feasibility and efficacy. *Haemophilia* 2012; **18**(6): 855–9.

22 Ljung R. Hemophilia and prophylaxis. *Pediatr Blood Cancer* 2013; **60** (Suppl. 1): S23–6.

23 Björkman S. Prophylactic dosing of factor VIII and IX from a clinical pharmacokinetic perspective. *Haemophilia* 2003; **9**(Suppl. 1): 101–10.

24 Björkman S, Oh M, Spotts G, *et al.* Population pharmacokinetics of recombinant factor VIII: the relationships of pharmacokinetics to age and body weight. *Blood* 2012; **119**(2): 612–18.

25 Hilliard P, Funk S, Zourikian N, *et al.* Hemophilia joint health score reliability study. *Haemophilia* 2006; **12**: 518–25.

26 Pettersson H, Ahlberg A, Nilsson IM. A radiologic classification of hemophilic arthropathy. *Clin Orthop* 1980; **149**: 153–9.

27 Manco-Johnson M, Nuss R, Funk S, Murphy J. Joint evaluation instruments for children and adults. *Haemophilia* 2000; **6**: 649–57.

28 Kilcoyne R, Nuss R. Radiological assessment of haemophilic arthropathy with emphasis on MRI findings. *Haemophilia* 2003; **9**(Suppl. 1): 57–64.

29 Lundin B, Babyn P, Doria AS, *et al.* Compatible scales for progressive and additive MRI assessments of haemophilic arthropathy. *Haemophilia* 2005; **11**: 109–15.

30 Lundin B, Manco-Johnson ML, Ignas DM, *et al.*, and the International Prophylaxis Study Group. An MRI scale for assessment of haemophilic arthropathy from the International Prophylaxis Study Group. *Haemophilia* 2012; **18**(6): 962–70.

31 Martinoli C, Della Casa Alberighi O, di Minno G, *et al.* Development and definition of a simplified scanning procedure and scoring method for Haemophilia Early Arthropathy Detection with Ultrasound (HEAD-US). *Thromb Haemost* 2013; **109**(6): 1170–9.

32 Bullinger M, Von Mackensen S. Quality of life in children and families with bleeding disorders. *J Pediatr Hematol Oncol* 2003; **25**(Suppl. 1): S64–7.

33 Poonnoose PM, Manigandan C, Thomas R, *et al.* functional independence score in haemophilia: a new performance-based instrument to measure disability. *Haemophilia* 2005; **11**: 598–602.

34 van Genderen FR, van Meeteren NL, van der Bom JG, *et al.* Functional consequences of haemophilia in adults: The development of the Haemophilia Activities List. *Haemophilia* 2004; **10**: 565–71.

35 Ljung R. The risk associated with indwelling catheters in children with haemophilia. *Br J Haematol* 2007; **138**: 580–6.

36 Price VE, Carcao M, Connolly B, *et al.* A prospective, longitudinal study of central venous catheter-related deep venous thrombosis in boys with hemophilia. *J Thromb Haemost* 2004; **2**: 737–42.

37 Ettingshausen C, Kurnik K, Schobess R, *et al.* Catheter related thrombosis in children with haemophilia A. Evidence of a multifactorial disease. *Blood* 2002; **99**: 449–500.

38 Santagostino E, Gringeri A, Berardinelli L, Beretta C, Muca-Perja M, Mannucci PM. Long-term safety and feasibility of arteriovenous fistulae as vascular accesses in children with haemophilia: A prospective study. *Br J Haematol* 2003; **123**: 502–6.

39 Chambost H, Ljung R. Changing pattern of care of boys with haemophilia in western European centres. *Haemophilia* 2005; **11**: 92–9.

40 Björkman S, Oh M, Spotts G, *et al.* Population pharmacokinetics of recombinant factor VIII: the relationships of pharmacokinetics to age and body weight. *Blood* 2012; **119**(2): 612–18.

CHAPTER 21

Hemophilia in adolescence

Pia Petrini

Karolinska University Hospital, Stockholm, Sweden

Introduction

Although the terms puberty and adolescence are often used interchangeably, and have some chronological overlap, these terms do not mean the same thing. Puberty is a distinct stage of development marked by substantial hormonal and somatic changes (Figure 21.1 and 21.2).

Adolescence, however, is a broader term used for the time of rapid physical, social, and cognitive development that occurs during the transition from childhood to adulthood, usually between the ages of 10 and 22 years.

The physical aspects of maturation are well characterized in early adolescence and are necessary for the start of psychosocial maturation. Male puberty is characterized by a huge variation between healthy individuals. The average time schedule of male pubertal development is entirely different from that of females. In girls, puberty and growth spurt proceed and continue in a parallel fashion. On average, boys start puberty almost 2 years later and the maximum growth spurt in body height starts even later at mid-puberty, which is 3–3.5 years later than in girls (Figure 21.1). At this age (13–14 years), the developmental differences are the greatest between girls and boys and also between boys. A delayed start of puberty is common in boys in contrast to girls. Duration of pubertal development may also vary from 2 to 5 years. Knowledge about variations in normal puberty in males is crucial to be able to give support during this demanding time when most boys are concerned about their body image and peer acceptance [1].

Psychological changes include identity development. The development of one's identity may include development of body image, personal preferences, and vocational goals. During adolescence, emotional separation from parents and autonomy develop. Peers have a central role in building up the personality during these years. Psychosocial maturation is a slow process usually taking twice the time of physical development. This is a challenging time for any teenager and even more so for those with a chronic disease. For them it is often harder to break family ties, harder to feel accepted by their peer group, and to be realistic about their future.

One unique phenomenon of adolescence is the simultaneous psychosocial progression and regression (Figure 21.2). This phenomenon culminates during mid puberty and is clearly seen in the boy's relation with his parents. During regression, child-like features are again emphasized. Language is often coarse and vulgar with short sentences. Academic performance at school often declines. Clashes with parents and other authority figures are common. In contrast, basic intellectual abilities reach adult levels around the age of 16 years, long before the process of psychosocial maturation is completed. Risk taking and novelty seeking are hallmarks of typical adolescent behavior. Adolescents seek new experiences and higher levels of rewarding stimulation without considering future outcomes or consequences. Indeed, the risk of injury or death is higher during the adolescent period than in childhood or adulthood, and the incidence of depression, anxiety, drug use and addiction, and eating disorders increases Alcohol use may be an expression of their developmental drive to experiment and engage in behaviors with some risk and trying to increase peer socialization. These behaviors likely confer some evolutionary advantage. Increased novelty seeking is a path toward greater experience and knowledge, and increased risk taking may be part of the increased drive for independence during adolescence [2,3].

New brain research has shown connections between brain development and adolescent behavior. These findings indicate that adolescent brain development proceeds over a time period longer than previously thought. Magnetic resonance imaging (MRI) provides unique access to visualizing the brain. The prefrontal cortex is a critical area for higher-order cognitive processes and executive functioning. Executive functions include supervisory cognitive skills needed for goal-directed behavior such as planning and response inhibition. Many of the attributes commonly associated with adolescents, such as risky and impulsive decision-making, are now associated with this immature prefrontal cortex [4].

Textbook of Hemophilia, Third Edition. Edited by Christine A. Lee, Erik E. Berntorp and W. Keith Hoots.
© 2014 John Wiley & Sons, Ltd. Published 2014 by John Wiley & Sons, Ltd.

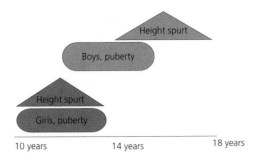

Figure 21.1 Average development of growth and puberty among healthy girls and boys. Girls start puberty at a younger age than boys and the growth spurt starts in a parallel fashion. In an average boy, puberty starts almost 2 years later and body growth start even later at 3–3.5 years after the girls. In an average large classroom, the differences between the largest and smallest boys are about 40 kg and 40 cm in weight and height, respectively. This happens at an age when everybody wants to be similar with their peers.

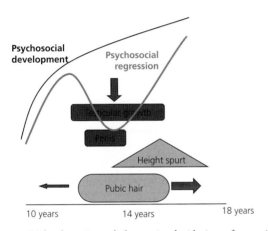

Figure 21.2 Mid-puberty is regularly associated with signs of regression. Regression represent the weakening or even failure of those qualities and skills established in childhood. It culminates during mid-puberty and is in most boys reversible. It is clearly seen in their relationship with their parents.

Issues affecting adolescents with hemophilia

Teens with hemophilia face all of the usual challenges of adolescence, but their life-long bleeding disorder can result in additional issues. Most pediatric services will be very aware of the challenges adolescents bring, and staff will have noticed a change from attentive child to provocative teenager. Before this time, from the preschool years, children should already have been spoken to directly about their treatment, and as they get older there is a greater emphasis and expectation that they will be knowledgeable about their condition and ideally take increasing responsibility for their own care. This includes learning how to mix and self-administer factor, understanding bodily functions: when and why bleeding occurs, how to treat, and when to seek advice and help.

A Scandinavian survey in young men with severe and moderate hemophilia showed that the average age for a patient to take over responsibility for their treatment was 14 years, but 25% of them required parental assistance in hemophilia-related care at the mean age of 17 years. A majority (68%) treated bleedings immediately and 60% used extra infusion when needed. Thus one-third of them did put themselves at risk for complications by their unwillingness to recognize the need for treatment [5].

Poor compliance with hemophilia therapy during adolescence in combination with risky behaviors may result in serious and recurrent bleeding episodes with impact on future outcomes. The teenager may for the first time question their medical regimen and deny the diagnosis. It is crucial to develop an understanding about the social issues regarding disclosure and learning how to balance privacy (i.e. do not tell anyone) versus trust (i.e. tell your friends about your condition) [6].

Normal adolescent development is characterized by experimentation, inconstant behaviour, and a sense of invincibility. Thus, long-term health outcomes promoted by clinical staff can have very little relevance when young people are more concerned about their body image and peer acceptance. It is hardly surprising that compliance reaches its lowest point in adolescence. It is recognized that adolescents are likely to reduce or stop prophylaxis. Teenagers may not perceive prevention of potential future joint disease as a high priority but tend to focus on the present. As short-term goals are more likely to be perceived as relevant substitution therapy to prevent bleeding episodes interfering with daily activities often are more acceptable by the maturing adolescent. Boys with hemophilia who are actively involved in the design of their own tailored prophylactic regimen around "risk periods" in their day-to-day lives (e.g. sport, evenings out, etc.) are more likely to continue treatment to prevent bleeding symptoms. Even daily infusion of factor concentrates can be accepted by young men with regular and frequent sport activities [7,8]. Participation in sporting activities has been shown to increase self-esteem and social adaptation. Better coordination and strength in muscles can reduce intra-articular hemorrhages in persons with hemophilia and physical activity should be encouraged in all adolescences [9,10]. The increasing problem with obesity in the young generation may also contribute to the problems with arthropathy in adults with hemophilia [11].

Prophylactic regimens designed by healthcare professionals are less likely to be complied with if not they do not recognize the individual needs of these boys. Caregivers can support compliance by education, encouragement, and helping these young men to integrate treatment into everyday life.

Transitional care

An increasing number of young people with a chronic illness or disability originating in childhood survive to adulthood, and ultimately these young people need transition to adult care.

Transition medicine is defined as the deliberate, coordinated process of moving a patient from pediatric-oriented to adult-oriented healthcare with the goal of optimizing the young adult's ability to assume adult roles and functions. Health transition is also part of the wider transition from dependent child to independent adult. The transfer of young people, particularly those with special health needs, from child to adult services requires specific attention. Young adults are usually transferred between the ages of 16 and 18 years, or around the time they graduate from secondary education. Moving to adult services is often desired by young people and seen as a logical step, while parents are more anxious [11].

Young people should be helped to take responsibility for medications from as early an age as possible, and should be seen by themselves in clinic visits during their teenage years (with parents invited to join the session later). Parents may find it difficult to step aside, even though they agree it is necessary. A schedule of likely timings and events should be given to young people in early adolescence. Transition guidelines such as those published by the Medical and Scientific Advisory Committee (MASAC) can be very helpful (Table 21.1) Support from peers with hemophilia during camps and meetings are of great impor-

Table 21.1 Checklist items from Medical and Scientific Advisory Committee (MASAC) Guidelines for Transition of People with Bleeding Disorders: Transition guidelines for 16–18 year olds in the category of "Self Advocacy and Self Esteem." (Source: MASAC Document #142: Transition Guidelines for People with Bleeding Disorders. http://hctransitions.ichp.ufl.edu/pdfs/TransitionGuidelines-BleedingDisorders.pdf)

Goals and objectives	Strategies
Young adult expresses medical, physical, and social needs to others	Discuss bleeding disorder/impact on daily living and plans for future
	Young adult should demonstrate and interaction with staff expected
Young adult will be able to advocate and negotiate for health care	Ensure young adult has skills to negotiate needs (travel letter, ER care, PT referral)
Young adult understands rights and responsibilities for health care	Discuss what is expected of the young adult and what can be expected from the health care staff
	Continue discussion re problems with peers or awkward situations (i.e. infusions at school)
Young adult seeks information/ services to ensure ongoing health	Discuss education support (regional, NHF, WFH, Internet)
Young adult understands utilization of the adult health care system	Discuss plans for transition to adult care (primary care/bleeding disorder care). Provide written material as needed
	HTC staff should facilitate introductory visi
	Pediatric staff support may be offered for the first few months of transition

tance and the internet should be recommended for information and communication.

There are cultural differences between the pediatric- and adult-oriented specialities that complicate transfer. Pediatric care is often described as familiar with a relaxed and child-friendly atmosphere where parents are closely involved, while adult care is more focused on responsibility and management. Many young men find it exciting to make a fresh start and build new relationships as they are transferred to the adult team [12].

Transition programs are necessary even when pediatric and adult services are in the same hospital, as geographic closeness often does not translate into a close professional relationship. A joint pediatric–adult clinic is very useful to introduce adolescents to adult physicians and to hand over clinical issues. Joint clinics between pediatric and adult healthcare teams can improve the transfer and help young people to communicate with the new team [13–16].

Poor transition processes can have a significantly negative effect on morbidity and mortality in young adults. Patients can become "lost in transition." For example, Kipps et al. described that attendance of young people at four diabetes services averaged 94% before transfer to an adult clinic, but fell to 57% 2 years after transfer [17]. Adult hemophilia care teams usually have a high level of medical expertise but may be unprepared to the noncompliance with treatment seen in adolescents. Particularly in diseases such as haemophilia, young people with few complications may get little attention from the adult team, who focus their time on older patients with more complications.

Barriers to successful transition are unwillingness of pediatric-oriented providers and parents to "let go" of their youngsters. Obstacles to successful transition may also arise from adolescents themselves, or their parents, if they feel excluded from all decision making in the new setting [18].

There are several ways of effecting transfer of care. None of them is proven to be better than any other, but the transfer should always be planned and expected by the patient and the parents. Future work will include research evaluating models of adolescent support, evaluating and refining the transition checklists, and ensuring that the time is right for each individual.

References

1 Siimes MA, Aalberg V, Petrini P. *Boys with Haemophilia: Physical and Psychosocial Development in Adolescence.* Helsinki, Finland: Nemo Publishers, 2006.
2 Eaton DK, Kann L, Kinchen S, et al. Youth risk behaviour surveillance–US 2009. *MMWR Surveill Summ* 2010; **4**: 59: 1–142.
3 Steinberg L. A dual systems model of adolescent risk-taking. *Curr Dir Psychol Sci* 2007; **16**(2): 55–9.
4 Moreno M. Adolescence extended: Implications of new brain research on medicine and policy. *Acta Paediatr* 2012; Nov 23.

5 Khair K, Colstrup L, Wollter IM, *et al.* The benefits of prophylaxis: views of adolescents with severe haemophilia. *Haemophilia* 2012; **18**: e286–9.

6 Young G. From boy to man: recommendations for the transition process in haemophilia. *Haemophilia* 2012; **18**(Suppl. 5): 27–32.

7 Petrini P, Seuser A. Haemophilia care in adolescence – compliance and lifestyle issues. *Haemophilia* 2009; **15**(Suppl. 1): 15–19.

8 Kadir K, Gibson F, Meerabeau L. Risks and benefits of sports and fitness activitiesfor people with haemophilia. *Haemophilia* 2004; **10**(Suppl. 4): 161–3.

9 Gomis M, Querol F, Gallach JE, *et al.* Exercise and sport in the treatment of haemophilic patients: a systematic review. *Haemophilia* 2009; **15**(1): 43–54.

10 Mulder K, Cassis F, Seuser DR, *et al.* Risks and benefits of sports and fitness activities for people with haemophilia. *Haemophilia* 2004; **10**(Suppl. 4): 161–3.

11 Hofstede FG, Fijnvandraat K, Plug I, Kamphuisen PW, Rosendaal FR, Peters M. Obesity: a new disaster for haemophilic patients? A nationwide survey. *Haemophilia* 2008; **14**: 1035–8.

12 van Staa AL, Jedeloo S, van Meeteren J, Latour JM. Crossing the transition chasm: experiences and recommendations for improving transitional care of young adults, parents and providers. *Child Care Health Dev* 2011; **37**(6): 821–32.

13 Kennedy A, Sloman F, Douglass JA, Sawyer SM. Young people with chronic illness; the approach to transition. *Intern Med J* 2007; **37**: 555–60.

14 Bryon M, Madge S. Transition from paediatric to adult care: psychological principles. *J Roy Soc Med* 2001; **94**(Suppl. 40): 5–7.

15 Mennito SH, Clark JK. Transition medicine: a review of current theory and practice. *Southern Med J* 2010; **103** (4).

16 Kyngas H. Patient education: perspective of adolescents with a chronic disease. *J Clin Nurs* 2003; **12**: 744–51.

17 Kipps S, Bahu T, Ong K, *et al.* Current methods of transfer of young people with type 1 diabetes to adult services. *Diabet Med* 2002; **19**: 649.

18 Tuchman LK. Cystic fibrosis and transition to adult medical care. *Pediatrics* 2010; **125**: 566–73.

CHAPTER 22

Old age medicine and hemophilia

Evelien P. Mauser-Bunschoten and Roger E.G. Schutgens
University Medical Center Utrecht, Utrecht, the Netherlands

Introduction

Life expectancy of patients with hemophilia in industrial countries increased to over 70 years in 2001 [1,2]. In the UK, life expectancy of patients with nonsevere hemophilia in 1999 was 75 years compared to 78 years for the general population; for severe hemophilia this was 63 years [1]. When excluding individuals infected with human immunodeficiency virus (HIV) and hepatitis C virus (HCV), life expectancy of Dutch patients with mild and moderate hemophilia approached that of the male population in general (75 years compared to 76 years), and life expectancy of patients with severe hemophilia increased from 63 years in 1972 to 71 years in 2001 [2].

This implies that hemophilia is no longer a disorder of children and young adolescents. Nowadays, almost half of all patients treated at the van Creveldkliniek, a large hemophilia treatment center for children and adults in the Netherlands, were born before 1967 (Figure 22.1).

Elderly hemophilia patients have different problems compared to the younger generations. They not only have to live with arthropathy, HCV, and/or HIV infection, but a growing number will suffer from comorbidity. Comorbidity is defined as the effect of all other diseases an individual patient might have, other than the primary disease of interest. In the case of the hemophilia patient, this includes internal and cardiovascular diseases, urologic problems, or cancer.

This chapter focuses on age-related comorbidity in the aging hemophilia patient and its consequences.

Internal diseases

Hypertension

Observational studies from the past have shown that hemophilia patients have a higher mean blood pressure, have hypertension twice as often, and use more antihypertensive medication compared to the general population [3]. Recent reports have confirmed these findings. In 709 adult hemophilia patients from the Netherlands and the UK, hypertension was documented in 49% of the patients, as compared to 40% in the general population [4]. Furthermore, the prevalence of hypertension was higher in patients with severe hemophilia as compared to the nonsevere type (odds ratio 1.75). The prevalence of hypertension appears to increase with age: in a cohort study from Italy, hypertension was found in 70% of hemophilia patients aged ≥ 65 years [5]. Similarly, in Dutch patients aged ≥ 59 years, hypertension was found in 76% as compared to 65% in the general population [6]. Another recent study in Dutch adult patients also demonstrated that concomitant obesity further increases the risk of hypertension [7]. In that study, the prevalence of hypertension between nonobese hemophilia patients and controls where 30% and 12%, respectively. In obese subjects, this prevalence increased to 55% and 41%, respectively.

The reason for this increased prevalence of hypertension in hemophilia is not clear. An explanation might be that the incidence of renal insufficiency is higher in patients with hemophilia [8]. This may be caused by renal bleeding in the past, HIV infection, or medication like tranexamic acid or protease inhibitors. Although no relation was found between hypertension and creatinine levels, a trend toward more hypertension in patients with a history of renal bleeding was found [4]. Hypertension increases the risk of myocardial infarction, and adequate treatment is obligatory. Furthermore, hypertension increases the risk of intracranial hemorrhage (ICH). The French ICH study group analyzed 123 ICH episodes in patients with hemophilia, and found that 20 (16.3%) of them occurred in patients >50 years of age [9]. Interestingly, the proportion of patients with severe hemophilia decreased with age (Table 22.1) [9], and in 12.5% of the ICH episodes hypertension was found. The presence of hypertension was not associated with an increased risk of death due to ICH.

Since they are at higher risk of developing hypertension, blood pressure in hemophilia patients should be regularly

Textbook of Hemophilia, Third Edition. Edited by Christine A. Lee, Erik E. Berntorp and W. Keith Hoots.
© 2014 John Wiley & Sons, Ltd. Published 2014 by John Wiley & Sons, Ltd.

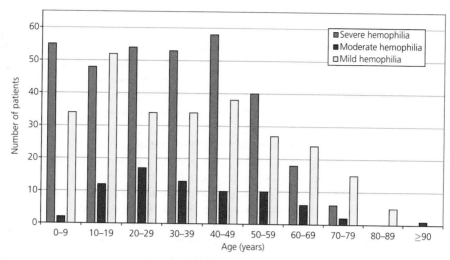

Figure 22.1 Number of patients, according to age and severity of hemophilia, treated at the van Creveldkliniek in 2011 ($n = 727$). Patients > 40 years: 318 (44%).

Table 22.1 Intracranial hemorrhage (ICH) according to age and hemophilia severity [9].

Age group	Proportion of ICH (%)	Proportion of severe hemophilia (%)
0–1 months	8.1	90.0
1–24 months	17.9	90.0
2–15 years	21.1	53.8
15–50 years	36.6	66.7
>50 years	16.3	50.0

checked and hypertension adequately treated. In the absence of other cardiovascular risk factors, a systolic blood pressure $\leq$140 mmHg and a diastolic pressure $\leq$90 mmHg should be pursued. In cases of increased risk for cardiovascular disease, such as in the presence of diabetes mellitus or a positive family history for cardiovascular events, a systolic pressure $\leq$130 mmHg and a diastolic pressure $\leq$80 mmHg should be aimed for.

Renal abnormalities

In the 1970s, renal abnormalities were studied by Prentice *et al.* and Beck and Evans [8,10]. The majority of lesions were seen in the upper renal tract and were apparently the result of clot formation. This may be negatively influenced by the use of tranexamic acid during hematuria. Abnormalities on intravenous pyelography and isotope renography were also found [8]. A more recent publication describes a strong association between hypertension and HIV, and chronic and acute renal disease in hemophilia patients [11]. An association with inhibitors and recent hematuria was described.

The prevalence of urolithiasis is higher in hemophilia patients as compared to controls (odds ratio 17.6) [12]. Furthermore, in this study it was documented that urolithiasis was the cause of recurrent hematuria in 33% of the cases. There is an on-going

multicenter trial (the H3 study) that documents renal function in adult hemophilia patients on a European level. Results are expected in 2013–2014.

Chronic kidney disease is an independent risk factor for cardiovascular disease and is associated with a worse prognosis of cardiovascular disease in nonhemophilic patients [13]. Furthermore, in nonhemophilic patients, traditional cardiovascular risk factors (including older age) are more prevalent in patients with chronic kidney disease.

In elderly hemophilia patients, especially those with hematuria in the past, renal function should be measured annually. In the case of renal dysfunction, referral to a renal specialist might be warranted.

Overweight

Overweight is an increasing problem in the industrial world in hemophilia as well in the general population. A Dutch study revealed that between 1992 and 2001, the prevalence of overweight (body mass index 25–30 kg/m^2) has increased from 27% to 35% in adult Dutch hemophilia patients [14]. However, overweight occurred significantly less frequently in hemophilia patients than in the general Dutch male population, in which the prevalence of overweight was 41% in 1992 and 50% in 2001. The prevalence of obesity (body mass index >30 kg/m^2) doubled from 4% to 8%, which was not significantly decreased compared to the general population (5% in 1992 and 8% in 2001) [14]. As described above, obesity has an impact on the development of hypertension, where prevalence increases from 41% to 55% [7].

A high body mass index is associated with a significant limitation in range of motion (ROM) and with a greater chance of developing a target joint [15]. Obese hemophilia patients score lower in activities of daily life compared to nonobese hemophilia patients [7]. In older patients, mobility is already reduced due to severe arthropathy caused by bleedings in the past [7].

The lack of activity in these patients might increase the body mass index, which in turn influences arthropathy. Overweight and obesity are also associated with hip abnormalities in hemophilia patients [16].

As the body mass index increases with age, the hemophilia patient has a longer life expectancy, and the prevalence of obesity in the general population is foreseen, it might be expected that obesity will occur more frequently within the aging hemophilia population. It is important for hemophilia patients not to be overweight, as increased body weight is a risk factor for the development of diabetes mellitus (DM), atherosclerosis, and cardiovascular disease, and may further damage arthropathic joints due to an increase in weight bearing, which affects activities of daily life. Therefore, regular physical activity should be advised. If functional limitations limit daily activities, a physical therapist familiar with hemophilia may be of help. In some cases referral to a dietitian may be indicated.

Diabetes mellitus

There are several reports on the prevalence of DM in hemophilia. In Canada, a prevalence of 24% in a cohort of hemophilia patients compared to 6.1% in control males was reported [3]. In Dutch hemophilia patients ≥59 years, DM was 9.5% [6]; another report from the Netherlands reported 2% in nonobese patients versus 14% in obese patients [7].

The largest study to date is on 709 adult hemophilia patients from the Netherlands and the UK. The prevalence of DM in hemophilia was 6.1% as compared to 6.3% in the general population and was equal in severe versus nonsevere hemophilia (7.0% vs 5.2%) and Dutch versus UK patients (5.9% vs 6.2%) [17]. In hemophilia patients infected with HIV, the use of highly active antiretroviral therapy (HAART) significantly increased the risk of DM as compared to the general population (24% vs 4%) [17].

Overall, in hemophilia patients not using HAART, there is no reason to assume that the prevalence of DM is different from that of the general population where in HAART-treated patients, the prevalence is increased. In aging hemophilia patients, especially those with overweight, glucose levels should be checked annually. If treatment with insulin is indicated, subcutaneous injections can be applied without bleeding complications.

Cholesterol

Elderly hemophilia patients show significantly lower cholesterol levels than the general population (5.1 vs 5.6 mmol/L) [6]. Lower cholesterol levels are also found in hemophilia patients infected with HIV [17] .

Patients with severe hemophilia have the lowest cholesterol levels, which would suggest an association between low cholesterol concentrations and the clotting factor deficiency or its treatment. Another hypothesis is that viral infections influence both the immune system and liver function, and therefore have an effect on cholesterol levels. This is supported by the observation that chronic HCV is associated with lower cholesterol concentrations [18].

In aging hemophilia patients, cholesterol levels (i.e. total cholesterol, high-density and low-density lipoprotein fraction) should be measured in those who are at risk of developing cardiovascular disease. If increased, treatment is indicated in line with general guidelines.

Osteoporosis

Osteoporosis is an important morbidity factor in patients with hemophilia; it has been primarily linked to arthropathy and reduced weight bearing and is more evident in patients who have had no access to optimal care for joint and muscle bleedings. Number and severity of arthropathic joints are associated with lower bone marrow density in the neck of the femur [19]. Painful hemophilic arthropathy with reduced mobility and lack of activity may lead to a reduction of bone mass. Additional risk factors are chronic HCV which is associated with lower vitamin D levels, HIV, low body mass index, and age [20]. Number and severity of arthropathic joints are associated with lower bone marrow density in the neck of the femur. A correlation was found between long-term prophylaxis and physical activity and bone density.

Osteoporosis can be prevented by adequate exercise with the aim of developing maximum bone marrow density in early adolescence. In older hemophilia patients, a regular exercise programme that incorporates aerobics, strength training, and balance and flexibility activities is helpful in improving functional mobility and reducing the risk of falls, osteoporosis, and osteoporotic fractures [21]. Prophylaxis to prevent joint bleeding, weight-bearing physical activity (sports), physical therapy, surgery to remobilize patients, and calcium and vitamin D supplementation are recommended [22].

Cardiovascular disease

Although several studies report a reduced mortality rate due to ischemic cardiovascular disease in hemophilia patients compared to the general age-matched male population, the number of deaths due to ischemic heart disease is increasing [1,2,23]. In the Netherlands between 1972 and 2001, death caused by ischemic heart disease increased from 2% to 6% [2]. An American study demonstrated that the age-specific prevalence of ischemic heart disease in hemophilia patients ranged from 0.05% in those aged under 30 years to 15.2% in those aged 60 years or older [24].

Although hemophilia patients have a more unfavorable cardiovascular risk profile and hypertension is more frequently seen in this patient group, hemophilia seems to protect against cardiovascular disease [4,17]. Hospital discharge rates for ischemic heart disease in the US were lower compared to age-matched males [24]. A recent study found a lower incidence of nonfatal myocardial infarction in severe hemophilia as compared to controls (1.7% vs 4.0%), where it was similar for nonsevere hemophilia (3.6%) [25]. Other studies, however, found a similar or higher prevalence of heart disease compared to a control group [3,26]. The lower incidence of ischemic heart disease in patients with hemophilia has been attributed to the hypocoaguable state of these patients compared to the general population, leading to a decreased tendency to form occlusive thrombi. Whether the deficiency of coagulation factor VIII or IX also exerts a protective effect on the development of atherosclerosis has been the subject of many trials. Studies concerning intima-media thickness (IMT) in hemophilia patients report conflicting results [27,28]. Using B-mode ultrasound, Srámek *et al.* found no differences in IMT of the carotid artery among patients with bleeding disorders and healthy controls. IMT of the femoral artery was minimally reduced in patients with bleeding disorders compared to controls (adjusted difference 0.078 mm; 95% CI 0.17–0.018 mm). Femoral artery walls were thinnest in individuals with moderate to severe hemophilia [28]. Another study, however, showed that the mean IMT was significantly lower in 50 patients with hemophilia (38 severe, 12 moderate) compared to control subjects [27].

Recently, however, two studies have irrefutably demonstrated that factor VIII deficiency does not protect against the development of atherosclerosis. The first was a study in elderly patients, aged ≥59 years and therefore at high risk for developing atherosclerosis [6]. Forty-two patients were matched with 613 controls and coronary artery calcification (CAC) was measured with a multidetector computed tomography (CT) scan. The amount of CAC was measured in terms of Agatston scores. It appeared that there was no difference between CAC scores of hemophilia patients and controls, nor was there any influence of the severity of hemophilia on the CAC scores.

The second was a study measuring IMT and flow-mediated dilatation (FMD) in 51 obese and 47 nonobese patients and 42 obese and 50 nonobese controls [29]. There were no differences between the groups.

In summary, as hemophilia patients develop atherosclerosis in a similar way as the general population and have an unfavorable cardiovascular risk profile, prevention of cardiovascular disease in hemophilia is of great importance, especially for the nonsevere population. Regular screening programs should be offered to the aging patient, with a focus on hypertension and obesity.

Management

The management of cardiovascular disease is a major challenge. We developed a guideline for the management of cardiovascular disease in 2009. Recently, this guideline has been prospectively evaluated and has proven to be safe and feasible [30]. The main issues are summarized in Table 22.2.

When *cardiac intervention* is needed for coronary syndromes, percutaneous coronary intervention (PCI) with stenting is feasible in hemophilic patients. Adequate clotting factor concentrate (CFC) correction in combination with an adapted anticoagulant

Table 22.2 Decision making in cardiovascular management in hemophilia [30]. Reproduced with permission of John Wiley and Sons.

Antiplatelet therapy	Not in severe patients without prophylaxis
	Dual antiplatelet therapy only when trough levels >0.25 U/L
Therapeutic heparin or vitamin K antagonists	Only when trough levels >0.25 U/L
Access site for coronary intervention	Radial preferred over femoral
Stenting	Bare metal stent preferred over drug-eluting stent
Clotting factor replacement	Peak 0.8 U/L during intervention Trough 0.25 U/L during dual antiplatelet therapy

and antiplatelet therapeutic schedule tailored to the individual patient profile is required, taking into account severity of hemophilia, severity of cardiovascular disease, age, inhibitor status, and renal function. The balance between thrombosis and hemostasis requires a tight cooperation between hemophilia specialists and cardiologists. Both short- and long-term treatment with antiplatelet drugs should be weighed against the increased bleeding risk. In general, antiplatelet medication in patients with hemophilia is feasible, but may sometimes require an adjusted prophylaxis with CFC [27,31].

Stable angina pectoris in patients with mild and moderate hemophilia can be treated with 80 mg aspirin daily. In patients with severe hemophilia using prophylaxis aiming at trough levels of 1%, aspirin can be tried. The use of aspirin should be carefully balanced against the bleeding phenotype of the patient. When bleeding frequency increases, aspirin should be stopped. In our center, we have used aspirin in moderate hemophilia and severe hemophilia patients on prophylaxis successfully without bleeding complications.

Acute coronary syndromes in need of PCI require adequate correction with CFC. We recommend pursuing peak levels of 0.8 U/L and trough levels of 0.45 U/L before PCI and until 48 h after PCI. Higher levels should be avoided in order to prevent occlusive thrombi. During complete CFC correction, heparin can be administered according to standard cardiologic treatment protocols. Glycoprotein IIb/IIIa inhibitors (e.g. abciximab, tirofiban) are used in PCI with stenting and have been used in hemophilia patients [32]. However bivalirudin is reported to be safer than the combination of heparin and glycoprotein IIb/IIIa inhibitors [33].

We prefer to use a radial artery access site for PCI instead of femoral, in order to minimize retroperitoneal or groin bleeds. If a stent is needed, we recommend a bare metal stent (BMS) instead of a drug-eluting stent, as the latter requires prolonged dual antiplatelet therapy with aspirin and clopidogrel. As dual antiplatelet therapy, we recommend an oral loading dose of 600 mg clopidogrel in hemophilia patients before PCI, followed by 75 mg clopidogrel daily for a minimum of 2 weeks after

BMS, in addition to 80 mg aspirin. If possible, a duration of 4 weeks should be pursued. These dosages are the same as in nonhemophilic patients. However, this necessitates the use of CFC aiming at trough levels of 0.25 U/L as long as dual antiplatelet therapy is given. Regular clotting factor level measurements are required to optimize dosing. Once monotherapy with aspirin is continued, replacement therapy is required in patients with severe hemophilia with 12–13 U per kilogram of body weight of factor VIII three times per week or 25 U per kilogram of body weight of factor IX twice a week, aiming at trough levels of >0.01 U/L.

Atrial fibrillation

A European survey among 29 patients showed that the prevalence of atrial fibrillation in hemophilia increases with age: 1.7% in patients >40 years and 3.6% in patients >60 years [34]. Anticoagulation management in these patients is complex. The European Society of Cardiology recommends to anticoagulate based upon the CHADSVASc score: simplified this implicates that a patient with a score of 0 receives no anticoagulation and a patient with 2 or more receives a vitamin K antagonist (VKA) or a new oral anticoagulant. In patients with a score of 1, anticoagulation is preferred over nothing. The mean CHADSVASc score in the European hemophilia survey was 1.3, indicating that hemophilia patients have a generally good risk profile.

Taken together, the assumed lesser thrombotic risk in hemophilia as compared to the general population, the standard use of oral anticoagulation with VKA is not as straightforward as in the general population. We recommend to anticoagulate based upon trough level and CHADS2 risk score. The use of VKA is only recommended in patients with a CHADS2 score of 2 or more, and with high enough trough levels [35]. In all other cases, the patient should either receive aspirin or no anticoagulation at all, depending on hemophilia severity and stroke risk.

Malignancy and surgical interventions

In a large study of hemophilia patients from the USA, prevalence of leukemia, lymphoma, and liver cancer was significantly higher than among American males [36]. This may be due to viral infections. Other studies found a lower rate of fatal malignancies in hemophilia patients not infected with HCV or HIV [37]. With increasing age, patients with hemophilia will develop malignancies and other diseases like prostate hyperplasia, which require biopsy and in some cases surgical intervention. Although information on the management of hemostasis in patients with various malignancies is sparse, in general, treatment is the same as for other patients. When chemotherapy is required, blood counts should be regularly performed and in the case of thrombocytopenia intensive prophylaxis with clotting factor may be indicated [38].

Hemophilia is not a contraindication for medical intervention or surgery, but adequate clotting factor correction is required. Duration and dosage depend on the type of intervention or surgery and severity of hemophilia. Daily measurement of clotting factor levels helps to optimize therapy with CFC. Early mobilization is indicated, not only to prevent deep venous thrombosis, but also to prevent deterioration of pre-existing arthropathy.

Prevention of deep venous thrombosis

Deep venous thrombosis is described in hemophilia patients receiving high doses of CFC during surgical interventions [39,40].

According to local hospital guidelines patients undergoing surgery could be treated with thrombosis prophylaxis with low-molecular-weight heparin according to local protocols, as in patients without hemophilia. Thrombosis prophylaxis should always start *after* complete CFC correction! In addition, compression stockings can be used perioperatively until the patient is fully mobilized.

Tooth extraction

Many elderly hemophilia patients lacked good dental care during their youth, due to their clotting factor deficiencies, and have teeth which are in bad condition, often necessitating tooth extractions. This requires good coordination between dentist or oral surgeon and hematologist.

Clotting factor concentrate correction depends on the number of extractions, the health of the gingiva, and complications during extraction. For uncomplicated extractions, a single infusion with CFC, aiming at a peak level of 50%, in combination with tranexamic acid in a dosage of 1 g four times a day, will do. In patients with severe or moderate hemophilia, CFC should be repeated on the first and fifth day after extraction to prevent late bleeding. To avoid upper airway hematoma, nerve trunk infiltration and general anesthesia may only be given after complete CFC correction. Local application of antifibrinolytics, like Spongostan oral, and silk suturing may further prevent bleeding.

Sexuality

For many people, sexuality is an essential part of wellbeing. People will continue trying to find satisfactory sexual expression and intimacy. Being old is no reason to give up sex. Hemophilia can be accompanied by sexual dysfunction which may include lack of sexual desire or excitement (erection), or sexual response (ejaculation) [41,42].

Pain, or fear of pain, may affect sexual desire. Hemophilic arthropathy may place limitations on sexual intercourse as well. Chronic HCV or HIV itself, or its treatment, can influence sexuality. Fear of transmission, or use of condoms, may decrease sexual desire in a patient or his partner. Hypertension, kidney disease, and heart disease may also have a negative effect.

Communication between healthcare professionals and the patient is important to detect sexual dysfunction. As patients are mostly too shy to bring up the subject, hemophilia caregivers should proactively do so. For counseling the PLISSIT model (permission, limited information, specific suggestions, and intensive therapy) can be used [42]. Analgesics before sexual contact, and specific advice, including positions suitable for various joint problems, may further improve sexual expression. Erection-enhancing medication (e.g. tadalafil, sildenafil, vardefafil) may be useful, but may cause severe nose bleeds. Local application of alprostadil, MUSE (medicated urethral system for erection), or gentle stimulation with a vibrator may be good alternatives. However, intracavernous injections should be avoided and there is a contraindication for vacuum therapy in hemophilia as this may cause penile bleeding.

Psychological problems

Associated with the physical aspects of arthropathy and aging, hemophilia patients become aware of, or suffer from, psychosocial problems. These may be triggered by loss of work, early retirement, decline in health, or altered family dynamics. The patients' network may shrink and informal care may become a problem. Adaptations at home, increased caregiver support, and eligibility of formal caregivers may help the patient to maintain their home situation. But sometimes they have to give up independent life and move to a nursing home. For hemophilia patients, who have fought for self-determination for many years, this can be very dramatic. Conversely, many hemophilia patients have learned to overcome problems with their disease during their youths. These experiences will help them tackle the problems that they may meet when getting older.

Fear during hospitalization

During hospitalization, patients may be confronted with unexpected emotional problems, due to negative experiences in their youth. This may be aggravated by fear. As most patients are manager of their own disease, lack of control, especially during hospitalization, may cause additional stress and emotions. Furthermore, the fact that patients are used to self-infusion may be confusing for medical staff unfamiliar with hemophilia patients. Good information and education by a hemophilia nurse is mandatory.

Quality of life

Quality of life is an important issue in aging hemophilia patients. Several studies indicate that quality of life, especially regarding physical functioning, is reduced compared to the general population, even in patients with mild hemophilia [3,43]. Factors that negatively influence quality of life in these patients are increasing age, severity of hemophilia, the presence of arthropathy, HCV infection, HIV infection, and unemployment. Health-related quality of life (HRQoL) was determined in a cohort of 602 Dutch hemophilia patients [44]. Figure 22.2 shows HRQoL in the general population and in hemophilia patients aged <40 years or >40 years, with or without HCV infection. HRQoL was measured using the RAND-36 questionnaire, assessing eight domains of HRQoL: physical functioning, social functioning, physical wellbeing (e.g. difficulties in daily activities due to physical health problems), emotional wellbeing (e.g. difficulties in daily activities due to emotional problems), mental health, vitality, bodily pain, and general health. Higher scores indicate better quality of life. In hemophilia patients in general, HRQoL was significantly lower for patients aged 40 years or older than for patients aged <40 years in all domains (P value of the Mann–Whitney U test ≤0.001). In patients with a current HCV infection, the only nonsignificant difference between the two age groups occurred in the mental health domain (P value 0.07). All other domains showed significantly worse HRQoL in HCV-infected patients aged 40 years or older, than in patients aged <40 years (adjusted from Posthouwer et al. [44]).

Pain

Pain has a negative effect on quality of life. Wallny et al. studied pain in a group of 91 adult hemophilia patients with a mean age of 43 years. On average, they had four joints with major pain: ankle (45%), knee (39%), elbow (7%), and hip (6%) [45]. Fourteen percent of patients complained of distressing pain in the spine. Fifty per cent of patients had pain throughout the day, when no treatment was given. These findings were confirmed by van Genderen et al. who found that 36% of patients with pain used analgesics [46].

Since pain has an impact not only on quality of life, but also on daily functioning, it has to be addressed adequately. Treatment consists of pain medication, distal traction, transcutaneous electrical nerve stimulation (TENS), and hot packs. Adequate pain medication can be prescribed according to the guideline in Box 22.1 [47]. Since codeine and morphine often lead to constipation, prescription of a laxative is mandatory. Morphine may cause nausea, which improves with time and can be treated with rectal metoclopramide.

Diclophenac and other nonsteroidal anti-inflammatory drugs are theoretically contraindicated and should, in general, be avoided, because they may affect platelet function and may increase bleeding tendency. However, some patients with chronic arthropathic pain may benefit from ibuprofen, without bleeding complications. Rattray et al. reported a positive effect for cyclo-oxygenase 2 (COX-2) inhibitors in chronic pain in a small group of patients with hemophilia [48]. When given in commonly used doses, COX-2 inhibitors do not increase the risk of cardiovascular disease [49].

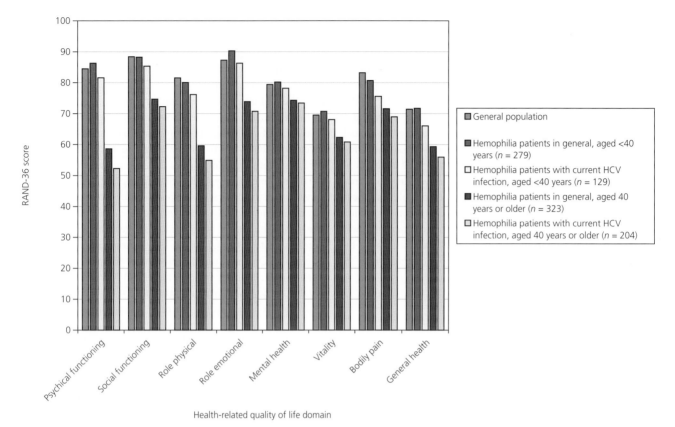

Health-related quality of life domain

Figure 22.2 Health-related quality of life in hemophilia patients in general, and in a subgroup of hemophilia patients with a current hepatitis C (HCV) infection, divided in different age groups, compared with the general population. Adapted from [44]. Obtained from *Haematologica*/the *Hematology Journal* website http://www.haematologica.org). Higher RAND-36 scores indicate better quality of life.

Box 22.1 Strategies for pain management in patients with hemophilia [47]. Reproduced with permission of John Wiley and Sons.

1. Paracetamol/acetaminophen
   If not effective
2. COX-2 inhibitor (e.g. celecoxib, meloxicam, nimesulid)
   OR
   Paracetamol/acetaminophen plus codeine (3–4 times/day)
   OR
   Paracetamol/acetaminophen plus tramadol (3–4 times/day)
3. Morphine: use a slow-release product with an rapid release. Increase the Slow-release product if the rapid release product is used more than 4 times/day

---

Balance dysfunctions and risk of falls

Falls are associated with increased morbidity, mortality, and referral to nursing homes. So far, there is little literature on the problem of falling in patients with hemophilia. According to Rao *et al.*, risk factors for falls include muscle weakness, a history of falls, arthritis (especially of the knee), and

impairment in gait and activities in daily living [50]. In general, patients with hemophilic arthropathy have several of these risk factors.

The most effective preventive strategies are multifactorial interventions targeting identified risk factors, balance training, and exercises for muscle strength.

Conclusion

Comorbidity is quite common in the latter phase of human life, and hemophilia patients are no exception. It may lead to an increase in functional limitations, psychosocial complaints and symptoms, social and societal problems, and a decrease in quality of life. Besides adequate treatment of hemophilic arthropathy, HCV and HIV infection, it is important to look for ways to prevent or reduce comorbidity and improve quality of life. Hemophilia caregivers should play a role in this and during annual check-ups not only pay attention to hematologic aspects of hemophilia, but also to age-related comorbidity, sexuality, and psychosocial problems.

Comorbidity in hemophilia patients may lead to complex treatment. Lack of coordination between various healthcare

In a Nordic multicenter PMS study, 57 patients were enrolled and studied for safety, and 39 of these were evaluated for the efficacy of BDD-rFVIII over a period of 24 months. The hemostatic effect was excellent in 74% and good in 26%. Among patients on regular prophylaxis, 6/30 patients (20%) were free of bleeding during the study term. The median number of bleeding episodes during the 24 months was 4 (range 0–30) [23].

PMS investigations with a newer BDD-rFVIII (Moroctocog alfa, AF-CC, albumin free cell culture) were carried out in 204 subjects [24]. These were double-blind randomized pharmacokinetic cross-over studies. Part 1 targeted PTPs with >150 EDs, and demonstrated equivalence of BDD-rFVIII and a full-length rFVIII (FL-rFVIII, Advate) with respect to pharmacokinetics and the development inhibitors. The half-life of BDD-rFVIII was 11.2 ± 5.0 h and *in-vivo* recovery was $103 \pm 21\%$. A total of 94 patients received regular prophylaxis using a protocol-defined regimen (30 IU/kg, three times a week). Among these, 43 subjects (45.7%) were free of bleeding and 14 subjects did not have spontaneous bleeding. Three subjects developed *de-novo* inhibitors (1.5% in all subjects). They were low titer and transient antibodies.

In addition, a careful retrospective analysis of pharmacokinetic performance, efficacy, and safety in patients switching from FL-rFVIII to BDD-rFVIII was conducted in the UK [37]. No significant differences were observed between half-life measurements during the switch from FL-rFVIII (half-life median 9.15 h, range 6.4–22) to BDD-rFVIII (half-life median 9.7, range 4.7–16.8) and back to FL-rFVIII (half-life median 9.0, range 5.0–19.5). Furthermore, there were no significant differences in the usage of product type or in bleeding [25].

Efficacy for surgical treatment

An open-label clinical study of BDD-rFVIII, administered by either bolus infusion or continuous infusion for hemostatic treatment during surgery, was assessed in 25 patients. Efficacy was rated to be "excellent" or "good" in all cases. The total units of BDD-rFVIII in bolus infusion and continuous infusion were 92 608 and 66 247, respectively. The median preoperative doses for bolus infusion and continuous infusion were 49.3 (range 21.3–72.9) IU/kg and 49.8 (22.9–52.2) IU/kg, respectively. [26]

Incidence of *de-novo* inhibitors using FL-rFVIII and BDD-rFVIII

Reported differences in immunogenicity between FL-rFVIII and BDD-rFVIII are controversial. PTPs are the most appropriate patients to assess the effects of new FVIII therapies on inhibitor development, and Aledort *et al.* conducted a metaanalysis of 29 prospective clinical studies of 3012 PTPs, to examine the incidence of *de-novo* inhibitors in patients treated with the FL or BDD products [27]. A total of 35 *de-novo* inhibitors were observed, and the cumulative hazard for all was 1.25% with a 95% confidence interval of 0.63–1.88%. The rate of high-titer inhibitors (>5 BU) was 0.29% (confidence interval 0.01–0.57%). The risk of *de-novo* inhibitors was higher with exposure to BDD-rFVIII than with FL-rFVIII, and the authors concluded that rFVIII products may differ in immunogenicity.

Recombinant factor VIII concentrates with a longer half-life

The need for frequent infusions of therapeutic products remains a major issue for patients with hemophilia. New rFVIII products with a longer half-life would therefore be a major advance in clinical management. Several strategies have been attempted, including, initially, formulation with pegylated liposomes. Long-acting effects were identified in preclinical and phase I/II studies, but unfortunately, phase III studies did not convincingly confirm the improved efficacy. Recently new technologies based on site-directed pegylation [28], fusion protein linked to the Fc domain of human immunoglobulin [29,30], or the production of single-chain FVIII have been applied to the development of longer acting FVIII concentrates. These various products are currently being assessed in preclinical and clinical investigations. The long-acting effect is reported to be less than that of equivalent rFIX products (see below), but infusion frequency is expected to be reduced to perhaps twice every week or to infusions at night.

More recently, different and novel concepts of hemostatic treatment based on recombinant immunoglobulin have been proposed. For example, antibodies to antitissue factor pathway inhibitor (TFPI) [31] and FVIII mimetic, bi-specific antibodies recognizing FIXa and FX [32] could have dramatic effects of hemostasis in hemophilia *in vivo*. Humanized recombinant antibodies of this nature could have several advantages in overcoming the unresolved issues of classic replacement therapy. The products could be administered by subcutaneous injection, and a longer half-life, up to 2–3 weeks would be expected. In addition, and very importantly, the hemostatic effects of these products would not be restricted in hemophilia A patients with inhibitor.

Recombinant factor IX (BeneFIX)

The unique challenge in the development of rFIX protein for clinical use was the need for post-translational modifications, such as γ-carboxylation, sulfation, and propeptide cleavage. The manufacturing process designed by the Genetics Institute uses a CHO cell line that has been cotransfected with an rFIX cDNA expression plasmid and a cDNA expression plasmid encoding an engineered form of the protease PACE (paired basic amino acid cleaving enzyme). PACE is necessary for the proper cleavage of the signal peptide and secretion of FIX [33].

Another challenge has been to develop a method to eliminate foreign proteins from the production process. Now all CHO cells used in the synthesis of rFIX are grown in serum free medium containing only sucrose, amino acids, salts, recombinant human (rh) insulin, and vitamin K. Thus, a major advantage of the product, nonacog alfa (BeneFIX), is that it is virtually risk free in terms of transmission of bloodborne viruses and spongiform agents [33].

Pharmacokinetic studies

A double-blind randomized cross-over study was conducted in 11 patients with hemophilia B. The elimination half-lives of the rFIX and monoclonal antibody-purified pdFIX were 17.7 and 18.1 h, respectively. *In-vivo* recovery of rFIX, however, was 28% lower than that of pdFIX ($P < 0.05$). This difference was probably due to differences in sulfation of Tyrl55 and phosphorylation of Ser158, suggesting that these residues are important in the clearance of FIX. There was no evidence of increased thrombogenicity using the rFIX in this study [33].

Clinical trials in previously treated patients

An open-label multicenter study to evaluate the long-term safety, efficacy, and pharmacokinetics of rFIX concentrate has been performed. In 55/56 patients, hemostatic efficacy was rated as excellent or good in the majority of bleeding episodes and surgical procedures. Eighty per cent (854/1070) of new bleeding episodes were treated with a single infusion of rFIX. One subject discontinued the study after 1 month of treatment because of repeated bleeding episodes that were difficult to control. This subject's dose appears not to have been adequately titrated.

Another patient developed a low-titer FIX inhibitor after 39 EDs to rFIX. The peak titer was 1 BU/mL and the inhibitor disappeared after 11 months [34]. Clinical responses during 13 different surgical procedures ($n = 24$), including orthotropic liver transplantation, were rated as excellent or good in 97% of cases [34].

Clinical trials in previously untreated patients

By June 1999, 60 PUPs were enrolled in an open-label multinational multicenter study to evaluate safety and efficacy. Seventy-five per cent of all bleeding episodes were managed with a single infusion of *BeneFIX*. In 50 PUPs with follow-up inhibitor assays, two developed high-titer inhibitors (maximum 42 and 18 BU/mL) with anaphylactoid reactions. Complications of this nature are well known to be a unique feature of the FIX inhibitor response in 50% of patients after exposure to any FIX-containing product [35]. In view of the lower *in-vivo* recovery of FIX activity following rFIX infusion, dosage recommendations for BeneFIX are as follows:

Number of FIX units required

$$= \text{body weight (kg)} \times \text{desired FIX increase (\%)} \times 1.2$$

It should be noted that even lower recoveries may be seen in infants and young children.

Postmarketing clinical studies

Nonacog alfa, rFIX, was approved for use in the USA in 1997, in Europe in 1998, and is now universally commercialized. In 2007, reformulated rFIX with iso-osmotic diluent containing 0.234% sodium chloride for minimizing the risk of red blood cell agglutination and reducing the volume to 5 mL was approved.

In accordance with the requirements of the European Medicines Agency an open-label noninterventional prospective observational cohort study (registry) involving 52 sites in nine European countries was conducted between 2002 and 2009. The registry included PMS data for both the original and reformulated rFIX. Two patients developed inhibitors. One was a recurrent inhibitor and had been previously detected in this patient. The other was a *de-novo* inhibitor which developed in a patient with severe hemophilia B after 9 EDs. Eight patients experienced allergic reactions. Two of these were considered to be serious. One patient had a history of anaphylaxis after infusions plasma-derived FIX concentrates in the presence of a FIX inhibitor. The other had no history of allergic reactions or inhibitor. One 71-year-old patient experienced deep venous thrombosis in association with hemostatic therapy after the surgery for spinal stenosis [36].

In general, allergic reactions appear to be associated with the development of a FIX inhibitor. This is not always the case, however. A retrospective study of the incidence of allergic reactions to FIX in the patients with hemophilia B examined the records from 163 patients who had received rFIX. Of these, 88 received pdFIX and 71 received both product types. In total, seven patients (3.89%) experienced allergic reactions. Four of these had been treated with rFIX (3.41%) and three had been treated with pdFIX (1.84%). The allergic reaction in three of those patients who had received rFIX was associated with a FIX inhibitor. Similarly, the adverse event in two of those patients treated with pdFIX appeared to be associated with an inhibitor. These data tended to confirm that allergic reactions were more frequent in those who developed an inhibitor (although not exclusively). The 95% confidence intervals for the incidence of allergic reactions to rFIX and pdFIX were 0.0–3.9% and 1.2–7.5%, respectively, and there were no statistical differences between rFIX and pdFIX in this respect [37].

Longer acting recombinant factor IX products

The strategies devised for producing longer acting rFIX products are basically similar to those for rFVIII, as typified by pegylation [38,39] and fusion with Fc [40,41] or albumin [42]. In preclinical and clinical studies, the half-lives of modified rFIX appeared to be 3–5-fold longer than with nonmodified rFIX. This represents a substantial improvement compared with modified rFVIII (approximately 1.5-fold increase in half-life),

Table 23.2 Current status of clinical studies of longer acting products for hemophilia A and B.

	Name of product	Modification process	Indication	Company	Current status
FVIII	N8-GP (NN7088)	Site-specific pegylation at *O*-glycan site in BDD-rFVIII	HA	NovoNordisk	Phase III
	BAX-855	Random pegylation via lysine residues in full-length rFVIII	HA	Baxter	Phase II/III
	peg rFVIII (BAY 94-9027)	Site-specific cysteine-directed pegylation at cystein residue introduced on BDD-rFVIII	HA	Bayer	Phase III
	rFVIIIFc	BDD-rFVIII linked with Fc of immunoglobulin	HA	Biogen/Idec	Phase III
	CSL 627 rFVIII-SC	Single-chain rFVIII by covalent bond between heavy and light chains	HA	CSL Behring	Phase I/III
FIX	N9-GP (NN7999)	Site-specific pegylation at *O*-glycan site in rFIX	HB	NovoNordisk	Phase III
	rFIXFc	rFIX linked with Fc of immunoglobulin	HB	Biogen/Idec	phase III
	CSL654 rFIX-FP	rFIX linked with albumin	HB	CSL/Behring	Phase II/III
Others	NN7415	Humanized anti-TFPI monoclonal antibodies	HA, HB (inhibitors)	NovoNordisk	Phase I
	ACE910	FVIII mimetic humanized bi-specific antibodies to FIXa and FX	HA (inhibitors)	Chugai	Phase I

BDD, B-domain deleted; FIXa, activated factor IX; FX, factor X; HA/B, haemophilia A/B; rFVIII, recombinant factor VIII; rFIX, recombinant factor IX.

and it is possible that infusions of, for example, rFIXFc or glyco-PEGylated rFIX (N9 GP) every 2 weeks may be sufficient to maintain trough FIX activity levels greater than 1–2 IU/dL. Initial phase III studies of longer acting rFVIII and rFIX products have been completed (Table 23.2).

Future prospects

The impact of the improved effect *in vivo* of longer acting proteins is more evident with rFIX (3–5 times longer half-life) than with rFVIII (1.5 times longer half-life). The classicl concept of hemostatic treatment for patients with hemophilia may not be entirely appropriate for the new products, and major changes in therapeutic protocols seem likely to be required when these longer acting concentrates, especially modified rFIX, are produced commercially on a larger scale. Levels of 5–10 IU/dL FIX activity may be readily achieved, and simple overall protocols may not be practical in view of the wide variation in specific clinical symptoms and individual physical activity. More personalized and tailor-made dosing protocols will be required. Furthermore, some of the greatest difficulties that have emerged with the increasing use of recombinant proteins for the treatment of hemophilia have been associated with cost and currency exchange rates. These have led to a complex debate, especially regarding the limited availability of these products in less developed countries. Finally, the relationship between inhibitor development and product type in particular remains controversial, and immunogenicity should be carefully and thoroughly investigated in well-organized protocols when the new FVIII or FIX therapeutic materials become more widely available.

Acknowledgments

The authors of this chapter are supported by grants both from the Ministry of Health, Labour and Welfare, Research on Regulatory Science of Pharmaceuticals and Medical Devices, and the Blood Products Research Organization, Japan.

References

1 White GC, McMillan CW, Kingdon HS, Shoemaker CB. Use of recombinant antihemophilic factor in the treatment of two patients with classic hemophilia. *N Engl J Med* 1989; **320**: 166–70.

2 Schwartz RS, Abildgaard CF, Aledort LM, *et al.* Human recombinant DNA-derived antihemophilic factor (factor VIII) in the treatment of hemophilia A. *N Engl J Med* 1990; **323**: 1800–5.

3 Abshire TC, Brackmann H-H, Scharrer I, *et al.* Sucrose formulated recombinant human antihemophilic factor FVIII is safe and efficacious for treatment of hemophilia A in home therapy. *Thromb Haemost* 2000; **83**: 811–16.

4 Musso R, Santagostino E, Faradji A, *et al.* Safety and efficacy of sucrose-formulated full-length recombinant factor VIII; experience in the standard clinical setting. *Thromb Haemost* 2008; **99**: 52–8.

5 Giangrande PLF, for the Kogenate Bayer Study Group. Safety and efficacy of Kogenate Bayer in previously untreated patients (PUPs) and minimally treated patients (MTPs). *Haemophilia* 2002; **8**(Suppl. 2): 19–22.

6 Kreuz W, Gill JC, Rothschild C, *et al.* Full-length sucrose-formulated recombinant factor VIII for treatment of previously untreated or minimally treated young children with severe hemophilia A: Results of an international clinical investigation. *Thromb Haemost* 2005; **93**: 457–67.

7 Delumeau JC, Ikegawa C, Yokoyama C, Haupt V. An observational study of sucrose-formulated recombinant factor VIII for Japanese patients with hemophilia A. *Thromb Haemost* 2008; **100**: 32–7.

8 Rubinger M, Lillicrap D, Rivard GE, *et al.* A prospective surveillance study of factor VIII inhibitor development in the Canadian hemophilia A population following the switch to a recombinant factor VIII product formulated with sucrose. *Haemophilia* 2008; **14**: 281–6.

9 Lusher JM, Scharrer I. Evolution of recombinant factor VIII safety: KOGENATE and Kogenate FS/Bayer. *Int J Hematol* 2009; **90**: 446–54.

10 White GC, Courter S, Bray GL, *et al.* A multicenter study of recombinant factor VIII (Recombinate) in previously treated patients with hemophilia A. *Thromb Haemost* 1997; **77**: 660–7.

11 Blanchette VS, Shapiro AD, Liesner RJ, *et al.* Plasma and albumin-free recombinant factor VIII: Pharmacokinetics, efficacy and safety in previously treated pediatric patients. *J Thromb Haemost* 2008; **6**: 1319–26.

12 Negrier C, Shapiro A, Berntorp E, *et al.* Surgical evaluation of recombinant factor VIII prepared using a plasm/albumin-free method: Efficacy and safety of Advate in previously treated patients. *Thromb Haemost* 2008; **100**: 217–23.

13 Bray GL, Gomperts ED, Courter S, *et al.* A multicenter study of recombinant factor VIII (Recombinate): Safety, efficacy, and inhibitor risk in previously untreated patients with hemophilia A. *Blood* 1994; **83**: 2428–35.

14 Tarantino MD, Collins PW, Hay CR, *et al.* Clinical evaluation of an advanced category antihaemophilic factor prepared using a plasma/albumin-free method: pharmacokinetics, efficacy, and safety in previously treated patients with hemophilia A. *Haemophilia* 2004; **10**: 428–37.

15 Blanchette VS, Shapiro AD, Liesner RJ, *et al.* Plasma and albumin-free recombinant factor VIII: pharmacokinetics, efficacy and safety in previously treated pediatric patients. *J Thromb Haemost* 2008; **6**: 1319–26.

16 Oldenburg J, Goudemand J, Valentino L, *et al.* Postauthorization safety surveillance of ADVATE [antihaemophilic factor (recombinant), plasma/albumin-free method] demonstrates efficacy, safety and low-risk for immunogenicity in routine clinical practice. *Haemophilia* 2010; **16**: 866–77.

17 Kelley B, Jankowski M, Booth J. An improved manufacturing process for Xyntha/ReFacto AF. *Haemophilia* 2010; **16**: 717–25.

18 Lusher JM, Lee CA, Kessler CM, Bedrosian CL, for the Refacto 3 Study Group. The safety and efficacy of B domain deleted recombinant factor VIII concentrate in patients with severe hemophilia A. *Haemophilia* 2003; **9**: 38–49.

19 Recht M, Abshire T, Lusher J, *et al.* Results of a single-dose randomized, double-blind, 2-period crossover pharmacokinetic study of b-domain deleted recombinant FVIII (BDDrFVIII), current manufacturing process (REFACTO) and BDDrFVIII, Albumin-free manufacturing process (REFACTO AF). *Blood* 2003; **102**: Abstract 2942.

20 Recht M, Nemes L, O'Brein AC, *et al.* ReFacto AF is effective and safe in previously treated patients with hemophilia A: Final results of a pivotal phase III study. *Blood* 2007; **110**: Abstract 1151.

21 Smith MP, Giangrande P, Pollman H, *et al.* A postmarketing surveillance study of the safety and efficacy of ReFacto (St Louis-derived active substance) in patients with hemophilia A. *Haemophilia* 2005; **11**: 444–51.

22 Di Paola J, Smith MP, Klamroth R, *et al.* ReFacto and Advate: a single-dose, randomized, two-period crossover pharmacokinetics study in subjects with hemophilia A. *Haemophilia* 2007; **13**: 124–30.

23 Petrini P, Rylander C. Clinical safety surveillance study of the safety and efficacy of long-term home treatment with ReFacto utilizing a computer-aided diary: a Nordic multicentre study. *Haemophilia* 2009; **15**: 175–83.

24 Recht M, Nemes L, Matysiak M, *et al.* Clinical evaluation of moroctocog alfa (AF-CC), a new generation of B-domain deleted recombinant factor VIII (BDDrFVIII) for treatment of hemophilia A: demonstration of safety, efficacy, and pharmacokinetic equivalence to full-length recombinant factor VIII. *Haemophilia* 2009; **15**: 869–80.

25 Rea C, Dunkerley A, Sørensen B, Rangarajan S. Pharmacokinetics, coagulation factor consumption and clinical efficacy in patients being switched from full-length FVIII treatment to B-domain-deleted r-FVIII and back to full-length FVIII. *Haemophilia* 2009; **15**: 1237–42.

26 Windyga J, Rusen L, Gruppo R, *et al.* BDDrFVIII (Moroctocog alfa [AF-CC]) for surgical hemostasis in patients with hemophilia A: results of a pivotal study. *Haemophilia* 2010; **16**: 731–9.

27 Aledort LM, Navickis RJ, Wilkes MM. Can B-domain deletion alter the immunogenicity of recombinant factor VIII? A meta-analysis of prospective clinical studies. *J Thromb Haemost* 2011; **9**: 2180–92.

28 Mei B, Pan C, Jiang H, *et al.* Rational design of a fully active, long-acting PEGylated factor VIII for hemophilia A treatment. *Blood.* 2010; **116**: 270–9.

29 Powell JS, Josephson NC, Quon D, *et al.* Safety and prolonged activity of recombinant factor VIII Fc fusion protein in hemophilia A patients. *Blood* 2012; **119**: 3031–7.

30 Dumont JA, Liu T, Low SC, *et al.* Prolonged activity of a recombinant factor VIII-Fc fusion protein in hemophilia A mice and dogs. *Blood* 2012; **119**: 3024–30.

31 Hilden I, Lauritzen B, Sørensen BB *et al.* Hemostatic effect of a monoclonal antibody mAb 2021 blocking the interaction between FXa and TFPI in a rabbit hemophilia model. *Blood* 2012; **119**(24): 5871–8.

32 Kitazawa T, Igawa T, Sampei Z, *et al.* A bispecific antibody to factors IXa and X restores factor VIII hemostatic activity in a hemophilia A model. *Nat Med* 2012; **18**: 1570–4.

33 White GC, Beebe A, Nielsen B. Recombinant factor IX. *Thromb Haemost* 1997; **78**: 261–5.

34 White GC, Shapiro A, Ragni M, *et al.* Clinical evaluation of recombinant factor IX. *Semin Hematol* 1998; **35**(Suppl. 2):33–8.

35 Warrier I. Factor IX inhibitor and anaphylaxis. In: Rodriguez-Merchan EC, Lee CA (eds.) *Inhibitors in Patients with Hemophilia.* Oxford: Blackwell Science, 2002: 87–91.

36 Berntorp E, Keeling D, Makris M, *et al.* A prospective registry of European hemophilia B patients receiving nonacog alfa, recombinant human factor IX, for usual use. *Haemophilia* 2012; **18**: 503–9.

37 Recht M, Pollmann H, Tagliaferri A, *et al.* A retrospective study to describe the incidence of moderate to severe allergic reactions to factor IX in subjects with hemophilia B. *Haemophilia* 2011; **17**: 494–9.

38 Østergaard H, Bjelke JR, Hansen L, *et al.* Prolonged half-life and preserved enzymatic properties of factor IX selectively PEGylated

on native N-glycans in the activation peptide. *Blood* 2011; **118**: 2333–41.

39 Negrier C, Knobe K, Tiede A, Giangrande P, Møss J. Enhanced pharmacokinetic properties of a glycoPEGylated recombinant factor IX: a first human dose trial in patients with hemophilia B. *Blood* 2011; **118**: 2695–701.

40 Peters RT, Low SC, Kamphaus GD, *et al.* Prolonged activity of factor IX as a monomeric Fc fusion protein. *Blood* 2010; **115**: 2057–64.

41 Shapiro AD, Ragni MV, Valentino LA, *et al.* Recombinant factor IX-Fc fusion protein (rFIXFc) demonstrates safety and prolonged activity in a phase 1/2a study in hemophilia B patients. *Blood* 2012; **119**: 666–72.

42 Metzner HJ, Weimer T, Kronthaler U, Lang W, Schulte S. Genetic fusion to albumin improves the pharmacokinetic properties of factor IX. *Thromb Haemost* 2009; **102**: 634–44.

CHAPTER 24

Products used to treat hemophilia: plasma-derived coagulation factor concentrates

Paul L.F. Giangrande
Churchill Hospital, Oxford, UK

Introduction

The development of blood products for the treatment of hemophilia has dramatically altered the prognosis for those patients who live in affluent countries and have regular access to safe products. The median life expectancy for people with severe hemophilia increased fivefold from only 11 years during the period 1831–1920 to 56.8 years during the period 1961–1980 [1]. In more recent years, infection with human immunodeficiency virus (HIV) and hepatitis C virus (HCV) has had a significant negative impact. Access to treatment also improves the quality of life of patients, at least in part by facilitating access to normal education and employment [2].

In recent years, the relative merits of plasma versus recombinant products have been a major topic of debate. The arguments focus primarily on safety with regard to transmission of pathogens which must be of prime concern in the selection of products for the treatment of hemophilia. However, the relative immunogenicity of the two classes of product has also been a subject of controversy. It has also been suggested that plasma-derived products may be more effective than recombinant products in achieving immune tolerance in patients with inhibitors.

The cost of recombinant factor VIII concentrates has fallen significantly in recent years, and is now similar to that of plasma products. A recent survey conducted in Europe showed that plasma-derived products are still used more widely than recombinant ones [3]. It is clear that there will continue to be a global requirement for plasma-derived as well recombinant coagulation factor concentrates for many years to come. One important positive consequence of the gradual but progressive switch to recombinant products in developed countries is that this has helped to secure effective and safe treatment for people in developing countries. As patients in more affluent parts of the world as North America, Europe, Australia, and Japan switch to recombinant products, manufacturers of plasma-derived products are seeking new markets in the developing world where concentrates have needed to be competitively priced.

Cryoprecipitate

Although coagulation factor concentrates are now regarded as the treatment of choice for hemophilia in developed countries, it must be recognized that cryoprecipitate still forms the mainstay of treatment for patients in many less affluent countries around the world. The discovery by Judith Pool in 1965 that a fraction of thawed plasma contained factor VIII was a major landmark in the development of products for the treatment of hemophilia [4].

Cryoprecipitate is prepared by slow thawing of fresh frozen plasma (FFP) at 4°C for 24 h, when cryoprecipitate appears as an insoluble precipitate and separated by centrifugation. It contains significant quantities of factor VIII, von Willebrand factor (VWF), fibrinogen, and factor XIII (but not factor IX or XI). Current AABB (American Association of Blood Banks) standards call for a minimum standard of 80 IU factor VIII per pack (and 150 mg fibrinogen). However, in practise the coagulation factor content of individual packs in developing countries is variable and is usually not controlled.

The most significant problem with cryoprecipitate is that it cannot be easily subjected to viral inactivation procedures (such as heat or solvent/detergent treatment) and this inevitably translates into a risk of transmission of viral pathogens which is not insignificant with repeated exposure. For example, a study based on data from Venezuela estimated a cumulative risk of 40% for HIV and almost 100% for HCV over a lifetime (60 years) of treatment with cryoprecipitate [5]. The use of this product in the treatment of congenital bleeding disorders cannot therefore be recommended in countries which can afford coagulation factor concentrates.

Textbook of Hemophilia, Third Edition. Edited by Christine A. Lee, Erik E. Berntorp and W. Keith Hoots.
© 2014 John Wiley & Sons, Ltd. Published 2014 by John Wiley & Sons, Ltd.

Certain steps can at least be taken to minimize the risk of transmission of viral pathogens. These include careful selection of donors to eliminate and producing packs from single donors. Once collected, the plasma should be quarantined until the donor has been recalled and retested for markers of infection: if the donor does not return, the plasma should not be used. Polymerase chain reaction (PCR) testing is a technology which has a potentially much greater relevance for the production of cryoprecipitate than concentrates, as the latter are subjected to viral inactivation steps. Quality control, involving the monitoring of factor VIII content, is also very important. A method for solvent/detergent treatment of cryoprecipitate has recently been developed for application in the developing world which should help to make this product safer [6].

Much of what has been written about cryoprecipitate applies to the use of FFP, which is a source of all coagulation factors. As it contains factor IX, it is still used for the treatment of hemophilia B in countries unable to afford the use of plasma-derived factor IX concentrate. Packs of FFP subjected to some form of virucidal treatment (including solvent/detergent treatment) are already available. The possibility of severe allergic reactions to infused plasma, including transfusion-related acute lung injury (TRALI) attributed to cytotoxic antibodies of donor origin in the infused plasma, have been recognized for some time [7,8]. An additional benefit of solvent/detergent treated FFP is a significant decrease in the incidence of such allergic reactions [9].

Principles of manufacture

There are some common steps involved in the manufacture of coagulation factor concentrates. Plasma proteins such as albumin, coagulation factor concentrates, and immune globulin preparations are manufactured from large pools of human plasma, primarily by the Cohn cold ethanol fractionation method. This method, developed by Edwin Cohn in Boston in the 1940's, involves the sequential precipitation of specific proteins under varying conditions of ethanol and pH conditions.

In the case of factor VIII, cryoprecipitate is produced using a standard ethanol/dry ice process for snap freezing and the cryoprecipitate is extracted by thawing in a 4°C. Antihemophilic factor (AHF) is extracted from the cryoprecipitate by dissolving in a buffer. Fibrinogen is removed from the resulting supernatant by precipitation, followed by precipitation of factor VIII from supernatant. Factor VIII is then purified by chromatographic techniques, either using ion-exchange chromatography or immunoaffinity chromatography.

Factor IX is prepared by anion-exchange chromatography in the presence of heparin, applied to cryoprecipitate-depleted plasma, or the use of immunoaffinity chromatography.

The coagulation protein (factor VIII or IX) protein is then freeze-dried and lyophilized concentrate bottled under sterile conditions. At some stage, either as a final step or during the manufacturing process, a specific virucidal step such as heat treatment and/or solvent/detergent treatment is applied (see below).

Quality control is an essential element in the manufacturing process, and each batch of product is randomly sampled and analysed for factor VIII (or IX) clotting activity, electrolyte concentration, pyrogenicity, sterility, and toxicity. The bottles are labelled with a batch number and bottle number before being issued for use only if all release parameters are satisfied. Regulatory agencies such as the American Food and Drug Administration (FDA) and the European Medicines Agency (EMA) generally conduct some form of independent oversight of this process by routine monitoring of the manufacturers' test results or by conducting their own tests.

The plasma used for fractionation may be recovered plasma, typically derived from whole blood procured from volunteer donors, or source plasma, usually collected form paid donors who undergo periodic plasmapheresis. In the past, plasma for fractionation from paid donors was considered to be at higher risk of viral infection than plasma from voluntary donors drawn from the same population. However, this can no longer be considered to be the case. Donor selection procedures are designed to identify and exclude donors at risk of being infected with pathogenic viruses. Exclusion criteria include a history of bloodborne infection, intravenous drug use, and high risk sexual behavior. The quarantining of plasma until a donor appears for retesting (inventory hold) is an additional precaution which may be taken. Nucleic acid testing (NAT) is now routinely employed by an increasing number of manufacturers for detection of a wide range of viruses including HIV, HCV, parvovirus B19, and both hepatitis A and B.

The establishment of a "plasma master file" for plasma-derived products is a concept which has been pioneered by the European regulatory authorities (EMA). This contains details of all donations in a batch of products. This permits tracing of blood donations through the screening procedure right up to intravenous administration. Within Europe, the plasma master file replaces that part of the marketing authorization application (MAA) describing the raw material plasma and makes the arrangements for movement of plasma, intermediates, and products across member states both easier and more transparent. Two particular issues deserve further consideration: purity of product and the number of virucidal steps.

Product purity

Product purity should not be confused with concentrate safety or efficacy. Purity simply refers to the percentage of the desired ingredient (e.g. factor VIII) in concentrates relative to other ingredients present. Concentrates on the market vary widely in their purity from around 5.0 IU factor VIII/mg protein in intermediate-purity concentrates to 2000 in the case of high-purity concentrates. Generally, products which are produced at higher purity tend to be associated with low manufacturing yields and therefore cost more. High-purity products are more readily soluble, which is more convenient for home treatment and also facilitates administration by continuous infusion if desired in the setting of surgery. The incidence of allergic reactions is also probably lower with high-purity products. However, there is no clear evidence that modern high-purity concentrates offer a higher margin of safety with regard to transmission of pathogens.

The relative immunogenicity of recombinant and plasma-derived factor VIII concentrates has been a source of ongoing debate and controversy. It is clear that the principal determinant of inhibitor development is the underlying molecular abnormality, with large deletions and nonsense mutations being associated with a particularly high risk. It has been hypothesized that the presence of VWF and other proteins in plasma-derived products may confer beneficial immunomodulatory benefits on such products [10]. A large retrospective systematic review found no clear incidence of an increased risk of inhibitor development amongst previously untreated patients who received recombinant products [11]. An ongoing international prospective study of previously untreated patients aims to provide a definitive answer to this question [12]. For similar reasons, it has also been suggested that plasma-derived products may be more effective in achieving immune tolerance in patients who develop inhibitors [13]. The Rescue Immune Tolerance Study (RESIST) study will compare the outcome of immune tolerance in relation to the purity of the product used. A separate analysis in the study will focus specifically on the outcome of using plasma products in the subset of patients who have already failed to achieve tolerance with high-purity products [13,14].

Several studies have suggested that the use of high-purity concentrates retards the decline in CD4+ lymphocyte counts in HIV individuals, but this has not been a consistent finding [15,16]. However, it has not been clearly demonstrated that any resulting change in CD4+ lymphocyte numbers is associated with a slowing in the rate of progression to acquired immune deficiency syndrome (AIDS) or death and any such positive effect of high-purity products is insignificant when compared to the immune reconstitution associated with antiretroviral therapy.

None of the brands of high-purity plasma-derived factor VIII or recombinant concentrates contain VWF. The fact that less pure factor VIII concentrates usually contain significant quantities of VWF means that it may also be useful in the treatment of von Willebrand disease. Examples of concentrates suitable for the treatment of von Willebrand disease include Optivate and 8Y (BPL), Alphanate and Fanhdi (Grifols), Haemate P (CSL Behring), Wilate (Octpharma), and Wilfactin (LFB) [17].

In the case of factor IX concentrates, high-purity concentrates have been shown to induce less activation of coagulation than prothrombin complex concentrates [18]. The latter should no longer be employed in the routine management of hemo-

philia B in view of case reports of thrombosis (including venous thromboembolism, disseminated intravascular coagulation, and myocardial infarction) associated with their use [19,20]. There is no suggestion of an increased risk of inhibitor development associated with recombinant factor IX compared to that seen with plasma-derived factor IX [21].

Methods of viral inactivation and elimination

The introduction of heat treatment and solvent/detergent treatment using such agents as tri(n-butyl)phosphate (TNBP) and Triton X-100 in the mid-1980s effectively eliminated the risk of transmission of HIV and HCV through the use of plasma-derived products [22,23]. It has since proved to be highly effective against a wide range of newly emerged viral pathogens with a lipid envelope such as West Nile virus, the severe acute respiratory syndrome (SARS) coronavirus and avian influenza [24,25]. However, solvent/detergent treatment with such agents as TNBP and Triton X-100 does not inactivate nonenveloped viruses such as hepatitis A [26]. Furthermore, some viruses (such as human parvovirus B19 virus) are relatively resistant to both types of physical process. Whilst infection with parvovirus is rarely of clinical significance, it is naturally of concern that this hardy DNA virus is resistant to physical virucidal treatments [27].

All virus inactivation and removal steps have their limitations. It is recommended that two distinct and effective steps that are complementary be incorporated into the plasma product manufacturing process [28]. European guidelines recommend that at least one step effectively inactivates or removes nonenveloped viruses. A 2001 recommendation from the Committee for Proprietary Medicinal Products (CPMP) states that: "for all plasma-derived medicinal products, it is an objective to incorporate effective steps for inactivation/removal of a wide range of viruses of diverse physico-chemical characteristics. In order to achieve this, it will be desirable in many cases to incorporate two distinct effective steps which complement each other in their mode of action such that any virus surviving the first step would be effectively inactivated/removed by the second. At least one of the steps should be effective against non-enveloped viruses. Where a process step is shown to be reliably effective in inactivating or removing a wide range of viruses including enveloped and non-enveloped viruses of diverse physico-chemical characteristics and the process contains additional stages reliably contributing to the inactivation/removal of viruses, a second effective step would not be required" [28]. It is recommended that all patients receiving plasma-derived concentrates be vaccinated against hepatitis A and B as an additional precaution [29].

The UK was the center of a large outbreak of bovine spongiform encephalopathy (BSE) in cattle which started in 1985. It is now accepted that variant Creutzfeldt–Jakob (vCJD) in humans

Table 25.1 Treatment of hemarthrosis with low doses of factor VIII and IX. Reproduced from [1].

Dose (U/kg body weight)	Factor plasma level (%)	Number of treated episodes	Success rate (%)	Therapeutic material	Type of bleed	References
23	24–33	25	56–64	Cryo	Hemarthrosis	[27]
20–30	40–50	51	92	FVIII, other	Hemarthrosis	[26]
10		51	96	FVIII	Hemarthrosis	[13]
7–9		106	90	FVIII	Hemarthrosis	[28]
11–13		173	79			
15–17		64	94			
8–12		62	100	FVIII	Hemarthrosis, other	[29]
7.5–12.5	15–25	196	89	FVIII	Hemarthrosis, other	[30]
12.5–20	25–40	349	94			
3–7		60	100	FVIII/FIX	Hemarthrosis	[31]
31	53	144	99	Cryo	Hemarthrosis, other	[32]
7		119	73	FVIII, other	Hemarthrosis	[33]
14		134	75			
28		86	64			
11–16		144	78	FVIII, other	Hemarthrosis	[34]
7		95	89	FVIII	Hemarthrosis	[35]
14		106	77			

Table 25.2 Guidelines for factor replacement in severe and moderate hemophilia A and B. Reproduced from [1].

Site of hemorrhage	Optimal factor level (%)	Dose (U/kg body weight)		Duration (days)
		Factor VIII	Factor IX	
Joint	30–50	15–25	30–50	1–2
Muscle	30–50	15–25	30–50	1–2
Gastrointestinal tract	40–60	30–40	40–60	7–10
Oral mucosa	30–50	15–25	30–50	Until healing
Epistaxis	30–50	15–25	30–50	Until healing
Hematuria	30–50	15–25	30–50	Until healing
Central nervous system	80–100	50	80–100	10–21
Retroperitoneal	50–100	30–50	60–100	7–14
Trauma or surgery	50–100	30–50	60–100	Until healing

kilogram of body weight will raise the plasma FIX by 0.01 U/mL. Much of the difference in expected recovery between FVIII and FIX is a result of variable volumes of distribution. FVIII circulates almost exclusively intravascularly and FIX diffuses into the extracellular water space [14]. Thus, to correct for interpatient variability after infusion of FVIII and FIX products, individual pharmacokinetic studies can be performed to optimize dosing.

The dose needed to achieve hemostasis varies widely and choice of dose needs to be calculated taking into account a number of parameters: severity of the bleeding episode; pharmacologic properties of the clotting factors, which include the half-life; and the *in-vivo* recovery based on the volume of distribution within the vascular compartments. The doses suggested in Table 25.2 serve as a guide to calculate the approximate amount required and are not based on randomized clinical trials. Therapeutic infusion of replacement factor should be administered as early as possible in an attempt to prevent permanent damage to joints and soft tissues and

should continue until adequate hemostasis has been achieved or wound healing is complete. Bleeding complications in association with surgical procedures can be seen in 4–23% of cases, usually in the postoperative period rather than during the surgery [15–18].

Factor replacement can be administered by either intermittent bolus or continuous infusion (CI). Some advantages of the latter include: total factor use may decrease by as much as 30% [19,20]; achievement of a faster steady state in plasma; maintenance of a constant therapeutic factor level; and avoidance of peaks and troughs, which facilitates laboratory monitoring [21]. Of note, when CI is started, the dose needed is often higher during the first few postoperative days because of the rapid clearance of the factor in the immediate postoperative period [22].

Ideally, for individuals who must undergo elective major surgical procedures, an *in-vivo* recovery and half-life study should be performed during a non-bleeding state with a 3–5 half-life wash-out period. A dose of the therapeutic product to increase the plasma level to 100% should be used and samples for factor activity should be drawn at times 0, 30 min, 60 min, 3 h, 6 h, 9 h, 24 h, 28 h, 32 h, and 48 h postinfusion. For FIX, additional time points at 50 and 72 h should be drawn given the longer half-life [23].

Based on the pharmacokinetic study of the individual, an initial "loading" dose and subsequent doses can be calculated. For example, in an individual with FVIII deficiency and a normal recovery and half-life, factor dosing can be calculated as follows. Assuming that 8–12 h after the initial bolus the plasma level will decrease by about 50%, further doses can be given of one-half of the loading dose every 8–12 h. If CI is employed, the initial loading dose should be divided by 12, which is equal to the number of units per hour of FVIII concentrate. CI is usually started immediately following the initial bolus administration. For example, to raise the FVIII level to 100% in a 70-kg individual with <1% activity, the initial loading dose will be 3500 units followed by boluses of 1750 units every 8–12 h. For CI, 292 units/h will be the calculated loading dose. FVIII levels should be monitored at least once a day and dosing adjusted accordingly.

The dose calculations for FIX concentrates are different from those used in FVIII deficiency because the recovery of infused FIX is lower (~50%) owing to the diffusion over a larger volume. In addition, there is some evidence to suggest that FIX binds to elements on the vessel wall, more specifically to collagen type IV [24]. Thus, to raise to 100% of normal a 70-kg severely affected patient, 7000 units should be given as a bolus, followed by half this amount every 12–18 h. The CI dosing for this is calculated by dividing the loading dose by 24, i.e. approximately 292 units of FIX per hour [25].

For those individuals with a rapid initial phase decay or consumption (>50% decline in 6 h), a second bolus of FVIII or FIX can be given (approximately 50% of initial bolus) within 3–6 h of starting the surgery to avoid excessive intraoperative and immediate postoperative hemorrhage. Thereafter, half or more of the initial loading dose should be readministered every 12 h in order to maintain nadir factor levels greater than 50%. Factor activity should be measured daily and adjusted to maintain the desired level (Table 25.2). In emergency situations when a pharmacokinetic evaluation is not available an initial dose of 50 IU/kg of FVIII or 100 IU/kg of FIX can be administered followed by a CI of approximately 3–5 IU/kg/h.

Home treatment

In the 1970s, home therapy was introduced as supplies of factor production became more widely available and as self-infusion was taught more commonly. This made a great impact on the treatment of hemophilia. This mode of treatment has substantially improved the quality of life of these individuals, especially those with severe hemophilia, as it reduces visits to the hospital and prevents long-term complications, such as arthropathy, when early treatment is initiated. As an indication

for home infusion, a minimal spontaneous bleeding episode is defined as any symptom of pain or distress recognized by the patient in a joint or soft-tissue space. Minimal bleeding or hemarthrosis at an early stage may not be associated with significant edema, erythema, or heat, and usually there is no known trauma [13]. Doses as small as 10 U/kg of FVIII or FIX have been proven to be effective in this type of bleeding and theoretically will lead to a plasma level of approximately 20% in FVIII or 10% in FIX activity. Such dosing proved successful in the management of 49/51 early joint hemorrhages in hemophilia A patients described by Abildgaard in 1975 [13]. It should be noted that this dose is not adequate for full-blown hemarthroses or for bleeding in critical anatomic areas (e.g. head and neck, throat, wrists, hand, foot, abdomen, or gastrointestinal tract).

Moderate bleeding episodes (e.g. hemarthrosis, advanced soft-tissue hemorrhage) often respond to an early infusion of 20–25 U/kg, which will correspond to a plasma level of 40–50% FVIII activity or 20–25% FIX activity. Honig *et al.* [26] reported successful treatment of acute hemarthrosis in 48/51 episodes using a single dose of 20–30 U of FVIII per kilogram of body weight. In many of these individuals, a single infusion is sufficient to control the bleeding; however, if no improvement is noted in 12–24 h or if significant symptoms persist, a second infusion should be administered.

During severe bleeding episodes (e.g. central nervous system, surgical procedures, and severe trauma) larger doses of replacement therapy are necessary. In addition, maintenance doses are needed to sustain hemostatic levels until bleeding is controlled or, if surgery is required, until the wound is well healed. This may take up to 10–20 days of replacement therapy depending on the surgery. For FVIII-deficient individuals, an initial infusion of 40–50 U/kg should be sufficient to obtain hemostasis in this context and levels should be maintained by repeated doses of at least 20–25 U/kg at approximately 12-h intervals to maintain physiologic circulating levels of the deficient clotting factor for a specified duration (Table 25.2). FIX replacement should be started with an initial bolus of 80–100 U/kg followed by repeated doses of 40–50 U/kg every 18–24 h.

Treatment guidelines for specific bleeding episodes

Mouth and neck region

Bleeding from the floor of the mouth, pharynx, or epiglottic area can result in partial or complete airway obstruction. External compression of the airway because of hemorrhage can also be seen after the placement of neck or subclavian catheters in hemophilic individuals. Hence, such bleeding should be treated with aggressive replacement therapy of the deficient factor until complete resolution of the bleeding is established. Doses to maintain factor levels above 80% should be the goal of treatment.

Complicated joint bleeds

Hip joint or acetabular hemorrhages are of major concern because of increased intra-articular pressure from accumulated blood. The concomitant inflammation may lead to aseptic necrosis of the femoral head. Replacement therapy should start promptly. These individuals can be treated with twice-daily infusions to sustain a factor level above 30% for at least 3 days, along with enforced bed rest.

Iliopsoas hemorrhages

Iliopsoas bleeds are less frequently encountered in young children. Together with pain, common clinical manifestations of iliopsoas bleeding are upward flexion of the thigh, discomfort on passive extension, and decreased sensation over the ipsilateral thigh owing to compression of the sacral plexus root of the femoral nerve. Twice-daily infusion should be administered to maintain a factor level above 20% for about 3 days followed with daily infusions until symptoms decrease. Bed rest should be enforced.

Compartment syndrome

Bleeding into closed-compartment muscle and tissue areas, such as the hand, wrist, forearm, and anterior or posterior tibial compartments, may result in compression of the nerves and blood vessels. Initial symptoms such as pain and edema can be preceded by paresthesias and loss of distal pulses. Prompt treatment with replacement factor is indicated to maintain levels of around 50–100% of normal. If replacement therapy fails to stop the progression, surgical decompression may be indicated.

Central nervous system hemorrhages

These are usually traumatic in origin and should be considered an emergency until proven otherwise by imaging studies. Factor infusion should be given immediately, even prior to imaging studies and neurologic consultation. FVIII or FIX levels should be kept at 80–100% of normal. Late bleeding after head trauma can manifest as long as 3–4 weeks after the injury. Hence, patients with head trauma should be infused immediately unless the injury is proven insignificant.

Following treatment of the acute episode, which usually is of approximately 2 weeks duration, prophylactic treatment for about 6 months is usually indicated to decrease the possibility of a recurrent intracerebral hemorrhage. Doses of about 40 U/kg of FVIII every other day and 50 U/kg of FIX twice weekly should be given [22].

Hematuria

Gross spontaneous and asymptomatic hematuria is not uncommon in the hemophilic population. Trauma, calculi, and infections should be ruled out, and treatment with increased oral or intravenous fluids, bed rest, and a short course of corticosteroids (i.e. prednisone 0.5 mg/kg/day) for 3–4 days is usually sufficient to arrest the bleeding. If symptoms persist then therapy with the deficient factor should be given at a dose to keep plasma levels of about 30–50% of normal until complete resolution of the hematuria. Antifibrinolytic agents, such as tranexamic acid or ε-aminocaproic acid, are contraindicated in individuals with hematuria because of the risk of forming clots in the urinary tract and producing obstruction.

Other

For certain particular circumstances, such as aggressive rehabilitation after orthopedic surgery, prophylactic replacement therapy is indicated. Doses of 20–30 U/kg of FVIII or 40–60 U/kg of FIX on the day of therapy should be sufficient to prevent hemorrhages.

Conclusion

The replacement of FVIII and FIX in the management of hemophilia is not based on randomized studies but mostly on trial and error from clinical experiences. Adequate calculations for the administration of FVIII/FIX can be made based on pharmacokinetic studies to improve the outcome of care in hemophilia.

References

1 Escobar MA. Treatment on demand—in vivo dose finding studies. *Haemophilia* 2003; **9**: 360–7.

2 Swanton MC. Hemophilic arthropathy in dogs. *Lab Invest* 1959; **8**: 1269.

3 Brinkhous KM, Swanton MC, Webster WP, Roberts HR. In: Vanderfield IR (ed.) *Dosing. Hemophilic arthropathy transfusion therapy in its amelioration—canine and human studies.* Sydney, Australia: The Haemophilia Society of NSW, 1966: 18–21.

4 Brinkhous KM, Langdell RD, Penick G, *et al.* Newer approaches to the study of haemophilia and haemophilioid states. *J Am Med Assoc* 1954; **154**: 481.

5 Biggs R, Macfarlane RG. Haemophilia, Christmas disease and related conditions. In: Biggs R, Macfarlane RG (eds.) *Human Blood Coagulation and its Disorders*, 2nd edn. Springfield, IL: Charles C Thomas, 1957: 239–74.

6 Pool JG, Hershgold EJ, Pappenhagen AR. High-potency antihaemophilic factor concentrate prepared from cryoglobulin precipitate. *Nature (London)* 1964; **203**: 312–13.

7 McMillan CW, Diamond LK, Surgenor DM. Treatment of classic hemophilia: The use of fibrinogen rich in factor VIII for hemorrhage and for surgery. *N Engl J Med* 1961; **265**: 277.

8 Ramgren O. Haemophilia in Sweden, III. Symptomatology, with special reference to differences between haemophilia A and B. *Acta Med Scand* 1962; **171**: 237.

9 Biggs R, Macfarlane RG. Haemophilia and related conditions: A survey of 187 cases. *Br J Haematol* 1958; **4**: 1.

10 Kasper CK, Dietrich SL, Rapaport SI. Hemophilia Prophylaxis with AHF Concentrate. XII Congress International Society of Hematology. New York, 1968: 176.

11 Aronstam A, Wassef M, Hamad Z, *et al.* A double-blind controlled trial of two dose levels of factor VIII in the treatment of high risk

haemarthroses in haemophilia A. *Clin Lab Haematol* 1983; **5**: 157–63.

12 Aronstam A. Prevention of haemophilic arthropathy. *Folia Haematol* 1990; **117**: 499–504.

13 Abildgaard CF. Current concepts in the management of hemophilia. *Semin Hematol* 1975; **12**: 223–32.

14 Berntorp E, Bjorkman S. The pharmacokinetics of clotting factor therapy. *Haemophilia* 2003; **9**: 353–9.

15 Kasper CK, Boylen AL, Ewing NP, *et al.* Hematologic management of hemophilia A for surgery. *J Am Med Assoc* 1985; **253**: 1279–83.

16 Lachiewicz PF, Inglis AE, Insall JN, *et al.* Total knee arthroplasty in hemophilia. *J Bone Joint Surg Am* 1985; **67**: 1361–6.

17 Kitchens CS. Surgery in hemophilia and related disorders. A prospective study of 100 consecutive procedures. *Medicine (Baltimore)* 1986; **65**: 34–45.

18 Rudowski WJ, Scharf R, Ziemski JM. Is major surgery in hemophiliac patients safe? *World J Surg* 1987; **11**: 378–86.

19 Hathaway WE, Christian MJ, Clarke SL, Hasiba U. Comparison of continuous and intermittent Factor VIII concentrate therapy in hemophilia A. *Am J Hematol* 1984; **17**: 85–8.

20 Rochat C, McFadyen ML, Schwyzer R, *et al.* Continuous infusion of intermediate-purity factor VIII in haemophilia A patients undergoing elective surgery. *Haemophilia* 1999; **5**: 181–6.

21 Goldsmith JC. Rationale and indications for continuous infusion of antihemophilic factor (factor VIII). *Blood Coag Fibrinol* 1996; **7**(Suppl. 1): S3–6.

22 Lusher J. Hemophilia A and B. In: Lilleyman JS, Hann IM, Blanchette VS (eds.) *Pediatric Hematology*, 2nd edn. London: Churchill Livingstone, 1999: 585–600.

23 Lee M, Morfini M, Schulman S, Ingerslev J, and the Factor VIII/ Factor IX Scientific and Standardization Committee of the International Society for Thrombosis and Haemostasis. Scientific and Standardization Committee Communication. The design and analysis of pharmacokinetic studies of coagulation factors. International Society on Thrombosis and Haemostasis. Available at: https://c ymcdn.com/sites/www.isth.org/resource/group/d4a6f49a-f4ec-450f-9e0f-7be9f0c2ab2e/official_communications/fviiiphar maco.pdf

24 Wolberg A, Stafford DW, Erie DA. Human factor IX binds to specific sites on the collagenous domain of collagen IV. *J Biol Chem* 1997; **272**: 16717–20.

25 Roberts HR, Escobar MA. Other coagulation factor deficiencies. In: Loscalzo J, Schafer AI (eds.) *Thrombosis and Hemorrhage*, 3rd edn. Philadelphia: Lippincott Williams & Wilkins, 2003: 575–98.

26 Honig GR, Forman EN, Johnston CA, *et al.* Administration of single doses of AHF (factor VIII) concentrates in the treatment of hemophilic hemarthroses. *Pediatrics* 1969; **43**: 26–33.

27 Brown DL, Hardisty RM, Kosoy MH, Bracken C. Antihaemophilic globulin: Preparation by an improved cryoprecipitation method and clinical use. *Br Med J* 1967; **2**: 79–85.

28 Penner JA, Kelly PE. Lower doses of factor VIII for hemophilia. *N Engl J Med* 1977; **297**: 401.

29 Ashenhurst JB, Langehannig PL, Seeler RA. Early treatment of bleeding episodes with 10 U/kg of factor VIII. *Blood* 1977; **50**: 181–2.

30 Weiss AE. Doses of Factor VIII for hemophilic bleeding. *N Engl J Med* 1977; **297**: 1237–8.

31 Ripa T, Scaraggi FA, Ciavarella N. Early treatment of hemophilia with minimal doses of factor VIII or factor IX. *Blood* 1978; **51**: 763.

32 Allain JP. Dose requirement for replacement therapy in hemophilia A. *Thromb Haemost* 1979; **42**: 825–31.

33 Aronstam A, Wasssef M, Choudhury DP, *et al.* Double-blind controlled trial of three dosage regimens in treatment of haemarthroses in haemophilia A. *Lancet* 1980; **i**: 169–71.

34 Aronstam A, Wassef M, Hamad Z, Aston DL. The identification of high-risk elbow hemorrhages in adolescents with severe hemophilia A. *J Pediatr* 1981; **98**: 776–8.

35 Aronstam A, Wassef M, Hamad Z. Low doses of factor VIII for selected ankle bleeds in severe haemophilia A. *Br Med J* 1982; **284**: 790.

CHAPTER 26

Products used to treat hemophilia: regulation

Albert Farrugia
University of Western Australia, Perth, Australia

Introduction

Hemophilia care consists of many components [1]. The provision of concentrates of the deficient coagulation factors is an essential component and their safety, quality, and efficacy need to be assured independently of the measures dictated by the market and the individual manufacturers. Over the past 20 years, this assurance has become the role of regulatory authorities. Compared to other products of pharmaceutical manufacture, the regulation of hemophilia products is a relatively recent phenomenon. The products of industrial scale plasma fractionation have been subject to the oversight of the American Food and Drugs Administration (FDA) since the 1940s, because of the products' status as biologics subject to a regulatory framework which is over a century old. In Europe, the evolution of a system of harmonized and centralized approval of medicinal products in the European Union initially exempted plasma derivatives [2] and only commenced their incorporation in 1989 [3]. The factors contributing to the significant heightening of this oversight over the past 20 years have been reviewed [4].

These factors have resulted in a regulatory framework in the developed world which assesses hemophilia products as medicines in the highest category of risk relative to other therapeutic agents. It is noteworthy that systems of official regulation mandating standards and other measures are now coupled with voluntary standards adopted by industry bodies as additional features of a comprehensive nexus of arrangements contributing to product quality and risk minimization [5]. While the requirements now in place in the European Union demonstrate the comprehensive range of measures now in place in that market (Figure 26.1), they are fairly representative of the systems in place worldwide in terms of the aspects of product manufacture which they address and the target outcomes. The principles underlying these product-related measures have been discussed [6], and while the principal focus has been on the products of industrial plasma fractionation, the lessons learned through these products are now reflected in the requirements for the products of recombinant technology.

Underpinning these measures is the unspoken but practiced concept of "zero risk" in blood product manufacture and delivery. While this is a natural outcome of past failures, it has led to a regulatory framework which appears to be detached from the standard risk management and cost-effective, evidence-based principles which shape modern healthcare delivery. While product safety is paramount, some of the measures introduced and embedded in current practise are difficult to quantify in terms of safety, while their effect on supply and delivery can be profound.

Products of local and blood bank production

The option of delivering product from local production in mainstream blood banking environments generally only exists for hemophilia A through the production of cryoprecipitate (cryo). Cryoprecipiate in blood banks may be produced in a closed system of blood bags and then lyophilized to increase its convenience [7]. The following features of the product need to be kept in mind:

- Cryo is a crude product which will not meet criteria for high-purity plasma concentrates, such as potency, purity, and solubility. However, this is not a significant problem in terms of its safety.
- The ability to characterize the product through representative batch sampling is limited. That is, it is not possible to label a vial of freeze-dried cryo for potency. Hence, accurate dosage for procedures such as surgery and prophylaxis is problematic.
- Viral reduction techniques are not easily applied to the manufacture of cryo. This is because they are based on technology not easily adapted to blood centers, and because the low purity of the product prevents inactivation through heat.

The issues underpinning access to cryo have been reviewed [8]. In particular, the safety aspects have been emphasized by Evatt *et al.* [9], who have shown that in the absence of

Textbook of Hemophilia, Third Edition. Edited by Christine A. Lee, Erik E. Berntorp and W. Keith Hoots.
© 2014 John Wiley & Sons, Ltd. Published 2014 by John Wiley & Sons, Ltd.

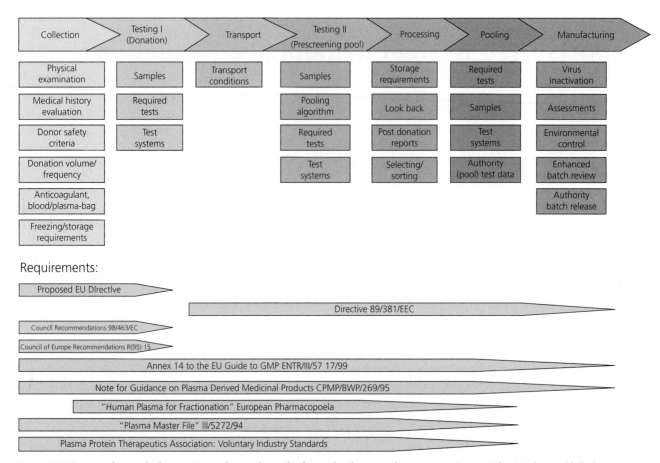

Figure 26.1 Systems of oversight for assuring product quality and safety in the plasma products sector in Europe. After J. Bult, unpublished observations.

Table 26.1 Risk (%) that a person with hemophilia in Venezuela or the USA will be exposed to human immunodeficiency virus (HIV)-contaminated blood product based on years of treatment and risk of an HIV-infected donation. From [9]. Reproduced with permission of John Wiley and Sons.

Years of treatment	Venezuela			USA
	Lower (1/25 700)[a]	Mid (1/21 200)[a]	Upper (1/17 500)[a]	Mid (1/545 100)[a]
5	3.4	4.2	5.0	0.16
10	6.8	5.1	9.8	0.33
15	10.0	12.0	14.3	0.49
20	13.1	15.6	18.6	0.66
30	19.0	22.5	26.6	0.99
40	24.4	28.8	33.7	1.3
50	29.5	34.6	40.2	1.6
60	34.3	39.9	46.0	2.0

[a]Estimated risk for HIV-infected donation.

additional safety measures, the risk of human immunodeficiency virus (HIV) infection in individuals with hemophilia exposed to cryo over a lifetime is significant (Table 26.1). Enhancement of cryo safety could include the selection of donors from low-risk populations, whose plasma could be quarantined until the donor has been recalled and retested for markers of infection. All such testing should be done with the most sensitive tests possible and using intervals which allow donors to seroconvert for the transfusion-transmitted viruses in case they were infected at the time of donation. Using nucleic acid testing (NAT), the viral window period for the important viruses can be substantially decreased. Pools of dedicated plasma donors, carefully selected and repeatedly tested, can in time become a source of very safe raw material, compared to first-time donors.

Some approaches to the viral inactivation of cryo have been described [10]. Any level of viral inactivation will result in a drop in factor VIII (FVIII) yield, and therefore the optimization of yields using improved plasma handling techniques is necessary if the safety and supply of cryo are to be enhanced. The pharmacologic stimulation of donors to produce more FVIII may be worth considering as a means of improving yields [11]. Over the past 5 years, a technique developed by El Ekiaby *et al.* [12] has shown great promise in producing cryo within a closed plastic bag blood bank system allowing the introduction and removal of solvent/detergent chemicals for the inactivation of viruses. Such a system will obviate the risks of enveloped viral transmission concerning Evatt *et al.* [9]. However, the nature of the manufacturing process for cryo results in a limitation in the ability to exert many of the standard features of pharmaceutical quality control which are possible for concentrates. In particular, the absence of sizeable batches makes homogenous batch sampling, characterization, and labeling of ingredients of interest (active and impurities) difficult. Nevertheless, the ability to impose quality system management and adherence to good manufacturing practises is considered to be universally applicable. There are several standards and regulations in the international regulatory environment, which are applied for the manufacture and characterization of cryo. The US Code of Federal Regulations (CFR) [13] includes requirements for cryoprecipitate which ensure that the measures underpinning whole blood transfusion safety in the USA will be reflected in cryo. These measures include NAT testing which will enhance cryo safety as discussed above. In Europe, centralized oversight of blood components including cryo is established through the Blood Directive of the European Commission [14] which will replace and override the current European Union national member states' requirements for these products. This Directive is underpinned by technical standards for safety and quality which are reflective of those recommended by the Council of Europe [15] and currently do not include NAT testing. Hence, this important measure for the safety of cryo is not in universal use in the European environment. Therefore, alignments to the evolving European regulatory framework will not, as currently perceived by this author, enhance the safety of cryo to the level found in the US.

In summary, cryo may be subjected to a level of regulatory oversight which, while unable to assure safety and quality to the standards available for concentrates, can result in these properties being reflective of the safety of the local blood supply. Any additional measures such as the introduction of viral inactivation for cryo are limited. Therefore, while much can be done to improve the safety of cryo as a therapeutic modality in the developing world, it can never substitute for concentrates in terms of safety and quality which can be assured by regulatory oversight.

Products of large-scale plasma fractionation

Plasma concentrates are similar to conventional pharmaceuticals in that they are produced in large batches from a homogenous pool of starting material, through well-defined processes subject to the tenets of standard pharmaceutical quality control. However, biologic drugs such as factor concentrates cannot be considered as generic agents and each manufacturing process requires individual assessment with full product specification. While general properties leading to quality and safety may be reflected in standards of the pharmacopeia, the range of approaches to the manufacture of FVIII and factor IX (FIX) concentrates developed over the past 40 years results in significant differences between products which require thorough evaluation for their potential effect on the factors of interest and the impurities in the products.

Regulatory agencies oversee the introduction and maintenance of factor concentrates on the market through a set of well-defined principles which are common across the developed world. These include:
- Facility licensure (good manufacturing practise or GMP).
- Premarket product assessment.
- Postmarket surveillance.

Facility licensure

Licensure of plasma fractionation plants is done through reference to codes of GMP which are generally generic documents specifying quality standards for manufacture which are common for all medicinal products. Such GMPs seek to ensure that manufacture is done consistently to high standards such that product safety, quality, and consistency are assured. Following inspections which may identify deficiencies, the regulator and the manufacturer generally collaborate to ensure the issue of a manufacturing license which will allow production to a high standard. The Pharmaceutical Inspectorate Convention has adopted a GMP for medicinal products which includes a chapter specifically addressing plasma-derived products [16]. The requirements of this chapter are shown in Box 26.1.

The importance of GMP in assuring product safety is recognized by the regulator and product manufacturer alike. The ability of the latter to manufacture product consistently to a

---

Box 26.1 Principles of good manufacturing practise for plasma fractionation agencies. Pharmaceutical Inspectors Convention Scheme 2003.

- Quality management
- Premises and equipment
- Blood and plasma collection
- Traceability and postcollection measures
- Production and quality control
- Retention of samples
- Disposal of rejected blood, plasma, or intermediates

similar, predefined, and high manufacturing standard is pivotal to safety and depends on GMP. Examples of breakdowns in GMP impacting on product safety are now rare due to the high standards of manufacture evolved over the past 20 years, but such incidents have been implied in product safety problems including viral transmission due to inadequate segregation between previral and postviral inactivation streams [17]. With viral inactivation processes, it is impossible to subject product batches to final testing to assure adequate viral elimination, and reliance on GMP for this is absolute. The whole of the manufacturing chain requires adherence to GMP, and its presence in collection and testing procedures is strictly enforced by regulators [18]. Voluntary industry standards have been introduced for ensuring that the minimal measures enforced by regulators are buttressed by additional measures for areas such as the processing of fractionation intermediates from different sources [19].

Premarket product approval

The assessment of the manufacturing process and the features of the product are done through the submission of product dossiers which describe these in great detail. The main agencies the FDA and the European Union's European Medicines Agency (EMA; formerly EMEA) have standard formats for the submission of data for manufacturing, preclinical, and clinical assessment. A crucial component for these is the data for the description and validation of the viral inactivation steps incorporated into the manufacture. The EMA has issued detailed guidance for the performance of such studies [20]. Such guidances are a feature of the regulatory framework of all the major agencies, and provide the industry with regulator's assessment of the state of the art in the safety, quality, and efficacy of plasma derivatives.

International efforts for the harmonization of regulatory procedures have included the development of standardized approaches for the collation and presentation of data for regulatory review, through the so-called Common Technical Document (CTD). The International Conference for Harmonisation (ICH) has developed CTDs for the assessment of several aspects of safety, quality, and efficacy [21]. These documents provide a structured path for manufacturers to compile data in a form which is easily assessable, and their use for plasma derivatives, while still at an early stage, should contribute to further streamlining the regulatory process.

An essential component of the premarket approval process is the demonstration of product pharmacokinetics and efficacy through the conduct of appropriate clinical trials. It is necessary to demonstrate that a product will show the established pharmacokinetic profile for the relevant coagulation factors, i.e. *in-vivo* recovery and half-life. Proof of efficacy to a clinical endpoint under the various indications sought, e.g. prophylaxis, treatment of episodic bleeds, and surgery, is also needed.

Clinical requirements for the assessment of adverse events such as viral transmission and inhibitor development demand patient numbers which are considerably larger than is feasible if conventional assurance based on statistical principles is to be generated. Given these limitations, the EMA has revised its requirements for the clinical efficacy of FVIII and FIX to allow efficacy and adverse event assessment to be reviewed through lower patient numbers than previously required [22]. Similar flexibility has been shown on the need for previously untreated patients (PUPs) and nonbleeding patients, both scarce groups to access. It is still not possible for regulators to fully exempt plasma concentrates from the requirements of clinical studies on the basis of so-called "comparability" with similar products [23]. The level of characterization possible for these products, particularly in relation to potential predictors of efficacy and adverse events, is necessarily limited, and surrogates for clinical studies are not yet available. Hence, the continuing debate on "biosimilar" biologic products has seen the EMA exempt hemophilia and similar products from the concept, but normal standards of safety, quality, and efficacy are required [24].

While the pressure is on regulators to avoid "over-regulation," there are still some areas of plasma product regulation where provisions could be strengthened. The European system mandates centralized—and rigorous—oversight for these products if they are manufactured using certain biotechnologic techniques, e.g. monoclonal antibody affinity chromatography. Products produced with earlier technology are regulated through the Mutual Recognition Procedure [25] emanating from review by one authority in a single member state. Considering that these products were developed and placed on the market prior to the modern era of stringent regulation, the maintenance, in individual European states, of hemophilia products which are not reflective of current best practise in the field, demands review if patient care and safety are to be ensured. This is especially important as many of these products have been succeeded in the market by more developed products but still have a presence in emerging countries lacking a sophisticated regulatory system.

Postmarket surveillance

Once products are approved and on the market, it is essential that their quality, safety, and efficacy are maintained throughout their market lifetime. This is achieved through postmarket activities which include:

- Maintenance of GMP through regular inspections after the introduction of the products.
- Testing of batches prerelease in order to ensure conformance to specifications.
- Appropriate recording and reporting mechanisms for adverse events.

The importance of these measures needs to reflect the fact that novel plasma-derived hemophilia concentrates are now rare,

PART IX

Surgical management

CHAPTER 28

General surgical management of patients with hemophilia

Cindy Leissinger and Rebecca Kruse-Jarres

Tulane University School of Medicine, Louisiana, USA

Introduction

Since the introduction of factor replacement therapy, surgery has been performed with reliable success in hemophilia patients. Orthopedic procedures have traditionally accounted for the majority of these surgeries, owing to the high prevalence of hemophilia-associated joint disease. However, as the hemophilia population ages, the need for nonorthopedic procedures is growing, and these are now routinely performed at most comprehensive hemophilia treatment centers (HTCs).

Despite technical advances and the wide availability of clotting factor concentrates, surgery remains challenging for patients with hemophilia because of uncertainty regarding the optimal level and duration of replacement therapy needed to maintain hemostasis. This is particularly true during the postoperative period, when variability in hemostatic demands and healing rates is highest. To date, there has been a paucity of clinical trials looking at best treatment practises for surgery in hemophilia patients. Consequently, hemostatic management is primarily guided by individual and collective clinical experience, consensus guidelines, and anecdotal reports in the literature.

This chapter focuses on bleed management during major and minor nonorthopedic surgeries in patients with hemophilia, discusses special considerations in persons with mild or moderate hemophilia undergoing surgery, and describes potential nonbleeding complications associated with invasive procedures.

General considerations

The keys to success in hemophilia patients undergoing surgery are a multidisciplinary approach to care and a hospital with the experience and capability to care for patients with complex bleeding problems. Open communication among the surgeon, anesthesiologist, hematologist, and other hemophilia team members is critical. Additionally, the hospital must provide immediate access to appropriate clotting factor concentrates, and the hospital laboratory must have the ability to perform factor levels with a rapid turnaround time (e.g. results available in <2 h).

Preoperative preparation for the hematologist includes verifying the absence of a factor inhibitor, confirming the patient's response to the factor concentrate that will be used during surgery, and assessing other potential bleeding problems (particularly important for patients with human immunodeficiency virus and/or chronic hepatitis). The goal of perioperative factor replacement therapy is to achieve and maintain factor levels in the normal (hemostatic) range and to continue factor infusions until wound healing has occurred. Immediately before the start of surgery, the patient's factor level should be raised to the desired target, typically 80–100%. Subsequent factor doses are administered as scheduled bolus doses or as a continuous infusion. Periodic intraoperative and postoperative monitoring of the patient's factor levels ensure an adequate response to treatment.

Major surgery

The most common general surgeries reported from one HTC included hernia repair, cholecystectomy, and gastrointestinal procedures (representing 30%, 28%, and 18%, respectively, of all general surgeries performed) [1]. Other procedures, such as splenectomy, kidney and liver transplantation, and vascular and cardiac surgeries, although less frequent, are done routinely in many centers.

A comprehensive literature review conducted by Hermans *et al.* examined 35 clinical studies published between 1965 and 2007 that collectively described 1114 patients with severe, moderate, or mild hemophilia A ($n = 862$) or B ($n = 241$) who

Textbook of Hemophilia, Third Edition. Edited by Christine A. Lee, Erik E. Berntorp and W. Keith Hoots.
© 2014 John Wiley & Sons, Ltd. Published 2014 by John Wiley & Sons, Ltd.

underwent a total of 1328 major surgical procedures, including 621 nonorthopedic surgeries [2]. Perioperative hemostasis was provided by a variety of plasma-derived and recombinant factor concentrates administered via bolus dosing, continuous infusion, or both, and antifibrinolytic therapy was used adjunctively in approximately 25% of the procedures. The target preoperative factor level reported was generally 80–100% (range >50–100%). Postoperatively, the majority of studies used target factor levels exceeding 50% during the first postoperative week, and greater than 30% in postoperative week 2. The duration of treatment, although variable, was generally between 9 and 16 days (range 3–54 days). Bleeding complications occurred in 10% of the procedures, with the vast majority of these complications (and two bleed-related fatalities) reported in articles published before 1990.

Results from a 2009 survey of practise patterns conducted at 26 HTCs in 15 European countries showed that perioperative target factor levels were similar to those reported in the literature review [2]. However, perioperative clotting factor was more likely to be administered via continuous infusion for major surgery procedures: ~50% rate in the survey versus 16% reported in the older literature review. These findings are consistent with current US practise patterns, where major surgeries are frequently performed with continuous factor infusion using the target goals for factor replacement previously described.

Although formal pharmacokinetic evaluation and factor recovery studies performed before major surgery can accurately predict appropriate perioperative factor dosing for an individual patient, this time-consuming approach has largely been replaced by the frequent measurement of intraoperative and postoperative factor levels, followed by immediate adjustment of factor dosing.

The survey of HTCs found that antifibrinolytic therapy is used as an adjunct to hemostasis in more than two-thirds of major orthopedic surgeries and a substantial number of nonorthopedic procedures [2]. Tranexamic acid (TXA) and the less potent antifibrinolytic ε-aminocaproic acid (EACA) reduce blood loss by inhibiting the conversion of plasminogen to plasmin [3]. One study found the combination of antifibrinolytic therapy plus continuous factor infusion could potentially enhance the cost-effectiveness of treatment by reducing factor concentrate requirements [4].

Cardiac surgery

Although severe clotting factor deficiency may provide some protection from atherosclerotic cardiovascular disease [5–7], patients with hemophilia, particularly those with mild or moderate hemophilia [8], are increasingly diagnosed with coronary artery disease (CAD) and undergoing coronary angioplasty or coronary artery bypass grafting. The frequency of valve replacement surgery and to a lesser extent, repair of congenital cardiac abnormalities, is also growing in this patient population.

Hemophilia patients undergoing cardiopulmonary bypass (CPB) surgery require target replacement levels of 100%. Continuous factor infusion is preferred to bolus dosing throughout the early postoperative period to avoid fluctuations in factor levels that may result in bleeding (low troughs) or increase thrombotic risk (high peaks). Factor levels should be routinely checked before CPB and again immediately after the patient comes off the pump, when an additional factor bolus may be needed. Heparinization during CPB is safe, but it interferes with laboratory testing of factor levels using a standard partial thromboplastin time (PTT)-based assay. Such testing is typically not necessary in uncomplicated procedures, but when it is, a chromogenic assay can be used for this purpose. Factor levels should be checked daily after surgery, with target factor levels gradually tapered over 2 weeks [8,9]. Antifibrinolytics are commonly used for the first 7–10 postoperative days to augment hemostasis [8,10].

Cardiac surgery in individuals with bleeding disorders is challenging because it often requires concomitant antiplatelet and anticoagulant therapy [8]. In hemophilia patients undergoing coronary angioplasty with stent placement, bare metal stents are preferred because the duration of dual antiplatelet therapy is shorter than is needed with drug-eluting stents (4 weeks vs 6–12 months) [11]. When valve replacement is necessary, bioprosthetic valves are preferred to mechanical valves to reduce the need of ongoing antithrombotic therapy [12].

Minor surgery

In patients with hemophilia, even "minor" procedures have the potential for life-threatening bleeding complications and require a well-constructed plan for hemostatic management.

The initial therapeutic goal is to achieve a factor level between 50% and 100%, depending on the procedure. Maintenance replacement therapy postprocedure is usually less intense than with major surgery and is administered for 1–10 days.

Minor procedures involving mucosal surfaces may result in an eschar that falls off in 7–10 days and, without adequate hemostasis, can cause late bleeding. In some patients, early factor coverage followed by antifibrinolytic therapy may be sufficient to prevent bleeding resulting from eschar separation. For those with mild hemophilia A who respond to desmopressin (deamino-D-arginine vasopressin; DDAVP), its use may achieve and maintain the desired target factor VIII (FVIII) level before and for 1–2 days after the procedure, but tachyphylaxis limits repetitive use [13]. Antifibrinolytics can be safely and effectively used in conjunction with DDAVP [14].

Dental surgery

Dental surgeries are the most frequently performed procedures in hemophilia patients. In the previously described comprehensive literature review, a total of 1470 dental surgeries were reported in more than 20 separate studies [2]. Factor replacement therapy was used in 71% of procedures, a preoperative factor level of 50% was targeted for most of the patients, and the duration of replacement therapy ranged between 5 and 7 days. Antifibrinolytic therapy was used adjunctively for a median of 7 days in a majority of the studies, and fibrin glue was used for local hemostatic control at the extraction site in approximately half of the studies.

Randomized controlled trials have shown that both TXA and EACA significantly reduce bleeding after dental surgery in patients with hemophilia [15,16]. World Federation of Hemophilia guidelines recommend starting oral antifibrinolytic therapy the day before dental surgery (EACA 50 mg/kg four times daily or TXA 1g three times daily) and continuing treatment for total of 7 days [17]. Fibrin glue, which consists mainly of fibrinogen and thrombin and mimics the final steps of the coagulation cascade where fibrinogen is converted into fibrin, can be useful for local hemostasis during dental procedures [17].

Liver biopsy
Up to 98% of persons with hemophilia treated with plasma-derived clotting factor concentrate before 1985, when viral inactivation was introduced into the manufacturing process, were infected with one or more forms of hepatitis, most notably hepatitis C virus [18]. Liver biopsy is often useful for determining the activity of hepatitis-related liver disease, predicting prognosis, guiding treatment decisions, and monitoring therapeutic efficacy [19,20]. For the 778 liver biopsies included in the comprehensive literature review, a prebiopsy target factor level of 100% was used in the majority, regardless of the type of biopsy (i.e. percutaneous, laparoscopic, transjugular) [2]. Postbiopsy target levels were 70–100% for the first 24h, 50–70% for the next 24–48h, and >50% for the following 48–72h. When factor replacement was extended for 5–7 days, the target level was >30%. Concomitant use of antifibrinolytic agents was uncommon.

Endoscopy
Endoscopy, particularly of the gastrointestinal tract, may be performed for routine screening, diagnosis, and therapy. For screening endoscopy that does not involve biopsy or other mucosal disruption, target factor levels preprocedure of 50–80% are generally considered sufficient. When biopsy or polypectomy is anticipated, a target preprocedure factor level of 80–100% is reasonable and postprocedure bleeding prophylaxis is necessary. Factor replacement is typically continued for a minimum of 3 days postendoscopy to maintain factor levels >25%; adjunctive antifibrinolytic therapy is maintained for at least 7 days [21]. When endoscopy is more extensive (e.g. multiple biopsies, sclerotherapy, sphincterotomy), factor levels exceeding 30% should be maintained for up to 14 days to prevent significant or delayed bleeding [22,23]. Antifibrinolytics may be a helpful adjunct for bleeding prophylaxis associated with gastrointestinal endoscopic procedures.

Urologic procedures
Growing numbers of older men with hemophilia are undergoing prostate biopsy to rule-out cancer. A prebiopsy target dose of 100% followed by daily factor infusions to maintain levels >25–50% for 7 days are recommended [24]. Minimal postprocedure hematuria and hematospermia for a week or more is common in men without a bleeding disorder and does not necessarily indicate inadequate factor replacement in patients with hemophilia. Antifibrinolytic therapy has been associated with the development of obstructing clots when given to hemophilia patients with urinary tract bleeding [25] and is probably best avoided in those undergoing genitourinary instrumentation or surgery.

Surgery in children

The most frequently performed invasive procedures in children with hemophilia are dentistry, which is usually not as traumatic as in adults and can be treated less intensively; circumcision; insertion of a central venous access device (CVAD); and tonsillectomy/adenoidectomy.

Circumcision
Included in the comprehensive review by Hermans *et al.* were five studies that reported on factor replacement therapy in 197 children undergoing circumcision [2]. The target preoperative factor level was 50–100%, and replacement therapy was continued for 2–12 days postprocedure to maintain levels >30% for at least the first 4 days after circumcision. Antifibrinolytic therapy and fibrin glue were used in most of the procedures.

Central venous access device insertion
Central venous access devices are commonly used to facilitate factor replacement in children with hemophilia. Subcutaneously tunneled, fully implantable ports are the most common CVAD, used in more than 75% of patients who receive an indwelling catheter [26]. A major review by Valentino *et al.* of 48 studies collectively described 2973 CVAD insertions in 2704 hemophilia patients [26]. Among the patients treated with FVIII or factor IX (FIX), the target level before surgery (reported for 13 studies) was 100%. Follow-up doses were designed to maintain levels >50% for 2–3 days, after which the dose was tapered to maintain levels of 30–75% for an additional 1–5 days. In the Hermans *et al.* literature review, concomitant antifibrinolytics were used infrequently (<25% of the reports) [2].

Tonsillectomy/adenoidectomy
Bleeding is common after tonsillectomy/adenoidectomy, occurring in up to 7% of children without a coagulopathy [27]. Three retrospective studies involving 24 children with hemophilia who underwent tonsillectomy/adenoidectomy were included in the comprehensive literature review [2]. The preoperative target factor level varied between 80% and 100%, and factor

replacement was maintained for 5–11 days after surgery. Antifibrinolytic therapy, used in more than 90% of the patients, was also continued for 5–11 days postoperatively.

Special considerations in patients with mild hemophilia

The principles of factor replacement therapy and target factor levels for surgery are the same regardless of hemophilia severity, although the dose required to reach this target level decreases with increasing baseline levels of the deficient factor [28]. However, additional hemostatic options are available to some patients with mild hemophilia undergoing surgery.

DDAVP

DDAVP, which elevates FVIII about threefold over baseline, is an important alternative to factor replacement in patients with mild hemophilia A undergoing minor surgical procedures [28,29]. Because of substantial interpatient variation in FVIII increase following DDAVP administration, patients with mild hemophilia A should undergo DDAVP challenge to evaluate their response to treatment [28]. Predictors of a good response are higher baseline factor level and older age [30]. An FVIII level ≥50% after DDAVP administration suffices for most minor surgical procedures.

Caveats to the use of DDAVP include the risk for fluid retention, seizures associated with hyponatremia, and the potential for tachyphylaxis after two to three doses [14]. DDAVP is not recommended for children under the age of 2 years, and fluid intake should be closely regulated in all patients. Additionally, DDAVP should be used with caution in persons with medical disorders associated with sodium abnormalities, such as heart failure and renal disorders.

Antifibrinolytic therapy

For patients with very mild forms of hemophilia (baseline factor levels >30%), monotherapy with a systemic or topical antifibrinolytic agent may be sufficient for minor surgery, particularly for procedures involving the oral mucosa [2,3,28].

Potential nonbleeding complications of surgery

The development of inhibitory antibodies that neutralize the clotting function of FVIII or FIX is the most serious nonbleeding complication associated with surgery in patients with hemophilia. Tissue damage that occurs with surgery increases immunologic danger signals that, when combined with intense factor replacement, appears to raise the risk of inhibitor development [31]. A systematic review conducted by Eckhardt et al. found that patients with severe hemophilia A whose first exposure to FVIII was intensive replacement therapy during surgery

had a fourfold higher inhibitor risk than patients who initially received factor concentrate to treat acute bleeding [31]. Currently, elective surgery in very young children with hemophilia is often delayed until they are older and have had repeated exposure to factor concentrates, in an attempt to reduce their risk for an inhibitor.

Studies in patients with mild and moderate hemophilia A have also shown an association between high-intensity factor exposure and increased inhibitor risk [32]. Moreover, this risk does not appear to diminish with previous FVIII exposures or age. Several investigators have suggested an association between continuous factor infusion used for surgery and inhibitor development [32,33]. Consequently, many treaters now use bolus dosing for surgery in nonsevere hemophilia patients and in those with limited exposure to factor concentrates to potentially reduce the risk of inhibitor formation [34]. The preferential use of DDAVP rather than FVIII in DDAVP-responsive patients is another strategy that may reduce inhibitor risk in patients with mild and moderate hemophilia A.

Deep venous thrombosis (DVT) appears to be a very rare occurrence in hemophilia patients undergoing major surgery [35], and DVT chemoprophylaxis is not generally used. However, mechanical DVT prophylaxis, early ambulation, and avoidance of excess factor replacement (with blood levels exceeding 150%) should be important goals during the postoperative course.

Summary

Surgery is an increasingly necessary component of care for patients with hemophilia. Surgery requires a specialized team approach and a hospital capable of supporting intense factor concentrate use and timely laboratory monitoring. The optimal approach utilizes the coordination and resources of the comprehensive HTC team. With planning, teamwork, and careful postoperative follow-up, both major and minor nonorthopedic procedures can be performed with high rates of success.

Acknowledgments

The authors wish to thank Michele Grygotis for her expert editorial assistance.

References

1 Aryal KR, Wiseman D, Siriwardena AK, Bolton-Maggs PH, Hay CR, Hill J. General surgery in patients with a bleeding diathesis: how we do it. *World J Surg* 2011; **35**(12): 2603–10.

2 Hermans C, Altisent C, Batorova A, *et al*. Replacement therapy for invasive procedures in patients with haemophilia: literature review, European survey and recommendations. *Haemophilia* 2009; **15**(3): 639–58.

3 Tengborn L. Fibrinolytic inhibitors in the management of bleeding disorders. World Federation of Hemophilia. Treatment of Hemophilia Series; November 2012, no. 42. Available at: http://www.wfh.org/en/page.aspx?pid=1270

4 Schulman S, Loogna J, Wallensten R. Minimizing factor requirements for surgery without increased risk. *Haemophilia* 2004; **10** (Suppl. 4): 35–40.

5 Rosendaal FR, Varekamp I, Smit C, *et al.* Mortality and causes of death in Dutch haemophiliacs, 1973–86. *Br J Hematol* 1989; **71**(1): 71–6.

6 Triemstra M, Rosendaal FR, Smit C, Van der Ploeg HM, Briet E. Mortality in patients with hemophilia. Changes in a Dutch population from 1986 to 1992 and 1973 to 1986. *Ann Int Med* 19951; **123**(11): 823–7.

7 Darby SC, Kan SW, Spooner RJ, *et al.* Mortality rates, life expectancy, and causes of death in people with hemophilia A or B in the United Kingdom who were not infected with HIV. *Blood* 2007; **110**(3): 815–25.

8 Rossi M, Javaram R, Sayeed R. Do patients with hemophilia undergoing cardiac surgery have good surgical outcomes? *Interact Cardiovasc Thorac Surg* 2011; **13**: 320–31.

9 MacKinlay N, Taper J, Renisson F, Rickard K. Cardiac surgery and catheterization in patients with haemophilia. *Haemophilia* 2000; **6**(2): 84–8.

10 Tang M, Wierup P, Terp K, Ingerslev J, Sorensen B. Cardiac surgery in patients with haemophilia. *Haemophilia* 2009; **15**(1): 101–7.

11 Helft G, Gilard M, Le Feuvre C, Zaman AG. Drug insight: antithrombotic therapy after percutaneous coronary intervention in patients with an indication for anticoagulation. *Nat Clin Pract Cardiovasc Med* 2006; **3**(12): 673–80.

12 Benzadon MN, Thierer JM, Trivi M, *et al.* Is early anticoagulation necessary after biological aortic valve replacement? *Int J Cardiol* 2008; **128**(3): 422–3.

13 Kaufmann JE, Vischer UM. Cellular mechanisms of the hemostatic effects of desmopressin (DDAVP). *J Thromb Haemost* 2003; **1**(4): 682–9.

14 Dunn AL, Powers JR, Ribeiro MJ, Rickles FR, Abshire TC. Adverse events during use of intranasal desmopressin acetate for haemophilia A and von Willebrand disease: a case report and review of 40 patients. *Haemophilia* 2000; **6**(1): 11–14.

15 Forbes CD, Barr RD, Reid G, *et al.* Tranexamic acid in control of haemorrhage after dental extraction in haemophilia and Christmas disease. *Br Med J* 1972; **2**(5809): 311–13.

16 Walsh PN, Rizza CR, Matthews JM, *et al.* Epsilon-Aminocaproic acid therapy for dental extractions in haemophilia and Christmas disease: a double blind controlled trial. *Br J Haematol* 1971; **20**(5): 463–75.

17 Brewer A, Correa ME. Guidelines for dental treatment of patients with inherited bleeding disorders. World Federation of Hemophilia. Treatment of Hemophilia Series; May 2006, no. 40. Available at: www.lhsc.on.ca/Health.../Bleeding.../TOH-40_Dental_treatment .pdf

18 Makris M, Preston FE, Rosendaal FR, Underwood JC, Rice KM, Triger DR. The natural history of chronic hepatitis C in haemophiliacs. *Br J Haematol* 1996; **94**(4): 746–52.

19 Bravo AA, Sheth SG, Chopra S. Liver biopsy. *N Engl J Med* 2001; **344**(7): 495–500.

20 DiMichele DM, Mirani G, Wilfredo Canchis P, Trost DW, Talal AH. Transjugular liver biopsy is safe and diagnostic for patients with congenital bleeding disorders and hepatitis C infection. *Haemophilia* 2003; **9**(5): 613–18.

21 Fogarty PF, Kouides P. How we treat: patients with haemophilia undergoing screening colonoscopy. *Haemophilia* 2010; **16**(2): 363–5.

22 Katsinelos P, Pilpilidis I, Paroutoglou G, *et al.* Endoscopic sphincterotomy in adult hemophiliac patients with choledocholithiasis. *Gastrointest Endosc* 2003; **58**(5): 788–91.

23 Van Os EC, Kamath PS, Gostout CJ, Heit JA. Gastroenterological procedures among patients with disorders of hemostasis: evaluation and management recommendations. *Gastrointest Endosc* 1999; **50**(4): 536–43.

24 Fogarty PF, Kouides P. How we manage prostate biopsy and prostate cancer therapy in men with haemophilia. *Haemophilia* 2012; **18**(3): e88–90.

25 Ashrani AA, Green D. Overview of cancer and thrombosis. In: Green DKH, (ed.) *Coagulation in Cancer.* Dordrecht, Netherlands: Springer Science + Business Media, LLC; 2009.

26 Valentino LA, Ewenstein B, Navickis RJ, Wilkes MM. Central venous access devices in haemophilia. *Haemophilia* 2004; **10**(2): 134–46.

27 Krishna P, Lee D. Post-tonsillectomy bleeding: a meta-analysis. *Laryngoscope* 2001; **111**(8): 1358–61.

28 Schulman S. Mild hemophilia. Revised edition. World Federation of Hemophilia. Treatment of Hemophilia Series; November 2012, no. 41. Available at: http://www.wfh.org/en/page.aspx?pid=492

29 Mariana G, Ciavarella N, Mazzucconi MG, *et al.* Evaluation of the effectiveness of DDAVP in surgery and in bleeding episodes in haemophilia and von Willebrand's disease. A study on 43 patients. *Clin Lab Haematol* 1984; **6**(3): 229–38.

30 Revel-Vilk S, Blanchette VS, Sparling C, Stain AM, Carcao MD. DDAVP challenge tests in boys with mild/moderate haemophilia A. *Br J Haematol* 2002; **117**(4): 947–51.

31 Eckhardt CL, van der Bom JG, van der Naald M, Peters M, Kamphuisen PW, Fijnvandraat K. Surgery and inhibitor development in hemophilia A: a systematic review. *J Thromb Haemost* 2011; **9**(10): 1948–58.

32 Sharathkumar A, Lillicrap D, Blanchette VS, *et al.* Intensive exposure to factor VIII is a risk factor for inhibitor development in mild hemophilia A. *J Thromb Haemost* 2003; **1**(6): 1228–36.

33 Eckhardt CL, Menke LA, van Ommen CH, *et al.* Intensive perioperative use of factor VIII and the Arg593->Cys mutation are risk factors for inhibitor development in mild/moderate hemophilia A. *J Thromb Haemost* 2009; **7**(6): 930–7.

34 Kempton CL, Soucie JM, Miller CH, *et al.* In non-severe hemophilia A the risk of inhibitor after intensive factor treatment is greater in older patients: a case–control study. *J Thromb Haemost* 2010; **8**(10): 2224–31.

35 Girolami A, Scandellari R, Zanon E, Sartori R, Girolami B. Non-catheter associated venous thrombosis in hemophilia A and B. A critical review of all reported cases. *J Thromb Thrombolysis* 2006; **21**: 279–84.

CHAPTER 29

Continuous infusion of coagulation products in hemophilia

Angelika Batorova[1] and Uri Martinowitz[2]

[1] Medical School of Comenius University, University Hospital, Bratislava, Slovakia
[2] Sackler School of Medicine, Tel Aviv, Israel

Introduction

People with hemophilia often require intensive factor replacement aimed at maintaining hemostatic factor levels over prolonged periods. Continuous infusion (CI) of factors VIII (FVIII) and IX (FIX) is an effective alternative to conventional intermittent bolus injections (BI), now widely used particularly in settings of surgery and major bleeding. Continuous administration of the missing factor maintains a steady hemostatic factor level within the circulation, avoiding dangerous troughs below the hemostatic minimum and unnecessary high peaks, associated with traditional intermittent injections of coagulation factors. Owing to a gradual decrease in clearance of infused coagulation factors during CI, in addition to efficient hemostasis this method has a potential for significant reduction of product requirements associated with intensive hemophilia therapy [1,2]. Clinical studies employing CI have demonstrated this method to be a safe and effective, both hemostatically and in terms of cost, treatment modality [2–7].

The use of CI is only possible if all essential requirements are met, including stability of coagulation products to be administered during extended time periods, availability of reliable infusion devices and employment of measures for aseptic preparation of concentrate.

The chapter deals with the principles of CI and actual issues of this effective modality of factor replacement in hemophilia.

Historical background and rationale for continuous infusion

The idea to normalize hemostasis by continuous administration of missing coagulation factor was suggested by Brinkhous in 1994 [8]. Hermens [9], in his mathematical model for administration of FVIII and FIX, demonstrated that the dose needed to keep the plasma level above the hemostatic minimum increases with the interval between injections. The theoretical differences between continuous infusion and intermittent bolus injections is shown in Figure 29.1. The area under the curve (AUC) which corresponds with the total amount of FVIII required, is about one-third less if continuous infusion is used [2]. Thus, CI has a potential to markedly reduce factor consumption. Hathaway et al. [10], in one of the first clinical observations with CI, could not confirm the expected 30% reduction in requirements by CI. Using a fixed rate of FVIII, he observed unexpected progressive increase of FVIII levels. His data, however, served as the ground for the development of the adjusted-dose CI [1,2]. We found that this elevation was the result of gradual decrease in the clearance after a steady hemostatic factor level has been achieved [1,2]. The reason for this phenomenon is still obscure; however, it provides a potential for additional saving of factor concentrates by adjustment of the rate of infusion proportionally to the decreasing clearance. A simple steady-state equation was adopted to calculate the required rate of infusion adjusted to the rate of the decreasing clearance. The guidelines for the administration of the adjusted-dose CI of coagulation factors were introduced in 1992 [1] and they are still in use.

Stability of concentrates and continuous infusion technique

An essential prerequisite for CI is factor concentrate maintaining its extended stability in the clinical settings of its use, i.e. after reconstitution, in the reservoir of the infusion pump at room temperature. Extensive stability studies conducted in the early 1990s demonstrated that most plasma-derived concentrates (pdFVIII/FIX) available at that time remained stable for several days after their reconstitution, and sometimes even for weeks [1,11]. Subsequently, many new-generation products

Textbook of Hemophilia, Third Edition. Edited by Christine A. Lee, Erik E. Berntorp and W. Keith Hoots.

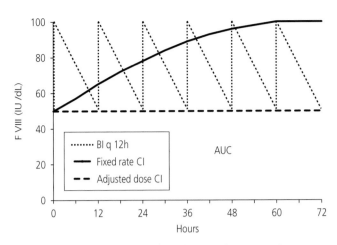

Figure 29.1 Factor VIII levels obtained during replacement with intermittent bolus injections (BI) and continuous infusion (CI) of fixed or adjusted doses. AUC, area under the curve; FVIII, factor VIII. From [1]. Reproduced with permission of John Wiley and Sons.

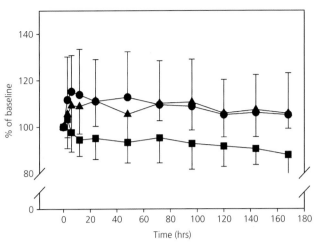

Figure 29.2 Stability of recombinant factor FVIII full length (rFVIII-FS) activity for 7 days at room temperature in both WalkMed and CADD infusion bags. Mean per cent recovery ±SD for rFVIII-FS activity based on activity from the time zero level following reconstitution of the concentrate. Lines represent concentrate without additives (squares), with addition of unfractionated heparin (triangles), and with addition of low- molecular- weight heparin (circles). From [16]. Reproduced with permission of John Wiley and Sons.

have been tested and proven to comply with the stability requirements for CI [12–17]. A good stability and low volume of concentrates allow to employ comfortable portable mini-pumps [18] with the exchange of infusion bags with concentrated products at intervals of 1–3 days (and longer), making this treatment convenient [1]. Nevertheless, in the USA and Canada, 59% and 80% of hemophilia centers employing the CI method, respectively, further dilute the concentrates with 60–500 mL of normal saline, and only 41% of US centers use the products up to 24 h after reconstitution [5,19,20].

Continuous infusion of new-generation recombinant products

An expanding use of CI encouraged the manufacturers to prove the stability of new-generation concentrates and their compatibility with the devices commonly employed in CI procedures. Despite proven extended stability of new recombinant products (rFVIII, rFIX, rFVIIa), the manufacturers still recommend to infuse the concentrates within a few hours after reconstitution. However, the product monographs of plasma/albumin-free recombinant human FVIII-rAHF-PFM (Advate), full-length rFVIII (Kogenate FS), and rFIX (BeneFIX) provide information about extended stability of product and feasibility for CI, employing low-volume infusion pumps which provide low infusion speeds. However, these products should not be further diluted for continuous infusion. A technical problem arises from the reduced volume (2.5–5.0 mL) of reconstituted highly concentrated products and relatively large dead space of current infusion devices. This is the reason why some clinicians further dilute the reconstituted concentrates, particularly for CI in children who require very small amounts of concentrate or, when the mini-pumps are not available. As shown by

in-vitro experiments, the dilution of B-domain deleted rFVIII and rAHF-PFM did not affect their stability [13,15]. However, in contrast to an excellent stability of undiluted rFVIII-FS for more than 7 days (Figure 29.2) [16], the dilution further than by the regular reconstitution resulted in initial loss of activity and decreased stability of product stored in the vials or syringes (Figure 29.3) [21,22]. Revel-Vilk et al. [22] demonstrated that these in-vitro losses of FVIII did not diminish the efficacy of CI in vivo. CI of rFVIII-FS diluted to 80 U/mL with 0.9% saline administered with a syringe pump to a boy with severe hemophilia postsurgically resulted in stable FVIII activity levels within the target range [22]. Nevertheless, before initiating CI it is advisable to test the stability of each concentrate type and to assay its compatibility with the particular infusion set to be used for CI.

Bacteriologic safety of continuous infusion

To ensure the bacteriologic safety of CI, a multidisciplinary initiative involving pharmacists, physicians, and nurses should be implemented [23]. The preparation and filling of the containers for CI must be done under sterile conditions, e.g. under laminar air flow.

The experiments focused on the risk of contamination and bacterial overgrowth during prolonged incubation of concentrates in the pump reservoir and proved that many FVIII and FIX concentrates are poor growth mediums for most bacterial strains [1,2,11]. Inoculation of the reservoirs of mini-pumps, containing factor concentrates, with common contaminants did

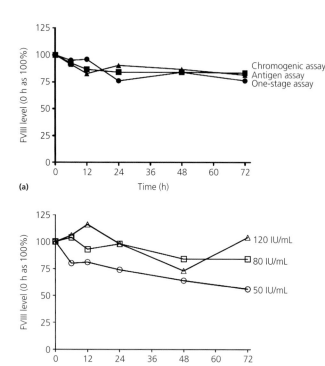

(a)

(b)

Figure 29.3 Stability of recombinant factor VIII full length (rFVIII-FS) in samples stored in polypropylene syringes at room temperature for up to 72 h, expressing the FVIII level immediately upon reconstitution or dilution (i.e. at 0 h) as 100%. **(a)** Undiluted rFVIII-FS assayed with the one-stage FVIII:C assay (closed circles), the chromogenic FVIII:C assay (closed squares), and the FVIII antigen assay (closed triangles). **(b)** rFVIII-FS diluted with 0.9% saline to 120 (open triangles), 80 (open squares), and 50 (open circles) U/mL, respectively. From [22]. Reproduced with permission of John Wiley and Sons.

not cause bacterial overgrowth and the thousands of cultures performed from mini-pump reservoirs after completion of the infusion were all negative [1,4,11,18]. Similarly, studies employing simulated CI with mini-pumps failed to find any microbial contamination of the infusion sets used for up to 6–7 days [1,15], and the bacterial safety of CI is also confirmed by clinical trials [4,16].

Prevention of thrombophlebitis

Thrombophlebitis at the site of venous access is a frequent adverse event of CI of undiluted FVIII concentrates, probably because of their high osmolarity [2]. This complication occurring in 2–11% of CI treatments [24] can be avoided by adding of heparin (5 U/mL) to the concentrate [1,2]. Such minor amounts of heparin neither influence the stability of the reconstituted FVIII and FIX [1,25] nor affect *in-vivo* hemostasis achieved by CI. In some products, addition of heparin may even improve stability, as in the case of rFVIII-FS [16]. In contrast, the addition of unfractionated heparin (UH) to rFVIIa leads to

immediate loss of activity of 20–30%, and the addition of low-molecular weight heparin (LMWH) causes aggregate formation without loss of activity [17,26]. Currently, the most widely adopted method of preventing local phlebitis during CI of rFVIIa is the parallel infusion of saline (10–20 mL/h) through a three-way connector [26–28].

Modes of continuous infusion and treatment protocols

The dosing of factor replacement is based on both the clinical experience of the treating hematologist and specific pharmacologic calculations that take into account the basic pharmacokinetics of clotting factors, such as *in-vivo* recovery and biologic half-life. The main goal of CI is to ensure adequate hemostasis by the maintenance of safe steady-state levels of the coagulation factor in circulation, eliminating unnecessary high peaks as well as trough levels which may fall below the minimum hemostatic level. However, although the factor level is accepted by the regulatory agencies as a surrogate parameter for efficacy, the hemostatic minimum for particular clinical situations still remains to be empirical rather than evidence based. A secondary, but no less important, goal of CI is to reduce the amount of factor required for the maintenance of desired hemostatic levels.

Adjusted-dose continuous infusion

This method employs pharmacokinetic dosing and takes advantage of decreasing clearance of coagulation factor during CI. The simple protocol for this method is based on the following set of principles [1]:

1 Pharmacokinetic evaluation prior to a planned CI is recommended but not mandatory. Pharmacokinetic testing is based on a bolus administration of approximately 50 IU/kg of factor and measurement of factor levels before infusion and then at nine postinfusion time points over the following 36–48 h [29]. The most important pharmacokinetic parameter for calculating the ideal rate of continuous infusion is the clearance.

2 The loading dose is calculated using *in-vivo* recovery (IU/dL per IU/kg). A dose is selected that will raise the factor level to the level appropriate for the specific situation; for major bleeds and surgery the level of 1.0 IU/mL is required.

3 CI is initiated immediately following bolus administration of the loading dose. The initial rate is calculated using the clearance obtained in the pre-procedure pharmacokinetic evaluation according to the following steady-state equation:

$$\text{Rate of infusion (IU/kg/h)} = \text{clearance (mL/kg/h)} \times \text{desired level (IU/mL)}$$

4 From the second day, the CI maintenance dose is adjusted using the same equation according to actual clearance, which is calculated from the daily factor level measurements.

5 Acceptable target minimum FVIII levels for major surgery are 0.7–0.8 IU/mL, 0.5 IU/mL, and 0.3 IU/mL for postoperative days 1–3, 4–6, and 7–10, respectively.

6 Perioperative hemostatic demands may increase factor consumption beyond that expected. In order to prevent an undesired drop in the factor level, it is advisable to check factor activity, or at least the activated partial thromboplastin time (aPTT), 6–8 h after the start of CI, and to increase the rate if necessary.

7 In most patients who require treatment for more than 1 week, a significant decrease in FVIII clearance is observed during the first 5–6 days of CI, followed by a plateau at a significantly lower level than that observed in the first days postoperatively [1,4,30]. This allows one to reduce the maintenance dose progressively and results in a significant sparing of concentrate.

In the absence of preoperative pharmacokinetic evaluation or, in particular, in emergency situations, the initial maintenance dose may be calculated using the mean of a hemophilia population-based clearance, which is approximately 3.5 mL/kg/h for FVIII and 4.5 mL/kg/h for FIX. However, one has to be aware of possible interindividual variations in clearance, which may be influenced by age, body weight, laboratory assay employed, and even the type of factor concentrate used [29,31]. Higher levels of clearance are physiologically observed in children.

Preoperative pharmacokinetic evaluation is a valuable tool to optimize CI, particularly if a major surgical procedure is planned. Pharmacokinetic testing may also alert one to an unsuspected low-titer inhibitor that may not be detectable by conventional inhibitor testing methods.

Fixed-rate continuous infusion

Some authors, aiming at FVIII/IX maintenance levels of 1.0 IU/mL for the first few postoperative days, have shown that this may be achieved with a fixed rate of FVIII and FIX of 4–5 IU/kg/h and ≥4–6 IU/kg/h, respectively, on average [6,20,32–34]. However, at this regimen often much higher levels are observed than those required to achieve satisfactory postoperative hemostasis [5–7,10,20,33]; further, during fixed-rate CI, the levels would be expected to rise gradually over the first 4–6 days owing to the decrease in clearance, which may result in unnecessarily high factor consumption unless appropriate adjustments are made daily, as described above.

Clinical indications for continuous infusion

Continuous infusion of coagulation factors in hemophilia A and B is indicated in situations that require the maintenance of efficient hemostatic factor levels for a period longer than 3–5 days. Such situations include the treatment of major bleeds, minor and major surgical procedures, management of bleeding in some patients with low-titer or low-affinity inhibitors, and,

rarely, short- and/or long-term prophylaxis. CI has been used also in home therapy settings for large bleeds requiring the maintenance of adequate and sustained FVIII levels over several days [2,3], or after minor surgeries not requiring hospital admission.

Continuous infusion of factor VIII

Continuous infusion using a variety of pdFVIII and rFVIII products has been introduced into common practise of hemophilia management worldwide, with 61% and 59% of comprehensive care centers employing CI in the US and Europe, respectively [19,20,24]. The Japanese guideline for hemophilia treatment suggest to use CI for major surgery [35,36]. Many reports demonstrated CI to be safe and hemostatically effective for all indications mentioned above, including the most demanding surgical procedures [1,2,4–7,20,34–38]. Most recently Takedani [37], Rahmé et al. [38], and Chevalier et al. [39] reported on successful use of CI in 28, 20, and 72 total knee replacements, respectively. A prospective controlled study comparing CI and BI for major surgery using protocols that were similar regarding the surgical technique and postoperative target minimum levels demonstrated that efficacy and safety were better with CI than with BI in terms of minimum factor levels achieved, blood loss (as measured by a decrease in hemoglobin level), blood transfusion requirements, and bleeding complications (Table 29.1) [4]. The clearance of FVIII decreased over 6 days of CI from initial rates of 3.89 ± 0.86 mL/kg/h to a plateau at a minimum of 2.1 ± 0.54 mL/kg/h ($P < 0.01$). FVIII consumption was 36% lower in the CI group (total dose of FVIII for 13 days 467 ± 104 IU/kg vs 733 ± 126 IU/kg; $P < 0.01$). High efficacy and similar level of FVIII saving (30%) was observed by Bidlingmaier et al. [6] who compared prospectively two groups of age- and procedure-matched patients treated with CI and BI (563.2 vs 812.8 IU/kg; $P < 0.006$). Nyshiya et al. [35] observed product saving of 24.4% with CI in 30 major surgical procedures compared to BI. Takedani [37] employing three different concentrates for CI observed the interproduct variability with significantly higher infusion rate required to maintain the same factor level (Figure 29.4) and higher total consumption of Advate (652 ± 183.0 IU/kg) when compared with Kogenate-FS (395.1 ± 65.0 IU/kg, $P < 0.01$) and Cross-Eight M pdFVIII (519.1 ± 68.0 IU/kg, $P < 0.05$). A recent survey on CI practise in 22 European hemophilia centers showed 13/59% centers using CI, all employing adjusted-dose CI of undiluted concentrates, however, with a wide range of FVIII levels targeted in the settings of major surgery: a median (range) target FVIII levels were of 1.0 (0.7–1.0) IU/mL, 0.8 (0.5–1.0) IU/mL, and 0.5 (0.4–0.8) IU/mL for the day of surgery, days 1–3 and 4–7, respectively [24]. The incidence of postoperative bleeding among the centers was only 1.8% (range 0–7.0%). Eight centers reported cost savings over traditional bolus therapy ranging from 15% to 36% [24]. Table 29.2 presents the characteristics of recent studies on CI with rFVIII products; the difference in

Table 29.1 Continuous infusion versus intermittent injections of factor VIII in severe hemophilia A patients undergoing major surgery [4]. Reproduced with permission of John Wiley and Sons.

	Bolus injections	Continuous infusion	P
Number (patients/operations)	18/18	22/25	
Age (years)	24 ± 14	26 ± 14	NS
Body weight (kg)	60 ± 17	58 ± 25	NS
Treatment period (days)	13 ± 1	13 ± 1	NS
FVIII levels[a]—first week (IU/mL)	0.43 ± 0.09	0.54 ± 0.09	<0.01
Nadir of FVIII—first week (IU/mL)	0.31 ± 0.09	0.44 ± 0.06	<0.01
Major bleeding complications	3/18	0/25	NS
Postoperative drop of hemoglobin (g/L)	30.1 ± 21.3	15.6 ± 12.1	<0.05
Patients requiring blood transfusion	7/18	3/25	<0.01
Factor consumption—first week (IU/kg)	493 ± 81	342 ± 69	<0.01
Total factor consumption (IU/kg)	733 ± 126	467 ± 104	<0.01

Values expressed as mean ± SD.
NS, not significant.
[a]Constant levels in continuous infusion and trough levels in bolus injection.

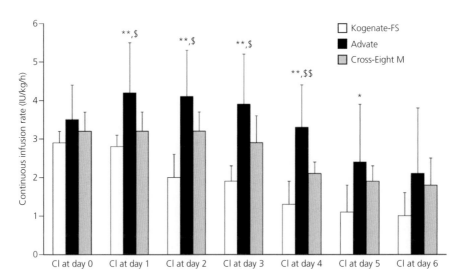

Figure 29.4 Continuous infusion rate. The continuous infusion rate of Advate is significantly greater than that of other concentrates ($*P < 0.05$; $**P < 0.01$ compared with Kogenate-FS; $\$P < 0.05$; $\$\$P < 0.01$ compared with Cross-Eight M). From [36]. Reproduced with permission of John Wiley and Sons.

the study design and duration of CI preclude comparison of the outcomes regarding the final factor consumption.

Continuous infusion of factor VIII for long-term prophylaxis

With regard to theoretical calculations [40] continuous infusion could have the potential for remarkable product savings in conditions of regular prophylaxis. However, there are still many limitations, mainly technical, for this indication. Nevertheless, CI was used for prolonged periods of 6–24 months in three of our patients after partial resection of a giant pseudotumor, in whom bleeding from the pseudotumor occurred when the FVIII level dropped below 10–20% [41]. The recent development of ultraconcentrated rFVIII with extended stability and

development of tiny implantable mini-pumps might be promising, especially for long-term prophylactic treatment.

Continuous infusion of factor IX

Hoots *et al.* [32], in a prospective multicenter study demonstrated CI of pdFIX Mononine to be safe and hemostatically effective in patients with hemophilia B undergoing surgery. Preoperative median clearance was 4.06 mL/kg/h (range 2.45–9.65 mL/kg/h) and hemostasis was achieved by infusion rate of 3.84 IU/kg/h (1.74–7.33 IU/kg/h). pdFIX and rFIX have different pharmacokinetics [32,33,42]. Poon *et al.* [42] observed *in-vivo* recovery of 1.05 ± 0.26 IU/dL per IU/kg and 0.77 ± 0.19 IU/dL per IU/kg for pdFIX and rFIX, respectively, with no significant difference in half-life. In the CI setting the clearance

CHAPTER 30

Surgery in inhibitor patients

Pål Andrè Holme

Oslo University Hospital, Oslo, Norway

Introduction

Surgery in persons with hemophilia and high-titer inhibitors is a clinical challenge and was for a long time considered almost impossible. However, experience during the last 10–15 years using bypassing agents has shown that, despite increased bleeding risk compared to noninhibitor patients, the results are in general good [1–12]. Consequently, patients with inhibitors should not be denied surgical procedures. Nevertheless, surgery continues to pose a major challenge in these patients as the costs are significantly higher than in patients without inhibitors in addition to a higher risk of bleeding.

At present, bypassing agents, such as activated prothrombin complex concentrate (aPCC) and activated recombinant factor VII (rFVIIa) are the only coagulation factor concentrates available for the treatment of inhibitor patients if the inhibitor titer is above 5 Bethesda units (BU). Bypassing agents require proper management since none of the products can guarantee sustained hemostasis. Clinical experience indicates that both products are effective in most patients, but in some patients one or the other seems to be superior. If first-line therapy fails, then the alternative bypassing agent should be used [14].

In hemophilia patients without inhibitors, there is a close relationship between the level of factor VIII (FVIII) or factor IX (FIX) measured *ex vivo* and the hemostatic efficacy in the patients. However, in inhibitor patients there is no such relationship using bypassing treatment as there is no established laboratory assay to monitor efficacy and optimal dosing.

All surgery in patients should be conducted in a hemophilia comprehensive care center (HCCC).

Products available for surgery

Activated prothrombin complex concentrate and activated recombinant activated factor VII

The bypassing agents, aPCC—factor eight inhibitor bypass activity (FEIBA, Baxter AG, Vienna, Austria) and rFVIIa (NovoSeven, NovoNordisk A/S, Bagsvaerd, Denmark)—are the treatment of choice in patients with inhibitors if the inhibitor level exceeds 5 BU. Which one to use depends on several factors such as the age of the patient, prior history of efficacy with a particular product, cost, and safety. aPCC has been used extensively for a long period of time and has the advantage of dosing every 8–12 h, whereas rVIIa must be infused every 2–3 h. rFVIIa offers the advantage of being a recombinant protein, and therefore is unlikely to be contaminated with infectious agents, as opposed to aPCC which is plasma derived. However, the risk is minimized as aPCC is now double virus inactivated and no transmission of bloodborne infectious agents has been reported since these precautions were undertaken. Both products are effective in achieving hemostasis in the majority of patients, and one should switch to the other product if the first choice fails. Side-effects including venous thrombotic events, disseminated intravascular coagulation (DIC) and myocardial infarction have been reported using both aPCC and rFVIIa [15–17], although at a very low rate, if doses within the manufacturers' recommended range are used. The main disadvantages of rFVIIa compared to aPCC are high cost and frequent infusions [3,18].

Preoperative planning

Due to the increased risk of bleeding complications during surgery, thorough planning should be undertaken prior to surgery in these patients. Coordinated standard pre-, intra-, and postoperative assessment and planning are intended to optimize surgical outcome and utilization of resources, while minimizing the risk of bleeding and other adverse events during and after surgery. It is recommended that any surgery in patients with hemophilia and inhibitors be planned in conjunction with an HCCC where there is a concentration of expertise and experience and performed in a hospital that incorporates an HCCC [19].

Prior to surgery, several aspects should be explored such as previous response to bypassing agents, outcome of prior surgery, and type of surgical procedure. The patient's expectations regarding surgical outcome and recovery are also important to

Textbook of Hemophilia, Third Edition. Edited by Christine A. Lee, Erik E. Berntorp and W. Keith Hoots.
© 2014 John Wiley & Sons, Ltd. Published 2014 by John Wiley & Sons, Ltd.

make clear prior to surgery. The hematologist should provide a written detailed treatment plan including duration and dosage of the hemostatic treatment.

In the preoperative planning for the patient, it is advisable to routinely assess for any sign of coronary heart disease as this might increase the risk of thromboembolic events using bypassing agents.

Relevant laboratory testing including a full blood cell count, fibrinogen, activated partial thromboplastin time, prothrombin time, and D-dimer should regularly be performed in the postoperative phase. However, frequent monitoring for anamnesis is not required as a rise in BU would not alter the management of a patient with a high-titer inhibitor using bypassing agents.

There are no standardized laboratory assays to monitor the efficacy and optimal dosing of bypassing products following surgery. However, preoperative evaluation of hemostatic response to bypassing agents using thrombin generation test (TGT) or thromboelastography (TEG) has been reported as a means to predict and optimize hemostatic outcome during the peri- and postoperative phase [20–22]. Dargaud *et al.* reported a small prospective study of 10 elective invasive procedures using a three-step protocol to individually tailor the use of the bypassing agent [20]. TGT were used *in vitro* to assess the dose-dependent response to each product, and the patients were then followed intra- and postoperatively, and it was reported that the thrombin generation correlated with clinical hemostasis. Preliminary findings suggest that these assays might be helpful to tailor the treatment for each patient, but it remains to be established if such tests are applicable during daily practise. However, due to high interlaboratory variations these laboratory assays need to be standardized and validated in the near future and further studies are needed to assess their ability to predict hemostatic outcome in patients with inhibitors undergoing surgical procedures.

Management of substitution therapy in the peri- and postoperative phase

In patients with a low-titer (<5 BU) or a low-responding inhibitor, the use of high-dose FVIII or FIX concentrates to overcome the inhibitors might be applicable in the initial phase. However, an anamnestic response may occur, and the hematologist should be prepared to switch to a bypassing agent at any time.

As there are no comparative studies of rVIIa and aPCC in surgery, personal experience, previous hemostatic response in the particular patient, and availability of products may guide the choice of bypassing agent [23].

Activated prothrombin complex concentrate–Feiba

During the last 15 years, more than 200 surgical procedures have been reported in nine case series each with more than 10

procedures performed using aPCC as replacement therapy in patients with inhibitors [2–10]. The hemostatic efficacy in these case series have been reported from 78% to 100%. Variable initial doses, frequency of infusions, and duration of treatment have been reported; however, continuous infusion (CI) has not been studied.

The Norwegian experience using aPCC for surgery accounts for 37 surgical procedures: 17 major and 20 minor [3,5]. aPCC was delivered by short-time infusions (15–20 min) three times daily. A preoperative loading dose of 100 U/kg was given. The following doses were adjusted to a total daily dose of 200 U/kg/day. Following the third postoperative day, the dose of aPCC was tapered to a daily dose of 150 U/kg and from the 7th postoperative day tapered gradually to 100 U/kg every 8 h. A further 50 U/kg every second day was given as postsurgical prophylaxis and prior to physiotherapy. A good or excellent hemostatic outcome was observed for all minor procedures and in 15/17 (88%) of the major procedures. A few consensus reports on the use of aPCC as replacement therapy in inhibitor patients undergoing surgery have been published [23–26]. Common to these recommendations are a preoperative bolus infusion of 50–100 U/kg, then a dose of 75–100 U/kg every 8–12 h for a maximum daily dose of 200 U/kg and depending on the clinical condition and type of surgery the dose may be tapered until discharge (Table 30.1).

Table 30.1 Recommended dosage of activated recombinant factor VIIa (rFVIIa) and activated prothrombin complex concentrate (aPCC) for surgery in patients with hemophilia and inhibitors.

		Preoperative dose	Postoperative management
rFVIIa			
	Minor surgery	90 μg/kg	90 μg/kg every 2 h up to four times, then every 3–6 h until discharge
	Major surgery	90–120 μg/kg	90 μg/kg every 2 h the first 48 h, then 90 μg/kg every 3, 4, then 6 h on days 3, 5, and 8, respectively, until discharge CI 50 μg/kg/h
aPCC			
	Minor surgery	50–100 U/kg	50–75 U/kg every 8–12 h until discharge
	Major surgery	75–100 U/kg	70 U/kg every 8 h for at least 3 days with a maximum daily dose of 200 U/kg. Dose may be tapered for day 4 to 50 U/kg every 8 h.

CI: continuous infusion.

Recombinant factor VIIa (NovoSeven)

A review of many small case series using rFVIIa for different surgical procedures in hemophilia patients with inhibitors has reported good hemostatic outcomes [11]. However, variable doses and protocols have been used, and only two small prospective randomized studies have addressed the dose and mode of administration. Shapiro *et al.* compared the effect of two doses of rFVIIa in 29 patients during minor and major surgical procedures [1]. The patients were randomized to either 35 µg/kg vs 90 µg/kg every 2 h for 2 days, then every 2–6 h for a total of 5 days. With respect to major surgery, the effectiveness at day 5 was found to be 40% for the low dose compared to 83% for the high dose. The authors concluded that rFVIIa at 90 µg/kg is an effective first-line option for major surgery in patients with inhibitors. With respect to minor surgery, hemostasis was effective in 70% and 100% of the procedures for the low dose and high dose, respectively.

The use of rFVIIa given as CI in a surgical setting in inhibitor patients has been reported with a good hemostatic outcome [27,28]. Pruthi *et al.* studied the efficacy and safety of administering rFVIIa, after an initial bolus dose of 90 µg/kg, either as repetitive bolus infusions (BI) (90 µg/kg) every 2 h or CI 50 µg/kg/h for 5 days in 22 major surgical procedures in a randomized prospective study [12]. It was found that there was comparable hemostatic efficacy and safety of BI and CI although the treatment was considered ineffective in three subjects in each arm of the trial.

Valentino *et al.* reported from the Hemophilia and Thrombosis Research Registry and literature, which also incorporated a small number of medical procedures (*n* = 45) in addition to surgical and dental procedures, and found rFVIIa to be effective in 333 (84%) of 395 procedures [16]. Thromboembolic complications attributable to rFVIIa were reported in 0.025% of these procedures.

Based on the present literature, a few general expert recommendations have been published for the use of rFVIIa in surgical procedures [23,26,29–31] (Table 30.1). The initial bolus dose should at least be 90 µg/kg given immediately preoperatively and then every 2 h for at least 48 h. However, due to observed bleeding complications in a minority of procedures, an initial dose of 120–180 µg/kg have been proposed [29]. After 2 days, the dose interval may be increased to 3, 4, and 6 h on days 3, 5, and 8, respectively, and continued until discharge. CI (50 µg/kg/h) after initial bolus therapy appears to be a promising modality based on one prospective study [12]. However, it is premature to recommend this mode of administration for routine use as further evidence is lacking and some treaters believe that the burst of thrombin generated after bolus administration is important for hemostasis.

Infusion of rFVIIa at 90 µg/kg is recommended before every physiotherapy session.

In case of unexpected peri- or postoperative bleeding episodes using bypassing agent one should increase the dose of the bypassing agent in use to the maximum dose (rFVIIa up to 270 µg/kg or aPCC up to 200 U/kg/day). If hemostasis is still not achieved, the alternative bypassing agent should be rapidly implemented similarly to unresponsive severe bleeding episodes [32] (Figure 30.1). When monotherapy with either of the products at maximum doses have been ineffective, sequential or concomitant treatment might be considered for salvage treatment.

Although the documentation for such treatment is sparse, one report on sequential therapy in five adults who had significant bleeding following major surgery suggests that sequential treatment is feasible and effective [33]. No clinical adverse events were observed in these patients. However, a significant increase in D-dimer levels was observed in three of the five patients.

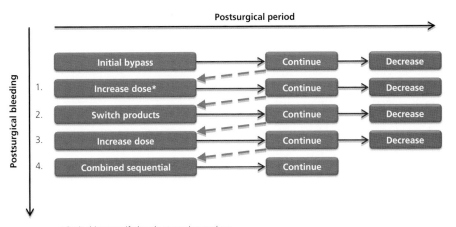

*Omit this stage if already at maximum dose

Figure 30.1 Algorithm to manage postsurgical bleeding episodes in patients with high-titer inhibitors. Modified from [13]. Reproduced with permission of Elsevier.

Concomitant infusion of rFVIIa (30–70 μg/kg) and aPCC (20–30 U/kg) in patients with bleeds unresponsive to monotherapy to treat 400 bleeds in five patients has also been published [34]. Concomitant treatment has never been reported in a surgical setting.

Bypassing agents and antifibrinolytics

The antifibrinolytic agent tranexamic acid (TXA) increases clot stability and is used concomitantly with coagulation factor replacement to improve hemostasis in hemophilia patients without inhibitors. It is not considered contraindicated to combine rFVIIa with TXA to improve hemostasis although it has not been systematically studied. In contrast, aPCC has not been recommended to be given together with TXA unless a time lag of 6 h between the administration of the two drugs. The reason for this precaution is safety concerns due to an estimated increased risk of thrombotic events and DIC. However, strong evidence supporting this precaution is lacking. An in-vitro study demonstrated that the combination of TXA and aPCC improved clot stability in FVIII inhibitor plasma without additional increase in thrombin generation [35]. Further, a recent clinical study showed good hemostatic efficacy and no episodes of thromboembolic events, DIC, or hypercoagulability in inhibitor patients following the concomitant use of TXA and aPCC where some previously had been refractory to monotherapy treatment [21]. The dose of TXA commonly used is 10 mg/kg intravenously or 20 mg/kg orally 3–4 times daily for 7–10 days.

When applied locally either as a mouth rinse or moistened dressings, the combination of TXA and aPCC is considered safe. This combination is highly recommended.

Postoperative management

Adequate pain control is an important factor in successful postoperative management and rehabilitation. However, in general, postoperative spinal and epidural anesthesia are contraindicated due to the risk of bleeds and lack of evidence supporting the safety of bypassing products for such procedures [23]. However, nerve blocks may be used in this patient group with caution [25]. Acetylsalicylic acid and cyclooxygenase-1 inhibitors should also be avoided since they induce platelet dysfunction and thereby contribute to impaired hemostasis.

A physiotherapy plan to support postoperative rehabilitation is advisable in patients undergoing elective orthopedic surgery in particular, and the physiotherapist should be experienced in the management of hemophilia and be in frequent communication with the other members of the hemophilia treatment team. Treatment with bypassing agents before each therapy session is recommended for 2–4 weeks after surgery [36,37].

Bypassing agents and thromboprophylaxis

Although thrombosis might be a concern using bypassing agents, postoperative anticoagulation (e.g. low-molecular-weight heparin) is not recommended in patients with inhibitors [19,38,39]. For the majority of patients, the use of gradated compression stockings and early mobilization are sufficient to prevent venous thromboembolism.

Economic considerations

Surgery in inhibitor patients is expensive and the concentrate costs is a 5–10-fold higher than in noninhibitor patients. However, aPCC has been shown to provide a cost benefit over rFVIIa [3,18].

Conclusion

In hemophilia patients with inhibitors, bypassing agent is safe and efficacious in maintaining hemostatic control and minimizing the risk of major bleeding complications during and following surgery. Consequently, no patients with inhibitors should be denied surgical intervention. However, it requires thorough planning, experience, and proper management since no product can guarantee sustained hemostasis. There is a great demand for standardized laboratory assays reflecting the hemostatic efficacy of bypassing agents.

References

1 Shapiro AD, Gilchrist GS, Hoots WK, Cooper HA, Gastineau DA. Prospective, randomised trial of two doses of rFVIIa (NovoSeven) in haemophilia patients with inhibitors undergoing surgery. *Thromb Haemost* 1998; **80**(5): 773–8.

2 Negrier C, Goudemand J, Sultan Y, Bertrand M, Rothschild C, Lauroua P. Multicenter retrospective study on the utilization of FEIBA in France in patients with factor VIII and factor IX inhibitors. French FEIBA Study Group. Factor Eight Bypassing Activity. *Thromb Haemost* 1997; **77**(6): 1113–19.

3 Tjonnfjord GE, Brinch L, Gedde-Dahl T, Brosstad FR. Activated prothrombin complex concentrate (FEIBA) treatment during surgery in patients with inhibitors to FVIII/IX. *Haemophilia* 2004; **10**(2): 174–8.

4 Dimichele D, Negrier C. A retrospective postlicensure survey of FEIBA efficacy and safety. *Haemophilia* 2006; **12**(4): 352–62.

5 Holme P, Tran H, Paus A, Tjonnfjord G. Surgery in haemophilia patients with inhibitors to FVIII/FIX: the Norwegian single centre study. *Thromb Haemost* 2011; **9**(Suppl. 2): 0-WE-028.

6 Stine KC, Shrum D, Becton DL. Use of FEIBA for invasive or surgical procedures in patients with severe hemophilia A or B with inhibitors. *J Pediatr Hematol Oncol* 2007; **29**(4): 216–21.

7 Rodriguez-Merchan EC, Jimenez-Yuste V, Gomez-Cardero P, Alvarez-Roman M, Martin-Salces M, Rodriguez de la Rua A. Surgery in haemophilia patients with inhibitors, with special emphasis on orthopaedics: Madrid experience. *Haemophilia* 2010; **16**(102): 84–8.

8 Lauroua P, Ferrer AM, Guerin V. Successful major and minor surgery using factor VIII inhibitor bypassing activity in patients with haemophilia A and inhibitors. *Haemophilia* 2009; **15**(6): 1300–7.

9 Rangarajan S, Yee TT, Wilde J. Experience of four UK comprehensive care centres using FEIBA(R) for surgeries in patients with inhibitors. *Haemophilia* 2011; **17**(1): 28–34.

10 Zulfikar B, Aydogan G, Salcioglu Z, *et al.* Efficacy of FEIBA for acute bleeding and surgical haemostasis in haemophilia A patients with inhibitors: a multicentre registry in Turkey. *Haemophilia* 2012; **18**(3): 383–91.

11 Obergfell A, Auvinen MK, Mathew P. Recombinant activated factor VII for haemophilia patients with inhibitors undergoing orthopaedic surgery: a review of the literature. *Haemophilia* 2008; **14**(2): 233–41.

12 Pruthi RK, Mathew P, Valentino LA, Sumner MJ, Seremetis S, Hoots WK. Haemostatic efficacy and safety of bolus and continuous infusion of recombinant factor VIIa are comparable in haemophilia patients with inhibitors undergoing major surgery. Results from an open-label, randomized, multicenter trial. *Thromb Haemost* 2007; **98**(4): 726–32.

13 Gomperts ED, Astermark J, Gringeri A, Teitel J. From theory to practice: applying current clinical knowledge and treatment strategies to the care of hemophilia a patients with inhibitors. *Blood Rev* 2008; **22** (Suppl. 1): S1–11.

14 Hay CR, Brown S, Collins PW, Keeling DM, Liesner R. The diagnosis and management of factor VIII and IX inhibitors: a guideline from the United Kingdom Haemophilia Centre Doctors Organisation. *Br J Haematol* 2006; **133**(6): 591–605.

15 Aledort LM. Comparative thrombotic event incidence after infusion of recombinant factor VIIa versus factor VIII inhibit bypass activity. *J Thromb Haemost* 2004; **2**(10): 1700–8.

16 Valentino LA, Cooper DL, Goldstein B. Surgical experience with rFVIIa (NovoSeven) in congenital haemophilia A and B patients with inhibitors to factors VIII or IX. *Haemophilia* 2011; **17**(4): 579–89.

17 Ehrlich HJ, Henzl MJ, Gomperts ED. Safety of factor VIII inhibitor bypass activity (FEIBA): 10-year compilation of thrombotic adverse events. *Haemophilia* 2002; **8**(2): 83–90.

18 Bonnet PO, Yoon BS, Wong WY, Boswell K, Ewenstein BM. Cost minimization analysis to compare activated prothrombin complex concentrate (aPCC) and recombinant factor VIIa for haemophilia patients with inhibitors undergoing major orthopaedic surgeries. *Haemophilia* 2009; **15**(5): 1083–9.

19 Kulkarni R. Comprehensive care of the patient with haemophilia and inhibitors undergoing surgery: practical aspects. *Haemophilia* 2013; **19**(1): 2–10.

20 Dargaud Y, Lienhart A, Negrier C. Prospective assessment of thrombin generation test for dose monitoring of bypassing therapy in hemophilia patients with inhibitors undergoing elective surgery. *Blood* 2010; **116**(25): 5734–7.

21 Holmstrom M, Tran HT, Holme PA. Combined treatment with APCC (FEIBA(R)) and tranexamic acid in patients with haemophilia A with inhibitors and in patients with acquired haemophilia A—a two-centre experience. *Haemophilia* 2012; **18**(4): 544–9.

22 Pivalizza EG, Escobar MA. Thrombelastography-guided factor VIIa therapy in a surgical patient with severe hemophilia and factor VIII inhibitor. *Anesth Analg* 2008; **107**(2): 398–401.

23 Teitel JM, Carcao M, Lillicrap D, *et al.* Orthopaedic surgery in haemophilia patients with inhibitors: a practical guide to haemostatic, surgical and rehabilitative care. *Haemophilia* 2009; **15**(1): 227–39.

24 Rodriguez-Merchan EC, Rocino A, Ewenstein B, *et al.* Consensus perspectives on surgery in haemophilia patients with inhibitors: summary statement. *Haemophilia* 2004; **10** (Suppl. 2): 50–2.

25 Rangarajan S, Austin S, Goddard NJ, *et al.* Consensus recommendations for the use of FEIBA(®) in haemophilia A patients with inhibitors undergoing elective orthopaedic and non-orthopaedic surgery. *Haemophilia* 2013; **19**(2): 294–303.

26 Makris M, Hay CR, Gringeri A, D'Oiron R. How I treat inhibitors in haemophilia. *Haemophilia* 2012; **18** (Suppl. 4): 48–53.

27 Schulman S. Safety, efficacy and lessons from continuous infusion with rFVIIa. rFVIIa-CI Group. *Haemophilia* 1998; **4**(4): 564–7.

28 Santagostino E, Morfini M, Rocino A, Baudo F, Scaraggi FA, Gringeri A. Relationship between factor VII activity and clinical efficacy of recombinant factor VIIa given by continuous infusion to patients with factor VIII inhibitors. *Thromb Haemost* 2001; **86**(4): 954–8.

29 Giangrande PL, Wilde JT, Madan B, *et al.* Consensus protocol for the use of recombinant activated factor VII [eptacog alfa (activated); NovoSeven] in elective orthopaedic surgery in haemophilic patients with inhibitors. *Haemophilia* 2009; **15**(2): 501–8.

30 Ljung RC, Knobe K. How to manage invasive procedures in children with haemophilia. *Br J Haematol* 2012; **157**(5): 519–28.

31 Berntorp E, Shapiro AD. Modern haemophilia care. *Lancet* 2012; **379**(9824): 1447–56.

32 Teitel J, Berntorp E, Collins P, *et al.* A systematic approach to controlling problem bleeds in patients with severe congenital haemophilia A and high-titre inhibitors. *Haemophilia* 2007; **13**(3): 256–63.

33 Gringeri A, Fischer K, Karafoulidou A, Klamroth R, Lopez-Fernandez MF, Mancuso E. Sequential combined bypassing therapy is safe and effective in the treatment of unresponsive bleeding in adults and children with haemophilia and inhibitors. *Haemophilia* 2011; **17**(4): 630–5.

34 Martinowitz U, Livnat T, Zivelin A, Kenet G. Concomitant infusion of low doses of rFVIIa and FEIBA in haemophilia patients with inhibitors. *Haemophilia* 2009; **15**(4): 904–10.

35 Dai L, Bevan D, Rangarajan S, Sorensen B, Mitchell M. Stabilization of fibrin clots by activated prothrombin complex concentrate and tranexamic acid in FVIII inhibitor plasma. *Haemophilia* 2009; **17**(5): e944–8.

36 Konkle BA, Nelson C, Forsyth A, Hume E. Approaches to successful total knee arthroplasty in haemophilia A patients with inhibitors. *Haemophilia* 2002; **8**(5): 706–10.

37 Solimeno LP, Perfetto OS, Pasta G, Santagostino E. Total joint replacement in patients with inhibitors. *Haemophilia* 2006; **12** (Suppl. 3): 113–16.

38 Mannucci PM, Schutgens RE, Santagostino E, Mauser-Bunschoten EP. How I treat age-related morbidities in elderly persons with hemophilia. *Blood* 2009; **114**(26): 5256–63.

39 Philipp C. The aging patient with hemophilia: complications, comorbidities, and management issues. *Hematol Am Soc Hematol Educ Program* 2010; 191–6.

PART X

Musculoskeletal

PART 2

Musculoskeletal

CHAPTER 33

Pseudotumors in patients with hemophilia

Michael Heim[1] and Uri Martinowitz[2]

[1] University of Tel Aviv, Tel Aviv, Israel
[2] Sackler School of Medicine, Tel Aviv, Israel

Introduction

Pseudotumor, an expending destructive encapsulated cyst/hematoma, is a rare but serious complication in persons with hemophilia (PWH). Its estimated incidence is reported at about 1%.

Only anecdotal reports and a few small case series have been published in the literature. Historically, these reports originated mainly from countries with limited resources where replacement therapy was not adequate. An assumption was thus made that there is a connection between the lack of factor replacement therapy and the development of pseudotumors. This suspicion has been strengthened by reports of the occurrence of pseudotumors in patients who have developed an antibody to the missing coagulation factor. There is no established standard approach to the management of pseudotumors and the treatment is based on clinical rationale and the opinion of experts with limited experience.

Pathogenesis of pseudotumors

There are two distinct pathologic forms that have been noted and categorized under the heading of pseudotumors. The first form occurs within the peripheral long bones and very often in the developing skeleton, while the second has a predilection particularly for the area of and around the pelvis. The former starts as an intraosseous expansion that can perforate the cortex, while the latter begins its growth in the soft tissues and may erode skeletal structures. Some authors believe that the pathology starts in Sharpey's fibers (the tissue connecting muscles to the periosteum).

Anatomically, this situation exists extensively around the pelvis and the thighs [1]. The intraosseous form is more aggressive then a simple bone cyst, for it actively expands, and yet is amenable to conservative treatment [2]. The soft-tissue masses have a distinct histologic structure [3]. The contents comprise necrotic blood but may also contain large quantities of blood and other liquefied tissue products. The pseudotumor has a thick capsule wherein blood vessels are encased and infuse the entire pseudotumor. The mass is expansive and hence has the ability to cause pressure necrosis of the surrounding tissues, which can include the cortex of bone (Figures 33.1, 33.2, 33.3, and 33.4). The pseudotumor may expand around structures such as the ureters, blood vessels, and nerves. These structures are not invaded by the tumoral growth but encircled, and upon gross anatomy would appear to be within the tumor mass [4].

Clinical presentation

There are two forms of pseudotumors. The peripheral pathology is generally amenable to early diagnosis in view of the anatomic deformation of fingers and toes, and/or the perceivable swelling noted over the dorsum of the hand or foot. Radiographic evidence is easily obtained and treatment can then be instituted.

The second form is usually intra-abdominal and slow growing. Early diagnosis rarely occurs as the expanding mass slowly fills up the area of the abdomen and/or the pelvis and retroperitoneum. Patients may note a general discomfort, but in the light of their experiences with intra-articular hemarthroses and muscle bleeds, these generalized symptoms are often ignored. Radiologic plates may show a displacement of viscera and/or bone erosion, and a more extensive investigation is then indicated to assess the extent of the pseudotumor.

Investigations prior to treatment

Although usually arising in the area of the pelvis, large pseudotumors can theoretically appear anywhere in the body. It must be appreciated that not only are the dimensions of the

---

Textbook of Hemophilia, Third Edition. Edited by Christine A. Lee, Erik E. Berntorp and W. Keith Hoots.
© 2014 John Wiley & Sons, Ltd. Published 2014 by John Wiley & Sons, Ltd.

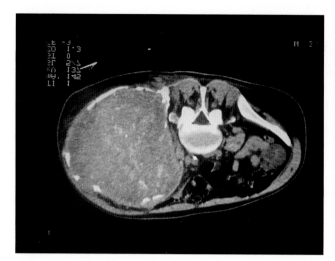

Figure 33.1 Computed tomography section through the level of the lumbar spine. A huge round pseudotumor can be noted. The pseudotumor has destroyed and fragmented the ileum and the mass extends almost to the midline.

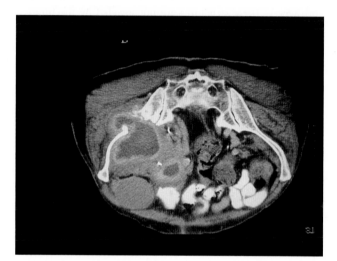

Figure 33.2 This computed tomography section shows a large pseudotumor mass that has expanded through the ileum. The mass can clearly be seen in the destroyed bone and on both sides of the ileum.

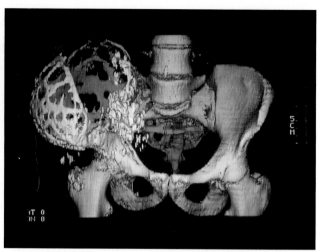

Figure 33.3 This figure clearly shows a computed tomography reconstruction of the pseudotumor, which has fragments of the ileum surrounding the mass. Note the encroachment onto the sacrum and the destroyed sacroiliac articulation.

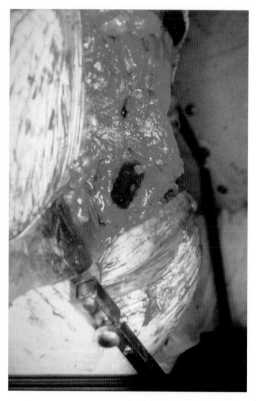

Figure 33.4 This intraoperative view clearly demonstrates a large hole in the ileum where the pseudotumor penetrated the cortex. (See also Plate 33.4.)

mass relevant, but also the contents and the anatomy of the surrounding area. The following investigations should be considered:

- Radiologic assessment to ascertain the osseous extent of the damage (regular radiographs and computed tomography usually suffice).
- The assessment of the structure and nature of the soft tissues and their relations to the bone can be mapped out by ultrasound and magnetic resonance imaging (MRI). Intravenous injection of gadolinium in conjunction with the MRI is suggested. The gadolinium helps to detect pathologic blood vessels and also helps to delineate the pseudotumor capsule.
- Intravenous pyelography should be considered if the growth is in the region of the kidney and its draining apparatus.
- It is important to evaluate the anatomy of major blood vessels in or close to the mass on arteriogram to plan the best surgical approach.

The planning of the operation should comprise a multidisciplinary team of experts, including an expert in invasive radiology, orthopedic and vascular surgeons, a urologist if the pelvis is involved, and—if required—spine specialists, liver specialists, general neurosurgeons, and any other specialist, depending on the expanse of the pseudotumor. It is of the utmost importance to appoint a coordinator (usually a surgeon, but could also be an experienced hemophilia expert) to coordinate the rotation of the various experts according to the progress of the surgery. Experts may be needed several times during surgery and the postoperative period, therefore members of the multidisciplinary team should be informed to be available during the whole surgical procedure, which may take several hours.

Hematologic assessment of the patients is essential and should include inhibitor testing and full pharmacokinetic evaluation to find the individual recovery, half-life, and clearance of the patient's missing factor prior to the surgery.

There should be a coagulation team and laboratory service available during the surgery and postoperative care planned. Sufficient concentrates should be reserved for the surgery and postsurgical period. High trough levels should be maintained over a period of 10 days to 3 weeks. According to our limited experience with four giant pseudotumors (two in Israel and two abroad with our participation and guidance) [5], the levels drop below the planned trough owing to high consumption. All four patients had diffuse bleeding from the extensive tissue damage. Fibrin glue was sprayed over the surfaces to assist local hemostasis but was ineffective in two operations because of the active bleeding that washed away the glue before clotting had occurred. Recombinant factor VIIa (rFVIIa) immediately stopped the diffuse bleed and allowed the use of fibrin glue (to prevent a rebleed). The most appropriate approach is to deliver the replacement therapy by continuous infusion. In the event of partial resection of the giant pseudotumor, an extended period of replacement treatment with higher trough levels may be necessary. Two of our four patients mentioned above required trough levels of factor VIII (FVIII) above 10% for periods of 6 months and 2 years, respectively. Any attempt to reduce the levels ended in retroperitoneal bleeding. One patient was living in another country (about an hour's flying time away), and once a week he sent a plasma sample by plane. His FVIII level was tested and in the evening he received instructions on the new rate of infusion required to maintain the desired level. The patient had a mini-pump and the necessary disposable sets and was trained to perform continuous home infusion [6].

Additional hemostatic measure

Owing to the extensive surgery, factor replacement alone may not be sufficient to control the diffuse and massive bleeding. The addition of fibrinolytic inhibitor is optional (high doses similar to cardiac surgery, as tranexamic acid 2 g every 4 h). The use of fibrin glue is recommended.

Prior to surgery

The pseudotumor receives its blood supply from vessels that are present within the capsule that surrounds the mass. These vessels have a number of "feeding" arteries, and if they can be thrombosed the risk of massive intraoperative bleeding can be reduced [7] and the pseudotumor mass may be reduced in size. Arteries have the ability of recanalization and hence the thrombosis should be carried out 7–10 days before surgery.

Realistic aims

The intention should be the entire eradication of the pseudotumor and reconstruction of the normal anatomy. This is not always possible as there may be destroyed bone. The displaced viscera are not usually a problem. Bony structures, e.g. the iliac bone, should be left in a stable condition [8], and if large bone fragments remain viable, but free floating after the tumor has been excised, it is suggested that fixation methods be implemented [9]. "Dead space" can be "plugged" by the insertion of the omentum [10]. Bone allografts and/or bone substitutes can be used together with fibrin glue in the reconstruction of skeletal integrity. The peripheral pseudotumors are easily treated by the opening of a bone window, the drainage and curettage of the contents and then the packing of the pseudotumor space with bone and/or bone substitutes [11] mixed with glue [12].

Total excision is the intention, but is not always possible. The dissection is carried out around the capsule of the pseudotumor, but vital structures, although completely surrounded by the capsule, may be very deeply "embedded" within the contents of the pseudotumor. Structures such as the ureter can be damaged easily even though a catheter may have been inserted previously. It is probably safer to leave a small fragment of the pseudotumor wall attached to the vital structure than to risk damaging it. Abdominal pseudotumors may be enormous, and the authors have managed a case in which 6 L of liquid contents was drained out of the pseudotumor.

Complications

The complications may be divided into two groups, intra- and perioperative, and late complications. The former relates to the surgical procedure, which may require a multidisciplinary surgical team to conduct complicated surgery in a very protracted procedure. Infection is always a risk but even more so in the late recovery phase. The formation of a constantly draining sinus creates a situation wherein an open canal exists between the exterior, the bowel [13], and the abdominal cavity. This situation inevitably results in a purulent discharge and may lead to death.

Another complication is the regrowth or regeneration of a pseudotumor. Intra-abdominal pseudotumors are usually only diagnosed at a late stage, when huge expansion and destruction has taken place. If the pseudotumor is recognized early, excision can be less complicated. Excision causes extensive alteration in the soft-tissue anatomy owing to the extensive healing fibrosis and adhesions. Postexcision follow-up is necessary to document and discover whether the pseudotumor has reformed and started growing once again.

The use of radiotherapy for the management of pseudotumors is not needed. Hilgartner and Arnold [14] reported using this modality in 1975. Espandar et al. [15] retested the use of radiotherapy suggesting doses between 6 and 23.5 Gy by delivery in small fragments. It was postulated [14] that the radiotherapy affects the feeding blood vessels to the growth and hence its curative effect. Kapoor et al. [16] questioned and reviewed the results of radiotherapy treatment. Post-therapy recurrences of pseudotumors were reported. From the analysis of the literature review, it appears that the results of treatment with radiotherapy and factor replacement versus radiotherapy alone produce similar results.

Gilbert [17] described two types of pseudotumors: proximal and distal. The proximal involve the pelvis and long bones while the distal are in the small bones of the hands and feet. The latter group has been successfully managed by factor replacement only.

It is important to note that the hematologic control of the coagulation status of these patients may be complicated by acute hemorrhaging (requiring massive blood replacement), large oozing areas, and the fact that the patient may have an inhibitor to the missing coagulation factor. Factor assays should be carried out during the preoperative period, and ample supplies of relevant clotting factor should be present and not just on standby elsewhere.

The physical rehabilitation of patients after such massive surgery requires the dedication of the rehabilitation team. Initially, the patient requires intensive nursing care. Wound dressing and general nursing guides the patient from the postoperative catabolic state into an anabolic phase. Psychological support is essential for the patient and the family. Progress is slow and the physical therapist and the occupational therapist enhance joint movements and muscle strengthening. Once the wounds have healed, hydrotherapy is added to the therapeutic regime and more intensive physical therapy. During this rehabilitation period, which starts initially on an inpatient basis and progresses to an ambulatory service, the authors have found it necessary from time to time to remind the patient of his physical status prior to the surgery. This reinforcement assists the patient in appreciating the improvement in the quality of life.

In conclusion, where surgery is necessary, it should be carried out in a tertiary medical center by the most experienced multidisciplinary team. For more information, a short list of the key references has been provided. There are many case reports in the older medical literature that have been omitted from this list. The major issues are covered by the references.

References

1 Duthie R, Matthews J, Rizza C, Steel W. Haemophilic cysts and pseudotumours. In: Duthie R, Matthews J, Rizza C, Steel W (eds.) *The Management of Musculoskeletal Problems in the Haemophilias.* Oxford: Blackwell Scientific Publications, 1972; 84–98.

2 Gilbert MS, Forster A. A rational approach to the treatment of haemophilic blood cysts (pseudotumours) in patients with inhibitors. In: Rodrigues-Merchan EC, Lee CA (eds.) *Inhibitors in Patients with Haemophilia.* Oxford: Blackwell Science, 2002; 142–5.

3 Rodrigues-Merchan EC. The haemophilia pseudotumour. *Haemophilia* 2002; **8**: 12–16.

4 Heim M, Luboshitz J, Amit Y, Martinowitz U. The management of giant haemophilic pseudotumours. In: Rodrigues-Merchan EC, Goddard NJ, Lee CA (eds.) *Musculoskeletal Aspects of Haemophilia.* Oxford: Blackwell Science, 2000; 105–11.

5 Valentino LA, Martinowitz U, Doolas A, Murali P. Surgical excision of a giant pelvic pseudotumour in a patient with haemophilia A. *Haemophilia* 2006; **12**: 541–4.

6 Martinowitz U, Schulman S, Gitel S, et al. Continuous infusion of factor concentrates in children. In: Pettersson H, Gilbert MS (eds.) *Handbook of Hemophilia.* New York: American Elsevier Publishing, 1975; 569–89.

7 Sevilla J, Alvarez MT, Hernandez D, et al. Therapeutic embolization and surgical excision of haemophilic pseudotumour. *Haemophilia* 1999; **5**: 360–3.

8 Heeg M, Van Smit M, de Meer J, Van Horn JR. Excision of a haemophilic pseudotumour of the ileum complicated by fistulation. *Haemophilia* 1998; **4**: 132–5.

9 Ishiguro N, Iwahosi Y, Kato T, et al. The surgical treatment of haemophilic pseudotumours on an extremity: a report of three cases with pathological fractures. *Haemophilia* 1998; **4**: 126–31.

10 Bellinazzo P, Silvello L, Caimi T, et al. Long-term evaluation of a novel surgical approach to the pseudotumour of the ileum in haemophilia: Exeresis and transposition of the omentum in the residual cavity. *Haemophilia* 2000; **6**: 702–4.

11 Sagarra M, Lucas M, de La Torre G, et al. Successful surgical treatment of haemophilic pseudotumour, filling the defect with hydroxyapatite. *Haemophilia* 2000; **6**: 55–6.

12 Caviglia HA, Fernandez-Palazzi F, Galatro G, et al. Percutaneous treatment of haemophilic pseudotumours. In: Rodrigues-Merchan EC, Goddard NJ, Lee CA (eds.) *Musculoskeletal Aspects of Haemophilia.* Oxford: Blackwell Science, 2000; 97–104.

13 Heaton D, Robertson R, Rothwell A. Iliopsoas haemophilic pseudotumour with bowel fistulation. *Haemophilia* 2000; **6**: 41–3.

14 Hilgartner M, Arnold W. Hemophilic pseudotumor treated with replacement therapy and radiation. *J Bone Joint Surg* 1975; **57A**: 1145–6.

15 Espandar R, Heidaic P, Rodriguez-Merchan EC. Management of haemophilic pseudotumours with special earplysis on radiotherapy and arterial embolization. *Haemophilia* 2009; **15**: 448–57.

16 Kappor R, Sastric J, Malhotra P, Kumar V, Singh P. Hemophilic pseudotumour—is there a role of radiotherapy? A case report with review of the literature. *Turk J Hematol* 2006; **23**: 53–8.

17 Gilbert MS. Characterizing the hemophilic pseudotumor. *Ann NY Acad Sci* 1975; **240**: 313–15.

muscle girth [21]. It is a stimulating environment and an excellent aerobic exercise; however, it may entail some low risk for patients with severe hemophilia who experience hemarthroses in their elbows and shoulders.

Pain associated with hemophilic arthropathy and age-related musculoskeletal comorbidities is a challenge in the management of PWH. Advice and education on distinguishing between chronic arthritic pain and acute bleeding pain is important. Effective pain management strategies including analgesia, anti-inflammatory medications, TENS (transcutaneous electrical nerve stimulation), graded exercise activity, and pain education, together with conservative and surgical approaches to address the underlying mechanisms are thus crucial to improve functional capacity.

In individuals with advanced single or multiple joint arthropathy, maximizing function and adapting to limitations with appropriate strategies such as pacing activities, exercise programs, provision of aids to activities of daily living, and avoiding aggravating activities needs to be considered. If the limitation of movement is as a result of contractures and the end feel of the joint is hard and bony, manual physiotherapy techniques may have limited benefit. In the presence of chronic synovitis, the end range limitation of ROM must be respected. Approaching the closed packed position, where the synovium could become impinged or when the bony surfaces are coming into contact, should be avoided [22].

Adaptive and corrective splints and orthoses may be considered for joint instability and deformity. PWH and valgus/varus malalignment of the hind foot and flat/cavus foot often experience discomfort while walking or standing for long periods. The use of foot insoles and shoes has been shown to reduce pain and improve ankle propulsion in patients with endstage ankle arthropathy [23]. There is no consensus with respect to the best type of foot orthoses for managing foot pain in PWH; however, Lobet *et al.* proposed insoles as the first option for patients with moderate ankle arthropathy or partially correctable rear foot, whereas orthopedic shoes can be used for those with more severe pain or poor ROM [23].

Although physiotherapy can be provided without factor cover with care, it does enhance confidence for both the patient and physiotherapist, particularly when introducing new techniques and exercise regimes. If, following physiotherapy treatment, the symptoms are unchanged, the patient should be referred for an orthopedic opinion. Joint clinics attended by all members of the team can be very valuable as shared discussions with the patient can ensure the most appropriate management strategy.

Physical activity and sport

Participation in appropriate sports and physical activity should be encouraged as part of the global approach to the management of hemophilia as they provide numerous physical benefits, as well as supporting the emotional and social wellbeing of PWH. An active lifestyle is associated with the prevention of cardiovascular disease, diabetes, cancer, hypertension, obesity, depression, and osteoporosis; this also holds true for those suffering from chronic health conditions such as PWH.

Physical activity for PWH is associated with specific challenges, such as the risk of injury, overloading, and potential bleeds, but correctly managed participation in physical activity and exercise can improve strength, proprioception, and joint ROM, together with reducing frequency of bleeding [24]. The WFH have produced guidelines for physical activity programs, and the safety of sports has been classified according to risk [25]. Additionally, a five-item fitness check has been developed to assess physical ability so that the most appropriate sport can be chosen for the individual [26].

Physical activity should be encouraged from as young an age as practical to help establish a positive attitude and develop a lifelong habit of participation. Care needs to be taken to avoid introducing children to activities that place undue stress and strains upon their joints whilst recognizing that activity choices can be expanded as children age and coordination and strength develop [26]. Activities of interest should be identified and realistic goals set, based on capability, previous experience, and severity of hemophilia. Because each PWH is unique, the choice of the most suitable sport or exercise program needs be made collaboratively between the multidisciplinary team, and should take into account the individual patient's physical status, interests, and social requirements. Before starting a new physical activity, a thorough evaluation of musculoskeletal function should be performed. Advice on appropriate safe activities should be given on an individual basis. The physiotherapist can advise on the adaptations or modifications to a sport that are needed for a PWH to safely participate.

Sports and physical activities should ideally be performed under the cover of factor replacement and more intense physical activity, particularly competition, should be matched to the days that factor prophylaxis is administered. In situations of limited or no factor availability, it is still beneficial for PWH to participate in physical activity appropriate to their individual circumstances although the potential risk of injury should be carefully considered. If factor replacement is limited, use should be carefully matched to planned activities and, where possible, on-demand treatment should be provided.

Elective orthopedic procedures

Progression of arthropathy to a painful, severe stage with functional limitations can be an indication for elective orthopedic procedures. Provided that appropriate clotting factor levels are maintained postsurgery, the rehabilitation of PWH largely mirrors that of their counterparts without a coagulopathy with some specific considerations [27].

Total knee replacement

Due to the presence of arthrofibrosis and bone deformities in the preoperative stage, stiffness and loss of ROM continue to be a complication after total knee replacement in PWH [28]. The degree of preoperative flexion contracture is the most important variable influencing the postoperative ROM after total knee replacement [28]. To improve outcome, early postoperative knee mobilization, both passive using the continuous passive mobilization device, and active, should be performed as soon as possible both in flexion and in extension. Muscle isometric contractions and low-intensity open kinetic chain exercises should also be started in order to restore the quadriceps control to prevent the persistence of an extension lag which has detrimental effects on the patient's posture. Weight bearing as pain allows should be started once hemostasis has been achieved. Outpatient physiotherapy sessions focus on the continuity of ROM exercises for flexion and extension, restoration of balance with the help of proprioceptive exercises, and alternating specific muscle strengthening in open kinetic chain and more functional exercises in closed kinetic chain.

Ankle arthrodesis

In patients with arthropathy of the ankle joint, arthrodesis has been found to eliminate pain, recurrent bleeding, and correct deformity [29]. After surgery, the ankle is generally immobilized in a plaster cast for 8–12 weeks. Progressive weight bearing in 25% increments is usually commenced after 6–8 weeks with full weight bearing achieved at approximately 10–12 weeks; however, this will depend on the surgeon. Isometric exercises can begin on the day of surgery. Strengthening of the lower extremity, low-level proprioceptive exercises, and control of swelling are part of the treatment. In the later phases of rehabilitation, emphasis is placed on developing maximum efficiency of gait as well as maximizing ROM of nonfused joints of the forefoot and midfoot.

Synovectomy

Synovectomies are advocated in PWH to stop repetitive cycles of intra-articular bleeds and/or chronic synovitis. Radioactive synovectomies (synoviorthesis) are relatively quick, noninvasive, and less painful compared with chemical synovectomies, surgical arthrotomies, or arthroscopies. The synovectomy itself, however, does not solve the muscle atrophy, loss of ROM and instability, often developed during many years. The key is in taking advantage of the subsequent, relatively safe, bleed-free period to address these important issues [27].

Patients with inhibitors

In PWH and inhibitors, physiotherapy treatment should be carefully timed to occur with the administration of replacement factor concentrates. The underlying principles for managing acute bleeding and arthropathy in patient with inhibitors remain the same as previously discussed for noninhibitor patients. Exercises should be started and progressed more slowly. A carefully controlled, graded exercise program, starting with isometric exercises with low repetitions and progressing slowly based on response to exercises and patient comfort is advised. Hydrotherapy and sports such as tai chi may still be enjoyed, facilitating muscle strength and good postural control as well as promoting the psychological benefits of exercise [30]. While no direct comparison has been made regarding the frequency of bleeds in PWH with and without inhibitors following participation in sports, exercise for PWH with inhibitors remains a challenge. High-risk sports are not suitable. Some sports can be performed in sitting rather than standing positions, thus reducing the weight-bearing stresses on lower limb joints affected by arthropathy [31].

The aging hemophilic individual

People with hemophilia are living longer and it has been shown that joint damage increases linearly with age in those with the disorder and remains the main comorbidity associated with the older PWH [32,33]. Increasing pain, muscle weakness, and atrophy along with an increased risk of falling are key features of advanced hemophilic arthropathy and aging [34].

Research in the nonhemophilic population has shown that age-related effects on the musculoskeletal system can be curtailed by exercise. Multicomponent weight-bearing and nonweight-bearing exercise programs undertaken two to three times per week for at least 12 weeks and targeting gait and balance training, functional tasks, muscle strengthening, and three-dimensional exercise such as tai chi, yoga, and dance seem most effective in the older person [35,36]. Age alone should not be seen as a barrier to physical activity, particularly for low-impact activities such as swimming and cycling. Rehabilitation and preventative physiotherapy are essential to preserve remaining joint function, to reduce the risk of falls, and to maintain or improve QoL in elderly PWH.

Emerging clinical assessment tools in hemophilia

Monitoring the biomechanical and functional status of hemophilic joints is the current challenge. Evaluation of bone and soft tissue with radiologic imaging together with clinical joint scoring are employed to monitor hemophilic arthropathy and these are discussed in detail in other chapters. However, clinical joint scoring may not be sensitive to early changes in joint status and does not provide an understanding of the causes underlying the impairments [2,4,37,38].

Recently, an interest in the biomechanical status of hemophilic joints has emerged. Recent work evaluating joint status and functional impairments associated with lower limb hemophilic arthropathy utilizing specialized laboratory equipment to study biomarkers of human motor performance has shown that when young preadolescent boys with hemophilia and a history of ankle joint bleeding are compared to age- and size-matched typically developing peers, lower limb muscle strength and size is reduced in hemophilic boys [3]. Alterations in balance [5], spatiotemporal parameters [4], and kinematic and kinetic gait patterns [2,26] have also been observed. Muscle strength and atrophy appear to underlie these biomechanical changes [3,39].

In adults, Lobet *et al.* [40] used three-dimensional gait analysis to quantitatively describe the kinematics, metabolic cost, mechanical work, and efficiency of walking in 31 PWH with multiple lower limb arthropathy. The authors reported that the net metabolic cost of transport was greater in PWH and directly correlated to the loss in active joint ROM calculated during walking. Furthermore, Lobet *et al.* [38] found moderately strong relationships between ankle plantar flexion ROM, plantar flexion moment, calf muscle power, and self-reported pain and stiffness in those with arthropathy of the ankle. Radiologic together with WFH orthopedic scores were compared with ankle muscle power and no significant associations were found between the clinical and radiologic scores and ankle power. This discordance highlight discrepancies between functional alterations detected by these new biomechanical assessment tools and the structural changes assessed using "classic" X-ray or clinical scoring.

There is a need for clinicians to become updated on the evaluation of biomechanical joint function and consider tools such as ultrasound, static and dynamic myometry, three-dimensional motion analysis and timed function tests [41]. Integrating biomechanical research with clinical research has the potential to improve our monitoring of the early blood-induced changes in the physical status of the hemophilic joint.

References

1 Manco-Johnson MJ, Abshire TC, *et al.* Prophylaxis versus episodic treatment to prevent joint disease in boys with severe hemophilia. *N Engl J Med* 2007; **357**(6): 535–44.

2 Stephensen D, Drechsler W, Winter M, Scott O. Comparison of biomechanical gait parameters of young children with haemophilia and those of age-matched peers. *Haemophilia* 2009; **15**(2): 509–18.

3 Stephensen D, Drechsler W, Scott O. Comparison of muscle strength and in-vivo muscle morphology in young children with haemophilia and those of age-matched peers. *Haemophilia* 2012; **18**(3): e302–10.

4 Bladen M, Alderson L, Khair K, Liesner R, Green J, Main E. Can early subclinical gait changes in children with haemophilia be identified using the GAITRite walkway. *Haemophilia* 2007; **13**(5): 542–7.

5 De Souza FM, Pereira RP, Minuque NP, *et al.* Postural adjustment after an unexpected perturbation in children with haemophilia. *Haemophilia* 2012; **18**(3): e311–15.

6 Gallach JE, Querol F, Gonzalez LM, Pardo A, Aznar JA. Posturographic analysis of balance control in patients with haemophilic arthropathy. *Haemophilia* 2008; **14**(2): 329–35.

7 World Health Organization (WHO). *International Classification of Functioning, Disability and Health*. Geneva: WHO, 2001.

8 Zourikian N, Forsyth AL. Physiotherapy evaluation and intervention in the acute hemarthrosis: Challenging the paradigm. In: Rodiriguez-Merchan EC, Valentino LA (eds.) *Current and Future Issues in Hemophilia Care*, 1st edn. Oxford: Blackwell Publishing, 2011; 156–61.

9 Forsyth AL, Rivard GE, Valentino LA, *et al.* Consequences of intra-articular bleeding in haemophilia: science to clinical practice and beyond. *Haemophilia* 2012; **18**(Suppl. 4): 112–19.

10 Forsyth AL, Zourikian N, Valentino LA, Rivard GE. The effect of cooling on coagulation and haemostasis: Should "Ice" be part of treatment of acute haemarthrosis in haemophilia? *Haemophilia* 2012; **18**(6): 843–50.

11 Wolberg AS, Meng ZH, Monroe DM, III, Hoffman M. A systematic evaluation of the effect of temperature on coagulation enzyme activity and platelet function. *J Trauma* 2004; **56**(6): 1221–8.

12 Hoffman M. Animal models of bleeding and tissue repair. *Haemophilia* 2008; **14**(Suppl. 3): 62–7.

13 Hakobyan N, Kazarian T, Valentino LA. Synovitis in a murine model of human factor VIII deficiency. *Haemophilia* 2005; **11**(3): 227–32.

14 Acharya SS. Exploration of the pathogenesis of haemophilic joint arthropathy: understanding implications for optimal clinical management. *Br J Haematol* 2012; **156**(1): 13–23.

15 Charalambides C, Beer M, Melhuish J, Williams RJ, Cobb AG. Bandaging technique after knee replacement. *Acta Orthop* 2005; **76**(1): 89–94.

16 Sorensen B, Benson GM, Bladen M, *et al.* Management of muscle haematomas in patients with severe haemophilia in an evidence-poor world. *Haemophilia* 2012; **18**(4): 598–606.

17 Collins NC. Is ice right? Does cryotherapy improve outcome for acute soft tissue injury? *Emerg Med J* 2008; **25**(2): 65–8.

18 Blamey G, Forsyth A, Zourikian N, *et al.* Comprehensive elements of a physiotherapy exercise programme in haemophilia–a global perspective. *Haemophilia* 2010; **16**(Suppl. 5): 136–45.

19 Gomis M, Gonzalez LM, Querol F, Gallach JE, Toca-Herrera JL. Effects of electrical stimulation on muscle trophism in patients with hemophilic arthropathy. *Arch Phys Med Rehabil* 2009; **90**(11): 1924–30.

20 Mulder K. *Exercises for People with Haemophilia*. Montreal, Canada: World Federation of Haemophilia, 2006.

21 Garcia MK, Capusso A, Montans D, Massad E, Battistella LR. Variations of the articular mobility of elbows, knees and ankles in patients with severe haemophilia submitted to free active movimentation in a pool with warm water. *Haemophilia* 2009; **15**(1): 386–9.

22 Gurcay E, Eksioglu E, Ezer U, Cakir B, Cakci A. A prospective series of musculoskeletal system rehabilitation of arthropathic joints in young male hemophilic patients. *Rheumatol Int* 2008; **28**(6): 541–5.

23 Lobet S, Detrembleur C, Lantin AC, Haenecour L, Hermans C. Functional impact of custom-made foot orthoses in patients with haemophilic ankle arthropathy. *Haemophilia* 2012; **18**(3): e227–35.

24 Souza JC, Simoes HG, Campbell CS, Pontes FL, Boullosa DA, Prestes J. Haemophilia and exercise. *Int J Sports Med* 2012; **33**(2): 83–8.

25 Wittmeier K, Mulder K. Enhancing lifestyle for individuals with haemophilia through physical activity and exercise: the role of physiotherapy. *Haemophilia* 2007; **13**(Suppl. 2): 31–7.

26 Seuser A, Boehm P, Kurme A, Schumpe G, Kurnik K. Orthopaedic issues in sports for persons with haemophilia. *Haemophilia* 2007; **13**(Suppl. 2): 47–52.

27 De Kleijn P, Blamey G, Zourikian N, Dalzell R, Lobet S. Physiotherapy following elective orthopaedic procedures. *Haemophilia* 2006; **12**(Suppl. 3): 108–12.

28 Lobet S, Pendeville E, Dalzell R, *et al*. The role of physiotherapy after total knee arthroplasty in patients with haemophilia. *Haemophilia* 2008; **14**(5): 989–98.

29 Gamble JG, Bellah J, Rinsky LA, Glader B. Arthropathy of the ankle in hemophilia. *J Bone Joint Surg Am* 1991; **73**(7): 1008–15.

30 Danusantoso H, Heijnen L. Tai Chi Chuan for people with haemophilia. *Haemophilia* 2001; **7**(4): 437–9.

31 Heijnen L. The role of rehabilitation and sports in haemophilia patients with inhibitors. *Haemophilia* 2008; **14**(Suppl. 6): 45–51.

32 Khleif AA, Rodriguez N, Brown D, Escobar MA. Multiple comorbid conditions among middle-aged and elderly hemophilia patients: prevalence estimates and implications for future care. *J Aging Res* 2011; doi: 10.4061/2011/985703. Epub 2011 Sep 7.

33 Siboni SM, Mannucci PM, Gringeri A, *et al*. Health status and quality of life of elderly persons with severe hemophilia born before the advent of modern replacement therapy. *J Thromb Haemost* 2009; **7**(5): 780–6.

34 Stephensen D, Rodriguez-Merchan EC. Orthopaedic co-morbidities in the elderly haemophilia population: a review. *Haemophilia* 2012; **19**(2): 166–73.

35 Gillespie LD, Robertson MC, Gillespie WJ, *et al*. Interventions for preventing falls in older people living in the community. *Cochrane Database Syst Rev* 2009; **2**: CD007146.

36 Liu CJ, Latham NK. Progressive resistance strength training for improving physical function in older adults. *Cochrane Database Syst Rev* 2009; **3**: CD002759.

37 Lobet S, Detrembleur C, Francq B, Hermans C. Natural progression of blood-induced joint damage in patients with haemophilia: clinical relevance and reproducibility of three-dimensional gait analysis. *Haemophilia* 2010; **16**(5): 813–21.

38 Lobet S, Hermans C, Pasta G, Detrembleur C. Body structure versus body function in haemophilia: the case of haemophilic ankle arthropathy. *Haemophilia* 2011; **17**(3): 508–15.

39 Groen W, van der NJ, Bos K, *et al*. Joint health and functional ability in children with haemophilia who receive intensive replacement therapy. *Haemophilia* 2011; **17**(5): 783–90.

40 Lobet S, Detrembleur C, Hermans C. Impact of multiple joint impairments on the energetics and mechanics of walking in patients with haemophilia. *Haemophilia* 2013; **19**: e66–72.

41 Stephensen D, Drechsler WI, Scott OM. Biomechanics of lower limb haemophilic arthropathy. *Blood Rev* 2012; **26**(5): 213–21.

CHAPTER 36

Outcome assessment in hemophilia

Pradeep M. Poonnoose and Alok Srivastava
Christian Medical College, Tamil Nadu, India

Introduction

In the management of chronic diseases, assessment of long-term outcome is important, not only to document the impact of the condition on the individual, but also to compare different treatment strategies. In the early 1980s, the Musculoskeletal Committee of the World Federation of Hemophilia (WFH) introduced the clinical and radiologic Pettersson score to assess musculoskeletal outcome in hemophilia [1,2]. In addition to being insensitive to early change, these scores failed to assess the impact of interventions on the overall health of the individual, in terms of activities of daily living, functional ability, schooling, work and social life, and quality of life (QoL) [3]. Over the years, there has been a shift in the philosophy of outcome measurement, from the "biomedical model"—where changes in structure was the primary outcome measure—to an assessment in terms of the disablement process as conceptualized by the "biopsychosocial model" [4]. In line with this paradigm shift, several haemophilia-specific tools have been developed to make a "holistic" assessment of musculoskeletal outcome [3]. With the array of tools available to assess the efficacy of therapeutic interventions, it is essential that the researcher is aware of the scope of these clinimetric instruments, as well as their psychometric properties (Box 36.1) [5].

Musculoskeletal assessment: outcome measurement

According to the International Classification of Functioning, Disability, and Health (ICF), evaluation of disability and health should focus on the impact of the disease on body structures and functions, activities, and participation (Figure 36.1) [6]. Body structures are parts of the body such as organs, limbs, and their components. Body functions are defined as the physiologic functions of these systems, such as range of motion (ROM), strength, and instability. Activities involve executing tasks or actions, and a range of activities that can be performed by the

individual are covered. Participation is defined as involvement in a life situation, such as sport, leisure, work, or social events. The ICF provides a single list of activities and participation in nine domains. According to their needs and purposes, investigators can designate some domains as activities and others as participation, without overlap; alternatively, they can designate all domains to be potentially both activities and participation, and use qualifiers to differentiate the data. The components of the list can be affected by contextual factors, which represent a person's background, and include both environmental and personal factors. Environmental factors comprise the physical, social, and attitudinal environment in which an individual lives and conducts day-to-day activities. They include social attitudes, architectural characteristics, and social and legal structures, as well as climate and terrain. Personal factors include aspects of an individual's life that are not necessarily part of the health condition or health status, such as age, sex, and indigenous status. The concept of QoL is complex, and embraces many characteristics of the social, economic, and physical environment, as well as the health and internal state of the individual [6].

In keeping with the ICF framework, the clinimetric instruments in hemophilia have been discussed under three broad sections: those that evaluate the structure and function of individual joints—the clinical and radiologic score; those that assess the limitation in activities and functional independence—both subjectively and objectively; and those that assess the individual's participation in life activities and QoL.

Musculoskeletal outcome: assessment of structure and function

Until recently, most long-term musculoskeletal outcome studies have used clinical and radiologic scores, in addition to the number and frequency of bleeding episodes, to determine the efficacy of different treatment regimes [7–10]. With the advent of early prophylaxis, the incidence of joint arthropathy has

Textbook of Hemophilia, Third Edition. Edited by Christine A. Lee, Erik E. Berntorp and W. Keith Hoots.
© 2014 John Wiley & Sons, Ltd. Published 2014 by John Wiley & Sons, Ltd.

Box 36.1 Psychometric properties: Definition of terms.

Reliability (reproducibility) of an instrument is the degree of consistency with which it measures the attribute it is measuring. Stability refers to the extent to which the instrument yields the same results on repeated administration (*test retest*). When the focus is on "equivalence" between observers, estimates of *interobserver reliability* may be obtained [16]. *Internal consistency* (Cronbach's α) estimates the extent to which the different subparts of the questionnaire/instrument assess the same attribute/characteristic [17]

Validity refers to the degree to which an instrument measures what it is supposed to be measuring
- *Content validity* refers to the extent to which the instrument covers all "domains" of the attribute being measured. This is based on judgment – either by a group of experts in the field or by the patients on whom it is being tested
- *Criterion validity* refers to the correlation between the instrument and some outside criterion. This can be *predictive*, i.e. the ability to predict a future condition/behavior; or *concurrent* validity, a measure of how well the test correlates with a previously validated instrument that measures the same attribute, both measures being taken at the same time[a]
- *Construct validity* measures the extent to which the instrument relates to other measures. This should be in keeping with the theoretical hypothesis concerning the relationship between the concepts being measured. Construct validity is considered whenever no single criterion is accepted as entirely adequate to define the quality to be measured.[b] This may be *convergent* or *discriminate*. Another method to study construct validity is using *factor analysis* which identifies clusters of related variables in the measured attribute

Responsiveness or sensitivity to change represents the ability of an instrument to detect a difference in the attribute following an intervention. This is measured using the standardized response mean (SRM), responsiveness index, or effect size index

[a]For example, correlation of a new IQ test with a standardized IQ test: HAL with FISH.
[b]For example, correlation between FISH and HJHS: both measure musculoskeletal outcome (but assess different domains) of structure and activity, respectively.

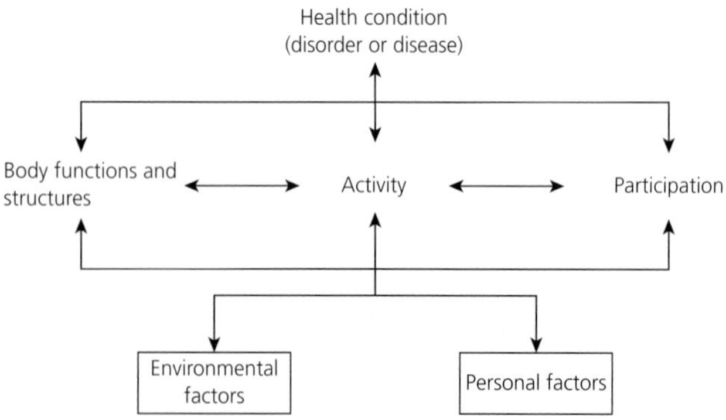

Figure 36.1 Interactions between the components of the International Classification of Functioning, Disability, and Health [6]. Reproduced with permission of the World Health Organization.

significantly reduced [7–10]. As the aim of therapy changed from preventing severe joint damage to maintenance of a normal joint with prophylactic therapy, it became necessary to improve these tools, and develop new ones, to make them more sensitive to early changes.

Physical examination scores

Physical joint assessment is commonly used in literature to measure structural and functional joint damage, as it is readily available and inexpensive. ROM has been the most commonly used physical outcome measure for evaluating the effects of intervention on joint health [11,12]. As more medical and surgical methods to improve function became available, it became necessary to develop an instrument that could assess a wider spectrum of physical changes that occur as a result of joint damage. Thus, the WFH endorsed the physical examination (PE) scale (Table 36.1). This scoring system, first described in 1985 [2,13], evaluates ROM, flexion deformity, swelling, crepitus, muscle wasting, instability, and axial deformity in the six major joints (i.e. ankles, knees, and elbows). A score of zero denotes a normal joint. The ankle and knees can score as high

Table 36.1 Physical joint examination score endorsed by the Orthopaedic Advisory Committee of the World Federation of Haemophilia (WFH) [2]. Reproduced with permission of Springer-Verlag.

Physical finding	Score	Scoring key
Swelling	0 or 2+ (S)	0 = None
		2 = Present
		S if chronic synovitis present
Muscle atrophy	0–1	0 = ≤1 cm
		1 = Present
Axial deformity (measured at knee and ankle only)		
Knee	0–2	0 = 0–7° valgus
		1 = 8–15° valgus or 0–5° varus
		2 = >15° valgus or >5° varus
Ankle	0–2	0 = No deformity
		1 = ≤10° valgus or ≤5° varus
		2 = >10° valgus or >5° varus
Crepitus on motion	0–1	0 = None
		1 = Present
Range of motion	0–2	0 = loss of <10% of total FROM (Full range of movement)
		1 = Loss of 10–33% of total FROM
		2 = Loss of >33% of total FROM
Fixed contracture	0 or 2	0 = <15% fixed flexion contracture
		2 = ≥15% fixed flexion contracture at hip and knee and equinus at ankle
Instability	0–2	0 = None
		1 = Present, but neither interferes with function nor requires bracing
		2 = Instability that creates a functional deficit or requires bracing
Total	0–12	Ankle or knee
	0–10	Elbow

Table 36.2 Pain instrument recommended by the Orthopaedic Advisory Committee of the World Federation of Haemophilia (WFH) [2]. Reproduced with permission of Springer-Verlag.

	Score	Scoring key
Pain	0–3	0 = No pain, no functional deficit, no analgesic use except with acute hemarthrosis
		1 = Mild pain, does not interfere with occupation nor with activities of daily living; may require occasional non-narcotic analgesics
		2 = moderate pain, partial or occasional interference with occupation or activities of daily living
		3 = Severe pain. Interferes with occupation or activities of daily living, requires frequent use of non-narcotic and narcotic medications

as 12 points, and the elbows a maximum of 10, giving a total of 68 for the six joints. Each joint is also scored for pain (0–3), and in some studies this has been added to the total score (Table 36.2). However, this scale was adopted and recommended for routine use at a time when most hemophilia patients in Western countries used much lower quantities of replacement therapy than now. As larger quantities of factor concentrates were used for replacement therapy, and as the frequency of bleeding was reduced with the use of primary prophylaxis, more joints maintained zero (normal) scores on the WFH PE scale [14]. In addition to this lack of sensitivity, the original WFH score does not take into account the normal physiologic changes that occur in children [15]. Furthermore, the score does not assess strength—an important function that affects physical activity.

These observations provided the impetus to develop new scoring systems. The Colorado PE instruments (full and half point) described by Manco-Johnson et al. [15] and the PedNet (Stockholm) instrument [16] were developed in an attempt to increase the sensitivity of physical assessment. Subsequently, these scores were combined by the International Prophylaxis Study Group (IPSG) to produce the Hemophilia Joint Health Score (HJHS). The aim was to produce a score that would be sensitive to early change, account for normal development in children, and be reliable, valid, and practical to administer. The reliability of HJHS version 1.0 was assessed in eight pediatric patients aged 4–12 years, and was found to be excellent with an interobserver coefficient of 0.83, and a test retest of 0.89 [17]. The Cronbach's α (internal consistency) was 0.86 [17]. Following a multicenter validation study, a second version was developed by removing/modifying redundant or less sensitive items [18]. The normative data for "range of motion" was also changed. In the latest version 2.1 (Table 36.3), each of the six joints has a total possible score of 20. There is an additional global gait assessment with scores from 0 to 4 that includes assessment of walking, hopping, running, and stair climbing, with a total possible score of 124. In version 1.0, a normal evaluation in all six joints gives a score of 0–6 [18]. The scores for a

"normal evaluation of the six joints" with HJHS version 2.1 has yet to be defined.

On assessing the validity of HJHS, version 1 had a moderate correlation of 0.42 with the "total physician score of joint health," but did not correlate with the modified C-HAQ (Childhood Health Assessment Questionnaire) [18]. Version 2.0 had a moderate correlation of –0.59 with Ped-HAL (pediatric version of the Haemophilia Activity List), a functional assessment tool [19]. Responsiveness was assessed by scoring the subjects before and after a physiotherapy program and the standardized response mean (SRM) was found to be excellent (–0.9) [19].

While the HJHS is better than the WFH in discriminating mild from severe hemophilia, as well as those on prophylaxis from those treated on demand [18], its usefulness in detecting early changes in joint arthropathy needs to be studied further. In a study from UK, 53% of 83 children aged 4–18 years with severe hemophilia, had a median score of 0 (version 2.1) [20]. In the study by Feldman et al., which included 226 subjects from North American and European centers, about 30% of the children had a HJHS score of 0 (version 1.0) [18]. In centers with children treated on demand, the scores were, however, higher. In a study from China, the median score of 20 children aged 5–17 years was 11 [21]. In another group of 20 children from Lithuania, the mean HJHS (version 2.1) score was 24.5, with none of the children having a score of 0 [22].

Radiologic scores

De Palma in 1956, and Jordan in 1958, described the characteristic X-ray abnormalities seen in hemophilic arthropathy [23]. De Palma proposed four classes of joint destruction based on a combination of roentgenographic and clinical manifestations [23]. In 1977, Arnold and Hilgartner refined this classification into five stages [24]. Wood et al. proposed a radiologic classification in 1969, but several parameters he described pertained to soft-tissue changes seen in the acute stage of hemarthrosis [25]. In 1980, Pettersson et al. created a scoring system based on the degree of joint destruction, as assessed by radiologic changes seen in the six most commonly affected joints (i.e. the knee, elbow, and ankle joints) [1]. This was incorporated into the first joint scoring system endorsed by the WFH [1,2,13]; a system that has so far been the standard for long-term outcome measurement in hemophilia (Table 36.4).

The introduction of more intensive prophylaxis in younger children enabled joints to be maintained at a stage where no radiologic changes could be detected [7,8]. As more patients maintained scores of 0 (normal joints), it became evident that conventional radiographs were insensitive to early changes in the hemophilic joint. Consequently, scoring systems based on magnetic resonance imaging (MRI) were developed. These could detect changes to the joint before they were apparent on X-rays. Changes observed by MRI were first described in 1986 by Kulkarni et al. [26], and several other reports of MRI use soon followed. The Denver scale [27], the European scale used by the Pediatric Network for Hemophilia Management

Table 36.3 Haemophilia Joint Health Score (HJHS) version 2.1. The HJHS was developed and validated by the Physical Therapy Expert Working Group of the International Prophylaxis Study Group (IPSG). From [59]. Reproduced with permission.

	Left elbow	Right elbow	Left knee	Right knee	Left ankle	Right ankle
Swelling	☐ NE	☐ NE	☐ NE	☐ NE	☐ NE	☐ NE
Duration (swelling)	☐ NE	☐ NE	☐ NE	☐ NE	☐ NE	☐ NE
Muscle atrophy	☐ NE	☐ NE	☐ NE	☐ NE	☐ NE	☐ NE
Crepitus on motion	☐ NE	☐ NE	☐ NE	☐ NE	☐ NE	☐ NE
Flexion loss	☐ NE	☐ NE	☐ NE	☐ NE	☐ NE	☐ NE
Extension loss	☐ NE	☐ NE	☐ NE	☐ NE	☐ NE	☐ NE
Joint pain	☐ NE	☐ NE	☐ NE	☐ NE	☐ NE	☐ NE
Strength	☐ NE	☐ NE	☐ NE	☐ NE	☐ NE	☐ NE
Joint total						

NE, non-evaluable

Sum of joint totals   +   [   ]
Global gait score   [   ]
(☐ NE included in gait items)

HJHS total score   =   [   ]

Swelling
0   No swelling
1   Mild
2   Moderate
3   Severe

Crepitus on motion
0   None
1   Mild
2   Severe

Strength (Using Daniel's & Worthingham's scale)
Within available ROM
0 = Holds test position against gravity with maximum resistance (gr.5)

1 = Holds test position against gravity with moderate resistance (but breaks with maximal resistance) (gr.4)

2 = Holds test position with minimal resistance (gr.3+) or holds test position against gravity (gr.3)

3 = Able to partially complete ROM against gravity (gr.3−/2+) or able to move through ROM gravity eliminated (gr.2) or through partial ROM gravity eliminated (gr.2−)

4 = Trace (gr1) or no muscle contraction (gr.0)
NE, non-evaluable

Duration
0   No swelling
    Or <6 months
1   >6 months

Flexion loss
Contralateral:
0 = <5°
1 = 5°–10°
2 = 11°–20°
3 = >20°

Normative tables:
0 = within range
1 = 1°–4°
2 = 5°–10°
3 = >10°

Muscle atrophy
0   None
1   Mild
2   Severe

Extension loss *(from hyperextension)*
Contralateral:
0 = <5°
1 = 5°–10°
2 = 11°–20°
3 = >20°

Normative tables:
0 = within range
1 = 1°–4°
2 = 5°–10°
3 = >10°

Global gait *(walking, stairs, running, hopping on 1 leg)*
0 = All skills are within normal limits
1 = One skill in not within normal limits
2 = Two skills are not within normal limits
3 = Three skills are not within normal limits
4 = No skills are within normal limits
NE, non-evaluable

Joint pain
0   No pain through active range of movement
1   No pain through active range—only pain on gentle overpressure or palpation
2   Pain through active range

40 Groen WG, Van der Net J, Helders PJ, *et al.* Development and preliminary testing of a Paediatric Version of the Haemophilia Activities List (pedhal). *Haemophilia* 2010; **16**: 281–9.

41 Poonnoose PM, Thomas R, Keshava SN, *et al.* Psychometric analysis of the Functional Independence Score in Haemophilia (FISH). *Haemophilia* 2007; **13**: 620–6.

42 Wittink H, Rogers W, Sukiennik A, Carr DB. Physical functioning: Self-report and performance measures are related but distinct. *Spine* 2003; **28**: 2407–13.

43 Isernhagen SJ. Functional capacity evaluation: Rationale, procedure, utility of the kinesiophysical approach. *J Occup Rehab* 1992; **2**: 157–68.

44 Hoeymans N, Feskens EJ, Van den Bos GA, Kromhout D. Measuring functional status: Cross-sectional and longitudinal associations between performance and self-report (Zutphen Elderly Study 1990–1993). *J Clin Epidemiol* 1996; **49**: 1103–10.

45 Hassan TH, Badr MA, El-Gerby KM. Correlation between musculoskeletal function and radiological joint scores in haemophilia A adolescents. *Haemophilia* 2011; **17**: 920–25.

46 Tlacuilo-Parra A, Villela-Rodriguez J, Garibaldi-Covarrubias R, Soto-Padilla J, Orozco-Alcala J. Functional Independence Score in Hemophilia: A cross-sectional study assessment of Mexican children. *Pediatr Blood Cancer* 2010; **54**: 394–97

47 Hassan TH, Badr MA, Fattah NR, Badawy SM. Assessment of musculoskeletal function and mood in haemophilia A adolescents: a cross-sectional study. *Haemophilia* 2011; **17**: 683–8.

48 McColl MA, Paterson M, Davis D, *et al.* Validity and community utility of the Canadian Occupational Performance Measure. *Can J Occup Therapy* 2000; **47**: 22–30.

49 Padankatti SM, Macaden AS, Cherian SM *et al.* A patient-prioritized ability assessment in haemophilia: the Canadian Occupational Performance Measure. *Haemophilia* 2011; **17**: 605–11.

50 Tanaka S, Hachisuka K, Okazaki T, Shirahata A, Ogata H. Health status and satisfaction of asymptomatic HIV-positive haemophiliacs in Kyushu, Japan. *Haemophilia* 1999; **5**: 56–62.

51 Trippoli S, Vaiani M, Linari S, Longo G, Morfini M, Messori A. Multivariate analysis of factors influencing quality of life and utility in patients with haemophilia. *Haematologica* 2001; **86**: 722–8.

52 von Mackensen S, Bullinger M, Haemo-QoL Group. Development and testing of an instrument to assess the Quality of Life of Children with Haemophilia in Europe (Haemo-QoL). *Haemophilia* 2004; **10**(Suppl. 1): 17–25.

53 Young NL, Bradley CS, Blanchette V, *et al.* Development of a health-related quality of life measure for boys with haemophilia: The Canadian Haemophilia Outcomes—Kids Life Assessment Tool (CHO-KLAT). *Haemophilia* 2004; **10**(Suppl. 1): 34–43.

54 Arranz P, Remor E, Quintana M, *et al.* Development of a new disease-specific quality-of-life questionnaire to adults living with haemophilia. *Haemophilia* 2004; **10**: 376–82.

55 Remor E, Young NL, von Mackensen S, Lopatina EG. Disease-specific quality-of-life measurement tools for haemophilia patients. *Haemophilia* 2004; **10**(Suppl. 4): 30–4.

56 Beeton K, Neal D, Lee C. An exploration of health related quality of life in adults with haemophilia—A qualitative perspective. *Haemophilia* 2005; **11**: 123–32.

57 Fischer K, Astermark J, Van der Bom JG, *et al.* Prophylactic treatment for severe haemophilia: Comparison of an intermediate-dose to a high-dose regimen. *Haemophilia* 2003; **8**: 753–60.

58 Manco-Johnson MK, Abshire TC, Shapiro AD, *et al.* Prophylaxis versus episodic treatment to prevent joint disease in boys with severe haemophilia. *N Engl J Med* 2007; **357**: 535–44.

59 International Prophylaxis Study Group (IPSG). Available at: http://www.ipsg.ca/

Transfusion-transmitted disease

CHAPTER 37

Viral hepatitis and hemophilia

Michael Makris[1] and Geoffrey Dusheiko[2]
[1] Royal Hallamshire Hospital, Sheffield, UK
[2] Royal Free Hospital, London, UK

Introduction

The introduction of clotting factor concentrates in the late 1960s and 1970s revolutionized the lives of persons with hemophilia, reducing the morbidity and mortality associated with their disease. This improvement was so marked that it was estimated that in the late 1970s the life expectancy of a person with hemophilia treated with concentrate approached that of the normal population. Unfortunately, this optimism was premature and the development of serious infections in the form of viral hepatitis and human immunodeficiency virus (HIV) led to new problems affecting the lives of persons with hemophilia. Table 37.1 lists the infections transmitted by concentrates, their physical characteristics, and the ability of viral inactivation processes to destroy them.

Clotting factor concentrates are prepared from plasma pools of up to 30 000 donations and prior to viral inactivation any infections present in the plasma donors could be transmitted to the recipient. The introduction of viral inactivation in 1985 largely eliminated the risk of hepatitis virus transmission by concentrates. Although some of the early viral inactivation methods were not 100% successful, there have been no hepatitis transmissions by concentrates since the early 1990s. All plasma-derived products in Europe now have to undergo viral inactivation by two different processes [1]. Concentrates produced by recombinant technology are free from the risk of hepatitis virus transmission.

Hepatitis viruses in hemophilia

Hepatitis A virus

Acute hepatitis A virus (HAV) infection can be demonstrated by the detection of immunoglobulin M (IgM) anti-HAV antibodies. HAV RNA testing in serum, stool, or liver by polymerase chain reaction (PCR) is a research tool. Past infection is confirmed by the detection of IgG anti-HAV.

As a result of donor screening, plasma pool testing, viral inactivation of concentrates, and vaccination of recipients, the risk of transmission of this virus by concentrates has been eliminated. In the early 1990s, there were a number of outbreaks of HAV in persons with hemophilia treated exclusively with solvent/detergent (S/D) treated concentrates [2]. This was not surprising because S/D does not inactivate viruses without a lipid envelope, such as HAV.

Hepatitis B virus

Hepatitis B virus (HBV) transmission was common prior to viral inactivation of concentrates with 50% of patients infected. Most adult patients cleared the virus spontaneously and developed immunity, and in countries where hepatitis B is not endemic, only 2–5% of persons with hemophilia are now chronically infected with hepatitis B. Because patients with bleeding disorders may receive non- or poorly virally inactivated blood products while visiting other (less developed) countries, it is recommended that all patients with inherited bleeding disorders who could be exposed to plasma-derived concentrates should be appropriately vaccinated against hepatitis B and hepatitis A.

Hepatitis C virus

Prior to 1985, hepatitis C virus (HCV) infection occurred in virtually all recipients of clotting factor concentrates at their first exposure [3]. Past exposure is indicated by the identification of anti-HCV antibodies while current infection is demonstrated by the detection of both anti-HCV and HCV RNA by PCR. All HCV RNA-positive patients should have their HCV genotype determined. A total of 80–90% of persons with hemophilia in Europe are infected with genotype 1, 10–15% with genotype 2 or 3, and ~5% with genotypes 4, 5, or 6 [4]. Surprisingly, despite the repeated infusion of infected concentrates prior to 1985, mixed infections are rare but this may be because of a methodologic problem where the PCR detects only the dominant genotype. Antibody testing can identify mixed infections but is not widely applied.

Textbook of Hemophilia, Third Edition. Edited by Christine A. Lee, Erik E. Berntorp and W. Keith Hoots.
© 2014 John Wiley & Sons, Ltd. Published 2014 by John Wiley & Sons, Ltd.

Table 37.1 The hepatitis viruses that can be transmitted by blood products, and their characteristics.

Virus	Genome	Lipid envelope	Size (nm)	Solvent/detergent resistant	Heat resistant
Hepatitis A	RNA	No	27	Yes	No
Hepatitis B	DNA	Yes	42	No	No
Hepatitis C	RNA	Yes	35–65	No	No
Hepatitis D	RNA	Yes	35	No	No

Monitoring of chronic hepatitis C

Chronic HCV is a relatively slowly progressive disease but the rate of hepatic fibrosis progression varies significantly between individuals. Monitoring is required to identify individuals with advanced disease. Monitoring methods can be subdivided into biochemical, radiologic, and histologic.

Biochemical monitoring

The most common method for monitoring the activity of HCV infection is via estimation of the serum aminotransferases [alanine aminotransferase (ALT) and aspartate aminotransferase (AST)], which can reflect inflammatory activity in the liver. It is also common to routinely measure serum albumin, bilirubin, and prothrombin time, but these do not become abnormal until there is advanced liver disease. ALT and AST estimation poorly reflect the stage of disease severity of liver disease and can be entirely normal in a proportion of patients with cirrhosis [5].

A number of algorithms based on biochemical testing are available, which claim to more accurately predict the severity of the liver disease. In one of these, the Fibrotest, the following are used in a patented algorithm to derive a score correlating liver disease severity: age, sex, α2-macroglobulin, haptoglobin, γ-glutamyl transferase (GT), total bilirubin, and apolipoprotein A1. In a study of persons with hemophilia from Israel, Maor *et al.* used the Fibrotest in 132 hemophiliacs [6] and were able to correctly identify the differing stage in patients who have cleared the virus and those with known advanced disease.

Hepatic imaging

The most commonly performed radiologic or imaging technique to evaluate hepatic fibrosis, architecture, or hepatic masses is ultrasound examination of the liver. Computed tomography (CT) and magnetic resonance imaging (MRI) may be used. The radiologic tests are quite sensitive for detecting HCClarger than 1 cm in size but are relatively poor at documenting liver fibrosis unless this is very advanced and portal hypertension is present.

Transient elastography, or Fibroscan, which uses a probe to measure propagation of an ultrasound shear wave and hence measures the elasticity of the liver, is particularly useful in hemophilia where liver biopsies are rarely performed. In a study in hemophilia, Posthouwer *et al.* [7] found that 18% of 124 unselected people with hemophilia with chronic HCV had severe fibrosis and 17% had cirrhosis. Only 7% of these patients were previously known to have cirrhosis by the other standard tests.

Histologic monitoring

Direct microscopic examination of liver tissue remains the gold standard in establishing disease stage, inflammation, and severity. Understandably, there is a reluctance to perform biopsies in patients with inherited bleeding disorders. Liver biopsy can be performed through the transcutaneous or preferably via the transjugular routes. Irrespective of the method used, biopsies should ideally be done under direct radiologic imaging.

Patients with hemophilia should have their bleeding disorder normalized with infused concentrate or desmopressin prior to liver biopsy. A number of protocols exist and the one recommended in the UK consists of:

- Immediately pre-biopsy: treat to 1.00 IU/mL, i.e. 100%.
- 12 h post-biopsy: measure level and treat to 1.00 IU/mL.
- 24 h post-biopsy: measure level and treat to 1.00 IU/mL.
- 48 h post-biopsy: measure level and treat to 1.00 IU/mL.

The fact that liver biopsies can now be performed in hemophilia relatively safely does not mean that liver biopsy is mandatory. Most patients can be treated for chronic hepatitis C with pegylated interferon (PEG-IFN) and ribavirin irrespective of their liver histology. Biopsies remain useful for patients with HCV RNA and normal transaminases where the hepatitis is mild, where the cause of the liver dysfunction is in doubt, or where cirrhosis needs to be established before transplantation or for surveillance for HCC.

Natural history of hepatitis C

Following acute HCV infection the disease leads to chronic infection (defined as HCV RNA positivity >6 months after acute infection) in 80–85%. Although deaths from fulminant hepatitis during acute infection have been reported in nonhemophilic patients, this is very rare, occurring in <1 in 10 000. Patients with chronic HCV seldom clear the virus spontaneously, but spontaneous resolution has been reported. Patients with active chronic hepatitis C may develop cirrhosis, decompensated cirrhosis, endstage liver failure, or HCC (Figure 37.1).

Spontaneous clearance

A total of 15–20% of patients infected with hepatitis C clear the virus spontaneously during the acute phase [8]. This is more

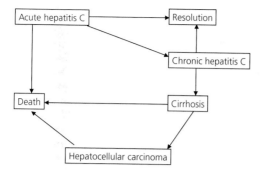

Figure 37.1 The natural history of hepatitis C.

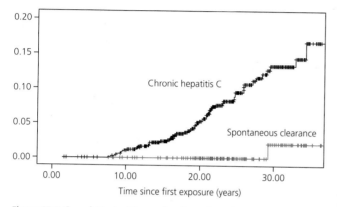

Figure 37.2 Cumulative incidence of endstage liver disease in 687 chronic hepatitis C virus (HCV) infected persons with hemophilia (PWH) and 160 PWH who cleared the HCV spontaneously.

> **Box 37.1** Definitions used in the assessment of hepatitis C treatment.
>
> Chronic hepatitis C virus (HCV): persisting infection (HCV RNA positive) 6 months or more after acute infection
> Rapid virological response (RVR): negative HCV RNA at 4 weeks
> Partial early virological response (pEVR): reduction of HCV RNA load by >2 logs (i.e. <1% level) 12 weeks after starting treatment
> Complete early virological response (cEVR): negative HCV RNA at 12 weeks
> End of treatment response (ETR): HCV RNA negative at treatment end
> Sustained virological response (SVR): HCV RNA negative 6 months after the end of treatment
> Transient response: reduction in HCV RNA by >2 logs during treatment but remaining positive at end of treatment
> Relapse: HCV RNA negative at end of treatment but relapse after this
> Nonresponse: no reduction of HCV RNA by >2 logs at any point during treatment

likely to occur when patients are infected in childhood. Once chronic hepatitis C is established 6 months after infection, spontaneous clearance rarely, if ever, occurs. Patients who clear the virus spontaneously prior to the onset of cirrhosis do not develop liver complications as a result of HCV in later life. Spontaneous clearance after acute hepatitis may be more common in patients with *IL28b* CC genotype [9].

Risks for disease progression

Patients who fail to clear the hepatitis C spontaneously or after treatment remain at risk for progression to liver failure and HCC (Figure 37.2). In one large hemophilia study which followed the cohorts from Sheffield, Utrecht, and the Royal Free Hospital in London, 15% of patients developed liver failure or HCC after 30 years. The risk was highest among HIV-positive patients who did not receive antiretroviral therapy, in whom the risk of liver failure was 40% at 30 years. Risk factors for liver disease progression in hemophilia include higher age at first exposure, longer length of time since infection, infection with genotype 1, high levels of alcohol intake, and HIV coinfection [7].

Extrahepatic manifestations of chronic hepatitis C

Several extrahepatic manifestations of HCV have been reported including mixed cryoglobulinemia, non-Hodgkin's lymphoma, porphyria cutanea tarda, lichen planus, hypothyroidism, and Sjögren's syndrome [10]. The presence of severe extrahepatic manifestations is an indication for HCV treatment even in the absence of marked liver disease.

Treatment

The first patients with hemophilia were treated with interferon in 1987, but response rates were low. The addition of ribavirin to interferon in 1995 and the subsequent pegylation of the interferon molecule have led to significant improvements in response rates [11]. A major recent development has been the introduction of the direct acting antiviral (DAA) drugs, telaprevir and boceprevir, which when used with PEG-IFN and ribavirin have increased the response rates in genotype 1 patients up to 70–80% [12–14].

The current standard of care for treatment of patients with hepatitis C is the combination of PEG-IFN and ribavirin with telaprevir or boceprevir for genotype 1. For patients with genotypes 2 and 3 PEG-IFN and ribavirin should be offered for 6 months while for individuals infected with genotypes 4, 5, and 6 treatment should be for 12 months. Telaprevir and boceprevir have limited activity against nontype 1 genotype. Activity in *in-vitro* cell culture systems revealed similar efficacy of protease inhibitors against genotypes 2a, 5a, and 6a and comparatively low but varying efficacy against genotype 3a isolates. Their use in genotypes other than 1 is not approved, however [15].

Box 37.1 shows the definitions used in the treatment of hepatitis C and Box 37.2 gives the recommended treatments for chronic HCV.

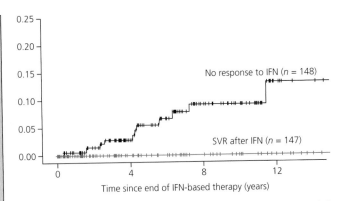

Box 37.2 Recommended treatment schedules for chronic hepatitis C (HCV).

Genotype 1

Treat with PEG-IFN and ribavirin for 48 weeks

Telaprevir or boceprevir should also be used

If HCV RNA level has not fallen by 2 logs by 12 weeks or not negative at 24 weeks, sustained viral response is unlikely and treatment can be stopped

Genotypes 2 or 3

Treat with PEG-IFN and ribavirin for 24 weeks

If HCV RNA is negative at 4 weeks, treatment can be reduced to 12–16 weeks

HIV/HCV coinfected patients: treat for 48 weeks irrespective of genotype

Figure 37.3 Risk of endstage liver disease in hemophilia. Patients who fail to respond to interferon (IFN) and ribavirin continue to have a high risk of liver failure. SVR, sustained virological response. Reproduced from [8] with permission of John Wiley & Sons.

Responses in people without hemophilia

In people without hemophilia the sustained virological response rate with PEG-IFN and ribavirin for genotype 1 is 40–50%, whereas for genotypes 2 and 3 it is 70–80%. Relapse rates remain relatively high (30% in patients with cirrhosis as a result of genotype 3 infection). PEG-IFN and ribavirin is available from two manufacturers (Roche and Schering-Plough) but there are no major differences in the response rates between these two interferons.

The addition of the DAA, telaprevir and boceprevir, to standard therapy leads to a more rapid decline in viral titers and significantly increases the response rates in genotype 1 patients. In phase 3 clinical trials, the combination of telaprevir/PEG-IFN/ribavirin led to a sustained virological response of 69% and 75% in treatment naive patients [12,13], respectively. Similarly, the combination of boceprevir/PEG-IFN/ribavirin led to a 65% response rate in the same group of patients. Individuals achieving a rapid virological response (undetectable virus in plasma at 4 weeks) are more likely to achieve sustained viral response (SVR) and in this group a total of 24 weeks' treatment appears to be as effective as 48 weeks. The presence of bridging fibrosis or cirrhosis reduces the SVR irrespective of treatment used.

Several potential viral targets of HCV have been identified. The next phase of therapy for hepatitis C will evolve to interferon-sparing or interferon-free antiviral regimens with new nonstructural protein 5b (NS5b) inhibitors, NS5a inhibitors, and a next generation of NS3 protease inhibitors [16–19].

Early virological response

The kinetics of response to treatment in the first 12 weeks of therapy are very useful in predicting SVR. Rapid virological response (RVR) is defined as a negative HCV RNA by PCR 28 days after commencing treatment. Complete early virological response (cEVR) is defined as a negative HCV RNA by PCR at 12 weeks. Partial EVR (pEVR) is defined as a >2 log decrease in viral load at week 12. RVR presages an SVR. Individuals with pEVR have a 75% chance of achieving SVR. Similarly, patients who do not achieve EVR have a >95% chance they will not achieve SVR.

Responses in people with hemophilia to treatment in treatment-naive patients

Responses to PEG-IFN and ribavirin in people with hemophilia are very similar to those in people without hemophilia. Posthouwer et al. reported a 59% SVR rate in people with hemophilia who had never been exposed to anti-HCV treatment previously. Although the response rate was lower in HIV-positive patients, it was still 32%, making this a very worthwhile subgroup to treat. Patients who clear the HCV with treatment have a dramatically reduced risk of progression of their liver disease. None of the 146 people with hemophilia in the Posthouwer study who obtained an SVR progressed up to 15 years of follow-up [11] (Figure 37.3).

At the time of writing, there have been no published reports of the response rates in patients with hemophilia being treated with telaprevir or boceprevir.

Responses to treatment in nonresponders, partial-responders, and responder-relapsers

Patients who have failed previous courses of therapy should be considered for retreatment with the DAA. In a phase 3 trial of telaprevir/PEG-IFN/ribavirin, the SVR was 86% for the responder-relapser group, 57% for the partial-responder, and 31% for the prior nonresponders [20]. Similarly, in another phase 3 study of boceprevir/PEG-IFN/ribavirin, the SVR was 72% in the responder-relapsers and 46% in the previous partial-responders [21]. Currently, there are no data available on the use of DAA in patients with hemophilia who failed previous therapies.

> **Box 37.3** Adverse events of treatment with PEG-IFN, ribavirin, telaprevir, and boceprevir. Only events occurring in >1% of patients are shown.
>
> Influenza-like symptoms (e.g. fever, malaise, myalgia, nausea, arthralgia, anorexia)
> Site of injection symptoms (e.g. pain, erythema)
> Neuropsychiatric (e.g. depression, anxiety, memory loss, insomnia, mood swings)
> Dermatologic (e.g. rash, reversible hair loss, photosensitivity)
> Hematologic (e.g. anemia, neutropenia, thrombocytopenia)
> Autoimmune (e.g. induction of autoantibodies, especially thyroid)

Adverse events of treatment

Adverse events during treatment are common and lead to premature discontinuation of treatment in 10–20% of patients. Box 37.3 lists the adverse effects occurring in >1% of treated patients. Influenza-like symptoms are seen most frequently and their tolerance can be increased by the use of paracetamol/acetaminophen and taking the interferon dose at times of reduced activity such as the weekends. Depression is frequently troublesome, especially in patients with a history of the disease. Antidepressant medication is very useful both as treatment and prophylaxis. Patients with a severe neuropsychiatric history should be assessed by a psychiatrist prior to treatment. Cytopenias are usually mild and can be managed by dose adjustment. In severe cytopenias, appropriate growth factors such as erythropoietin, granulocyte colony-stimulating factor, and eltrombopag can be used. Dysgeusia (altered or unpleasant taste sensations) and anemia are side-effects of boceprevir treatment. Telaprevir may cause are pruritus, rash, nausea, anemia and diarrhoea, and anorectal symptoms. Approximately 5% of patients experience severe dermatitis necessitating cessation of treatment, including drug rash with eosinophilia and systemic symptoms (DRESS) or even Stevens–Johnson syndrome. Severe dermatitis, however, is fortunately rare [22].

A rare but serious complication of particular interest to hemophilia is the development of antifactor VIII antibodies which can develop for the first time in patients with congenital hemophilia while having treatment or as autoantibodies (acquired hemophilia) in patients without a history of a bleeding disorder.

Treatment of patients with normal transaminases (ALT/AST)

Approximately a third of patients with chronic HCV have persistently normal aminotransferases; these individuals have less inflammation and fibrosis on liver biopsy and exhibit a more benign natural history. A total of 15–20% of these patients, however, have advanced fibrosis or cirrhosis and can develop liver failure and HCC [23]. Patients with normal ALT and AST have a similar response to antiviral therapy as other patients [24]. The decision to treat these patients is often difficult, especially in hemophilia where a liver biopsy is not usually available. This is actually one of the few situations where a liver biopsy does help in hemophilia because the identification of advanced disease would lead to a recommendation to treat. We would recommend that in the absence of treating all patients with normal serum aminotransferases, the following subgroups should be given priority: patients with advanced disease on biopsy or on noninvasive imaging/testing, patients with genotype 2/3 because of the high response rate, patients who wish to become pregnant, patients with symptomatic HCV such as those with severe tiredness or extrahepatic manifestations, and highly motivated individuals who wish to be hepatitis free.

Treatment of patients with cirrhosis

Patients with advanced liver disease may decompensate during treatment with interferon and ribavirin. It is, however, useful to treat patients with cirrhosis and monitor them carefully. Although only around 30% of patients achieve SVR, those who do so have an 80% less risk of liver failure or HCC development [25]. Despite this reduced risk for the development of complications, individuals with documented cirrhosis should continue to have surveillance for HCC.

Treatment of HIV-coinfected patients

Hepatitis C virus progresses more rapidly in HIV-coinfected patients, and these patients should be considered for treatment. Patients with hemophilia and HIV–HCV coinfection are likewise candidates for treatment with new direct-acting antivirals. Provisional data suggest that response rates are improved in coinfected patients (to 70%) but larger studies are required to confirm these findings. Treatment is best done in patients with a CD4 count of >200 × 10^6/L. Because of the risk of severe hemolysis, patients who are taking zidovudine (AZT), didanosine (ddI), or stavudine (d4T) should have their antiretroviral therapy modified so as to avoid these drugs during ribavirin therapy. The risk of adverse events in general is higher in coinfected patients. Coinfected patients should be treated for a total of 48 weeks irrespective of genotype. Drug–drug interactions between antiretroviral treatments and telaprevir or boceprevir are a potential problem and require appropriate management.

Hepatocellular carcinoma

Hepatocellular carcinoma is a malignant tumor arising in hepatocytes and is a complication occurring mainly in cirrhotic livers. HCC is increasingly seen in people with hemophilia. Regular monitoring for HCC should be performed in hemophilic patients with cirrhosis, but in the absence of liver biopsies it may be difficult to identify cirrhotic individuals. Noninvasive testing with the Fibrotest or Fibroscan may help refine the population for monitoring, but whether they identify all the patients at risk in hemophilia has not yet been confirmed. The two main means of monitoring for HCC are ultrasound scanning of the liver and measurement of serum α-fetoprotein. Ultrasound scanning is more sensitive for tumor detection. α-Fetoprotein may be elevated because of cirrhosis in the absence of HCC [26]. The most cost-effective surveillance strategy is ultrasound imaging and α-fetoprotein measurement every 6 months [27].

HCC, when isolated and not bridging the liver capsule, can be treated with resection or liver transplantation, which can be curative. Palliative treatments include ethanol injection into the tumor, radiofrequency ablation, and transarterial embolization [26].

Liver transplantation

Liver transplantation offers a cure to patients with hemophilia and liver failure or isolated HCC; these patients should be referred for the procedure in the same way as other patients with these complications. Because the liver is the site of production of factors VIII and IX, liver transplantation cures the hemophilia phenotypically, making it a highly cost-effective procedure, especially in patients with severe hemophilia [28,29]. Over 100 liver transplants have been carried out in persons with hemophilia worldwide. Factor VIII/IX concentrate is administered immediately before surgery either by bolus injection or continuous infusion and for the immediate postoperative period for 12–48 h, after which no further concentrate is required.

Liver transplantation is not contraindicated in HIV-positive individuals provided that the HIV is fully suppressed with highly active antiretroviral therapy (HAART) [30].

Postliver transplantation, the new liver is invariably reinfected with HCV if the recipient was HCV RNA positive going into transplantation, as is usually the case. Furthermore, the natural history of HCV post-transplant is altered and the median time to cirrhosis is abbreviated to only 10–12 years, with survival after decompensation of only 40% at 1 year [31]. Patients with established HCV infection postliver transplantation should be treated with interferon and ribavirin.

References

1 Committee for Proprietary Medicinal Products (CPMP). Note for guidance on plasma derived products. Document number CPMP/BWP/269/95 rev. 3, 2001.

2 Richardson LC, Evatt BL. Risk of hepatitis A virus infection in persons with hemophilia receiving plasma-derived products. *Transfus Med Rev* 2000; **14**: 64–73.

3 Rumi MG, Colombo M, Gringeri A, *et al*. High prevalence of antibody to hepatitis C virus in multitransfused hemophiliacs with normal transaminase levels. *Ann Intern Med* 1990; **112**: 379–80.

4 Preston FE, Jarvis LM, Makris M, Philp L, Underwood JC, Ludlam CA, Simmonds P. Heterogeneity of hepatitis C virus genotypes in hemophilia: relationship with chronic liver disease. *Blood* 1995; **85**: 1259–62.

5 Alberti A, Morsica G, Chemello L, *et al*. Hepatitis C viraemia and liver disease in symptom free individuals with anti-HCV. *Lancet* 1992; **340**: 697–8.

6 Maor Y, Bashari D, Kenet G, Lubetsky A, Luboshitz J, Shapiro JM. Non-invasive biomarkers of liver fibrosis in haemophilia patients with hepatitis C: can you avoid liver biopsy? *Haemophilia* 2006; **12**: 372–9.

7 Posthouwer D, Makris M, Yee TT, *et al*. Progression to end-stage liver disease in patients with inherited bleeding disorders and hepatitis C: an international, multicenter cohort study. *Blood* 2007; **109**: 3667–71.

8 Posthouwer D, Yee TT, Makris M, *et al*. Antiviral therapy for chronic hepatitis C in patients with inherited bleeding disorders: an international, multicenter cohort study. *J Thromb Haemost* 2007; **5**: 1624–9.

9 Thomas DL, Thio CL, Martin MP, *et al*. Genetic variation in IL28B and spontaneous clearance of hepatitis C virus. *Nature* 2009; **461**: 798–801.

10 Galossi A, Guarisco R, Bellis L, Puoti C. Extrahepatic manifestations of chronic HCV infection. *J Gastrointestin Liver Dis* 2007; **16**: 65–73.

11 Posthouwer D, Mauser-Bunschoten EP, Fischer K, Makris M. Treatment of chronic hepatitis C in patients with haemophilia: a review of the literature. *Haemophilia* 2006; **12**: 473–8.

12 Jacobson IM, McHutchison JG, Dusheiko G, *et al*. Telaprevir for previously untreated chronic hepatitis C virus infection. *N Engl J Med* 2011; **364**: 2405–16.

13 Sherman KE, Flamm SL, Afdhal N, *et al*. Telaprevir in combination with peginterferon alfa-2a and ribavirin for 24 or 48 weeks in treatment-naïve genotype 1 HCV patients who achieved an extended rapid viral response: final results of Phase III ILLUMINATE study. *Hepatology* 2011; **52**(Suppl. S): 401A–2.

14 Poordad F, McCone J Jr, Bacon BR, *et al*. Bocepravir for untreated chronic HCV genotype 1 infection. *N Engl J Med* 2011; **364**: 1195–206.

15 Silva MO, Treitel M, Graham DJ, *et al*. Antiviral activity of boceprevir monotherapy in treatment-naive subjects with chronic hepatitis C genotype 2/3. *J Hepatol* 2013; **59**: 31–7.

16 Sulkowski MS, Sherman KE, Soriano V, *et al*. Telaparevir in combination with peginterferon alfa-2a/ribavirin in HCV/HIV co-infected patients: SVR24 final study results. *Hepatology* 2012; **56**: 219A.

17 Sulkowski M, Pol S, Mallolas J, *et al*. Boceprevir versus placebo with pegylated interferon alfa-2b and ribavirin for treatment of hepatitis C virus genotype 1 in patients with HIV: a randomised, double-blind, controlled phase 2 trial. *Lancet Infect Dis* 2013; **13**: 597–605.

18 Osinusi A, Naggie S. Boceprevir for HCV in patients with HIV: where next? *Lancet Infect Dis* 2013; **13**: 563–4.

19 Dieterich D, *et al*. Simeprevir with pegylated interferon/ribavirin in patients co-infected with chronic hepatitis C virus and HIV-1: week-24 interim analysis of the TMC435-C212 study. Paper #154LB presented at the 20th Conference on Retroviruses and Opportunistic Infections (CROI), March 3–6 2013, Atlanta.

20 Zeuzem S, Andreone P, Pol S, *et al*. Telaprevir for retreatment of HCV infection. *N Engl J Med* 2011; **364**: 2417–28.

21 Bacon BR, Gordon SC, Lawitz E, *et al*. Bocepravir for previously treated chronic HCV genotype 1 infection. *N Engl J Med* 2011; **364**: 1207–17.

22 Sarrazin C, Hézode C, Zeuzem S, Pawlotsky J-M. Antiviral strategies in hepatitis C virus infection. *J Hepatol* 2012; **56**(Suppl. 1): S88–100.

23 Puoti C, Bellis L, Galossi A, *et al.* Antiviral treatment of HCV carriers with persistently normal ALT levels. *Mini Rev Med Chem* 2008; **8**: 150–2.

24 Jacobson IM, Ahmed F, Russo MW, *et al.* Interferon alpha-2b and ribavirin for patients with chronic hepatitis C and normal ALT. *Am J Gastroenterol* 2004; **99**: 1700–5.

25 Veldt BJ, Heathcote J, Wedemeyer H, *et al.* Sustained virologic response and clinical outcomes in patients with chronic hepatitis C and advanced fibrosis. *Ann Intern Med* 2007; **147**: 677–84.

26 Meijer K, Haagsma EB. HCV-related liver cancer in people with haemophilia. *Haemophilia* 2012; **18**: 17–24.

27 Thompson Coon J, Rogers G, Hewson P, *et al.* Surveillance of cirrhosis for hepatocellular carcinoma: systematic review and economic analysis. *Health Technol Assess* 2007; **11**: 1–206.

28 Gordon FH, Mistry PK, Sabin CA, Lee CA. Outcome of orthotopic liver transplantation in patients with haemophilia. *Gut* 1998; **42**: 744–9.

29 Wilde J, Teixeira P, Bramhall SR, Gunson B, Mutimer D, Mirza DF. Liver transplantation in haemophilia. *Br J Haematol* 2002; **117**: 952–6.

30 Ragni M, Devera ME, Roland ME, *et al.* Liver transplant outcomes in HIV (+) haemophilic men. *Haemophilia* 2013; **19**: 134–40.

31 Picciotto A. Antihepatitis C virus therapy in liver transplanted patients. *Ther Clin Risk Manag* 2006; **2**: 39–44.

CHAPTER 38

Transfusion-transmitted disease: emerging infections

Thomas R. Kreil

Baxter BioScience, Vienna, Austria

Introduction

For this chapter the discussion of emerging infectious agents with relevance to transfusion-transmitted diseases will be limited to those infectious agents which can be considered of potential relevance for the pathogen safety of plasma-derived hemophilia treatment products. As effective aseptic practises have long been embedded into the manufacturing processes of plasma derivatives, bacterial, fungal, and parasitic agents such as *Plasmodium*, *Babesia*, and *Borrelia*, that have been or potentially could be transfusion transmitted [1], will not be covered.

Human immunodeficiency virus (HIV) and the hepatitis B (HBV) and hepatitis C (HCV) viruses, clinically the most important causes of infectious adverse events associated with the treatment of hemophilia by plasma derivatives, are also excluded, as scientific knowledge about these viruses has advanced to a level that is hardly compatible with the "emerging" agent status any more, and, in addition, they are covered elsewhere in this book.

Finally, prion diseases and their impact on hemophilia treatment will be covered in a separate chapter, and thus they are not discussed here either.

The infectious agents that remain within scope are emerging viruses. During the last decade, several new viruses have been identified to occur in human blood, on occasion by equally novel molecular methods. For some of these viruses a causative association with a disease entity has yet to be revealed, so that their pathogenicity for humans remains unsubstantiated. During the same period, however, other viruses have caused epidemics or even a pandemic, facilitated by changes of these viruses or in the ecologic environment to favor zoonotic risk factors, or by the introduction of previously known agents into entirely naive populations by global commerce or travel.

In addition, the intimate link between labile blood products for transfusion and manufactured plasma products in general and for hemophilia treatment in particular, will be discussed in this chapter. While derived from human blood as a common source, pathogen safety concerns around these two product categories are intrinsically different: blood product safety margins are still to date limited to the selection of suitable donors and the testing of donations, whereas these measures are complemented by effective virus inactivation and removal steps, collectively virus reduction, during the manufacturing processes of plasma products. Despite this significant difference, during the emergence of infectious diseases when initial blood transfusion transmissions can become sentinel events that precipitate utmost public health attention, the level of concern and the felt need to implement additional safeguards are often quite similar for these two product classes: as additional information about the respective emerging agent is revealed or generated, such as the frequency of viremic donors and the level of viremia, as well as the specific reduction capacity for the virus of concern, more rational differentiation becomes possible.

Lipid-enveloped viruses

Some of the lipid-enveloped viruses detected in blood have not so far been found to be pathogenic for humans. For example, the GBV-C/hepatitis G virus (HGV) was shown to be transfusion transmissible [2], yet any pathogenic consequence of infection for humans has remained elusive [3]. In contrast, GBV-C/HGV infection was even shown to result in slower disease progression of HIV coinfection [4,5], possibly associated with reduced chronic immune- and T-cell activation as mediated by $CD3^+CD4^-CD8^-$ double-negative T cells (DNTC) [6].

The emergence of the severe acute respiratory syndrome (SARS) coronavirus in southern China represented a different level of challenge for human health, with 8.098 humans clinically infected, of whom 774 succumbed to their infection, in an epidemic that spread to 29 countries [7] within a matter of

Textbook of Hemophilia, Third Edition. Edited by Christine A. Lee, Erik E. Berntorp and W. Keith Hoots.
© 2014 John Wiley & Sons, Ltd. Published 2014 by John Wiley & Sons, Ltd.

weeks, before circulation of the virus could be halted by significant public health efforts. The demonstration of low-levelled viremia during the clinical stages of the disease [8] also raised concern about the safety of hemophilia treatment products, although transfusion transmission of the SARS virus was never reported. In addition, virus reduction studies using another coronavirus (Baxter GPS, unpublished), a physicochemically closely related so-called "model virus" [9], had established evidence that the SARS coronavirus would be inactivated during the manufacturing processes of plasma derivatives, which was later confirmed by limited investigations using the SARS coronavirus itself [10,11]. Long after the last case of SARS had been reported from China in May 2004, late September of 2012 has witnessed the detection of another novel coronavirus associated with human disease in Saudi Arabia, Quatar, and Jordan, at the time of writing still limited to nine human cases of which five were fatal. The public health response reflected the learning from the earlier SARS epidemic in an impressive way, with a specific assay for the detection of the new virus developed literally within days [12] and effectively deployed to diagnostic networks within a few weeks. The earlier investigations about the inactivation of coronavirus do, however, still provide adequate reassurance for the safety margins of plasma-derived hemophilia treatments against potential coronavirus contaminations of plasma for fractionation.

Other emerging lipid-enveloped viruses have actually caused blood transfusion transmissions, a situation reminiscent of earlier concerns for the safety of plasma derivatives.

After the 1999 introduction of West Nile virus (WNV) into the USA, the virus has emerged to endemicity across the nation, with seroconversion of approximately 1% of the entire population [13]. As a consequence of the first WNV blood transfusion transmissions, nationwide screening of the blood supply by nucleic acid amplification technology (NAT) was implemented. However, despite using the most modern technology available, the reduction of virus transmissions by blood transfusion was limited to a suboptimal 93% [14], testimony to the general limitation of any testing, i.e. a nonreactive test result not necessarily being equal to no virus present.

For plasma derivatives, the major contribution of virus reduction, i.e. virus inactivation and removal during the manufacturing process, has been verified as effective against WNV [15]. Consistent with these results, regulators differentiated between the safety margins of directly transfused blood products versus manufactured plasma products, and did not require the implementation of NAT for plasma for fractionation.

The demonstration of a substantial virus reduction capacity of plasma manufacturing processes for flaviviruses thus provides reassurance in a broader sense: despite the expanding geographic range of several flaviviruses and a certain level of blood transfusion transmissions of, for example, dengue virus [16], there is no concern for the safety of plasma derivatives, and new situations of emergence will likely not require changes in current testing practises for plasma for fractionation.

Another group of lipid-enveloped viruses that have been high on the global alert list are the (potentially) pandemic influenza virus candidates. Specifically, the highly pathogenic H5N1 virus, which has caused 608 reported human infections as of November 2012 (see WHO: http://www.who.int/influenza/human_animal_interface/HAI_Risk_Assessment/en/index.html), of which 359 (59%) have had a fatal outcome. Historic evidence for similar, and actually less pathogenic, influenza viruses supported the occurrence of preclinical viremia for influenza viruses [17], which has also been confirmed for the H5N1 virus itself [18]. In an attempt to achieve a more definitive understanding of virus behavior during the manufacturing processes of plasma derivatives, the H5N1 virus was studied in *verification* studies, and was shown to be effectively inactivated by the most commonly used virus inactivation techniques, such as vapor heating, solvent/detergent, and low pH treatment, as well as pasteurization [19]. And while the H5N1 pandemic has not occurred yet, the pandemic H1N1 virus that started to circulate in 2009 was not much of a concern for the safety of plasma products, based on these influenza H5N1 data.

The reported association of xenotropic murine leukemia virus-related virus (XMRV) with prostate cancer and chronic fatigue syndrome is also mentioned here. After these initial reports, a concern quickly grew that this newly recognized retrovirus could also be passed between humans through the blood supply. Additional donor deferral criteria were thus considered and partially implemented, whereas based on the state-of-the-art virus inactivation and removal procedures for plasma products, which because of their HIV history have to be evaluated for reduction of this retrovirus per the European Guideline on Plasma-derived Medicinal Products (EMA/CHMP/BWP/706271/2010), their safety margins were not questioned [20]. Increasingly, more solid scientific evidence does not ultimately seem to support XMRV as a virus of humans, and even less any causative role in human disease [21]. The episode is an important reminder though of how we base decisions on facts, unless in the absence of these the precautionary principle requires an alternative, and more conservative, course of action. Put differently, the generation of solid scientific evidence is the prime mandate in these situations of uncertainty, as only facts can support rational decision-making processes.

In general, lipid-enveloped viruses are now understood as rather an insignificant challenge to the safety margins of modern plasma derivatives, particularly given the widely demonstrated effectiveness of current virus inactivation and removal procedures.

Nonlipid-enveloped viruses

As generally the effectiveness of virus inactivation and certain removal technologies is more limited against nonlipid-enveloped viruses, owing to their typically higher physicochemical resistance and often smaller size, respectively, emerging viruses of this class can potentially be a more significant remaining concern. Fortunately, though, they have so far been associated with more moderate disease in humans, as compared to many of their lipid-enveloped counterparts. In fact, attempts at demonstrating an association with any clinical disease in humans has been difficult or unsuccessful for some of these viruses.

For example, the initial identification of Torque teno virus (TTV) [22] and the related SEN virus (SEN-V; reported on July 20, 1999, in the *New York Times*) as blood transfusion-transmissible viruses understandably sparked public health concerns. Specifically for hemophilia, it was later reported that at least TTV could also occur as a contaminant of plasma derivatives with less stringent purification processes [23]. Early reports even suggested that first-generation recombinant factor VIII (FVIII) products, through the albumin used as a stabilizer [24], could contain the virus nucleic acid, but this has been refuted by additional experiments [25]. However, no pathogenicity for humans has been substantiated to date, and so these viruses might be considered a commensal part of the microbiologic flora rather than a pathogen for humans.

The detection of the B19 parvovirus (B19V) in human plasma for fractionation was another concern for the treatment of hemophilia, particularly as the virus was suggested to reach uniquely high titers of up to 10E14 particles per milliliter [26], a number that would correspond to almost 0.1% of the blood volume. The virus was assumed to be mostly resistant to inactivation, based on studies conducted with animal parvoviruses as models.

Where virus reduction did not seem a promising approach, the implementation of NAT to limit the load of plasma pools for manufacturing, initially as voluntary industry standard developed by the Plasma Proteins Therapeutics Association (PPTA), was a first step to enhance safety margins. In retrospect, these testing interventions have been one of the most successful ever, as evidenced particularly by a comparison with the more recent introduction of WNV NAT. Using WNV NAT, the residual risk of WNV transfusion transmission was reduced to only 7% of the initial value, i.e. by approximately 10-fold, whereas B19V NAT has reduced the average plasma pool load from initially 10 000 000 to now only 100 copies/mL, i.e. a reduction by 100 000-fold.

The subsequent recognition of the closely related erythroviruses V9 [27] and A6 [28], now reclassified as B19V genotypes 2 and 3, has necessitated reliable detection of all genotypic variants and, therefore, been a challenge for the diagnostic tests used to reduce the virus load of plasma for fractionation.

The use of infectivity assays based on B19V-susceptible cell lines coupled with a molecular biology readout has more recently demonstrated the significantly greater sensitivity of the different B19 viruses to liquid heating [29], low pH [29,30], and vapor heating [31], as compared to earlier animal parvovirus models.

As already suggested by the clinical experience with plasma for transfusion, which occasionally transmitted B19V when it contained virus above a certain threshold concentration [32], antibody-mediated B19V neutralization provides additional safety margins [33]. Recent evidence may, however, suggest that particularly intermediate purity FVIII products as also used for the treatment of von Willebrand disease can still occasionally transmit the B19V [34].

Whether the more distantly related PARV4 and bocaviruses will turn out to be a challenge for the safety of hemophilia treatment products remains uncertain at present. These viruses are found in plasma for fractionation and even historic plasma derivatives [35], but clinically they have not been associated with major human health issues.

Reports from Japan have initially suggested the transfusion transmissibility of hepatitis E virus (HEV) [36], yet in the country foodborne zoonotic HEV infections had also been recognized. A significant prevalence of the virus in pig meat and even seroprevalence in humans has since become apparent in other countries, including several European countries and the USA (reviewed in [37]), also associated with several blood transfusion transmission cases as well as the demonstration of HEV RNA in individual plasma donations [38].

As yet, however, a practical virus infectivity assay that would enable the assessment of HEV reduction during the manufacturing processes of hemophilia treatment products has not become widely available; although limited investigation has shown the virus to be partially sensitive to liquid- and dry-heat inactivation [39]. Consistent with this finding, hemophilia patients treated with historic noninactivated plasma products carry HEV antibodies more often than those only treated with advanced virus-inactivated products [40].

Most importantly though, nonlipid-enveloped viruses are typically more resistant to a range of physiochemical conditions, and they have shown continued adaption. Therefore vigilance needs to be supported by continued research into the physicochemical nature of these agents and their corresponding behavior during plasma fractionation processes, so that informed decisions can be taken by industry and regulators in a timely fashion.

Future directions

The inception of hemophilia treatment, initially with plasma-derived clotting factor concentrates, has dramatically changed the life expectancy and quality of those affected. It has also brought about the risk of infectious disease transmission. With the implementation of effective virus inactivation/removal processes, supported by virus marker testing and donor selection, the safety margins of these products were significantly enhanced, and current plasma derivatives enjoy substantial safety margins with respect to known infectious agents. Given the particularly robust reduction capacity for lipid-enveloped viruses, one might predict that any future emerging viruses within this class will not represent a significant challenge. For nonlipid-enveloped viruses a higher level of vigilance and more frequent experimental work to verify assumptions will remain prudent, a task that many academic and industry research groups are focusing on every day.

The advent of an entirely different class of pathogens, i.e. prion agents, has emphasized that any use of an animal- or human-derived component anywhere in the manufacturing process may lead to concerns around the potential presence and transmissibility of a pathogenic agent contained in these, even when using recombinant production techniques.

Fortunately, advances in technology increasingly allow the production of recombinant proteins from production platforms entirely free of any exposure to human or animal proteins, thus potentially eliminating any infectious disease concerns associated with their medical use.

References

1 Alter HJ, Stramer SL, Dodd RY. Emerging infectious diseases that threaten the blood supply. *Semin Hematol* 2007; **44**: 32–41.

2 Linnen J, Wages J Jr, Zhang-Keck ZY, *et al*. Molecular cloning and disease association of hepatitis G virus: a transfusion-transmissible agent. *Science* 1996; **271**: 505–8.

3 Alter HJ. G-pers creepers, where'd you get those papers? A reassessment of the literature on the hepatitis G virus. *Transfusion* 1997; **37**: 569–72.

4 Lefrere JJ, Roudot-Thoraval F, Morand-Joubert L, *et al*. Carriage of GB virus C/hepatitis G virus RNA is associated with a slower immunologic, virologic, and clinical progression of human immunodeficiency virus disease in coinfected persons. *J Infect Dis* 1999; **179**: 783–9.

5 Tillmann HL, Heiken H, Knapik-Botor A, *et al*. Infection with GB virus C and reduced mortality among HIV-infected patients. *N Engl J Med* 2001; **345**: 715–24.

6 Bhattarai N, Rydze RT, Chivero ET, Stapleton JT. GB virus C viremia is associated with higher levels of double-negative T cells and lower T-cell activation in HIV-infected individuals receiving antiretroviral therapy. *J Infect Dis* 2012; **206**: 1469–72.

7 MMWR. Revised U.S. Surveillance Case Definition for severe acute respiratory syndrome (SARS) and update on SARS cases—United States and worldwide, December 2003. *MMWR* 2003; **52**: 1202–6.

8 Drosten C, Gunther S, Preiser W, *et al*. Identification of a novel coronavirus in patients with severe acute respiratory syndrome. *N Engl J Med* 2003; **348**: 1967–76.

9 EMEA. CPMP note for guidance on virus validation studies: the design, contribution and interpretation of studies validating the inactivation and removal of viruses (CPMP/BWP/268/95/rev). CPMP/BWP/268/95.

10 Darnell ME, Taylor DR. Evaluation of inactivation methods for severe acute respiratory syndrome coronavirus in noncellular blood products. *Transfusion* 2006; **46**: 1770–7.

11 Yunoki M, Urayama T, Yamamoto I, Abe S, Ikuta K. Heat sensitivity of a SARS-associated coronavirus introduced into plasma products. *Vox Sang* 2004; **87**: 302–3.

12 Corman VM, Eckerle I, Bleicker T, *et al*. Detection of a novel human coronavirus by real-time reverse-transcription polymerase chain reaction. *Eurosurveillance* 2012; **17/39**: pii=20285

13 Planitzer CB, Modrof J, Yu MYW, Kreil TR. West Nile virus infection in plasma of blood and plasma donors, United States. *Emerg Infect Dis* 2009; **15**: 1668–70.

14 Petersen LR, Epstein JS. Problem solved? West Nile virus and transfusion safety. *N Engl J Med* 2005; **353**: 516–17.

15 Kreil TR, Berting A, Kistner O, Kindermann J. West Nile virus and the safety of plasma derivatives: verification of high safety margins, and the validity of predictions based on model virus data. *Transfusion* 2003; **43**: 1023–8.

16 Tambyah PA, Koay ES, Poon ML, Lin RV, Ong BK. Dengue hemorrhagic fever transmitted by blood transfusion. *N Engl J Med* 2008; **359**: 1526–7.

17 Naficy K. Human influenza infection with proved viremia. Report of a case. *N Engl J Med* 1963; **269**: 964–6.

18 Chutinimitkul S, Bhattarakosol P, Srisuratanon S, *et al*. H5N1 influenza A virus and infected human plasma. *Emerg Infect Dis* 2006; **12**: 1041–3.

19 Kreil TR, Unger U, Orth SM, *et al*. H5N1 influenza virus and the safety of plasma products. *Transfusion* 2007; **47**: 452–9.

20 Klein HG, Dodd RY, Hollinger FB, *et al*. Xenotropic murine leukemia virus-related virus (XMRV) and blood transfusion: report of the AABB interorganizational XMRV task force. *Transfusion* 2011; **51**: 654–61.

21 Delviks-Frankenberry K, Cingöz O, Coffin JM, Pathak VK. Recombinant origin, contamination, and de-discovery of XMRV. *Curr Op Virol* 2012; **2**: 499–507.

22 Nishizawa T, Okamoto H, Konishi K, Yoshizawa H, Miyakawa Y, Mayumi M. A novel DNA virus (TTV) associated with elevated transaminase levels in posttransfusion hepatitis of unknown etiology. *Biochem Biophys Res Commun* 1997; **241**: 92–7.

23 Simmonds P, Davidson F, Lycett C, *et al*. Detection of a novel DNA virus (TTV) in blood donors and blood products. *Lancet* 1998; **352**: 191–5.

24 Azzi A, De SR, Morfini M, *et al*. TT virus contaminates first-generation recombinant factor VIII concentrates. *Blood* 2001; **98**: 2571–3.

25 Kreil TR, Zimmermann K, Pable S, Schwarz HP, Dorner F. TT virus does not contaminate first-generation recombinant factor VIII concentrate. *Blood* 2002; **100**: 2271–2.

26 Weimer T, Streichert S, Watson C, Groner A. High-titer screening PCR: a successful strategy for reducing the parvovirus B19 load in plasma pools for fractionation. *Transfusion* 2001; **41**: 1500–4.

27 Nguyen QT, Sifer C, Schneider V, *et al*. Novel human erythrovirus associated with transient aplastic anemia. *J Clin Microbiol* 1999; **37**: 2483–7.

28 Nguyen QT, Wong S, Heegaard ED, Brown KE. Identification and characterization of a second novel human erythrovirus variant, A6. *Virology* 2002; **301**: 374–80.

29 Blumel J, Schmidt I, Willkommen H, Lower J. Inactivation of parvovirus B19 during pasteurization of human serum albumin. *Transfusion* 2002; **42**: 1011–18.

30 Boschetti N, Niederhauser I, Kempf C, Stuhler A, Lower J, Blumel J. Different susceptibility of B19 virus and mice minute virus to low pH treatment. *Transfusion* 2004; **44**: 1079–86.

31 Berting A, Modrof J, Unger U, *et al.* Inactivation of parvovirus B19 during STIM-4 vapor heat treatment of three coagulation factor concentrates. *Transfusion* 2008; **48**: 1220–6.

32 Davenport RJ, Geohas G, Cohen S, *et al.* Phase IV study of Plas+SD: hepatitis A (HAV) and parvovirus B19 (B19) safety results. *Blood* 2000; **96**(Suppl.): 451a.

33 Modrof J, Berting A, Tille B, *et al.* Neutralization of human parvovirus B19 by plasma and intravenous immunoglobulins. *Transfusion* 2007; **48**: 178–86.

34 Soucie JM, De Staercke C, Monahan PE, *et al.* Evidence for the transmission of parvovirus B19 in patients with bleeding disorders treated with plasma-derived factor concentrates in the era of nucleic acid test screening. *Transfusion* 2012; **53**: 1217–25.

35 Fryer JF, Hubbard AR, Baylis SA. Human parvovirus PARV4 in clotting factor VIII concentrates. *Vox Sang* 2007; **93**: 341–7.

36 Mitsui T, Tsukamoto Y, Yamazaki C, *et al.* Prevalence of hepatitis E virus infection among hemodialysis patients in Japan: evidence for infection with a genotype 3 HEV by blood transfusion. *J Med Virol* 2004; **74**: 563–72.

37 Hoofnagle JH, Nelson KE, Purcell RH. Hepatitis E. *New Engl J Med* 2012; **367**: 1237–44.

38 Baylis SA, Gartner T, Nick S, Ovemyr J, Blumel. Occurrence of hepatitis E virus RNA in plasma donations from Sweden, Germany and the United States. *Vox Sang* 2012; **103**: 89–90.

39 Yunoki M, Yamamoto S, Tanaka H, *et al.* Extent of hepatitis E virus elimination is affected by stabilizers present in plasma products and pore size of nanofilters. *Vox Sang* 2008; **95**: 94–100.

40 Toyoda H, Honda T, Hayashi K, *et al.* Prevalence of hepatitis E virus IgG antibody in Japanese patients with hemophilia. *Intervirology* 2008; **51**: 21–5.

been identified. Within this patient cohort, autopsy material has been examined in seven patients and biopsy material in a further six [10]; no evidence of vCJD has been demonstrated in any of these samples although clearly this represents testing of only a very small proportion of the UK hemophilia population considered as being at risk of vCJD. Interestingly, it was treatment with nonimplicated FVIII concentrates that was identified as being the most likely source of vCJD infection in the hemophilic patient with presumed subclinical vCJD [10]. Considering the plasma pools from which clotting factor concentrates are manufactured each contain in the order of 20 000 donations, and based on the estimated prevalence of subclinical vCJD, it is likely that many pools have contained plasma from unidentified infected donors.

vCJD in other countries

Outside the UK, 49 cases of vCJD have been reported worldwide to date [4], 41 of which have been in Europe, the majority in France. While a small minority are understood to have acquired the disease in the UK, most patients are believed to have been infected in their country of origin. Other countries have adopted less precautionary approaches than the UK. Authorities in France concluded that the risk posed by implicated batches, even in the most pessimistic scenario, was very low and consequently continued to manufacture plasma sourced from their domestic blood supply, with the introduction of nano-filtration as an additional step in the process. In the United States, the Food and Drugs Administration have concluded that the risk of vCJD infection by plasma products ranges from 1 in 9.4 million to 1 in 15 000 [34].

Development of a screening test for vCJD

Improved evaluation of subclinical vCJD infection prevalence rates and the efficacy of the risk-reduction measures outlined in this chapter would be greatly facilitated by the availability of a blood test that reliably detects prion infectivity in asymptomatic individuals. However, the unique pathogenesis of prion diseases makes development of such tests very difficult for a number of reasons. The misfolded host cellular PrP^{sc} does not generate a humoral immune response, nor is there agent-specific nucleic acid. While immunoassays that detect PrP^{sc} in affected tissues use protease to degrade normal PrP, some protease-sensitive PrP^{sc} forms have also been reported [35]. Furthermore, to facilitate the successful identification of blood infectivity, an assay would be required that can detect much lower levels of PrP^{sc} than those found in tissues of clinical vCJD. Together with the higher $PrP:PrP^{sc}$ ratio found in blood compared to other tissue and the scarcity of blood samples from vCJD patients, these pose significant challenges to the development of a sufficiently sensitive and specific blood-based assay. Some of these have

been overcome by the demonstration of avid prion binding to surfaces such as metals [36], which have been used in the development of a quantitative blood-based assay for prion infectivity [37]. Levels of sensitivity and specificity of 71.4% and 100%, respectively, have been reported in a study of clinical vCJD cases [38]. This level of specificity can be interpreted as being sufficient for neurologic diagnostic use; however, extensive further validation would be required before these assays could be used as screening tests for the detection of subclinical vCJD infection and there is no currently available blood test for vCJD detection outwith the research setting.

References

1 Will RG, Ironside JW, Zeidler M, *et al.* A new variant of Creutzfeldt–Jakob disease in the UK. *Lancet* 1996; **347**(9006): 921–5.

2 Scott MR, Will RG, Ironside JW, *et al.* Compelling transgenetic evidence for transmission of bovine spongiform encephalopathy prions to humans. *Proc Natl Acad Sci USA* 1999; **96**(26): 15137–42.

3 Bruce ME, Will RG, Ironside JW, *et al.* Transmissions to mice indicate that "new variant" CJD is caused by the BSE agent. *Nature* 1997; **389**(6650): 498–501.

4 Andrews NJ. Incidence of variant Creutzfeldt–Jakob disease diagnosis and deaths in the UK, 2012. Available at: http://www.cjd.ed.ac.uk/documents/cjdq72.pdf

5 Llewelyn CA, Hewirr PE, Knight RS, *et al.* Possible transmission of variant Creutzfeldt–Jakob disease by blood transfusion. *Lancet* 2004; **363**(9407): 417–21.

6 Wroe SJ, Hewirr PE, Knight RS, *et al.* Clinical presentation and pre-mortem diagnosis of variant Creutzfeldt–Jakob disease associated with blood transfusion: a case report. *Lancet* 2006; **368**(9552): 2061–7.

7 Health Protection Agency (HPA). New case of transfusion-associated variant CJD. *Comm Dis Rep Weekly* 2006; **16**(6): 1.

8 Peden AH, Head MW, Ritchie DL, *et al.* Preclinical vCJD after blood transfusion in a PRNP codon 129 heterozygous patient. *Lancet* 2004; **364**(9433): 527–9.

9 Zaman SM, Hill FG, Palmer B, *et al.* The risk of variant Creutzfeldt–Jakob disease among UK patients with bleeding disorders, known to have received potentially contaminated plasma products. *Haemophilia* 2011; **17**(6): 931–7.

10 Peden A, McCardle L, Head MW, *et al.* Variant CJD infection in the spleen of a neurologically asymptomatic UK adult patient with haemophilia. *Haemophilia* 2010; **16**(2): 296–304.

11 Wadsworth JD, Joiner S, Hill AF, *et al.* Tissue distribution of protease resistant prion protein in variant Creutzfeldt–Jakob disease using a highly sensitive immunoblotting assay. *Lancet* 2001; **358**(9277): 171–80.

12 Head MW, Ritchie D, Smith N, *et al.* Peripheral tissue involvement in sporadic, iatrogenic, and variant Creutzfeldt–Jakob disease: an immunohistochemical, quantitative, and biochemical study. *Am J Pathol* 2004; **164**(1): 143–53.

13 Hilton DA, Ghani AC, Conyers L, *et al.* Prevalence of lymphoreticular prion protein accumulation in UK tissue samples. *J Pathol* 2004; **203**(3): 733–9.

14 Clewley JP, Kelly CM, Andrews N, *et al.* Prevalence of disease related prion protein in anonymous tonsil specimens in Britain: cross sectional opportunistic survey. *Br Med J* 2009; **338**: b1442.

15 Kaski D, Mead S, Hyare H, *et al.* Variant CJD in an individual heterozygous for PRNP codon 129. *Lancet* 2009; **374**(9707): 2128.

16 Foster PR. Assessment of the potential of plasma fractionation processes to remove causative agents of transmissible spongiform encephalopathy. *Transfus Med* 1999; **9**(1): 3–14.

17 Foster PR, Welch AG, McLean C, *et al.* Studies on the removal of abnormal prion protein by processes used in the manufacture of human plasma products. *Vox Sang* 2000; **78**(2): 86–95.

18 Reichl HE, Foster PR, Welch AG, *et al.* Studies on the removal of a bovine spongiform encephalopathy-derived agent by processes used in the manufacture of human immunoglobulin. *Vox Sang* 2002; **83**(2): 137–45.

19 Silveira JR, Raymond GJ, Hughson AG, *et al.* The most infectious prion protein particles. *Nature* 2005; **437**(7056): 257–61.

20 Truchot L, Arnaud D, Bloy C *et al.* CJD PrPsc removal by nanofiltration process: application to a therapeutic immunoglobulin solution (Lymphoglobuline). *Biologicals* 2006; **34**(3): 227–31.

21 Foster PR, Griffin BD, Bienek C, *et al.* Distribution of a bovine spongiform encephalopathy-derived agent over ion-exchange chromatography used in the preparation of concentrates of fibrinogen and factor VIII. *Vox Sang* 2004; **86**(2): 92–9.

22 Spongiform Encephalopathy Advisory Committee (SEAC), Position statement on TSE infectivity in blood, 2006. Available at: http://webarchive.nationalarchives.gov.uk/20110316162913/seac.gov.uk/statements/statement0806.htm

23 Boelle PY, Cesbron JY, Valleron AJ. Epidemiological evidence of higher susceptibility to vCJD in the young. *BMC Infect Dis* 2004; **4**: 26.

24 Swerdlow AJ, Higgins CD, Adlard P, *et al.* Creutzfeldt–Jakob disease in United Kingdom patients treated with human pituitary growth hormone. *Neurology* 2003; **61**(6): 783–91.

25 Brown KL, Wathne GJ, Sales J, *et al.* The effects of host age on follicular dendritic cell status dramatically impair scrapie agent neuroinvasion in aged mice. *J Immunol* 2009; **183**(8): 5199–207.

26 Houston F, Foster JD, Chong A, *et al.* Transmission of BSE by blood transfusion in sheep. *Lancet* 2000; **356**(9234): 999–1000.

27 Hunter N, Foster JD, Chong A, *et al.* Transmission of prion diseases by blood transfusion. *J Gen Virol* 2002; **83**(Pt 11): 2897–905.

28 UK Haemophilia Centre Doctors' Organisation (UKHCDO) Guidelines on therapeutic products to treat haemophilia and other hereditary coagulation disorders. *Haemophilia* 1997; **3**: 63–77.

29 Committee for Proprietary Medicinal Products (CPMP). Position statement on new variant CJD and plasma-derived medicinal products. 1998, European Agency for the Evaluation of Medicinal Products: London.

30 Millar CM, Connor N, Dolan G, *et al.* Risk reduction strategies for variant Creutzfeldt–Jakob disease transmission by UK plasma products and their impact on patients with inherited bleeding disorders. *Haemophilia* 2010; **16**(2): 305–15.

31 CJD Incidents Panel. Assessment of exposure to particular batches of variant Creutzfeldt–Jakob disease implicated plasma products, 2004.

32 Advisory Committee on Dangerous Pathogens. Guidance from the ACDP TSE Risk Management Subgroup, 2013. http://www.dh.gov.uk/health/2012/11/acdp-guidance/

33 Ghani AC, Donnelly CA, Ferguson NM, Anderson RM. Updated projections of future vCJD deaths in the UK. *BMC Infect Dis* 2003; **3**: 4.

34 Food and Drugs Administration. Draft quantitative risk assessment of vCJD risk potentially associated with the use of human plasma-derived factor VIII manufactured under United States license from plasma collected in the US, 2006. http://www.fda.gov/downloads/BiologicsBloodVaccines/SafetyAvailability/BloodSafety/UCM095104.pdf

35 Pastrana MA, Sajnani G, Onisko B, *et al.* Isolation and characterization of a proteinase K-sensitive PrPSc fraction. *Biochemistry* 2006; **45**(51): 15710–17.

36 Zobeley E, Flechsig E, Cozzio A, *et al.* Infectivity of scrapie prions bound to a stainless steel surface. *Mol Med* 1999; **5**(4): 240–3.

37 Edgeworth JA, Jackson GS, Clarke AR, *et al.* Highly sensitive, quantitative cell-based assay for prions adsorbed to solid surfaces. *Proc Natl Acad Sci USA* 2009; **106**(9): 3479–83.

38 Edgeworth JA, Farmer M, Sicilia A, *et al.* Detection of prion infection in variant Creutzfeldt–Jakob disease: a blood-based assay. *Lancet* 2011; **377**(9764): 487–93.

39 Millar CM, Makris M. Dealing with the uncertain risk of vCJD transmission by coagulation replacement products. *Br J Haematol* 2012; **158**: 442–52.

PART XII

Gene therapy

Table 41.1 Problems defined and solved in two adeno-associated virus-factor IX (AAV-FIX) trials.

Advances in first trial
- Vector transduces human liver and can direct therapeutic levels of expression
- The host immune response limits <u>duration</u> of expression through CD8+ T-cell response to AAV capsid
- Pre-existing antibodies to AAV capsid block transduction

Advances in second trial
- Cellular immune response to the vector can be managed by a course of high-dose steroids
- Use of a capsid serotype (AAV8) with strong tropism for liver allows vector to be infused intravenously

(Memphis, USA) collaborated to develop the protocol for the second AAV trial, which incorporated solutions to the problems identified in the first study (Table 41.1). To maximize the chances of efficacy, this trial excluded those with detectable neutralizing antibodies to AAV. Although this is not a viable long-term solution, given the number of adults with neutralizing antibodies to AAV, it did insure that each enrolled subject would be informative, since vector transduction would not be blocked by antibodies. Also, to address the risk of CD8+ T-cell-mediated destruction of the transduced cells, the investigators added a provision for a short course of prednisolone in the event of a rise in transaminases or a fall in FIX levels. In addition to these strategies for avoiding or managing the human immune response, the investigators also incorporated other recent advances in vector design, by switching to a serotype with strong liver tropism (AAV8) and by changing the conformation of the DNA expression cassette from single-stranded (ss), to self-complementary (sc) (essentially, a double-stranded cassette). Since ssDNA vectors must first be converted to a double-stranded form by host cell machinery in order to become transcriptionally active, it was hypothesized that this might lead to a more efficient expression cassette, able to achieve therapeutic FIX levels at lower doses. Animal studies [26] suggested that AAV8 had such strong tropism for liver that the vector could be infused intravenously, simplifying the administration procedure.

The scAAV8-LP1-FIXco trial began in London in March 2010 [1]. The first subjects, infused at doses of 2×10^{11} or 6×10^{11}, showed low but detectable levels of FIX postinfusion, ranging from 2 to 3%. These levels have been sustained since the initial infusions, effectively converting the subjects' severe disease to a moderately severe phenotype. The clinical outcomes are of interest and perhaps what one would have predicted—for younger subjects, with well-preserved joints based on improved therapy with concentrates over the past decades, elevation of FIX levels to the range of 2–3% was sufficient to allow a dramatic reduction in the use of clotting factor concentrates, and in the occurrence of spontaneous bleeding episodes. A subject in his 60s however, with substantial irreversible joint damage at the time he was infused, has

not been able to stop prophylaxis, despite attaining circulating levels of ∼2%. Infusion of the top dose, 2×10^{12} vg/kg, resulted initially in circulating levels of 8–10%, suggesting that this would be the therapeutic dose of product. However, at approximately 8 weeks post vector infusion, the transaminase levels rose sharply, and FIX levels declined; based on the protocol, the subject was begun on prednisolone at a dose of 60 mg daily, and this was tapered and stopped over the ensuing 8 weeks. The transaminases rapidly returned to normal, and the FIX level stabilized in the range of 1–2%. Subsequent studies of the subjects' peripheral blood mononucleated cells (PBMCs) again revealed a sharp increase in the numbers of circulating capsid-specific T cells, coinciding with the rise in liver enzymes, and disappearance of these cells from the circulation with the administration of prednisolone [1]. This set of findings supported the hypothesis that had been advanced after the first trial, and underscored the importance of the careful assessment of FIX levels and transaminases beginning at about 7 weeks. Thus with the next subject, these parameters were monitored frequently beginning at 7 weeks, and when the transaminases rose modestly, doubling within the normal range, at ∼8 weeks, the subject was immediately begun on prednisolone, which was tapered and stopped over a 4-week period. This subject's FIX level stabilized at 5%, converting his severe hemophilia to mild disease [1]. This level has been maintained for >2 years since the initial infusion, with observation ongoing. Four additional subjects have since been infused at this dose; based on changes in LFTs, two received the course of steroids beginning at about 8 weeks postinfusion, and two others never required them [27]. Of these four subjects, all have stabilized at FIX levels ranging from 3 to 7%, demonstrating that the result is reproducible.

One observation of note regarding the results in this study is the therapeutic dose, which was found to be 2×10^{12} vg/kg. This is of interest because it is identical to the dose that gave a level of 10–12% in the AAV2 trial. Thus, despite incorporating a number of features that were designed to build a more efficacious vector—use of AAV8 serotype, self-complementary DNA conformation, and codon optimization—the therapeutic doses were similar, raising questions about how readily dose finding in mouse models translates to humans. The dosing issues were at least partly related to problems in titering scAAV vectors, as it became clear that quantitative polymerase chain reaction (qPCR) titers underestimate the amount of vector present with sc vectors [28]. Although it was not possible to decrease the dose infused, the strong liver tropism of AAV8 allowed investigators to switch from a hepatic artery infusion to an intravenous infusion, greatly simplifying the infusion procedure. Also of interest is the difference in the timing of the transaminase elevation, which occurred at 3–4 weeks postvector infusion in the first trial (ssDNA in an AAV2 capsid) and at 7–9 weeks postvector infusion in the second trial (scDNA in an AAV8 capsid). Further studies will determine whether the capsid or the conformation of the DNA are primary

Table 41.2 Ongoing adeno-associated virus-factor IX (AAV-FIX) trials.

Sponsor	ClinicalTrials.gov Identifier	# Subjects	Transgene	Serotype
UCL/St Jude Children's Research Hospital	NCT00979238	10	Codon optimized wild type-sc	AAV8
Children's Hospital of Philadelphia	NCT01620801	15	Codon optimized wild-type-ss	AAV8
Asklepios Biopharmaceutical, Inc.	NCT01687608	16	Padua-sc	AAV8

sc: Self-complementary; ss: single-stranded.

Table 41.3 Typical inclusion criteria in adeno-associated virus-factor IX (AAV-FIX) gene therapy trials.

Inclusion
- Severe hemophilia B: FIX ≤2%
- Age ≥18 years
- HCV RNA viral load negative[a]
- HIV negative, or HIV positive and stable on HAART[b]
- No previous history of FIX inhibitor
- At least 20 exposure days to FIX concentrate
- Anti-AAV neutralizing antibody titer ≤1:5

[a]First trial included subjects who were HCV RNA viral load positive but they are now excluded because of potential need for course of steroids.
[b]Some trials may include HIV-positive individuals who are stable with adequate CD4 counts on highly active antiretroviral therapy (HAART).

determinants of the timing of this event, which is the signal for initiation of steroids.

Continuation of second trial, and additional trials now underway for hemophilia B

The success of the trial of Nathwani *et al.* now raises several questions, including whether it is possible to achieve even higher levels of expression, and whether the results can be extended to other groups of subjects who were excluded from the first round of trials (Tables 41.2 and 41.3). To address the first question, investigators will likely plan in the next phase of the trial to simply increase the vector dose. If the dosing scales linearly, one would predict that a 2.5-fold increase in dose would raise FIX levels to ~12.5%, an interesting target, given the natural history studies of Fischer *et al.* that document essentially *no* spontaneous bleeds in mild hemophilia A patients with FVIII levels ≥12% [29]. The major question for this approach is whether the CD8+ T-cell response to capsid, if it occurs, can still be controlled by steroids, as it is at the dose of 2×10^{12} vg/kg. Another strategy under investigation makes use of a high specific activity variant of FIX, FIX Padua [30]. The Padua variant of FIX was initially described in an Italian family in which the proband presented at age 23 years with a deep vein thrombosis, and was found to have a normal

FIX antigen level but a FIX activity level of 776%. Sequencing of the *FIX* gene and biochemical characterization of the variant showed that a point mutation that changed amino acid 338 from an arginine to a leucine resulted in a gain-of-function mutation that increased the specific activity by eightfold [31]. This trial is testing the safety and efficacy of intravenous infusion of an AAV8 capsid expressing a self-complementary construct encoding the Padua variant. One would predict that lower vector doses can be used to achieve similar FIX levels; the uncertainty is whether the nonwild-type Padua variant will be immunogenic. However, it should be noted that expression of any gene from an AAV vector in the liver tends to promote tolerance to the transgene product [32], so this is not likely to evoke an immune response.

Still another approach is being pursued by investigators at the Children's Hospital of Philadelphia [33]. In this study, the single-stranded expression cassette used in the first AAV2-FIX liver trial has been codon optimized and placed into an AAV8 capsid. The advantages of the ssDNA expression cassette are that manufacturing yields are higher. In addition, studies in mice suggest that single-stranded constructs are less immunogenic, since self-complementary DNA constructs evoke an innate immune response more efficiently than single-stranded constructs [34]. To achieve higher FIX levels, this trial will also increase doses up to 5×10^{12} vg/kg, and thus will provide data addressing whether prednisolone will suppress immune responses to capsid at this higher dose.

With respect to the second question, how to extend a successful approach to larger groups of subjects, ongoing trials will explore different strategies. One strategy being considered is to allow subjects who are HCV RNA viral load positive to enroll in studies. The rationale for excluding these subjects previously was that they are not good candidates for a course of high-dose steroids, which will almost certainly increase the HCV RNA viral load. Given the advent of the new direct-acting antivirals (DAAs), it is likely that this development could be controlled if it occurs. Of course, the number of hemophilia patients who are HCV RNA viral load positive is steadily dropping, not only as a function of aging of the population, but also as a function of therapy with the DAAs.

Another strategy is to use a method that allows inclusion of subjects with detectable neutralizing antibodies to AAV. Within the adult population, a substantial proportion of individuals, as many as 40% or more, carry neutralizing antibodies to AAV, developed as a result of exposure to the wild-type virus [25]. Studies in mice [24] and in nonhuman primates [23,35] have established that even modest titers of neutralizing antibodies, in the range of 1:5, block transduction of liver when vector is delivered through the circulation. Some investigators have explored plasmapheresis as an approach to reducing titers, but as one would predict, this strategy works better for low-titer inhibitors and is less effective at higher titers [36]. Mingozzi *et al.* have described a strategy in which empty capsids, a byproduct of most AAV manufacturing processes, can be used to absorb antibodies in the circulation, thereby allowing successful intravascular administration even in the presence of neutralizing antibody titers as high as 1:100 [37]. In this strategy, a patient's neutralizing antibody titer is used to determine a personalized final formulation of the injected product, in which empty capsids are added in the appropriate amount (to the full capsids which contain the therapeutic DNA) to counter the level of neutralizing antibodies in the patient's circulation. This strategy may allow successful vector administration to subjects who are currently excluded from all studies.

Extension of the approach to hemophilia A

Given the still early but nonetheless convincing success of AAV-mediated gene therapy for hemophilia B, attention has now turned to whether the same approach could be successful for hemophilia A. The size of the FVIII cDNA, ∼4.4 kb for the B-domain-deleted construct, presents an obstacle. Incorporation into the expression cassette of a promoter, an intron, and a polyadenylation signal results in a construct that is at the limits of what can be efficiently packaged. Recent studies by Sabatino *et al.* showed circulating canine FVIII levels of 3–8% in hemophilia A dogs following intravenous infusion of an AAV8 vector at a dose of 4×10^{13} vg/kg [38]. The data from the hemophilia B trials suggest the safety in humans of doses in the range of 2×10^{12} vg/kg, but do not provide information about doses that are 20-fold higher. (In fact, the data suggest that the immune response is dose dependent [1,14], raising questions about whether doses this high can be safely administered without risking an immune response that would not be controlled by prednisolone.) Ward *et al.* demonstrated in 2011 that codon optimization of the *F8* gene could, in the setting of a lentiviral vector, increase expression of FVIII by 30–40-fold [39]. McIntosh *et al.* further improved on this finding by generating a smaller codon-optimized sequence in which the 226 amino acid B-domain spacer that was found by Miao *et al.* to improve FVIII secretion [40,41] was replaced with a 14 amino acid sequence that retained the six *N*-linked glycosylation sites. This shorter expression cassette packaged efficiently, and in an AAV8 capsid, yielded plateau FVIII levels of ∼10–15% in nonhuman primates at a dose of 2×10^{12} vg/kg, a dose that can be administered to humans [41].

Based on these studies, plans are underway to develop clinical studies of AAV-FVIII.

Summary

The long-sought goal of gene therapy for hemophilia, continuous expression of levels of clotting factor sufficient to convert disease from severe to mild, has now been achieved for at least a few subjects in the setting of hemophilia B. Current work suggests that adults, who are HCV RNA viral load negative, and who do not have circulating antibodies to AAV, can undergo intravenous infusion of an AAV vector expressing wild-type FIX, and expect at least a few years (>36 months expression to date, with observation ongoing) of clotting factor levels in the range of 5%, provided that the cellular immune response that arises in most subjects is detected promptly and managed appropriately. This is a remarkable accomplishment, and clearly has the potential to revolutionize treatment for hemophilia worldwide. However, as with all novel therapies at the early stages, many questions remain, including the duration of expression from a single injection (>10 years in hemophilic dogs and in nonhuman primates but as yet unknown in humans), whether it will be possible to readminister vector, and whether there are any late side-effects that are not yet manifest. The primary concern in terms of late side-effects is the risk of insertional mutagenesis in the liver; although AAV is primarily nonintegrating, some level of vector integration clearly occurs in animal models at the doses being administered in the trials, and in some mice injected as neonates, has resulted in hepatocellular carcinoma when the mice reach advanced ages [42]. Long-term follow-up of subjects infused in the first AAV liver trial [43] has not shown evidence of similar events in human subjects infused as adults, but continued monitoring will be required. A goal of the next phase of the work is to determine whether additional groups of subjects, those with antibodies to AAV, those who are HCV RNA viral load positive, and those with hemophilia A, can be safely included in studies and can exhibit similar efficacy.

References

1 Nathwani AC, Tuddenham EG, Rangarajan S, *et al.* Adenovirus-associated virus vector-mediated gene transfer in hemophilia B. *N Engl J Med* 2011; **365**(25): 2357–65.

2 Mingozzi F, High KA. Therapeutic in vivo gene transfer for genetic disease using AAV: progress and challenges. *Nat Rev Genet* 2011; **12**(5): 341–55.

3 Blaese RM, Culver KW, Miller AD, *et al.* T lymphocyte-directed gene therapy for ADA- SCID: initial trial results after 4 years. Science. 1995; **270**(5235): 475–80.

4 Hacein-Bey-Abina S, von Kalle C, Schmidt M, *et al.* A serious adverse event after successful gene therapy for X-linked severe combined immunodeficiency. *N Engl J Med* 2003; **348**(3): 255–6.

5 Mingozzi F, High KA. Immune responses to AAV vectors: overcoming barriers to successful gene therapy. *Blood* 2013; **122**: 23–36.

6 High KA. Gene therapy in clinical medicine. In: Longo D, Fauci AS, Kaspar DL, Hauser SL, Jameson, JL, Loscalzo J (eds.) *Harrison's Principles of Internal Medicine*. New York: Mc-Graw Hill: 2011.

7 Murphy SL, High KA. Gene therapy for haemophilia. *Br J Haematol* 2008; **140**(5): 479–87.

8 Manno CS, Pierce GF, Arruda VR, *et al.* Successful transduction of liver in hemophilia by AAV–Factor IX and limitations imposed by the host immune response. *Nat Med* 2006; **12**(3): 342–7.

9 Mingozzi F, Maus MV, Hui DJ, *et al.* CD8(+) T-cell responses to adeno-associated virus capsid in humans. *Nat Med* 2007; **13**(4): 419–22.

10 Evans JP, Brinkhous KM, Brayer GD, Reisner HM, High KA. Canine hemophilia B resulting from a point mutation with unusual consequences. *Proc Natl Acad Sci USA* 1989; **86**(24): 10095–9.

11 Boyce N. Trial halted after gene shows up in semen. *Nature* 2001; **414**(6865): 677.

12 Arruda VR, Fields PA, Milner R, *et al.* Lack of germline transmission of vector sequences following systemic administration of recombinant AAV-2 vector in males. *Mol Ther* 2001; **4**(6): 586–92.

13 Favaro P, Downey HD, Zhou JS, *et al.* Host and vector-dependent effects on the risk of germline transmission of AAV vectors. *Mol Ther* 2009; **17**(6): 1022–30.

14 Finn JD, Hui D, Downey HD, *et al.* Proteasome inhibitors decrease AAV2 capsid derived peptide epitope presentation on MHC class I following transduction. *Mol Ther* 2010; **18**(1): 135–42.

15 Pien GC, Basner-Tschakarjan E, Hui DJ, *et al.* Capsid antigen presentation flags human hepatocytes for destruction after transduction by adeno-associated viral vectors. *J Clin Invest* 2009; **119**(6): 1688–95.

16 Office of Biotechnology Activities, Report on immune responses to adeno-associated virus (AAV) vectors. NIH Recombinant DNA Advisory Committee Meeting, June 19, 2007. Available at: http://oba.od.nih.gov/rdna_rac/rac_meetings.html

17 Chadeuf G, Ciron C, Moullier P, Salvetti A. Evidence for encapsidation of prokaryotic sequences during recombinant adeno-associated virus production and their in vivo persistence after vector delivery. *Mol Ther* 2005; **12**(4): 744–53.

18 Hauck B, Murphy SL, Smith PH, *et al.* Undetectable transcription of cap in a clinical AAV vector: implications for preformed capsid in immune responses. *Mol Ther* 2009; **17**(1): 144–52.

19 Li C, Goudy K, Hirsch M, *et al.* Cellular immune response to cryptic epitopes during therapeutic gene transfer. *Proc Natl Acad Sci USA* 2009; **106**(26): 10770–4.

20 Vandenberghe LH, Wang L, Sommanathan S, *et al.* Heparin binding directs activation of T cells against adeno-associated virus serotype 2 capsid. *Nat Med* 2006; **12**(8): 967–71.

21 Li H, Murphy SL, Giles-Davis W, *et al.* Pre-existing AAV capsid-specific CD8+ T cells are unable to eliminate AAV-transduced hepatocytes. *Mol Ther* 2007; **15**(4): 792–800.

22 Wang L, Figueredo J, Calcedo R, Lin J, Wilson JM. Cross-presentation of adeno-associated virus serotype 2 capsids activates cytotoxic T cells but does not render hepatocytes effective cytolytic targets. *Hum Gene Ther* 2007; **18**(3): 185–94.

23 Jiang H, Couto LB, Patarroyo-White S, *et al.* Effects of transient immunosuppression on adenoassociated, virus-mediated, liver-directed gene transfer in rhesus macaques and implications for human gene therapy. *Blood* 2006; **108**(10): 3321–8.

24 Scallan CD, Liu T, Parker AE, *et al.* Phenotypic correction of a mouse model of hemophilia A using AAV2 vectors encoding the heavy and light chains of FVIII. *Blood* 2003; **102**(12): 3919–26.

25 Calcedo R, Vandenberghe LH, Gao G, Lin J, Wilson JM. Worldwide epidemiology of neutralizing antibodies to adeno-associated viruses. *J Infect Dis* 2009; **199**(3): 381–90.

26 Nathwani AC, Rosales C, McIntosh J, *et al.* Long-term safety and efficacy following systemic administration of a self-complementary AAV vector encoding human FIX pseudotyped with serotype 5 and 8 capsid proteins. *Mol Ther* 2011; **19**(5): 876–85.

27 Davidoff A, Tuddenham EGD, Rangarajan, S, *et al.* Stable factor IX activity following AAV-mediated gene transfer in patients with severe hemophilia B. Proceedings of the American Society of Hematology, 54th Annual Meeting; December 10, 2012; Atlanta, GA.

28 Fagone P, Wright JF, Nathwani AC, Nienhuis AW, Davidoff AM, Gray JT. Systemic errors in quantitative polymerase chain reaction titration of self-complementary adeno-associated viral vectors and improved alternative methods. *Hum Gene Ther Methods* 2012; **23**(1): 1–7.

29 Den Uijl IE, Mauser Bunschoten EP, Roosendaal G, *et al.* Clinical severity of haemophilia A: does the classification of the 1950s still stand? *Haemophilia* 2011; **17**(6): 849–53.

30 ClinicalTrialsgov Identifier: NCT01687608. Open-label single ascending dose of adeno-associated virus serotype 8 factor IX gene therapy in adults with hemophilia B. 2012; Available at: http://clinicaltrials.gov/ct2/show/NCT01687608

31 Simioni P, Tormene D, Tognin, G. *et al.* X-linked thrombophilia with a mutant factor IX (factor IX Padua). *N Engl J Med* 2009; **361**(17): 1671–5.

32 Mingozzi F, Liu YL, Dobrzynski E, *et al.* Induction of immune tolerance to coagulation factor IX antigen by in vivo hepatic gene transfer. *J Clin Invest* 2003; **111**(9): 1347–56.

33 ClinicalTrialsgov Identifier: NCT01620801. Hemophilia B gene therapy-CCMT at CHOP. 2012; Available at: http://clinicaltrials.gov/ct2/show/NCT01620801

34 Martino AT, Suzuki M, Markusic DM, *et al.* The genome of self-complementary adeno-associated viral vectors increases toll-like receptor 9-dependent innate immune responses in the liver. *Blood* 2011; **117**(24): 6459–68.

35 Mingozzi F, Hasbrouck NC, Basner-Tschakarjan E, *et al.* Modulation of tolerance to the transgene product in a nonhuman primate model of AAV-mediated gene transfer to liver. *Blood* 2007; **110**(7): 2334–41.

36 Monteilhet V, Saheb S, Boutin S, *et al.* A 10 patient case report on the impact of plasmapheresis upon neutralizing factors against adeno-associated virus (AAV) types 1, 2, 6, and 8. *Mol Ther* 2011; **19**(11): 2084–91.

37 Mingozzi F, Anguela XM, Pavani G, *et al.* Overcoming pre-existing humoral immunity to AAV using capsid decoys. *Sci Transl Med* 2013; **5** (194): 194ra92. doi: 10.1126/scitranslmed.3005795.

38 Sabatino DE, Lange AM, Altynova ES, *et al.* Efficacy and safety of long-term prophylaxis in severe hemophilia A dogs following liver gene therapy using AAV vectors. *Mol Ther* 2011; **19**(3): 442–9.

39 Ward NJ, Buckley SM, Waddington SN, *et al.* Codon optimization of human factor VIII cDNAs leads to high-level expression. *Blood* 2011; **117**(3): 798–807.

40 Miao HZ, Sirachainan N, Palmer L, *et al.* Bioengineering of coagulation factor VIII for improved secretion. *Blood* 2004; **103**(9): 3412–19.

41 McIntosh J, Lenting PJ, Rosales C, *et al.* Therapeutic levels of FVIII following a single peripheral vein administration of rAAV vector encoding a novel human factor VIII variant. *Blood* 2013; **121**(17): 3335–44.

42 Donsante A, Miller DG, Li Y, *et al.* AAV vector integration sites in mouse hepatocellular carcinoma. *Science* 2007; **317**(5837): 477.

43 Wellman JA, Mingozzi F, Ozelo M, *et al.* Results from long-term follow-up of severe hemophilia B subjects previously enrolled in a clinical study of AAV2-FIX gene transfer to the liver. *Mol Ther* 2012; **20**(Suppl. 1): S28.

CHAPTER 42

Gene therapy: molecular engineering of factor VIII and factor IX

Sundar R. Selvaraj and Steven W. Pipe
University of Michigan, Michigan, USA

Introduction

Insights from recombinant DNA technology ushered in the gene therapy era. As the severe complications of hemophilia can be avoided with even a modest increase in plasma levels of factor VIII (FVIII) and factor IX (FIX), hemophilia became a popular target of gene therapy research. Most current gene therapy strategies rely on gene methodologies using vectors as delivery vehicles to provide a wild-type copy of the defective gene to a physiologically relevant target tissue. The most efficient vectors have proven to be engineered viruses, with known mechanisms for entering eukaryotic cells and harnessing their synthetic machinery to produce foreign proteins. Whereas this application to a wide range of preclinical animal models has demonstrated success for these strategies, there have been significant obstacles remaining for human clinical applications depending on the combination of vector used, expressed transgene, and target tissue chosen. This had resulted in only a few patients achieving transient low-level expression of either FVIII or FIX. However, promising clinical results have been observed recently in six adult males with severe hemophilia B in the UK. Expression of FIX at plateau levels ranging from 1 to 6% for periods of over 2 years were observed following an intravenous injection of an adeno-associated viral (AAV) vector encoding FIX under the control of a liver-restricted promoter [1]. This achievement, although in a small number of a relatively restricted subset of the hemophilia population, is still a major landmark in gene therapy for hemophilia and provides hope for long-term expression of therapeutic levels of FIX with potential applicability to FVIII and hemophilia A [2].

Continued advances in recombinant DNA technology remain a promising platform to address the remaining challenges for affordable and accessible recombinant clotting factors as well as gene therapy efforts. In particular, ongoing research has provided detailed structure and function characterizations for each phase of the lifecycles for FVIII (Figure 42.1) and FIX: biosynthesis, macromolecular interactions, activation/inactivation, and clearance. This has come through insights from the study of hemophilia mutations, site-directed mutagenesis, detailed structural models, and an expanded repertoire of animal models through molecular biology advances. This has opened up new frontiers for bioengineering strategies to overcome some of the remaining limitations inherent to current clotting factor concentrates. Partnering some of these bioengineering strategies with advances in gene therapy, vectorology, and immunology insights may increase the likelihood of a successful and broadly applicable gene therapy strategy.

Factor VIII with improved functional properties (Table 42.1)

Improved biosynthesis and secretion
Several mechanisms have been identified that limit FVIII expression:
- FVIII is susceptible to misfolding within the endoplasmic reticulum (ER), inducing transcription of ER stress-response genes through the unfolded protein response (UPR), a cellular adaptive response to regulate all levels of gene expression including transcription, translation, translocation into the ER lumen, and ER-associated degradation [3]
- FVIII forms nondisulfide-bonded high-molecular-weight aggregates that are retained within the ER through interactions with the protein chaperones immunoglobulin-binding protein (BiP/GRP78), calnexin and calreticulin.

FVIII also demonstrates a requirement for facilitated transport from the ER to the Golgi apparatus through interaction with the lectin LMAN1–MCFD2 complex. Although the study of FVIII synthesis and secretion in heterologous expression systems has its limitations, this is the method by which recombinant FVIII (rFVIII) is produced, and some gene therapy strategies are

Textbook of Hemophilia, Third Edition. Edited by Christine A. Lee, Erik E. Berntorp and W. Keith Hoots.
© 2014 John Wiley & Sons, Ltd. Published 2014 by John Wiley & Sons, Ltd.

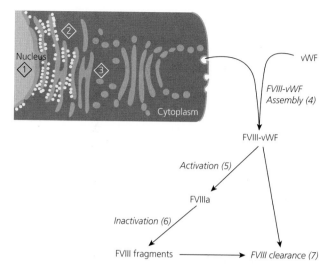

Figure 42.1 Overview of the factor VIII (FVIII) lifecycle and targets for bioengineering strategies. Schematic of FVIII biosynthesis from mRNA expression (1), chaperone-assisted folding with the endoplasmic reticulum (ER) (2), facilitated transport through the ER–Golgi intermediate compartment (3), secretion and assembly with von Willebrand factor (vWF) (4), activation (5), inactivation (6), and clearance from plasma (7). Numbers indicate realized targets of bioengineering.

presently directed to express FVIII in cells that do not normally produce the protein [4].

Increased mRNA expression

Early on in the study of rFVIII expression, it was demonstrated that the B domain of FVIII could be removed from the cDNA without loss of FVIII procoagulant activity. Removal of the B domain, the equivalent of approximately 38% of the primary cDNA sequence, significantly improved the yield of FVIII as a result of markedly increased levels of mRNA and increased translation [5]. The smaller size of the B-domain-deleted (BDD)-FVIII cDNA facilitated packaging within certain viral vectors that could not accommodate a full-length FVIII cDNA. Because BDD-FVIII has a biochemical profile similar to wild-type FVIII [6], there was enthusiasm to adopt it for gene therapy strategies. Clinical studies have shown the clinical efficacy of BDD-FVIII and rates of inhibitor formation in previously untreated patients with hemophilia A were similar to that observed with full-length rFVIII concentrates [6]. Thus, despite such a major modification of the FVIII protein, this bioengineered form of FVIII was not believed to likely be more immunogenic than wild-type FVIII. Although BDD-FVIII has been successfully expressed in several preclinical gene transfer applications in animal models, expression in human gene therapy applications has still been inefficient [7].

Introduction of a truncated intron 1 sequence of FIX within BDD-FVIII cDNA in place of introns 1 and 13 led to a 13-fold

Table 42.1 Summary of bioengineering strategies for factor VIII (FVIII) with improved functional properties.

Targeted functional improvement	Bioengineering strategy	References
Improved biosynthesis and secretion		
Increased mRNA expression	Removal of entire B domain	5
	Substitution with FIX intron 1	8
Reduced ER chaperone interactions	Phe309Ser	12
Improved ER–Golgi transport and Reduced ER stress	Shorter B-domain variants (226/N6)	20
Other	Codon optimization and B-domain spacer length optimization	25, 27
	Disulfide loop elimination	28
	Porcine–human hybrids	29
	Novel Asn-linked glycan in A1 domain of hFVIII	30
Improved functional activity		
Increased activation	des-(868-1562)-FVIII-HCII	32
Resistance to inactivation	Inactivation-resistant FVIII (IR8) (Arg336Ile/Arg562Lys/Arg740Ala/des-794-1689)	33
	A2-A3 disulfide-bridged FVIII (Cys664-Cys1826)	34
	FVIII-RH (single chain)	35
	Alteration of charged amino acids at A domain interfaces and disulfide/ hydrophobicity at A1–C2 interface	36
	(Ala/Val substitution at Glu272, Asp519, Glu665, Glu1984) Combination mutations	38
Improved plasma half-life		
	rVIII-single chain (stronger affinity to VWF, higher stability)	39
	LRP-binding site mutations (A2 domain residues 484-509 and C2 domain)	40
	Heparan sulfate proteoglycans-binding site mutations (A2 domain residues 558-565)	40
Reduced immunogenicity		
	Porcine–human FVIII hybrids	50

ER, endoplasmic reticulum; FIX, factor IX; HC, heavy chain; LRP, low-density lipoprotein receptor-related protein; VWF, von Willebrand factor.

increase in FVIII secretion that was associated with a dramatically higher level of FVIII mRNA accumulation in the cell [8]. Intron 13 in the *F8* gene was previously shown to code for part of a transcriptional silencer, which represses expression of *F8* [9]. This truncated intron 1 sequence of FIX has since been incorporated into gene transfer vectors that utilize BDD-FVIII cDNA with therapeutic FVIII plasma levels achieved within mice [10].

Reduced endoplasmic reticulum chaperone interactions

Secretion of FVIII requires its dissociation from the protein chaperone BiP, which resides in the ER and controls the transport of the FVIII primary translation product to the Golgi compartment by retaining misfolded protein molecules in the ER [11]. BiP possesses a peptide-stimulated adenosine triphosphatase (ATPase) activity. FVIII release from BiP and transport out of the ER requires high levels of intracellular adenosine triphosphate (ATP) and ATP hydrolysis by BiP [11]. A 110-amino acid region within the A1 domain of FVIII was identified, which inhibited its secretion [11]. A putative BiP-binding site was localized to a hydrophobic β-sheet within this 110-amino acid region, in which seven of 11 amino acid residues are Leu or Phe. Factor V (FV) has the identical domain structure to FVIII, and these proteins share ∼40% amino acid identity between their respective A and C domains. Curiously, FV is 20-fold more efficiently expressed compared with FVIII in mammalian expression systems, and does not interact with BiP. When the 110-amino acid region of FVIII bordered by residues 226–336 was replaced for the homologous residues from FV, the FV/FVIII hybrid exhibited a fivefold increase in the efficiency of secretion, most likely because of a decreased binding to BiP. However, the generated FV–FVIII hybrid did not retain a cofactor function. Further site-directed mutagenesis within the hydrophobic β-sheet within this 110-amino acid region of the FVIII A1 domain demonstrated that a single mutation of Phe309 to Ala or the homologous residue from FV (Ser) enhanced secretion of FVIII by threefold and the Phe309Ser mutant retained full cofactor function [12].

Improved endoplasmic reticulum–Golgi transport

The BDD-rFVIII modification produced a 20-fold increase in mRNA levels and expression of FVIII primary translation product [5]. However, despite this dramatic difference in accumulation of mRNA, secretion of BDD-rFVIII from the cell was only observed to be approximately twofold higher compared with full-length wild-type FVIII [6]. This was surprising and suggested that the rate of ER–Golgi transport for the BDD-rFVIII molecule was actually reduced compared with FVIII retaining the B domain. More insight into this followed the characterization of the molecular defect underlying the majority of patients with combined deficiency of FV and FVIII. First described in 1954 [13], patients with this rare autosomal recessive bleeding disorder have plasma levels of FV and FVIII (both antigen and activity) in the range of 5–30 U/dL. The disease-causing mutations have been limited to mutations in two proteins: LMAN1 [also known as ER–Golgi intermediate compartment (ERGIC) 53] and MCFD2 (multiple coagulation factor deficiency 2). LMAN1 is a homohexameric type 1 transmembrane protein. It was characterized as a mannose-binding lectin proposed to target specific glycoproteins to coat protein (COP)-II coated vesicles budding from the ER for transport to the Golgi [14]. Two-thirds of patients described with combined deficiency of FVIII and FV have null mutations of LMAN1, except for a single mutation that disrupts disulfide bond formation critical for its oligomerization [15]. LMAN1 has an N-terminal carbohydrate recognition domain (CRD) with a lectin-type fold consistent with a role in binding glycoproteins. Previous work demonstrated that LMAN1 is required for efficient secretion of FVIII and FV and that this is mediated by oligosaccharide structures within their respective B domains [16]. Almost another one-third of patients can be attributed to mutation in MCFD2, a small soluble protein with two calcium-binding EF-hand motifs in the C terminus, and interacts directly with LMAN1 to form a 1:1 stoichiometric complex [17]. Studies have demonstrated that proper folding of MCFD2 is dependent on the binding of Ca^{2+} to the EF-hand motifs and that its localization to the ERGIC is dependent on its ability to complex to LMAN1. Also, the C-terminal EF-hand domains of MCFD2 mediate interactions with both LMAN1 and FV/FVIII through separate binding sites. Interestingly, an MCFD2 mutant that does not complex with LMAN1 retains the ability to bind FVIII [18]. Similarly, the CRD of LMAN1 contains distinct, separable binding sites for both MCFD2, its partner protein and FV/FVIII, its cargo proteins, suggesting that MCFD2 is vital to cargo receptor formation and cargo loading in the ER and LMAN1 plays a central role in regulating the binding in the ER and the subsequent release of FV/FVIII in the ERGIC [19].

These insights on facilitated transport of FVIII within the secretion pathway have led to reconsideration of the functional role of the B domain and suggest a mechanism for the observed impaired rate of secretion with BDD-FVIII. Studies were conducted to determine the optimal oligosaccharide content required for efficient rate of secretion. When as few as 226 amino acid residues (encoding six potential asparagine-linked glycosylation sites) from the N-terminal portion of the B domain were added to a BDD-FVIII construct, this B-domain variant (226/N6) retained equal efficiency to BDD-FVIII in synthesis of the primary translation product (indicating efficient mRNA accumulation) yet secretion of this rFVIII protein was increased approximately 10-fold compared with BDD-FVIII (consistent with improved efficiency of ER–Golgi transport) [20]. Further, when this B-domain variant was combined with the Phe309Ser mutation, there was a further increase in the efficiency of secretion. This combined construct was then expressed *in vivo* utilizing hydrodynamic tail vein injection of naked plasmid DNA into the FVIII Exon

CHAPTER 43

Laboratory and quality control of assays

Steve Kitchen
Royal Hallamshire Hospital, Sheffield, UK

Pre-analytical variables

The quality of results of laboratory tests used in the diagnosis and management of hemophilia and allied bleeding disorders is very much dependent on the quality of the blood sample. Blood should be collected by clean venepuncture with minimal stasis using, where possible, a 21-gauge needle or butterfly avoiding heparin flushed venous lines and following published guidelines [1–3]. Patients do not need to be fasted [3] but should avoid strenuous exercise immediately prior to venepuncture [3] which may temporarily elevate the FVIII and von Willebrand factor (VWF) levels in plasma. If a patient is particularly stressed by sample collection there may be a temporary rise in FVIII/VWF.

The blood should be collected into 0.105–0.109 mol/L trisodium citrate maintaining a blood to citrate ratio of 9 : 1 [2]. If the tube contains less that its target volume, results may be affected. Tubes containing 90–110% of target volume are safe to test [2], though tubes with 80% of target volume can be analysed [3] subject to local validation [2]

After collection, the sample should not be stored at 2–8°C [1] since this can cause a progressive loss of FVIII and VWF to the extent that in one study approximately 50% of normal subjects would have been falsely classified as having hemophilia or von Willebrand disease (VWD) when their samples were stored at 2–8°C for 4 h prior to analysis [4]. Cold-related activation of factor VII (FVII) and factor XII (FXII) can also occur in blood or plasma stored at 2–8°C, which in turn shortens the prothrombin time (PT) and APTT.

Prolonged storage of blood or plasma prior to analysis leads to progressive loss of FVIII and false prolongation of APTT so tests should be performed within 4 h of sample collection [1,3].

The blood sample should be centrifuged for at least 10 min at room temperature (20–25°C) under a minimum of 1700 g [3]. If in-vitro hemolysis has occurred during sample collection or transport, this can have an important effect on several tests of hemostasis [5] including, particularly, APTT which may be falsely prolonged or falsely shortened.

Factor VIII or IX activity in such samples may be artificially elevated because of activation, and assays may be invalid due to nonparallel standard and test sample dose–response curves. Samples with visible in-vitro hemolysis should not be analysed.

If testing is not completed within 4 h of sample collection, platelet poor plasma can be stored deep frozen for more than 6 months at –70°C [6]. Frost-free freezers with automatic defrost cycles should not be used and storage in –20°C freezers is not recommended [3].

Internal quality control

Materials used for internal and external quality control should be similar in properties to test samples which is most easily achieved using human plasma. To ensure sufficient stability over a period of months, QC material can be frozen or lyophilized. Many tests of hemostasis are sufficiently stable for at least 18 months in samples stored at –70°C [6]. Lyophilized QC materials are buffered to improve stability and can be stored long term at –20°C or in some cases 2–8°C. For all nonmanual test systems, it has been recommended that the laboratory must include at least two levels of control material every 8 h of operation and each time a reagent is changed [7] and that more frequent QC testing should be performed if the volume of patient testing is high. One level of control should be tested at least every 4 h when continuous processing occurs [7].

If large numbers of samples are processed, the frequency of IQC testing should be set so that recall of erroneous patient results is avoided. For screening tests performed in laboratories processing >100 samples a day, testing every 2 h does not place too high a financial burden in relation to cost and can easily be achieved.

One of the two levels of control should be an abnormal or therapeutic level control near the clinically relevant range and the other should be within the normal range.

Results of PT and APTT are dependent on the reagent and instrument used for analysis, and target range for IQC should be specific for the method used. This can be set as mean ±2

Textbook of Hemophilia, Third Edition. Edited by Christine A. Lee, Erik E. Berntorp and W. Keith Hoots.
© 2014 John Wiley & Sons, Ltd. Published 2014 by John Wiley & Sons, Ltd.

standard deviations of 20 results obtained over a minimum of 10 sessions. For a full discussion of IQC in the hemostasis laboratory see Kitchen *et al.* [8].

Prothrombin time and activated partial thromboplastin time determination

Both PT and APTT can be dependent on the sample collection processing and storage, and by the reagent and instrument used for analysis. For this reason, each laboratory should establish a reference range locally [7]. For statistical validity, a minimum of 120 subjects has been recommended [7] but for practical purposes a close approximation can be obtained by testing samples from 20 to 30 subjects. Healthy hospital employees not receiving any medications, healthy blood donors, or asymptomatic partners of adult patients can be successfully used.

Hemophilia centers that were participants in the World Federation of Hemophilia (WFH) international External Quality Assessment Scheme (EQAS) were surveyed about their normal practise in relation to the source of their reference ranges in local use [9]. Approximately equal numbers of centers used blood donors or laboratory staff as a source of normal subjects. The programme includes two types of laboratory, namely international hemophilia training centers/established centers from twinning programmes or laboratories in emerging countries. More than 90% of participants in the latter group used manufacturers' literature as the source of their reference range, and only around one-quarter of UK National EQAS (NEQAS) participants reported using a locally determined reference range [9] indicating that guidelines recommending local establishment are not being followed.

Some recommendations in relation to establishing normal ranges for tests of hemostasis have been published [10] which included avoidance of intense physical exercise for 24 h prior to venepuncture, use of an environment that minimises physical and mental stress, and abstention from fatty foods and smoking on the morning of venepuncture. Published reference ranges should only be used as a guide. The normal samples should be collected, processed, and analysed using identical techniques to those used for patient samples. It is possible that a new lot number of reagent has a different associated normal range than previous lots from the same source but if results obtained on IQC materials before and after a change in lot number are unchanged it is unlikely that a new reference range is needed.

The distribution of PT and APTT results in normal subjects are usually normally distributed which can be confirmed by visual inspection in a graphic form (for an example see [10]). Clear outliers which are unexpectedly far from the other values can safely be excluded from further calculations. If the distribution is normal, the mean ±2 standard deviations can be used as a reference range. For a full discussion of reference ranges including construction of ranges with non-normally distributed data see [11].

Thromboplastin reagents used to determine PT vary in their sensitivity to deficiency of factor V (FV), FVII, or factor X (FX). In the presence of mild deficiencies in the range 20–50 IU/dL, the degree of prolongation may be minimal. In the case of factor II (FII) deficiencies in this range, the result may be within the normal range. The PT determined with reagents containing human tissue factor (extracted or recombinant) may be different from those obtained with reagents containing tissue factor of rabbit origin. In some subjects with FVII deficiency, the result may be grossly prolonged with one reagent and normal with another. The result obtained with human tissue factor reagents is likely to be more indicative of bleeding risk in such cases. Some PT reagents can be affected by the presence of some lupus anticoagulants, including some rare antibodies which prolong PT without prolonging APTT. Reagents with lower phospholipid concentrations such as those composed of lipidated recombinant tissue factor are more likely to be affected.

The APTT is markedly prolonged in the presence of moderate or severe deficiency of FVIII, factor IX (FIX), or factor XI (FXI) but results should be interpreted with caution when investigating subjects with possible mild bleeding disorders where factor levels may be close to normal. The degree of prolongation in the presence of 20–50 IU/dL levels of FVIII, FIX, and FXI is highly dependent on the reagent and instrument used for analysis. Normal APTT results will occur in some cases with 20–50 IU/dL levels of either FVIII, FIX, or FXI with currently used reagents. This means that factor assays are required if a patient has the appropriate personal or family history in order to exclude mild bleeding disorders even in the presence of a normal APTT.

Data comparing sensitivity of different APTT reagents to single factor deficiency are available through external quality assessment programs although caution is required in the interpretation of such data since the test samples are usually lyophilized, and an impact of sample preparation and processing on final APTT results cannot always be excluded. Data from recent UK NEQAS APTT surveys are shown in Table 43.1.

Centers are invited to submit an interpretation of their local result as normal, borderline or abnormal as assessed using their local reference range. For the April 2013 survey, the sample in Table 43.1 was from a donor with mild hemophilia B and FIX level of 37 IU/dL. Overall, 68% of centers interpreted their local APTT result as normal. These ranged from 43% of users of one reagent to 88% of users of another. Thus the successful detection of an abnormality was highly dependent on the reagent in use.

Elevated levels of one clotting factor can compensate for lower levels of another in APTT determinations. An elevated FVIII (e.g. caused by acute phase response) can lead to a normal APTT in the presence of mild FIX or FXI deficiency.

The presence of some therapeutic inhibitors of coagulation such as heparin, direct Xa inhibitors, or direct IIa inhibitors may prolong APTT [12]. The APTT may also be prolonged by FXII deficiency, high-molecular-weight kininogen deficiency or

Table 43.1 Activated partial thromboplastin time (APTT) results with different reagents. Data are from UK NEQAS surveys in which lyophilized samples from individual donors were analysed in >800 centers. Results are shown as the median ratio (test/mean normal APTT) for reagents used by more than 20 centers in all surveys.

Date of Survey	Sample	Reagents						
		APTT-SP IL	Synthasil IL	Actin FS Siemens	Actin FSL Siemens	Pathromptin Siemens	Cephascreen Stago	APTT HS TCoag
June 2012	FX 8 IU/dL	1.45	1.43	1.52	1.49	1.66	1.52	1.49
April 2012	FXII 5 U/dL	1.30	1.32	1.27	1.16	1.59	1.34	1.39
May 2012	FIX 4 IU/dL	1.11	1.16	1.25	1.18	1.25	1.24	1.16
Sept 2012	FVIII 40 IU/dL	1.35	1.30	1.28	1.26	1.48	1.33	1.40
Jan 2013	Normal	1.05	1.04	1.00	1.01	1.14	1.08	1.07
April 2013	FIX 37 IU/dL	1.10	1.11	1.19	1.15	1.22	1.20	1.12

prekallikrein deficiency, or by some lupus anticoagulants. APTT reagents vary markedly in their sensitivities to those defects depending on the phospholipid composition and concentration, and by the activator present in the reagent.

In relation to FXI deficiency, the APTT was prolonged when FXI was below 40 U/dL in one study [13] compared to 50–70 U/dL in another study [14]. Data from EQA programs and published studies indicate that currently most APTT reagents will have prolonged APTT results in patient samples when FXI is in the 25–60 U/dL range [15]. These differences in sensitivity mean that centers should be aware of the characteristics of the particular method in use locally. One way to assess sensitivity is to perform APTT on factor-deficient plasmas to which normal plasma has been added in increasing amounts to give a range of potencies, between <1 IU/dL and normal [7]. This approach has been questioned because the results obtained are influenced by the source of deficient and normal reference plasma used to construct these artificial mixtures, and because plasmas may be affected by the processing used in preparation of deficient plasmas [16].

When individuals with prolonged APTT arising out of routine screening are investigated, FXI deficiency was approximately five times more common than either FVIII of FIX deficiency [17] though this finding is likely to be dependent on the reagent used for screening.

One-stage factor assays

Currently, the most commonly performed factor assays are one-stage techniques. These are based on the APTT and, in the case of FVIII, depend on the ability of factor VIII in a patient sample to correct or shorten the delayed clotting of a deficient plasma which has a complete lack of FVIII. A reference plasma of known concentration is used with different dilutions (concentration) to construct a calibration curve in which the clotting time depends on the concentration of FVIII.

Dose–response curves constructed to calibrate factor assays can be plotted manually on graph paper but computer pro-

grams, which are often integrated in coagulation analyser software, improve the reliability, accuracy, and consistency of data handling. Validation is more easily achieved, usually by calculation of the correlation between clotting times and concentrations. Correlation coefficients (r) should be between 0.998 and 1.000 [1]. Some analysers perform parallelism checks using a slope ratio which should normally be in the range 0.9–1.1.

It is possible to store a calibration curve for particular lot numbers of reagents which is then used with test sample data generated at a later time. With care, this can give acceptable results but is not recommended in some guidelines [1,10] because test and calibration plasmas analysed together reduces variability in relation to stability of reagents and ambient temperature changes which would otherwise vary between the analysis of test and reference plasma and lead to increased assay imprecision. It has been shown that the between-center variability of FVIII results among centers using stored calibration can be more than twice that among centers making a calibration alongside test sample analysis [18].

In order for FVIII to be rate limiting in its influence on clotting time, the deficient plasma must provide an excess of all other relevant clotting factors, so the other factors need to be greater than 50 IU/dL in the deficient plasma [1,19]. Several guidelines recommend that at least three dilutions of test plasma should be analysed to improve precision and to ensure that the two important criteria for a valid assay have been met: (1) that there should be a straight line relationship between clotting times at different concentrations/dilutions; and (2) that the line through patient times is parallel to the calibration line.

Hemophilia center laboratories have been asked how many test plasma dilutions were analysed during FVIII and FIX assays performed in samples distributed by UK NEQAS on several occasions. Results grouped according to whether one, two, or three test plasma dilutions were used are shown in Table 43.2 which shows that precision of assay results is improved by the use of multiple test dilutions.

Use of a single test sample dilution can lead to gross underestimation of factor activity if lupus anticoagulant is present and

Table 43.2 Results of factor VIII (FVIII) and factor IX (FIX) assays obtained in UK hemophilia centers analysing the same external quality assessment UK NEQAS test sample. Results are grouped according to how many test sample dilutions were utilized. The CV results were statistically lower among centers using three dilutions compared to those using a single test sample dilution.

No. test sample dilutions	Factor IX Survey 2003			Factor VIII Survey 2009		
	n	Median IU/dL	CV (%)	*n*	Median IU/dL	CV (%)
1	22	6.3	54	39	6.6	96
2	17	6.5	29	18	5.8	28
3	42	6.0	23	49	6.1	29
Sample	Mild hemophilia B			Mild hemophilia A		

CV, coefficient of variation.

causes prolongation of clotting times that might be falsely interpreted as being due to low factor concentration. In extreme cases, powerful lupus antibodies can completely block the reaction even when test plasma is diluted in the assay which can give assay results of <1 IU/dL [20] in the presence of normal factor levels. More often, some clotting factor activity is detected but the measured activity increases at higher dilutions as the inhibitory effect of antibody is progressively lost. This manifests as nonparallelism between standard and test plasma lines provided multiple test plasma dilutions are included. A similar effect can occur in one-stage FIX and FXI assays when performed in the presence of potent anti-FVIII antibodies, when the anti-FVIII in the test plasma destroys FVIII in the FIX- or FXI-deficient plasma to different degrees in different test plasma dilutions. Chromogenic assays for FVIII or FIX utilize high initial plasma dilutions where the inhibiting effect of lupus anticoagulant (LAC) is usually diluted out [21]. The different phospholipids present in chromogenic assays reagents compared to one-stage methods may also play a role since no activity could be detected in a test plasma dilution of 1 in 80 in a one-stage technique whereas FVIII activity was normal in a chromogenic assay [22]. An alternative way to overcome this problem is to perform a one-stage assay using a reagent with high phospholipid concentration. Some data are available in relation to phospholipid concentrations of APTT reagents including evidence that one reagent has around 20 times more phospholipid than other reagents studied [23] and it has been recommended that the LAC-insensitive APTT reagents should be used for one-stage assays unless the presence of LAC has been excluded [1].

Factor VIII assay discrepancy

Several groups have reported an important minority of patients with mild hemophilia A who have a discrepancy between FVIII activity determined with different types of assay [24,25,26]. This includes 5–10% of patients with a normal one-stage FVIII (and normal APTT) but reduced activity by the two-stage clotting or chromogenic assay [26]. These subjects have a bleeding history consistent with hemophilia A and identifiable defects in the *F8* gene. Other cases have a reduced one-stage FVIII but normal two-stage or chromogenic activity [27], and in many of these the detection of abnormality has arisen during the investigation of a prolonged APTT as a chance finding during presurgical screening with only a small proportion arising from investigations for a possible bleeding disorder [25].

It is recommended that all hemophilia centers include a chromogenic or two-stage assay in addition to a one-stage technique, and that this should be performed in subjects with normal one-stage FVIII in the presence of a personal or family history consistent with mild hemophilia A [1,25].

Factor VIII assays after concentrate infusion

The recovery and half-life of FVIII and FIX can differ among patients, and may be less predictable in an individual during and after procedures. For optimal therapy, it is therefore useful to have laboratory assays available that can be used to determine plasma levels in order to inform patient management decisions. For plasma-derived FVIII concentrates, there can be differences between the results of one-stage and chromogenic assays in postinfusion plasma samples and the magnitude of these differences may depend on the test systems/reagents used [28]. For recombinant FVIII products, chromogenic assays give higher results than one-stage assays in the concentrate itself and in postinfusion samples from patients [29] for both full length recombinant and B-domain-deleted products. If postinfusion samples are assayed with the same type of assay as that used for potency labelling of the concentrate (both using one-stage assay or both using chromogenic), the observed factor levels in plasma are likely to be closer to the target. Since the chromogenic assay is currently less widely used than one-stage techniques, this issue is recognized more by centers using one-stage assays for postinfusion assays of concentrates whose potency was assigned by chromogenic assays (as recommended in Europe). Postinfusion samples from patients have traditionally been assayed using a plasma standard for calibration but one successful approach to avoid assay discrepancies is to use a product-specific concentrate standard to calibrate the FVIII assay. For one B-domain-deleted product used in different final formulations, the use of a product-specific standard to calibrate one-stage assays abolishes the difference between one-stage and chromogenic assay results that occurs if a plasma standard is used for calibration [30].

A number of products have been developed which contain FVIII and FIX proteins modified by pegylation, by fusion with other proteins, or in other ways in order to extend the half-time; these are in trials or in development. Guidance has been recently issued by the Scientific and Standardization Committee (SSC) of the International Society on Thrombosis and Hemophilia (ISTH) to assist concentrate manufacturers to define the quantity of active substance in the vial, and to guide physicians on the dose to be used for treatment that would correlate with recovery data measured in clinical laboratories [31]. This guidance proposes that the optimal approach to quantification in postinfusion assays will involve testing against a product reference composed of the same material as that which is infused. This will permit routine FVIII assay methods/reagents to be used for postinfusion testing provided the local assay system is included in manufacturers' guidance. It may be that postinfusion monitoring of some modified products will only be widely adopted if such product-specific standards are available, which would be facilitated by agreement between regulators, manufacturers, and standardization committees/bodies involved in the field. A laboratory providing assay data for patients under treatment with different products may have to maintain different assays or one assay with several standards for assay calibration and close liaison between laboratory and clinical colleagues in relation to the detail of a patient's treatment will continue to be vital for the safe and effective management of patients with hemophilia.

Factor VIII inhibitor testing

There is considerable variation in the reported incidence of FVIII inhibitors among patients with hemophilia A from <5% [32] to >50% [33], and it is likely that variations in assay sensitivity have contributed to this uncertainty. The first real standardization of inhibitor testing recognized that units of inhibitory activity were assay dependent and the proposed Bethesda assay and unit [34] were widely adopted. In this assay, normal plasma is used to construct a mixture of normal and patient plasma. After 2 h incubated at 37°C the loss of FVIII from this mixture is compared to the loss from a control mixture in which buffer replaces patient plasma. Due to problems of specificity and sensitivity, a modification was proposed by workers in Nijmegen: the normal plasma is buffered with imidazole and FVIII-deficient plasma replaces buffer in the control mixture [35,36]. There is marked interlaboratory variation in results of FVIII inhibitor assays when the same proficiency testing sample is analysed in different centers with coefficients of variation (CVs) usually in the 30–50% range [37–39] but sometimes more than 100% [37]. There are a number of reasons for the high variability.

By 2007, all centers returning FVIII inhibitor assays in the UK NEQAS exercises used plasma as the source of FVIII in their testing protocol [37]. This was mainly lyophilized material from commercial sources which was buffered but not according to the Nijmegen protocol and there was a significant difference between results obtained using the three most commonly used sources.

Another important source of variability between results is the FVIII-deficient plasma used to construct control mixtures and in the assay of residual FVIII. The results of FVIII inhibitor assays were 30–50% different depending on the FVIII-deficient plasma used [40]. Results were lower when FVIII-deficient plasma did not contain VWF. It is possible that other differences between the properties of the deficient plasmas used contributed to the differences observed. The same authors demonstrated that 4% bovine serum albumen solution could be substituted for FVIII-deficient plasma in the control mixture to reduce cost [41] so the VWF content of any deficient plasma used to construct the control mixture should not be relevant. It seems likely that the FVIII assay used for determination of residual FVIII activity is a major source of inhibitor result variability and if chromogenic or two-stage clotting assays are used the results may be different to those obtained with some one-stage assay techniques.

False-positive FVIII inhibitor results have been reported in the presence of the oral direct thrombin inhibitor dabigatran [42] so knowledge of current medication is important.

Inhibitors can develop in patients with mild hemophilia A and an inhibitor assay may be requested during a course of replacement therapy in moderate or severe cases. This means that the test sample may contain sufficient FVIII to influence the inhibitor results obtained in the assay. This problem can be overcome by inactivating residual FVIII activity in patient samples before mixing with normal plasma in the assay. Heating to 58°C for 1.5 h has been used in a procedure that will not dissociate any inhibitor that has complexed with FVIII prior to testing [43].

FVIII antibodies can also be quantified by immunologic assays which will detect inhibitors and also non-neutralizing antibodies that may be clinically relevant if they lead to increased clearance of FVIII without inhibiting FVIII in the FVIII assay performed as part of the Bethesda/Nijmegen assay [44].

References

1 Mackie I, Cooper P, Lawrie A, Kitchen S, Gray E, Laffan M, on behalf of the British Committee for Standards in Hematology. Guidelines on the laboratory aspects of assay used in hemostasis and thrombosis. *Int J Lab Hematol* 2013; **35**: 1–13.

2 Clinical and Laboratory Standards Institute (CLSI). Collection, transport and processing of blood specimens for testing plasma based coagulation assays and molecular hemostasis assays: approved guideline, 5th edn. 2008: H21–A5.

3 Srivastava A, Brewer AK, Mauser-Bunschoten EP, *et al.* Treatment guidelines working group on behalf of the World Federation of Hemophilia. Guidelines for the management of Hemophilia. *Hemophilia* 2013; **19**: 1–47.

4 Favaloro EJ, Soltani S, McDonald J. Potential laboratory misdiagnosis of Hemophilia and Von Willebrand owing to cold activation of blood samples for testing. *Am J Clin Pathol* 2004: **122**: 686–92.

5 Lippi G, Blanckaert N, Bonini P, *et al.* An overview of the leading cause of unsuitable specimens in clinical laboratories. *Clin Chem Lab Med* 2008: **46**: 764–72.

6 Woodhams B, Giradot O, Blanco M, Collese G, Gourmecin Y. Stability of coagulation proteins in frozen plasma. *Blood Coag Fibrinol* 2001: **12**: 229–36.

7 Clinical and Laboratory Standards Institute (CLSI). One stage prothrombin time test and activated partial thromboplastin time (APTT) test—Approved Guideline, 2nd edn. 2007; H47–A2.

8 Kitchen S, Preston FE, Olson JD. Internal quality control in the hemostasis laboratory. In: Kitchen S, Olson JD, Preston FE (eds) *Quality in Laboratory Hemostasis and Thrombosis*, 2nd edn. Wiley-Blackwell, Oxford, 2013: 57–64.

9 Jennings I, Kitchen DP, Woods TAL, Kitchen S, Walker ID, Preston FE. Laboratory performance in the World Federation of Hemophilia EQA programme 2003–2008. *Hemophilia* 2009; **15**: 571–7.

10 Kitchen S, McCraw A, Encheragucia M. Establishing a normal reference range. In: *Diagnosis of Hemophilia and Other Bleeding Disorders. A laboratory manual*, 2nd edn, 2010, www.wfh.org

11 Clinical and Laboratory Standards Institute (CLSI). How to define and determine reference intervals in the clinical laboratory: Approved guideline. 2000; C28–A2.

12 Baglin T, Keeling D, Kitchen S, and the British Committee for Standards in Hematology. Effects on routine coagulation screens and assessment of anticoagulant intensity of patients taking oral dabigatran or rivaroxaban: guidance from the British Committee for Standards in Haaematology. *Br J Hematol* 2012; **159**: 427–9.

13 Burns ER, Goldberg SN, Wenz B. Paradoxic effects of multiple mild coagulation factor deficiencies on the PT and APTT. *Am J Clin Pathol* 1993; **100**: 94–8.

14 Turi DC, Peerschke EI. Sensitivity of 3 APTT reagents to coagulation factor deficiencies. *Am J Clin Pathol* 1986; **85**: 43–9.

15 Bolton-Maggs PHB, Perry DJ, Chalmers EA, *et al.* The rare coagulation disorders – reviews with guidelines for management for the UK Hemophilia centre Doctors Organisation. *Hemophilia* 2004; **10**: 593–628.

16 Lawrie AS, Kitchen S, Efthymiou M, Mackie IJ, Machin SJ. Determination of APTT factor sensitivity: The misguiding guideline. *Int J Lab Hematol* 2013; **35**: 652–7.

17 Bowyer A, Smith J, Woolley AM, *et al.* The investigation of a prolonged APTT with specific clotting factor assays is unnecessary if an APTT with AFS is normal. *Int J Lab Hematol* 2011; **33**: 212–18.

18 Jennings I, Kitchen DP, Woods TAL, Kitchen S, Walker ID. Emerging technologies and quality assurance: the UK National External Quality Assessment Scheme perspective. *Semin Thromb Hemost* 2007; **33**: 243–9.

19 National Committee on Clinical Laboratory Standards (NCCLS). Determination of factor coagulant activities: approved guideline, 1997; H48–A.

20 Kazmi MA, Pickering W, Smith MP, Holland LJ, Savidge GF. Acquired hemophilia A : errors in the diagnosis. *Blood Coag Fibrinol* 1998; **9**: 623–8.

21 Chandler WL, Ferrell C, Lee J, Tun Tm Kha H. Comparison of three methods for measuring FVIII in plasma. *Am J Clin Pathol* 2003; **120**: 34–9.

22 De Maistre E, Wahl D, Perret-Guillaume C, *et al.* A chromogenic assay allows reliable measurement of FVIII levels in the presence of strong lupus anticoagulant. *Thromb Hemost* 1998; **79**: 237–8.

23 Kitchen Cartwright I, Woods TA, Jennings I, Preston FE. Lipid composition of seven APTT reagents in relation to heparin sensitivity. *Br J Hematol* 1999; **106**: 801–8.

24 Duncan EM, Duncan BM, Tunbridge LJ, Lloyd JV. Familial discrepancy between one stage and two stage factor VIII assay methods in a subgroup of patients with hemophilia A. *Br J Hematol* 1994; **87**: 846–8.

25 Kitchen S, Haywood C, Negrier C, Dargaud Y. New development in laboratory diagnosis and monitoring. *Hemophilia* 2010; **16** (Suppl. 5): 61–6.

26 Rodgers SE, Duncan EM, Sobieraj-Teague M, Lloyd JV. Evaluation of 3 automated chromogenic FVIII kits in the diagnosis of mild discrepant hemophilia A. *Int J Lab Hematol* 2009; **31**: 180–8.

27 Lyall H, Hill M, Westby J, Grimley C, Dolan G. Tyr346-Cys mutation results in factor VIII:C assay discrepancy and a normal bleeding phenotype—is this mild hemophilia A? *Hemophilia* 2008; **14**: 78–80.

28 Lee C, Barrowcliffe TW, Gray E, *et al.* Pharmacokinetic in vivo comparison using 1-stage and chromogenic substrate assays with two formulations of Hemofil-M. *Thromb Hameost* 1996; **76**: 950–6.

29 Barrowcliffe TW, Hubbard TW, Kitchen S. Standards and monitoring treatment. *Hemophilia* 2012; **18**(Suppl. 1): 61–5.

30 Pouplard C, Caron C, Aillaud MF, *et al.* The use of the new ReFacto AF laboratory standard allows reliable measurement of FVIII:C levels in ReFacto AF mock plasma samples by a one stage assay. *Hemophilia* 2011; **17**(5): e958–62. Erratum in: *Hemophilia* 2012; **18**(1): e42.

31 Hubbard AR, Dodt J, Lee T, *et al.,* on behalf of the FVIII and IX subcommittee of the Scientific and Standardisation Committee of the International Society on Thrombosis and Hemostasis. *J Thromb Hematol* 2013; **11**: 988–9.

32 McMillan CW, Shapiro SS, Whitehurst D, Hoyer LW, Rao AV, Lazerson J. The natural history of factor VIII:C inhibitors in patients with hemophilia A: a national cooperative study. II. Observations on the initial development of factor VIII:C inhibitors. *Blood* 1998; **71**(2): 344–8.

33 Ehrenforth S, Kreuz W, Scharrer I, *et al.* Incidence of development of factor VIII and factor IX inhibitors in hemophiliacs. *Lancet* 1992; **339**(8793): 594–8.

34 Kasper C, Aledort L, Counts R, *et al.* Letter: A more uniform measurement of factor VIII inhibitors. *Thromb Diath Hemorrah* 1975; **34**(3): 869–72.

35 Verbruggen B, Novakova I, Wessels H, *et al.* The Nijmegen modification of the Bethesda assay for factor VIII:C inhibitors: improved specificity and reliability. *Thromb Hemost* 1995; **73**(2): 247–51.

36 Giles AR, Verbruggen B, Rivard GE, Teitel J, Walker I, and the Association of Hemophilia Centre Directors of Canada. Factor VIII/IX Subcommittee of Scientific and Standardization Committee of International Society on Thrombosis and Hamostasis. A detailed

Standardization of von Willebrand factor assays

Assays for von Willebrand factor

The ristocetin cofactor method has continued to be the mainstay of assays of VWF, but it suffers from very high variability, both within and between laboratories. There are difficulties also with the preparation and stability of the platelet reagent, and the assay is labor intensive and difficult to automate. Because of these problems, alternative methods of measuring VWF function have been sought, and the collagen-binding method, which is much easier to perform and more reproducible, was introduced by Favorolo [44]. Although there has been some controversy over its clinical applicability, it is used in a number of clinical laboratories in conjunction with other methods such as multimer analysis, and is being considered also as a possible EP reference method for concentrates. The measurement of VWF antigen is also useful as an adjunct to the functional measurements; the original "rocket" electrophoresis method of Laurell has now been largely replaced by enzyme-linked immunoadsorbent assay (ELISA) assays.

Standards for von Willebrand factor

The course of standardization of VWF differed from that of FVIII and FIX in that, when the first IS for FVIII, plasma, was established in 1982, the same plasma was calibrated (against normal pools) for VWF [45]. Thus, a plasma standard was established before a concentrate standard, and in fact a separate concentrate IS for VWF concentrate was established only in 2002 [46]. The reason for this is the relatively slow development and licensing of VWF concentrates, with cryoprecipitate and fresh frozen plasma (FFP) continuing to be used for many years.

Standardization of bypassing agents

Activated prothrombin complex concentrates

FEIBA is an activated prothrombin complex concentrate (aPCC) produced by Baxter Healthcare in Austria, which is used to control spontaneous bleeding episodes or cover surgical interventions in hemophilia patients who develop inhibitors [47]. The in-vitro assay for FEIBA measures the ability of this product to shorten the aPTT of an FVIII-deficient plasma containing FVIII inhibitors. FEIBA is expressed in arbitrary units. One unit of FEIBA was originally defined as that amount of FEIBA which shortens the aPTT of high-titer FVIII inhibitor reference plasma to 50% of the blank value. There is a linear correlation between the logarithm of the FEIBA and the logarithm of the measured clotting time. The quantitative evaluation is made using a parallel line assay, or by using a calibration curve, relative to the manufacturer's own reference standard. These standards are produced by the manufacturer on a relatively small scale and are frequently replaced. They are generally calibrated relative to their predecessor. More recently, following concerns about the

reliability of this procedure, it was decided to develop a separate independent FEIBA reference standard (in relatively large quantities); this was established as a first NIBSC Working Standard for FEIBA after a collaborative study involving the manufacturers and three European control laboratories [48].

Clinical monitoring of patients undergoing FEIBA bypassing therapy, which would reflect achievement of hemostasis in vivo, has been difficult, although a thrombin generation assay [49] developed in 2003 seems to show some promise. Nevertheless, a truly standardized assay for ex-vivo monitoring has still been elusive.

Factor VIIa

Recombinant activated factor VII (rFVIIa; NovoSeven, Novo Nordisk, Denmark) has proved very successful in the treatment of inhibitor patients, although there are some patients who do not respond. The product was initially assayed against a plasma standard for FVII, but these assays proved quite variable, and a separate IS for FVIIa was developed [50].

FVIIa has a short half-life and considerable interindividual pharmacokinetic variability; consequently, many clinicians argue that treatment should be monitored, though the usefulness and practicality of such monitoring remain topics for debate. The injected FVIIa leads to a considerable increase in the patient's FVII clotting activity (FVII:C), and routine FVII:C assays can be used for monitoring. However, a specific assay for FVIIa has been developed by Morrissey et al. [51] and modified by Johannessen et al. to make it more reliable at low concentrations [52]. The reliability and clinical utility of FVII:C and FVIIa assays in monitoring rFVIIa treatment has been reviewed [53].

Standardization of assays of other coagulation factors

Assays of other coagulation factors are carried out only rarely in the context of congenital deficiencies, although they are performed more frequently in relation to acquired defects, population surveys, and by manufacturers of concentrates. In general, the same principles apply, as for FVIII and FIX, with plasma standards being used for plasma samples, and concentrate standards for assay of therapeutic concentrates (Table 44.1).

Standardization of global assays

In recent years there has been increasing recognition that specific assays may not be sufficiently informative to assess the patient's overall hemostatic state and that global tests may contribute useful additional information. Another reason for the revival of global assays is the development of technical innovations and more sophisticated methods of analysis, which have improved their reliability and reproducibility and led to more widespread use. Two tests developed in the 1950s that have recently undergone a renaissance are thromboelastography and the thrombin generation test (TGT). Both methods have been investigated for the assessment of patients with hemophilia; the TGT has been used more widely and appears to show the most promise.

Interest in the TGT was rekindled following a study by Hemker [54], in which the method was modified by the use of a chromogenic substrate to monitor the generated thrombin. This and other technical modifications provided much improved precision and sensitivity [55]. Subsequently, there have been other technical variations, notably the development of different chromogenic and fluorescent substrates that can be incorporated into the incubation mixture to give enhanced convenience and sample throughput [56]. Use of TGT for measuring activity of FVIII concentrates was investigated by McIntosh et al. [57]. Collaborative studies of the TGT on platelet poor plasma and hemophilic patient samples have been carried out [58,59]; however, at present there is insufficient understanding of the standardization of these assays to allow development of any recommendations by the ISTH/SSC.

References

1 Finney D. *Statistical Method in Biological Assay*. London: Charles Griffin, 1978.

2 Kirkwood TBL, Snape TJ. Biometric principles in clotting and clot lysis assays. *Clin Lab Haematol* 1980; **2**: 155–67.

3 Bangham DR, Biggs R, Brozovic M, *et al.* A biological standard for measurement of blood coagulation factor VIII activity. *Bull WHO* 1971; **45**: 337–51.

4 Kirkwood TBL, Barrowcliffe TW. Discrepancy between 1-stage and 2-stage assay of factor VIII:C. *Br J Haematol* 1978; **40**: 333–8.

5 Raut S, Heath A, Barrowcliffe TW. Establishment of the 6th International Standard for FVIII concentrate. *Thromb Haemost* 2001; **85**: 1071–8.

6 Barrowcliffe TW. Factor VIII and Factor IX Sub-committee. Recommendations for the assay of high-purity factor VIII concentrates. *Thromb Haemost* 1993; **70**: 876–7.

7 Barrowcliffe TW. The one-stage versus the two-stage factor VIII assay. In: Triplett DA (ed.) *Advances in Coagulation Testing*. Skokie, IL: College of American Pathologists, 1986: 47–62.

8 Hubbard AR, Curtis AD, Barrowcliffe TW, *et al.* Assay of factor VIII concentrates: comparison of chromogenic and 2-stage clotting assays. *Thromb Res* 1986; **44**: 887–91.

9 Raut S, Daniels S, Heath AB, on behalf of the SSC sub-committee on Factor VIII/FIX of the ISTH. Value assignment of the WHO 8th International Standard for factor VIII, concentrate (07-350). *J Thromb Haemost* 2012; **10**: 1175–6.

10 Albertengo ME, Barrowcliffe TW, Oliva L, Bevan S, Raut S. New recombinant standard for FVIII concentrate gives same results as previous plasma derived standards on a range of FVIII products. *Thromb Haemost* 2000; **83**: 789–90.

11 Barrowcliffe TW, Watton J, Tubbs JE, *et al.* Potency of high purity factor VIII concentrates (Letter). *Lancet* 1990; **ii**: 124.

12 Hubbard AR, Weller LJ, Bevan SA. A Survey of one-stage and chromogenic potencies in therapeutic FVIII concentrates. *Br J Haematol* 2002; **117**: 247–8.

13 Mikaelsson M, Oswaldsson U, Sandberg H. Influence of phospholipids on the assessment of factor VIII activity. *Haemophilia* 1998; **4**: 646–50.

14 Hubbard AR, Sands D, Sandberg E, *et al.* A multi-centre collaborative study on the potency estimation of ReFacto. *Thromb Haemost* 2003; **90**: 1088–93.

15 Raut S, Sands D, Heath AB, Barrowcliffe TW. Variability in factor VIII concentrate measurement: results from SSC field collaborative studies. *J Thromb Haemost* 2003; **1**: 1927–34.

16 Hubbard AR, Weller LJ, Bevan SA. Activation profiles of FVIII in concentrates reflect one-stage/chromogenic potency discrepancies. *Br J Haematol* 2002; **117**: 957–60.

17 Raut S, Heath AB, Lee M, Mertens K. Collaborative study on recombinant factor VIII concentrates: SSC/8/9—phase I & II field studies. Report to participants. An SSC working party study on behalf of the SSC FVIII/IX subcommittee. Unpublished report, 2007.

18 Pipe SW. The hope and reality of long-acting hemophilia products. *Am J Hematol* 2012; **87**, Issue S1, S33–9.

19 Peters RT, Low SC, Kamphaus GD, *et al.* Prolonged activity of factor IX as a monomeric Fc fusion protein. *Blood* 2010; **115**: 2057–64.

20 Metzner HJ, Weimer T, Kronthaler U, Lang W, Schulte S. Genetic fusion to albumin improves the pharmacokinetic properties of factor IX. *Thromb Haemost* 2009; **102**: 634–44.

21 Buyue Y, Liu T, Reidy T, *et al.* A novel single chain recombinant factor VIII Fc fusion protein is active in vitro and fully efficacious in an in vivo Hem A mouse bleeding model. *Blood* 2011; **118**: 1192.

22 Smolen J, Landewé RB, Mease P, *et al.* Efficacy and safety of certolizumab pegol plus methotrexate in active rheumatoid arthritis: the RAPID 2 study. A randomised controlled trial. *Ann Rheum Dis* 2009; **68**: 797–804.

23 Mei B, Pan C, Jiang H, *et al.* Rational design of a fully active, long-acting PEGylated factor VIII for hemophilia A treatment. *Blood* 2010; **116**: 270–9.

24 Leong L, Evans V, Ramsey P, *et al.* Evaluation of methods for potency testing of pegylated FVIII (PEG-FVIII, BAY 94-9027). *J Thromb Haemost* 2011; **9**(Suppl. 2): Poster P-TU-223.

25 Hubbard AR, Rigsby P, Barrowcliffe TW. Standardisation of Factor VIII and von Willebrand Factor in plasma: Calibration of the 4th International Standard (97/586). *Thromb Haemost* 2001: **85**: 634–8.

26 Hubbard AR, Bevan SA, Weller LJ. Potency estimation of recombinant factor VIII: effect of assay method and standard. *Br J Haematol* 2001; **113**: 533–6.

27 Lee CA, Owens D, Bray G, *et al.* Pharmacokinetics of recombinant factor VIII (Recombinate) using one-stage clotting and chromogenic factor VIII assay. *Thromb Haemost* 1999; **82**: 1644–7.

28 Lee CA, Barrowcliffe TW, Bray G, *et al.* Pharmacokinetic in vivo comparison using 1-stage and chromogenic substrate assays with two formulations of Hemofil-M. *Thromb Haemost* 1996; **76**: 950–6.

29 Ingerslev J, Jankowski, M, Weston SB, Charles LA. Collaborative field study on the utility of a BDD factor VIII concentrate standard in the estimation of BDD factor VIII:C activity in hemophilic plasma using one-stage clotting assays. *J Thromb Haemost* 2004; **2**: 623–8.

30 Hubbard AR, Dodt J, Lee T, *et al.*, and on behalf of the Factor VIII Factor IX Subcommittee of the Scientific and Standardisation Committee of the International Society on Thrombosis and Haemostasis. Recommendations on the potency labelling of factor VIII and factor IX concentrates. *J Thromb Haemost* 2013; **11**: 988–9.

31 Brozovic M, Bangham DR. Study of a proposed International Standard for factor IX. *Thromb Haemost* 1976; **35**: 222–36.

32 Barrowcliffe TW, Tydeman MS, Kirkwood TBL. Major effect of prediluent in factor IX clotting assay. *Lancet* 1979; **ii**: 192.

33 Barrowcliffe TW. Standardisation of factors II, VII, IX, and X in plasma and concentrates. *Thromb Haemost* 1987; **59**: 334.

34 Kasper CK, Aledort L, Aronson D, *et al.* Proceedings: A more uniform measurement of factor VIII inhibitors. *Thromb Diath Haemorrh* 1975; **34**: 612.

35 Austen DE, Lechner K, Rizza CR, Rhymes IL. A comparison of the Bethesda and New Oxford methods of factor VIII antibody assay. *Thromb Haemost* 1982; **47**: 72–5.

36 Barrowcliffe TW, Peake IR. Factor VIII inhibitor assays: NIBSC 3-day workshop. Report to participants. Unpublished report, 1982.

37 Verbruggen B, Novakova I, Wessels H, Boezeman J, van den Berg M, Mauser-Bunschoten E. The Nijmegen modification of the Bethesda assay for factor VIII:C inhibitors: improved specificity and reliability. *Thromb Haemost* 1995; **73**: 247–51.

38 Giles AR, Verbruggen B, Rivard GE, Teitel J, Walker I. A detailed comparison of the performance of the standard versus the Nijmegen modification of the Bethesda assay in detecting factor VIII:C inhibitors in the haemophilia A population of Canada. *Thromb Haemost* 1998; **79**: 872–5.

39 Peerschke EI, Castellone DD, Ledford-Kraemer M, Van Cott EM, Meijer P, and the NASCOLA Proficiency Testing Committee. Laboratory assessment of factor VIII inhibitor titer: the North American Specialized Coagulation Laboratory Association experience. *Am J Clin Pathol* 2009; **131**(4): 552–8.

40 Raut S, Sands D, Kitchen S, Preston FE, Barrowcliffe TW. Collaborative study on determination of FVIII Inhibitors. Report to participants. An SSC working party study on behalf of the SSC FVIII/IX subcommittee. Unpublished report, 2005.

41 Raut S, Faulkner L, Heath A. Collaborative study on proposed reference standard for FVIII Inhibitors. Report to participants. An SSC working party study on behalf of the SSC FVIII/IX subcommittee. Unpublished report, 2007.

42 Raut, S. SMIA: A new approach in FVIII inhibitor measurement and standardisation. Annual Meeting of the Scientific and the Standardization Committee of the ISTH, 2012. Section 2, Presentation CFBS09.

43 Daniels S, Heath A, McMullan N, Raut S. Development of a parallel-line-based assay for the assessment of factor VIII inhibitor Bethesda titers. *Haemophilia* 2012; **18**(Suppl.): 102.

44 Favorolo EJ. Collagen binding assay for von Willebrand factor (vWF:CBA): detection of von Willebrand's disease (vWD) and discrimination of vWD subtypes, depends on collagen source. *Thromb Haemost* 2000; **83**: 127–35.

45 Barrowcliffe TW. Standardization and assay. *Semin Thromb Haemost* 1993; **19**: 73–9.

46 Hubbard AR, Sands, Chang A, Mazurier C. Standardisation of von Willebrand factor in therapeutic concentrates: calibration of the 1st International Standard for von Willebrand factor concentrate (00/514). *Thromb Haemost* 2002; **88**: 380–6.

47 Hilgartner MW, Knatterud G, and the FEIBA Study Group. The use of factor-eight-inhibitor-by-passing-activity (FEIBA IMMUNO). Product for treatment of bleeding episodes in haemophiliacs with inhibitors. *Blood* 1983; **61**: 36–40.

48 Raut S, Daniels S, Gaertner P, Hunfeld A, Leitner M, Hockley J, Heath A. Factor VIII Bypassing Activity (FEIBA) assays: standardization and development of the 1st NIBSC Working Standard for FEIBA—results from a collaborative study. *Haemophilia* 2013; **19**: 304–9.

49 Varadi K, Negrier C, Berntorp E, *et al.* Monitoring the bioavailability of FEIBA with a thrombin generation assay. *J Thromb Haemost* 2003; **11**: 2374–80.

50 Hubbard AR, Weller LJ, Heath A. Calibration of the proposed WHO 2nd international standard factor VIIa concentrate (07/228). WHO ECBS Report 2008, WHO/BS/08.2090.

51 Morrissey JH, Macik BG, Neuenschwander PF, Comp PC. Quantitation of activated factor VII levels in plasma using a tissue factor mutant selectively deficient in promoting factor VII activation. *Blood* 1993; **81**: 734–44.

52 Johannessen M, Nielsen G, Nordfang O. Comparison of the factor VIII:C clot analysis and a modified activated factor VII analysis for monitoring factor VII activity in patients treated with recombinant activated factor VII (NovoSeven). *Blood Coagul Fibrinolysis* 2000; **11**(Suppl. 1): S159–64.

53 Barrowcliffe TW. Monitoring inhibitor patients with the right assays. *Semin Hematol* 2008; **45**(Suppl. 1): S25–30.

54 Hemker HC. The mode of action of heparin in plasma. In: Verstraete M, Vermylen J, Lijnen R, Arnout J (eds.) *Thrombosis and Haemostasis.* Leuven, Belgium: Leuven University Press, 1987: 17–36.

55 Hemker HC, Wielders S, Kessels H, Béguin S. Continuous registration of thrombin generation in plasma, its use for the determination of the thrombin potential. *Thromb Haemost* 1993; **70**: 617–24.

56 Hemker HC, Giesen P, Al Dieri R, *et al.* Calibrated automated thrombin generation measurement in clotting plasma. *Pathophysiol Haemost Thromb* 2003; **33**: 4–15.

57 McIntosh JH, Owens D, Lee CA, Raut S, Barrowcliffe TW. A modified thrombin generation test for the measurement of factor VIII concentrates. *J Thromb Haemost* 2003; **1**: 1005–11.

58 Gray E, Hogwood J, Rigsby P. Collaborative study on fluorogenic methods for thrombin generation tests. On behalf of the ISTH/SSC Working Party on Thrombin Generation Tests. Report to participants. Unpublished report, 2006.

59 Young G, Sørensen B, Dargaud Y, Negrier C, Brummel-Ziedins K, Key NS. Thrombin generation and whole blood viscoelastic assays in the management of hemophilia: current state of art and future perspective. *Blood* 2013; **121**: 1940–50.

CHAPTER 45

Global laboratory assays in hemophilia

Benny Sørensen[1] and Guy Young[2]

[1] Alnylam Pharmaceuticals, Massachusetts, USA
[2] University of Southern California Keck School of Medicine, California, USA

Introduction

An immediate consequence of a break in the vascular endothelium is exposure of extravascular tissue factor-bearing cells and platelet adhesion to the damaged vessel wall. Following activation via, for example, epinephrine, adenosine diphosphate (ADP), and collagen, the platelets aggregate and form a surface of negatively charged phospholipids where the coagulation factors can assemble and perform their enzymatic and catalytic functions [1]. The main purpose of the coagulation factors is to produce a timely, sufficient, and regulated amount of thrombin to cleave fibrinogen and activate factor XIII (FXIII) and thrombin activatable fibrinolysis inhibitor in order to produce a stable hemostatic plug and stop bleeding. Furthermore, the purpose of the hemostatic plug is to establish a matrix to facilitate repair and regeneration of the integrity of the vessel wall. Thrombin may be considered as the lead protein for stimulating and directing the generation of a hemostatic plug. That is, thrombin generation may be characterized as the momentum of the hemostatic system. Following production of less than 1% of the total thrombin generated in a healthy hemostatic system, a series of timely coordinated activation processes takes place: platelet activation, activation of factor V (FV) and FXIII, cleavage of fibrinogen, and activation of FVIII and factor XI (FXI) [2]. This initiation phase of thrombin generation is followed by a propagation phase of thrombin driven by the intrinsic tenase [factor IXa (FIXa) and activated factor VIIIa (FVIIIa)] and pro-thrombinase [factor Xa (FXa) and FVa] complexes [1]. The dynamic production of thrombin is regulated by natural anticoagulants, such as antithrombin and proteins C and S in order to prevent excessive production of thrombin that may result in thromboembolic events.

Thrombin is not the only determinant required to achieve hemostasis. Thrombin acts on substrates, such as fibrinogen and platelets, constituting the three-dimensional bricks of the hemostatic plug. Furthermore, hemostasis is also characterized by the formation of a clot structure being resistant to fibrinolysis and with physical strength to withstand blood pressure and flow of blood.

The hemostatic system is regulated by a coordinated interaction of coagulation proteins, natural anticoagulants, and cells. In particular, the platelets and the endothelium play an important role in the regulation of hemostasis; however, both white and red blood cells play supportive roles and impact thrombin generation and clot formation.

Limitations of standard coagulation assays

Standard coagulation assays such as the activated clotting time (aCT), prothrombin time [PT/INR (international normalized ratio)], or activated partial thromboplastin time (aPTT) provide information only of the initiation of clot formation. However, formation of a sufficient hemostatic plug is a continuous process with characteristic rate-specific properties. When there is a suspicion of hemophilia, the aPTT may be used to screen for potential factor deficiencies. If the aPTT is abnormal, levels of coagulation FVIII (hemophilia A) or FIX (hemophilia B) are evaluated by performing a one-stage clotting assay or a chromogenic assay. The one-stage clotting assay is also based on measurements of aPTT utilizing FVIII-deficient plasma, reference plasma, and patient plasma. Usually, these routine coagulation assays can provide a specific biochemical diagnosis to categorize patients as severe, moderate, or mild. However, the standard aPTT and single coagulation factor assays are only marginally correlated with the clinical phenotype of the coagulation disorder. Thus, some patients with severe hemophilia A (FVIII: C <1%) bleed frequently, whereas other patients bleed only occasionally despite similar biochemical diagnosis and comparable lifestyle.

Textbook of Hemophilia, Third Edition. Edited by Christine A. Lee, Erik E. Berntorp and W. Keith Hoots.
© 2014 John Wiley & Sons, Ltd. Published 2014 by John Wiley & Sons, Ltd.

Laboratory phenotyping of bleeding disorders and monitoring of hemostatic intervention

With respect to prediction of the clinical phenotype, a number of studies have demonstrated considerable heterogeneity in the baseline whole blood coagulation patterns among patients with verified FVIII levels <1% [23]. Furthermore, data have illustrated that patients diagnosed with severe hemophilia A (FVIII: C <1%) but having unusually good whole blood clotting profiles are associated with a less severe bleeding phenotype [26]. The low tissue factor assay has also been used to illustrate different response patterns to various levels of coagulation FVIII concentrate [23]. In addition, both *in-vitro* and *in-vivo* studies have demonstrated the ability of TEG to predict the clinical response to bypassing agents in patients with inhibitors [21,22,24,25]. So far, these studies represent single-center experiences. Nevertheless, the potential for TEG has been demonstrated. An *in-vivo* study demonstrated the ability of TEG to individualize therapy for three inhibitor patients, which led to more judicious use of bypassing agents as well as more convenient treatment regimens, ultimately reducing the cost of managing bleeds without compromising efficacy [27]. Additional studies are required to answer some of the questions raised by these initial studies, including which preanalytic methods provide the most sensitive, reliable, and reproducible results. In the near future, it is possible that TEG may be part of the tools used to design individual treatment regimens for patients with inhibitors. This will become increasingly important as new bypassing agents become available.

References

1 Mann KG. Biochemistry and physiology of blood coagulation. *Thromb Haemost* 1999; **82**: 165–74.

2 Brummel KE, Paradis SG, Butenas S, Mann KG. Thrombin functions during tissue factor-induced blood coagulation. *Blood* 2002; **100**: 148–52.

3 Young G, Sorensen B, Dargaud Y, Negrier C, Brummel-Ziedins K, Key NS. Thrombin generation and whole blood viscoelastic assays in hemophilia: current state-of-art and future perspectives. *Blood* 2013; **121**: 1944–50.

4 Hemker HC, Beguin S. Phenotyping the clotting system. *Thromb Haemost* 2000; **84**: 747–51.

5 Brummel-Ziedins KE, Vossen CY, Butenas S, Mann KG, Rosendaal FR. Thrombin generation profiles in deep venous thrombosis. *J Thromb Haemost* 2005; **3**: 2497–505.

6 Mann KG, Whelihan MF, Butenas S, Orfeo T. Citrate anticoagulation and the dynamics of thrombin generation. *J Thromb Haemost* 2007; **5**: 2055–61.

7 van Veen JJ, Gatt A, Cooper PC, Kitchen S, Bowyer AE, Makris M. Corn trypsin inhibitor in fluorogenic thrombin-generation measurements is only necessary at low tissue factor concentrations and influences the relationship between factor VIII coagulant activity and thrombogram parameters. *Blood Coag Fibrinol* 2008; **19**: 183–9.

8 Dielis AW, Castoldi E, Spronk HM, *et al.* Coagulation factors and the protein C system as determinants of thrombin generation in a normal population. *J Thromb Haemost* 2008; **6**: 125–31.

9 Kjalke M, Ezban M, Monroe DM, Hoffman M, Roberts HR, Hedner U. High-dose factor VIIa increases initial thrombin generation and mediates faster platelet activation in thrombocytopenia-like conditions in a cell-based model system. *Br J Haematol* 2001; **114**: 114–20.

10 Dargaud Y, Beguin S, Lienhart A, *et al.* Evaluation of thrombin generating capacity in plasma from patients with haemophilia A and B. *Thromb Haemost* 2005; **93**: 475–80.

11 Dargaud Y, Bordet JC, Lienhart A, Negrier C. Use of the thrombin generation test to evaluate response to treatment with recombinant activated factor VII. *Semin Hematol* 2008; **45**(Suppl. 1): S72–S73.

12 Dargaud Y, Lienhart A, Meunier S, *et al.* Major surgery in a severe haemophilia A patient with high titre inhibitor: use of the thrombin generation test in the therapeutic decision. *Haemophilia* 2005; **11**: 552–8.

13 Al Hawaj MA, Martin EJ, Venitz J, *et al.* Monitoring rFVIII prophylaxis dosing using global haemostasis assays. *Haemophilia* 2013; **19**: 409–14.

14 Dargaud Y, Lienhart A, Negrier C. Prospective assessment of thrombin generation test for monitoring of bypassing therapy in hemophilia patients with inhibitors. *Blood* 2010; **116**: 5734–7.

15 Jensen MS, Larsen OH, Christiansen K, Fenger-Eriksen C, Ingerslev J, Sorensen B. Platelet activation and aggregation: the importance of thrombin activity. A laboratory model. *Haemophilia* 2013; **19**: 403–8.

16 Gatt A, van Veen JJ, Woolley AM, Kitchen S, Cooper P, Makris M. Thrombin generation assays are superior to traditional tests in assessing anticoagulation reversal *in vitro*. *Thromb Haemost* 2008; **100**: 350–5.

17 Owen CA. *The History of Blood Coagulation*, 1st edn. Rochester: Mayo Foundation for Medical Education and Research, 2001.

18 Hartert H. Blutgerinnungsstudien mit der thrombelastographie, einem neuen untersuchungsverfahren. *Klin Wochenschr* 1948; **26**: 577–83.

19 Calatzis A, Fritzsche P, Calatzis A, Kling M, Hipp R, Stemberger A. A comparison of the technical principle of the roTEG coagulation analyser and conventional thromboelastographic systems. *Ann Haematol* 1996; **72**(Suppl. 1): P90 (abstract).

20 Sørensen B, Johansen P, Christiansen K, Wöelke M, Ingerslev J. Whole blood coagulation thromboelastographic profiles employing minimal tissue factor activation. *J Thromb Haemost* 2003; **1**: 551–8.

21 Sørensen B, Persson E, Ingerslev J. Factor VIIa analogue (V158D/E296V/M298Q-FVIIa) normalises clot formation in whole blood from patients with severe haemophilia A. *Br J Haematol* 2007; **137**: 158–65.

22 Ingerslev J, Poulsen LH, Sørensen B. Potential role of the dynamic properties of whole blood coagulation in assessment of dosage requirements in haemophilia. *Haemophilia* 2003; **9**: 348–52.

23 Sørensen B, Ingerslev J. Whole blood clot formation phenotypes in hemophilia A and rare coagulation disorders. Patterns of response to recombinant factor VIIa. *J Thromb Haemost* 2004; **2**: 102–10.

24 Sørensen B, Ingerslev J. Tailoring haemostatic treatment to patient requirements—an update on monitoring haemostatic response using thrombelastography. *Haemophilia* 2005; **11**(Suppl. 1): 1–6.

25 Chitlur M, Warrier I, Rajpurkar M, *et al.* Thromboelastography in children with coagulation factor deficiencies. *Br J Haematol* 2008; **142**: 250–6.

26 Rivard GE, Brummel-Ziedins KE, Mann KG, Fan L, Hofer A, Cohen E. Evaluation of the profile of thrombin generation during the process of whole blood clotting as assessed by thrombelastography. *J Thromb Haemost* 2005; **3**: 2039–43.

27 Young G, Blain R, Nakagawa P, Nugent DJ. Individualization of bypassing agent treatment for haemophilic patients with inhibitors utilizing thromboelastography. *Haemophilia* 2006; **12**: 598–604.

28 Ingerslev J, Christiansen K, Calatzis A, Holm M, Sabroe EL. Management and monitoring of recombinant activated factor VII. *Blood Coag Fibrinol* 2000; **11**(Suppl. 1): S25–30.

29 Sørensen B, Ingerslev J. Thromboelastography and recombinant factor VIIa—hemophilia and beyond. *Semin Hematol* 2004; **41**(Suppl. 1): 140–4.

Women and bleeding disorders

CHAPTER 47

Women and von Willebrand disease

Peter A. Kouides

University of Rochester School of Medicine, New York, USA

Introduction

Particularly in the past 15 years, studies have clearly documented a definite degree of obstetric [1,2] and gynecologic morbidity [3] in females with von Willebrand disease (VWD) [4] (Table 47.1). The vast majority of these patients over the course of their menstrual life will develop heavy menstrual bleeding (HMB) ($\geq$80%) [3,5]. Furthermore, up to a fifth of these patients have undergone surgical intervention such as hysterectomy for control of HMB refractory to medical management [3,5,6]. In addition, the constancy of the HMB clearly impairs quality of life (QOL) [3,5]. This chapter highlights and reviews the relevant gender-specific epidemiologic and clinical characteristics, and therapeutic issues in the patient with HMB and/or postpartum hemorrhage related to VWD.

Epidemiology

Understandably, case finding of VWD in women has focused on women presenting with HMB. Not surprisingly, women with unexplained HMB who test positive for VWD have a higher bleeding score based on the condensed Molecular and Clinical Markers for the Diagnosis and Management of Type 1 von Willebrand Disease (NMCMDM-1) VWD bleeding questionnaire [7]. A systematic review by Shankar *et al.* [8] has summarized the overall prevalence of the laboratory diagnosis of VWD in women presenting with HMB to be 13% [confidence intervals (CI) 11%, 15.6%] of a total of 988 women in 11 studies (Figure 47.1).

Regarding the younger patient with HMB [9], there has been few prevalence studies for an underlying bleeding disorder in the adolescent HMB population [9,10] and most of these studies have focused on the inpatient and emergency setting. In 61 adolescents referred for hemostasis evaluation to a hemophilia treatment center, a prevalence of VWD of 36% (22/61) (95% CI, 24–49%) was found [11]. Most recently in a single institution study of adolescents evaluated for HMB, approximately 10% of 235 patients had von Willebrand factor (VWF) ristocetin cofactor levels <50% [12]. A decision analysis model showed that testing for VWD in adolescents with HMB before the initiation of oral contraceptives is cost-effective [13].

Diagnostic aspects

The results of the epidemiologic studies reviewed above have led to relatively widespread VWD testing in the female population. However, the clinician must be aware that VWF and factor VIII (FVIII) levels can fluctuate [14]. Hormonal factors, both exogenous and endogenous, are a potential mechanism in part for such fluctuation. Consequently, there are several subtleties in the laboratory diagnosis of VWD that warrant clarification as follows:

1 Testing in relation to the menstrual cycle. A recent systematic review of 11 studies examining potential variation in the VWF levels in relation to the menstrual cycle noted that 5/11 studies reported the lowest VWF levels during menstruation or early follicular phase [15].

2 Testing in relation to combination oral contraceptive (OC) use. Historically, it has been felt that OC use can obscure the diagnosis of VWD based on an observation that estrogen can raise the VWF levels in VWD patients [16]. However, presently there is a lack of evidence demonstrating a definite effect on VWF levels of the current combination OCs (which are of lower dose potency than the estrogen preparations associated with the initial case reports of estrogen raising the VWF levels) wherein some studies have actually shown a dampening of the VWF levels among women on low-dose OCs [17,18].

3 Other laboratory issues. Other factors that may have an impact on the laboratory diagnosis of VWD in women are race and age. Studies have demonstrated significantly higher VWF levels in black women [17,19] even after adjusting for

Textbook of Hemophilia, Third Edition. Edited by Christine A. Lee, Erik E. Berntorp and W. Keith Hoots.

© 2014 John Wiley & Sons, Ltd. Published 2014 by John Wiley & Sons, Ltd.

Table 47.1 von Willebrand disease (VWD)-related complications in females.

Menstrual related	Other menstrual issues	Childbirth related
• Majority with heavy menstrual bleeding • Iron-deficiency anemia • Increased rate of surgical interventions: dilatation and curettage, hysterectomy • Decreased quality of life (increased time lost from school/work, ?increased anxiety/depression)	• Increased prevalence of midcycle pain (Mittelschmerz) and dysmenorrhea • Risk of hemoperitoneum • ?Increased incidence of endometriosis, polyps, fibroids	• Postpartum hemorrhage <24h • Postpartum hemorrhage >48h up to 4 weeks • Vulvar hematoma

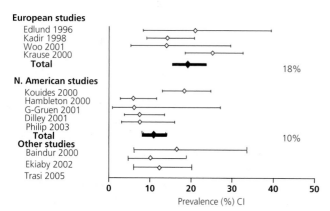

Figure 47.1 Prevalence of von Willebrand disease (VWD) in adult females presenting with heavy menstrual bleeding (HMB). CI, confidence intervals. The specific study citations can be found in [8]. Adapted from [8]. Reproduced with permission of John Wiley and Sons.

Table 47.2 Significant bleeding symptoms in women with von Willebrand disease (VWD).

	Study population	Symptoms more common in VWD patients than in non-VWD patients
Royal Free London, 1998 [21]	26/150 women presenting with heavy menstrual bleeding subsequently diagnosed with VWD (n = 26, presumed all type 1)	• Bruising • Dental-related bleeding • Surgical-related bleeding • Postpartum hemorrhage • Heavy menstrual bleeding since menarche • Multiple bleeding symptoms
Upstate NY Hemophilia Treatment Centers study, 2000 [5]	81 menstruating women registered at hemophilia treatment center, all type 1 VWD compared to a cohort of 150 menstruating volunteers	• Age (the younger the age, the higher the probability of VWD) • History of dental-related bleeding • Past or present history of anemia • A diminished quality of life during menses in relation to family activities
Centers for Disease Control, Atlanta, 2002 [22]	102 women with VWD registered at HTC compared to 88 controls	• Surgical-related bleeding • Excessive gum bleeding • Bleeding after minor injuries

the blood group. There is also an age-dependent increase in the VWF level independent of race [17]. However, the mean age of this study group was 26 ± 5.5 years so it is not known if this increase of VWF levels continues towards menopause.

Clinical characteristics

Women with VWD certainly have a very high relative risk of HMB compared to the general population and the prevalence of HMB by subjective report has been between 78% and 97% in women primarily with type 1 VWD [3,5]. Using the more objective pictorial blood assessment chart (PBAC) it has been reported that 78% of patients with VWD (primarily type 1) had evidence for HMB [3].

Women with VWD use more tampons and pads than non-VWD menstruating women and have frequent staining of

underclothes [5] and (28–66% [5,20]). Table 47.2 summarizes the prevalence of these bleeding symptoms in comparison to a control group of non-VWD women from several studies showing a higher prevalence of anemia and a much higher frequency of other mucocutaneous bleeding symptoms [5,21,22].

Women with type 2 and type 3 VWD have not been as extensively studied as the type 1 patients. A recent nationwide cross-sectional study of a total of 423 women with moderate to severe VWD in the Netherlands reported HMB in 81% and 20% necessitated a hysterectomy [23]. In the more common type 1 patient with even milder depression of the VWF level, there is still a relatively high rate (8–26%) of hysterectomy for control of HMB among type 1 patients [3,5,20,22]. In a case–control study of 102 women with VWD carried out by the American Centers for Disease Control (CDC), 26% had undergone hysterectomy compared with 9% of controls [22]. In two studies, there was also underlying uterine pathology noted in the hysterectomy specimen where it can be postulated that mild VWD may "unmask" a uterine fibroid [3,5]. In the CDC study, a statistically higher rate of fibroids compared to age-matched controls (32% vs 17%) was noted [22]. There may also be a higher prevalence of endometriosis (30% vs 10%), endometrial hyperplasia (10% vs 1%), and endometrial polyps (8% vs 1%) in VWD women compared to controls [22]. It has been hypothesized that VWD may exacerbate the presumed retrograde menstrual flow implicated in the pathophysiology of endometriosis [24]. The higher prevalence of endometrial hyperplasia and polyps in VWD women has been explained in terms of the VWD "unmasking" these lesions [24].

Regarding psychosocial aspects, several studies comprising over 300 patients with VWD compared to non-VWD women has shown unequivocally that these women do have impaired QOL [5,22,25]. Dysmenorrhea has been noted in approximately half [5,20]. A high rate of midcycle pain, termed "Mittelschmerz", has also been noted in women with VWD [5]; and these patients can develop an acute surgical abdomen from hemoperitoneum due to bleeding into the corpus luteum with subsequent rupture [26]. A report from Sweden showed that 9/136 women with VWD (6.8%) experienced hemorrhagic ovarian cysts [27]. There have also been reports of bleeding into the broad ligament with the patient presenting with a positive iliopsoas sign [28].

Management of von Willebrand disease-related heavy menstrual bleeding

An algorithm for the management of HMB adapted from a consensus panel is presented in Figure 47.2 [4].

Hemostatic agents (antifibrinolytic therapy, desmopressin, von Willebrand factor-containing plasma concentrates)

Since HMB is characterized by increased fibrinolysis of the menstrual fluid, tranexamic acid (TA) has been a mainstay of treatment for decades for the general HMB population [29]. There is also a new sustained-release formulation of TA available in the USA (Lysteda) that has been approved there for the general HMB population dosed at two tablets of 650 mg/tablet three times a day for the first 5 days of menses. Menstrual blood flow (MBL) was reduced 41% compared to 8% in the placebo arm accompanied by significant improvements in numerous QOL parameters [30].

Regarding desmopressin (DDAVP), in nonrandomized cohort studies, DDAVP has been reported by patient self-assessment as "excellent"/"very effective" in approximately two-thirds of patients with subcutaneous or intranasal (IN) use [31]. However, in 30 women with VWD-related HMB using the PBAC in a randomized control cross-over study, there was no difference in bleeding severity when IN-DDAVP was compared to placebo [32]. Regardless of whether the first treatment period involved the placebo or the IN-DDAVP, there was a reduction in the PBAC score that was statistically significant ($P = 0.01$). Similar results were noted in a related study of 20 women with HMB and a prolonged bleeding time comparing 300 mcg of IN-DDAVP with placebo [33]. There was no statistically significant decrease in MBL spectrophotometrically with DDAVP, compared with the placebo. However, there was a statistically significant decrease in bleeding when DDAVP was combined with TA [33].

In summary, more objective measurements of efficacy have not shown as great a benefit of IN-DDAVP for VWD-related HMB compared to prior studies using subjective assessment as the endpoint of efficacy. A relatively large multicenter US cross-over trial of women with abnormal laboratory hemostasis (including VWD) comparing IN-DDAVP and TA using the PBAC for assessment of MBL and four previously validated QOL measures were carried out [34]. Both medications reduced MBL and improved QOL among females with HMB and abnormal laboratory hemostasis, but TA proved to be more effective

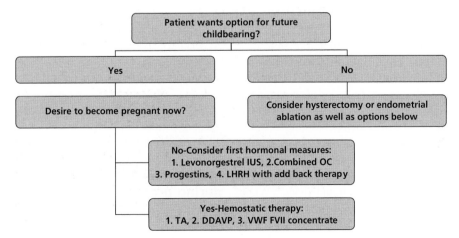

Figure 47.2 Algorithm of von Willebrand disease (VWD)-related heavy menstrual bleeding (HMB). DDAVP, desmopressin; FVII, factor VII; LHRH, lutenizing hormone releasing hormone; OC, oral contraceptive; TA, tranexamic acid; VWF, von Willebrand factor. Adapted from [4]. Reproduced with permission of Elsevier.

than IN-DDAVP [34]. In further improving the efficacy of these hemostatic agents for HMB, study of the efficacy and safety of combined therapy of IN-DDAVP and antifibrinolytic therapy or also hormonal therapy is in order. Interleukin-11 subcutaneously is also being studied as an option in women with mild VWD and HMB refractory to hemostatic or hormonal agents. A reduction in MBL by the PBAC >50% was observed in a pilot study of seven patients [35].

Approximately 10–15% of women with VWD will not respond to DDAVP because they either have severe type 1 VWD or type 2 or type 3 VWD. In those patients, for severe intractable HMB refractory to antifibrinolytic therapy and/or hormonal therapy or for prophylaxis before surgery, a plasma-derived VWF containing FVIII concentrate can be administered. The dosing is typically 40–60 units/kg of VWF:RCo units for major surgery and 20–40 u/kg of VWF:RCo units for HMB [36,37].

Hormonal therapy

Combined OC is useful for cycle regulation and inhibition of the growth and development of the endometrium. Conversely, the efficacy of OC in reducing menstrual loss in women with VWD or other bleeding disorders has not been well established [5]. Also, combined OCs have the added advantages of excellent contraception, good cycle control, and reduction in the incidence of dysmenorrhea, premenstrual tension, and cyst rupture. The latter is a rare but potentially life-threatening event (hemoperitoneum) in women with VWD [26]. In the light of those additional benefits, the 2008 National Heart Lung Blood Institute VWD treatment guidelines [36] advise front-line use of OC therapy for the adult or adolescent who does not desire pregnancy but may desire future childbearing. In a recent survey of 319 participants in the US Hemophilia Treatment Center network, OC was used most frequently to treat HMB followed by DDAVP [38].

Besides OCs, progestins may also be useful in high doses alone or in combination with DDAVP or factor concentrate to arrest acute HMB [4]. At this time, the best hormonal-based option for HMB in women with VWD may be the levonorgestrel intrauterine system, Mirena (LNG IUS). Long-term follow-up at the Royal Free Hospital in London of 26 women (of whom half had VWD) with inherited bleeding disorder-related HMB at a median duration of 33 months, showed a decrease in the median PBAC score from 235 (134–683) to 35 (0–89). Hemoglobin values and QOL scores also improved significantly [39]. Whether the underlying bleeding disorder promotes prolonged spotting (median 42 days, 30–90 days) as reported in one case [40] deserves further study as persistent spotting is an indication for removal. Similarly, whether there is a higher expulsion rate in women with underlying VWD is under study presently.

Lastly, endometrial ablation is another gynecologic option short of a hysterectomy [41]. An initial report, a decade ago, albeit of only seven patients with VWD-related HMB, reported a high failure rate in terms of 3/7 necessitating hysterectomy

within a year [42] but a recent study of 12 patients using the "newer" technique of bipolar radiofrequency ablation at a median follow-up of 32 months showed a decrease in the median PBAC from 1208 to 0 with hemoglobin values and QOL scores also improved significantly. None of the patients to date have failed to the point necessitating hysterectomy [43].

Obstetric aspects

It has been well established that part of the "physiologic response" in pregnancy is a progressive elevation of FVIII and VWF level [2]. However, it should be stressed that there is proportionately less elevation in the levels compared to those in the normal pregnant patient. Consequently and not surprisingly, a higher rate of postpartum hemorrhage (PPH) of 16–29% [1,5,28] vs 3–5% in the general population has been reported, in the first 24 h following delivery. This meets or exceeds the criteria for primary PPH [1]. Also, there appears to be a higher rate in type 2 (three patients) compared to type 1 patients [1,23,28]. This may result in the need for red cell transfusions in between 7% [1] and 17% [5] of type 1 patients.

In an analysis of the US Nationwide Inpatient Sample involving 4067 deliveries among women with VWD (1/4000 deliveries), James and Jamison observed that women with VWD were more likely to experience a PPH (OR 1.5; 95% CI: 1.1, 2.0), and had a fivefold increased risk of being transfused (OR 4.7; 95% CI: 3.2, 7.0). They also observed that women with VWD were more likely to experience antepartum bleeding (OR 10.2, 95% CI: 7.1, 14.6). Five of the 4067 women with VWD died, a maternal mortality rate 10 times higher than that for other women [44]. Besides an increased rate of PPH in VWD women, perineal hematomas appear to be more common [1,28].

The rise in FVIII and VWF levels occur in the second and third trimester so the clinician should not assume that there will not be excessive bleeding during amniocentesis or a first trimester abortion as levels may not have increased at this early gestational time point [45]. The presentation of VWD as transfusion-dependent bleeding at miscarriage has been reported [1]. VWF levels start to decline on day 3 postpartum [46], with excessive bleeding up to 5 weeks postpartum also being reported [5,47,48] with an average onset of delayed hemorrhage in one study of 15.7 ± 5.2 days. Consequently, it should be common practise to remind a postpartum patient of this possibility which may occur as late as 4–6 weeks postpartum.

Management of von Willebrand disease during pregnancy

As noted above, gestational palliation does occur during pregnancy so that if such patient needs a dental extraction during pregnancy or other invasive procedure, DDAVP is not necessary if the VWF levels have "normalized". In cases where the VWF

nucleotides that disrupt the protein reading frame and splice-site mutations that interrupt normal processing of *VWF* mRNA. Missense mutations often affect dimerization or multimerization and generally result in intracellular retention. The majority are located in exons 3–15 and 37–52. Heterozygous relatives of type 3 VWD patients are often asymptomatic even though more than 50% may have VWF levels <50 IU/dL [16] while some have symptoms similar to patients with type 1 VWD.

Type 1

A partial quantitative deficiency of VWF with a normal ∼1:1 ratio of functional activity (VWF:RCo) to quantity of VWF protein (VWF:Ag) and essentially normal HMW multimers characterize type 1 VWD [1]. A heterogeneous array of mutation types and disease mechanisms that are only beginning to be understood are responsible. Mutations have been identified in around 65% of patients examined by large multicenter studies undertaken in Canada, Europe, and the UK [10–13]. Index cases (IC) with lowest VWF levels, some with minor multimer abnormalities, had a detectable *VWF* mutation in virtually all cases; by contrast, of those with VWF levels close to the bottom of the normal range (50 IU/dL), only about 50% had a *VWF* mutation. Between 10% and 15% of IC had more than one candidate mutation (compound heterozygous or allelic mutations) but VWF levels in these individuals were not necessarily any lower than in those with a single heterozygous mutation [10,11,13]. Missense mutations predominated, but a wide range of other mutation types was present, including large in-frame deletions, splice, nonsense, small deletions and insertions, and candidate promoter mutations [9]. Similar mutation categories were seen as in type 3 VWD, but in very different proportions (Figure 48.2).

Two common mutations exemplify type 1 VWD: the fully penetrant dominant negative p.Arg1205His identified in 6% of IC [10–12] that results in very low VWF levels (VWF:RCo and VWF:Ag both often <10 IU/dL) as a result of normal synthesis and secretion but rapid clearance from the plasma. p.Tyr1584Cys, identified in 13% of IC [10–12] results in incompletely penetrant VWD, where VWD diagnosis is more common in individuals who also coinherit ABO blood group O. Slight enhancements to VWF clearance and ADAMTS13 proteolysis contribute to pathogenesis. p.Tyr1584Cys and similar mutations could be regarded as risk factors for bleeding. Blood group O is much more frequent in type 1 VWD cases (65% of European IC) than in the normal population [11], and contributes to reduced plasma VWF level through reduced residence time in comparison with other ABO blood groups.

Type 2

Type 2 VWD comprises qualitative disorders. These predominantly result from missense mutations and occasionally in-frame deletions or insertions that result in a VWF protein of slightly altered size. In addition to the secondary classification into types 2A, 2B, 2M, and 2N, type 2A can be further subclassified

by multimer profile to indicate specific disease mechanisms [1]. Mutation locations are summarized in Figure 48.1.

2A

Mutations in this VWD type lead to decreased VWF-dependent platelet adhesion and a deficiency of HMW multimers. Mutations act through a variety of different mechanisms and can be subclassified according to their multimeric profile, which correlate with different VWF locations. Classic type 2A mutations (2A(IIA)) [1] in or close to the A2 domain encoded by exon 28 enhance VWF cleavage by the metalloprotease ADAMTS13 through altering access to its cleavage site between amino acids (aa) p.Tyr1605-Met 1606, or result in reduced VWF secretion or may combine both mechanisms. A recently recognized location for 2A mutations in the D3 domain (exons 22–27) is reported to include around 30% of 2A defects. These individuals display a characteristic 2A(IIE) multimer profile where the intensity of "triplet" multimer satellite bands produced by ADAMTS13 cleavage of VWF is severely reduced [17]. Mutation mechanisms that may contribute to the phenotype include those affecting secretion, multimerization, clearance, and ADAMTS13 cleavage of VWF [17].

Smaller proportions of mutations are reported in diverse VWF domains. Mutations affecting disulfide bonding required for VWF CK domain dimerization yield aberrant multimer species terminated by VWF monomers. 2A(IID) VWD results from these mutations centered around p.Cys2771–Cys2773 (exon 52) [18]. Mutations in the D2 domain (exons 11–15, aa 404–625) can interfere with intersubunit disulfide bonding resulting in 2A(IIC) VWD [8,14]. Other type 2A missense mutations have been reported in the D1 domain (exons 6–7) [19] and very recently in the D4 and close to the B2 domain (exons 36 and 41) [20]. Additionally, an in-frame exon 9–10 duplication [21], exon 33–34 deletion and a splice mutation that may lead to skipping of exon 26 have been described in this disease type [20], so that full ascertainment of 2A mutations may require DNA sequence analysis of almost the entire VWF coding region along with dosage analysis for deletions/duplications. Most 2A mutations are dominantly inherited, but D2 and some CK mutations display recessive inheritance, requiring a second similar missense mutation or a null allele for symptoms to occur.

2B

2B mutations in this dominantly inherited VWD type have increased affinity for platelet GPIbα, evidenced in the laboratory through ristocetin-induced platelet aggregation (RIPA) at low ristocetin concentrations (≤0.7 mg/mL). This may be the only feature that identifies this disease type, but thrombocytopenia may be present in about 30% of cases, and this proportion increases with stress resulting from infection, surgery, pregnancy, and so on [22]. The transient appearance or aggravation of thrombocytopenia can result in increased bleeding risk. Following secretion, VWF may bind spontaneously to platelets through GPIbα which facilitates VWF cleavage by ADAMTS13, and can lead to loss of the HMW, most hemostatically active multimers. Occupation of platelet GPIbα receptors by soluble VWF leaves them unable to interact with VWF tethered to collagen at sites of blood vessel damage and this may contribute to symptoms. Mutations are within or close to the A1 domain and result in its conformational change. All are dominantly inherited missense changes with the exception of one reported in-frame insertion. The VWFdb lists 25 missense alterations affecting only 15 different aa between codons 1266 and 1461 [14]. Phenotypes associated with different mutations, including baseline and poststress platelet count and bleeding severity scores, have been investigated [22].

A genocopy (identical phenotype produced by two different genes) of the disorder, platelet-type VWD (PT-VWD) results from mutations in *GP1BA*, the gene encoding GPIbα. Missense mutations affecting only two different amino acids, p.Gly249 and p.Met255 along with a 27-bp in-frame deletion p.Pro449_Ser457del have been reported [23]. A variety of mixing tests to identify whether VWF or GPIbα is defective can be used for differential diagnosis, as can genetic analysis [23]. An international registry study analysed patients diagnosed with 2B VWD/PT-VWD and identified 2B VWD in 48% of 100 unrelated cases, other *VWF* exon 28 mutations in 8% and PT-VWD in 15%; misdiagnosis where no mutation was found in the targeted regions of either gene accounted for 26%, while one individual had acquired VWD [24].

2M

Patients with 2M VWD have decreased VWF-dependent platelet adhesion without deficiency of HMW multimers [1]. Dominantly inherited missense mutations that disrupt VWF binding to platelets or to subendothelium are responsible. This subtype is difficult to diagnose; good measurements of ability of VWF to bind GpIbα (VWF:RCo) or collagen (VWF:CB) relative to the quantity of VWF protein (VWF:Ag) along with a multimer profile demonstrating presence of HMW multimers are required. Missense mutations that reduce VWF:RCo are predominantly in the A1 domain (aa 1266–1549) while those few reported in the A3 domain reducing VWF:CB affect the short sequence between aa 1731 and 1786 [14,19,25]. There are also isolated case reports in the D3, A2, and CK domains. Differing sensitivities of VWF:CB assays to collagen-binding defects and lack of inclusion of VWF:CB assays in laboratory repertoire likely result in such patients being underrecognized.

2N

Mutations in VWD type 2N markedly decrease binding affinity for FVIII and result in low plasma FVIII, whilst VWF levels can be within the normal range. This disease type can be challenging to discriminate from mild hemophilia A in males and hemophilia A carriership in females unless a clear familial inheritance pattern is present, but the VWF-FVIII binding assay can

discriminate the disorders. The FVIII-binding domain was mapped to the first 272 residues of mature VWF (aa 764–1035) [1], but mutation location indicates that the area of VWF that can reduce FVIII binding extends further (aa 760–1225) [14]; 28 mutations affecting 24 different aa have been reported [14,19].

Two mutations are required for this recessively inherited VWD subtype: it can result from two missense mutations both of which disrupt FVIII binding or more commonly a missense plus a null allele. Mutations are predominantly in exons 18–20, with the remainder being in exons 17, 24, 25, and 27. A small proportion of mutations, notably those leading to loss of cysteine also result in loss of HMW multimers (e.g. p.Cys788Arg, p.Cys1060Arg/Tyr, p.Cys1225Gly) [14,19] whereas multimers in most cases are normal [26].

Mechanisms of mutation

Table 48.1 summarizes some of the characteristics of the *VWF* gene and protein which result in susceptibility to particular mutations. Many of these are common to other genes and proteins, whereas a few such as gene conversion represent more unusual mutation types. Some are described below.

Large deletions and duplications

Large deletions (of at least one *VWF* exon) were the first VWD mutation types identified. Southern blotting initially characterized deletions, but the exact size of the deleted region and mutation mechanism could not be ascertained. Furthermore, large deletions were underrecognized due to the difficulty of identifying them in heterozygotes in the presence of a non-deleted *VWF* allele.

Utilization of gene dosage techniques such as multiplex ligation-dependent probe amplification (MLPA) has allowed detection of dosage mutations affecting only one *VWF* allele. Large deletions contribute to all three VWD types: in type 3 VWD, deletions comprise 9% of reported mutations and most result in loss of VWF expression. In types 1 and 2 VWD, reported deletions are in-frame [27–30] and those expressed *in vitro* result in a dominant negative effect on VWF secretion and function [29,30]. Large deletions appear to also be fairly common in type 1 VWD; comprising 4% of mutations in the European type 1 VWD study [31]. Gene dosage analysis also allows detection of large duplication events. An in-frame duplication of exons 9–10 reported in type 2A(IIC) [21] suggests that other large duplications may contribute to VWD pathogenesis.

Recently identified deletions have been precisely mapped and their mechanism identified as homologous unequal recombination between *Alu* repeats [32]. Short mobile genetic elements that are very frequent in the human genome, initially recognized by the restriction enzyme *Alu* I, have been shown to be involved in the pathogenesis of some *VWF* deletions [30,33,34].

Table 48.1 von Willebrand factor (VWF) features resulting in susceptibility to particular mutations.

Feature	Detail	Result	Mutation location
Large gene size	Coding & flanking regions >180 kb	*VWF* presents a large target for mutations	*VWF*
Repetitive elements within introns	Repetitive elements including *Alu* repeats within *VWF* introns	Homologous recombination can result in large gene deletions	5' UTR & introns
Small nucleotide runs	Direct (particularly polypyrimidine) and inverted repeats susceptible to DNA polymerase replication errors	Nucleotide repeat sequences common site of small deletion & insertion mutations	Repeated nucleotides
CpG dinucleotides	Deamination of 5-methylcytosine to thymine results in C>T or G>A mutations being common	Many point mutations occur at CpG dinucleotides. Mutations affecting arginine codons (CGN) overrepresented	CpG sequences
Partial pseudogene	*VWFP* 97% similar to exons 23–34 & located on separate chromosome (22). *VWF* close to chromosome 12 telomere. Chi-like sequences in *VWF* and *VWFP*	Gene conversions affecting intron 27 & exon 28 are common	3' end of intron 27 to 5' end of exon 28
Transcription factor binding sites (TFBS)	Disruption of TFBS	Lack of/reduced mRNA transcription from one allele	5' UTR
Splice sites	Disruption of normal splicing	Can result in intron retention (null allele), exon skipping sometimes resulting in in-frame deletion, or cryptic splice site activation	Sequence surrounding splice junctions
Signal peptide cleavage by signal peptidase	Disruption/loss of cleavage	May result in VWF misfolding due to signal peptide retention	Not yet reported
VWF dimerization	VWF forms tail to tail dimers through disulfide bonds in the CK domain	Point mutation, particularly missense changes can disrupt VWF dimerization, (2A(IID))	CK domain
VWF multimerization	VWF forms head to head multimers through disulfide bonds between D3 domains	Point mutation, particularly missense changes can disrupt VWF multimerization, (2A (IIE & IIC))	D3 and D2 domains
Propeptide cleavage by Furin	Lack of propeptide cleavage from mature VWF	VWF-FVIII binding disrupted by steric hindrance	D' domain
Disulfide bonds	VWF contains 163 cysteines, all involved in intra- or interchain disulfide bonds	Cys loss or gain disrupts normal disulfide pairing. Mutations may result in lack of multimerization or multimer abnormalities	Cys residues, other residues which can be mutated to Cys
VWF cleavage by ADAMTS13	Enhancement of susceptibility to cleavage by VWF-cleaving metalloprotease, ADAMTS13	Missense changes in A domains enhance accessibility of p.Tyr1505-Met 1506 bond to cleavage	A2, also A1 & A3
VWF ligand binding sites	Disruption/enhancement of VWF binding to ligands including GpIbα, FVIII & collagen	Point mutations, particularly missense changes and in-frame deletions/insertions disrupt/enhance VWF function	Functional sites particularly in A, D' and D3 domains
VWF clearance from plasma	Enhanced VWF clearance from plasma	Missense changes, particularly in the D3 domain enhance VWF clearance by cells including macrophages [40]	Predominantly D3, D4 also reported

UTR, untranslated region.

von Willebrand factor pseudogene and gene conversion

Gene conversion is a reasonably common mutation mechanism in VWD. A short stretch of the *VWFP* sequence invades the gene sequence and replaces it [35], evidenced by sequential nucleotide substitutions that match pseudogene sequence. Chi-like 8-bp sequences in intron 27 and exon 28 are thought to promote conversion, as does the proximity of *VWF* to the chromosome 12 telomere and *VWFP* residing on a separate chromosome [35]. Two consecutive *VWF* nucleotide substitu-

tions corresponding to *VWFP* sequence can indicate that a conversion is likely to have occurred. Minimum and maximum extents of conversion can be deduced from examination of *VWF* and *VWFP* sequence differences and range from 8 bp to 517 bp [36], the latter having nine consecutive nucleotide substitutions originating in *VWFP* between c.3931C>T and c.4324A>G.

Phenotype resulting from gene conversion depends on the range of nucleotide replacements and consequent aa substitutions. Those incorporating p.Val1229Gly result in reduced VWF levels and have been classified as either type 1 or 2M VWD. Conversions including p.Pro1266Leu (or less frequently p.Pro1266Gln) result in mild type 2B (New York/Malmo variations) whereas those incorporating p.Gln1311* result in a nonsense mutation that has been reported in several type 3 VWD patients [14,19].

5' untranslated region

Recent type 1 VWD studies [10–12] were the first to examine the *VWF* untranslated region (5' UTR) in a significant number of patients and several single nucleotide variants have been identified (8% of type 1 cases on VWFdb); however, it is not yet known whether these affect *VWF* transcription significantly. However, the Canadian study identified a type 1 patient heterozygous for a deletion of 13 nucleotides from c.-1522_-1510, 48bp 5' of the mRNA transcription start site [12]. It disrupts a transcription factor binding site (TFBS) resulting in reduced VWF transcription [37]. Even though traditional *VWF* molecular analysis has mostly focused on protein coding exons and closely flanking intronic sequence, the 5' UTR may be an additional site that should be examined for candidate quantitative mutations.

Timing of genetic analysis

Where access to phenotype information is good and its results allow clear VWD categorization facilitating choice of appropriate treatment, genetic analysis is not required. For those patients where VWD type is unclear or where differential diagnosis is needed (e.g. between type 2N VWD and hemophilia A; between type 2B and PT-VWD), genetic analysis may be helpful in clarifying the cause of the patient's bleeding [38]. Additionally, identification of the causative mutation in an IC can facilitate analysis of family members and help to highlight their risk of bleeding associated with familial mutation(s). In type 3 VWD, genetic analysis can enable prenatal diagnosis.

Many laboratories currently offer targeted sequence analysis of selected exons when seeking mutations, particularly in type 2 VWD. In these instances, mutations may not be identified in all patients, especially where there are multiple possible mutation locations as in type 2A. In a recent analysis of *VWF* exon 28, the major location for mutations in types 2A, 2B, and 2M, mutations were detected in 41% of 56 patients with type 2 VWD [39]. Full analysis of patients with types 1 and 3 VWD for possible mutations currently consists of determination of the presence of large deletions/duplications using dosage analysis plus DNA sequence analysis of the proximal promoter, all 52 exons and intron/exon boundaries. In a recent study of German VWD patients where the entire coding region plus promoter were analysed and dosage analysis was undertaken for patients lacking clear causative mutations, mutation detection rates were 68% in 28 type 1 IC, 94% in 32 type 2 IC, and 94% in 18 type 3 IC [20].

Summary

The large multifunctional VWF protein is encoded by the extensive *VWF* gene. Gene structure and protein functional domains provide scope for many different mutation types, resulting in the diverse array of VWD types and mutation mechanisms responsible. Despite extensive analyses, these remain incompletely understood.

Acknowledgments

The author's research on VWD is funded by the NIH grant Zimmerman Program for the Molecular and Clinical Biology of von Willebrand Disease (ZPMCB-VWD); P01 HL81588.

References

1 Sadler JE, Budde U, Eikenboom JC, *et al*. Update on the pathophysiology and classification of von Willebrand disease: a report of the Subcommittee on von Willebrand Factor. *J Thromb Haemost* 2006; **4**: 2103–14.

2 Sadler JE. Biochemistry and genetics of von Willebrand factor. *Annu Rev Biochem* 1998; **67**: 395–424.

3 Zhou YF, Eng ET, Zhu J, *et al*. Sequence and structure relationships within von Willebrand factor. *Blood* 2012; **120**: 449–58.

4 Bloom AL. von Willebrand factor: clinical features of inherited and acquired disorders. *Mayo Clin Proc* 1991; **66**: 743–51.

5 Bowman M, Hopman WM, Rapson D, *et al*. The prevalence of symptomatic von Willebrand disease in primary care practice. *J Thromb Haemost* 2010; **8**: 213–16.

6 Rodeghiero F. von Willebrand disease: still an intriguing disorder in the era of molecular medicine. *Haemophilia* 2002; **8**: 292–300.

7 Hampshire DJ, Goodeve AC. The international society on thrombosis and haematosis von Willebrand disease database: an update. *Semin Thromb Hemost* 2011; **37**: 470–9.

8 Meyer D, Fressinaud E, Gaucher C, *et al*. Gene defects in 150 unrelated French cases with type 2 von Willebrand disease: from the patient to the gene. INSERM Network on Molecular Abnormalities in von Willebrand Disease. *Thromb Haemost* 1997; **78**: 451–6.

9 Goodeve AC. The genetic basis of von Willebrand disease. *Blood Rev* 2010; **24**: 123–34.

10 Cumming A, Grundy P, Keeney S, *et al*. An investigation of the von Willebrand factor genotype in UK patients diagnosed to have type 1 von Willebrand disease. *Thromb Haemost* 2006; **96**: 630–41.

11 Goodeve A, Eikenboom J, Castaman G, *et al*. Phenotype and genotype of a cohort of families historically diagnosed with type 1 von Willebrand disease in the European study, Molecular and Clinical Markers for the Diagnosis and Management of Type 1 von Willebrand Disease (MCMDM-1VWD). *Blood* 2007; **109**: 112–21.

12 James PD, Notley C, Hegadorn C, *et al*. The mutational spectrum of type 1 von Willebrand disease: Results from a Canadian cohort study. *Blood* 2007; **109**: 145–54.

13 Robertson JD, Yenson PR, Rand ML, *et al*. Expanded phenotype-genotype correlations in a pediatric population with type 1 von Willebrand disease. *J Thromb Haemost* 2011; **9**: 1752–60.

14 VWFdb. International Society on Thrombosis and Haemostasis Scientific and Standardization Committee VWF Information Homepage. Accessed 10 December 2012. Available from: www.vwf.group.shef.ac.uk

15 GeneTests Web site. Accessed 10 November 2012. Available from: http://www.ncbi.nlm.nih.gov/gtr/

16 Nichols WL, Hultin MB, James AH, *et al.* von Willebrand disease (VWD): evidence-based diagnosis and management guidelines, the National Heart, Lung, and Blood Institute (NHLBI) Expert Panel report (USA). *Haemophilia* 2008; **14**: 171–232.

17 Schneppenheim R, Michiels JJ, Obser T, *et al.* A cluster of mutations in the D3 domain of von Willebrand factor correlates with a distinct subgroup of von Willebrand disease: type 2A/IIE. *Blood* 2010; **115**: 4894–901.

18 Schneppenheim R, Brassard J, Krey S, *et al.* Defective dimerization of von Willebrand factor subunits due to a Cys-> Arg mutation in type IID von Willebrand disease. *Proc Natl Acad Sci USA* 1996; **93**: 3581–6.

19 HGMD. The Human Gene Mutation Database. Accessed 16 October 2012. Available from: http://www.biobase-international.com/product/hgmd

20 Yadegari H, Driesen J, Pavlova A, *et al.* Mutation distribution in the von Willebrand factor gene related to the different von Willebrand disease (VWD) types in a cohort of VWD patients. *Thromb Haemost* 2012; **108**: 662–71.

21 Schneppenheim R, Ledford-Kraemer M, Lavergne J-M, *et al.* Identification of the elusive mutation causing the historical von Willebrand disease type IIC miami. *J Thromb Haemost* 2011; **9**: (abstract P-WE-461).

22 Federici AB, Mannucci PM, Castaman G, *et al.* Clinical and molecular predictors of thrombocytopenia and risk of bleeding in patients with von Willebrand disease type 2B: a cohort study of 67 patients. *Blood* 2009; **113**: 526–34.

23 Othman M, Hamilton A. Platelet-type von Willebrand disease: results of a worldwide survey from the Canadian PT-VWD project. *Acta Haematol* 2010; **123**: 126–8.

24 Hamilton A, Ozelo M, Leggo J, *et al.* Frequency of platelet type versus type 2B von Willebrand disease. An international registry-based study. *Thromb Haemost* 2011; **105**: 501–8.

25 Keeling D, Beavis J, Marr R, *et al.* A family with type 2M VWD with normal VWF:RCo but reduced VWF:CB and a M1761K mutation in the A3 domain. *Haemophilia* 2012; **18**: e33.

26 Goodeve A. von Willebrand disease: molecular aspects. In: Lee C, Berntorp E, Hoots K (eds.) *Textbook of Haemophilia*, 2nd edn. Oxford: Wiley, 2010.

27 Yadegari H, Driesen J, Hass M, *et al.* Large deletions identified in patients with von Willebrand disease using multiple ligation-dependent probe amplification. *J Thromb Haemost* 2011; **9**: 1083–6.

28 Hampshire DJ, Bloomer LD, Al-Buhairan AM, *et al.* Investigation of the role of copy number variation in the pathogenesis of type 1 von Willebrand disease. *ASH Annual Meeting Abstracts* 2010; **116**: 2218.

29 Casari C, Pinotti M, Lancellotti S, *et al.* The dominant-negative von Willebrand factor gene deletion p.P1127_C1948delinsR: molecular mechanism and modulation. *Blood* 2010; **116**: 5371–6.

30 Sutherland MS, Cumming AM, Bowman M, *et al.* A novel deletion mutation is recurrent in von Willebrand disease types 1 and 3. *Blood* 2009; **114**: 1091–8.

31 Hampshire DJ, Cartwright A, Bloomer LD, *et al.* Copy number variation is a significant contributor to type 1 VWD pathogenesis in the EU MCMDM-1VWD cohort. *J Thromb Haemost* 2011; **9**: (abstract O-MO-138).

32 Cooper DN. Human gene mutation in pathology and evolution. *J Inherit Metab Dis* 2002; **25**: 157–82.

33 Xie F, Wang X, Cooper DN, *et al.* A novel Alu-mediated 61-kb deletion of the von Willebrand factor (VWF) gene whose breakpoints co-locate with putative matrix attachment regions. *Blood Cells Mol Dis* 2006; **36**: 385–91.

34 Mohl A, Marschalek R, Masszi T, *et al.* An Alu-mediated novel large deletion is the most frequent cause of type 3 von Willebrand disease in Hungary. *J Thromb Haemost* 2008; **6**: 1729–35.

35 Chen JM, Cooper DN, Chuzhanova N, *et al.* Gene conversion: mechanisms, evolution and human disease. *Nat Rev Genet* 2007; **8**: 762–75.

36 Sutherland MS, Keeney S, Bolton-Maggs PH, *et al.* The mutation spectrum associated with type 3 von Willebrand disease in a cohort of patients from the north west of England. *Haemophilia* 2009; **15**: 1048–57.

37 Othman M, Chirinian Y, Brown C, *et al.* Functional characterization of a 13-bp deletion (c.-1522_-1510del13) in the promoter of the von Willebrand factor gene in type 1 von Willebrand disease. *Blood* 2010; **116**: 3645–52.

38 Keeney S, Bowen D, Cumming A, *et al.* The molecular analysis of von Willebrand disease: a guideline from the UK Haemophilia Centre Doctors' Organisation Haemophilia Genetics Laboratory Network. *Haemophilia* 2008; **14**: 1099–111.

39 Ahmad F, Jan R, Kannan M, *et al.* Characterisation of mutations and molecular studies of type 2 von Willebrand disease. *Thromb Haemost* 2013; **109**: 39–46.

40 van Schooten CJ, Shahbazi S, Groot E, *et al.* Macrophages contribute to the cellular uptake of von Willebrand factor and factor VIII in vivo. *Blood* 2008; **112**: 1704–12.

CHAPTER 49

von Willebrand disease: epidemiology

Francesco Rodeghiero and Giancarlo Castaman
San Bortolo Hospital, Vicenza, Italy

Introduction

In 1926, Erik von Willebrand investigated a family with a new bleeding disorder, later universally known as von Willebrand disease (VWD) in recognition of his pioneering discovery [1]. At that time, he was probably unaware that he was studying what would be recognized 60 years later as the most frequent inherited hemorrhagic disorder. Indeed, VWD is high in the differential diagnosis of patients presenting with mild bleeding symptoms and a prevalence up to 1% has been estimated in a large epidemiologic investigation conducted by our group in 1987 [2]. However, a clear-cut diagnosis of VWD often remains difficult or elusive, because of the wide spectrum of clinical and laboratory manifestations and variable penetrance and expressivity in its inheritance. Unfortunately, in this regard recent molecular characterization of the disease does not provide practical guidance for diagnosis.

For these reasons, the actual prevalence of clinically significant cases of VWD is uncertain despite the ever-increasing number of diagnostic laboratory tools. Prevalence estimates are critically influenced by the clinical criteria used to select subjects and also by the laboratory criteria to confirm the diagnosis. Moreover, the assessment of the bleeding history is often more difficult in the epidemiologic than in the clinical setting. Physicians must rely on the patient's bleeding history, which is confounded by personal recollection (recall bias), unless subjects have suffered from severe hemorrhages, possibly leading to hospitalization. Until recently, no clinical methods were available to objectively quantitate mild or intermediate bleeding symptoms, with the possible exception of surgical bleeding and menorrhagia [3] which have validated methods for quantification of bleeding. The number of symptoms reported by a patient may be influenced by his/her education, family setting (e.g. some symptoms may be underreported by subjects belonging to a bleeding family) and personality, but also by the type of data ascertainment. For example, as many as 23% of Swedish girls reported three or more hemorrhagic symptoms when a self-reported questionnaire was used [4]. In contrast, when a physician-managed questionnaire was used to query these same young women, three or more hemorrhagic symptoms were reported in fewer than 1% of normal control subjects [5]. Hence, stringent clinical criteria and standardized questionnaires to assure interobserver reproducibility have the highest likelihood of achieving complete ascertainment [6]. Thus, it is important to understand the potential pitfalls that arise in prevalence estimation of VWD in relation to its clinical presentation. The use of different methods for prevalence estimation may indeed produce divergent results, with far lower prevalence figures obtained in hospital-based investigations in comparison with population-based investigations, since different categories of subjects are considered (Figure 49.1).

Ascertainment and validity of epidemiologic data

von Willebrand disease is usually classified into three types on the basis of clinical and laboratory phenotypes. Type 1, accounting for the large majority of cases, is represented by partial quantitative defects; type 2 by qualitative defects; and type 3 by virtual absence of von Willebrand factor (VWF) in plasma [7]. In practise, qualitative defects are suspected by measuring a significantly reduced VWF ristocetin cofactor activity to antigen ratio and confirmed by assessing the distribution of high/ intermediate/low-molecular-weight VWF multimers or more subtle abnormalities. This allows subclassification of type 2 into 2A (lack of high- and intermediate-molecular-weight multimers), 2B (lack of high-molecular-weight multimers), 2M (all species of multimers present), or more rare variants [8]. However, from the point of view of clinical presentation and diagnostic approach, three distinct groups of VWD patients may be considered (Table 49.1).

In the first group (*group A*), patients present with a life-long history of severe to moderate bleeding symptoms, often requiring hospitalization for transfusion, replacement therapy, surgical intervention (e.g. nose packing for epistaxis, dilatation and

Textbook of Hemophilia, Third Edition. Edited by Christine A. Lee, Erik E. Berntorp and W. Keith Hoots.
© 2014 John Wiley & Sons, Ltd. Published 2014 by John Wiley & Sons, Ltd.

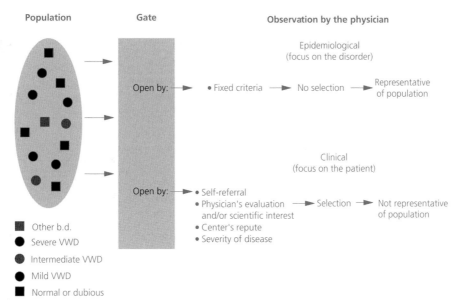

Figure 49.1 How the criteria used for the identification of patients to be investigated for von Willebrand disease (VWD) affects the prevalence estimates of the disease.

Table 49.1 Classification of von Willebrand disease (VWD) according to clinical presentation and diagnostic approach.

	Severe VWD (group A)	Intermediate VWD (group B)	Mild VWD (group C)
Symptoms	Manifest bleeding	Intermediate	Mild or very mild
Cosegregation (linkage) of symptoms with low VWF/haplotype	Invariable	Variable	Inconsistent
VWF levels	About 10 IU/dL or less	About 30 IU/dL	40–50 IU/dL
Diagnosis	Easy	Repeated testing needed	Not always possible; not clinically useful in most cases
Epidemiologic ascertainment	Referral-based: appropriate	Referral-based: underestimated	Cross-sectional: overestimated

VWF, von Willebrand factor.

curettage in women for menorrhagia). Iron-deficiency anemia is also common, especially in women. Laboratory investigations show VWF activity levels below or around 10 IU/dL. Linkage with a mutant VWF gene is usually complete as well as the likelihood of detecting a specific VWF mutation [9]. This group of patients includes recessive type 3 VWD, some dominant type 1 patients with full penetrance and expressivity (including the Vicenza type), and most type 2A and 2B VWD patients. Prevalence estimates for these patients may be reliably obtained from hospital-based cohorts, as it is highly unlikely that these patients have ever been referred to a specialized secondary coagulation center, at least in Western countries.

The second group of patients (*group B*) comprises subjects with a milder but still definite bleeding phenotype. These patients may have frequent spontaneous bleeding episodes (such as mucocutaneous bleeding) and may be referred for bleeding after trauma or minor surgery, especially when mucous membranes are involved. Laboratory investigations typically show VWF activity levels around 30 IU/dL. Linkage analysis

with mutations in the *VWF* gene is consistent with an autosomal dominant disease with variable penetrance in most cases [10,11]. Most subjects with type 1 and some with type 2 VWD are included in this group. Prevalence estimates for these patients are partly underestimated from hospital-based cohorts, because some patients may never seek hospital evaluation, resulting in a falsely low prevalence. Very large cross-sectional (population-based) investigations should be used to identify this cohort group.

The third group of patients (*group C*) comprises patients with a quite mild hemorrhagic phenotype (bleeding score around 1). Bleeding symptoms are occasional, sometimes absent even after trauma or minor surgery. Laboratory investigation shows VWF activity levels around 40–50 IU/dL, and repeated measurements and adjustment for ABO group to achieve an accurate diagnosis are often required. Linkage analysis fails to detect association with VWF haplotype in up to 50% of the families, indicating a possibly spurious association [12]. Family investigations and standardized diagnostic tools (e.g. bleeding questionnaire) are of utmost importance in trying to achieve a definite diagnosis. Indeed, in most group C patients, we could demonstrate by using a Bayesian approach developed by our group [13] that even in the presence of two family members (including the proband) with VWF levels just below 40 IU/dL), a final odds ratio of VWD of approximately 2.0 would be produced (false-positive equals true-positive rates). This creates a need for setting more stringent clinical criteria to achieve a "useful" diagnosis, thereby avoiding mislabeling with the stigmata of a definite genetic diagnosis on subjects with a small risk of minor bleeding.

Prevalence of severe von Willebrand disease (group A)

Most cases of clinically moderate to severe VWD are represented by type 3 and some cases with type 1, type 2A, and 2B VWD. The prevalence of type 3 VWD is very low, ranging from 0.1 to 5.3 per million in the population. Weiss *et al.* reported in 1982 a prevalence of 1.53 and 1.38 per million of severe VWD in Europe and North America, respectively, based on the report from 195 referral centers worldwide [14]. A subsequent re-evaluation of these subjects through measurement of VWF:Ag with a highly sensitive method (immunoradiometric assay) showed a prevalence of severe VWD (defined by an antigen level <1 U/dL) of 0.45 per million [15]. Significant differences in the prevalence of severe VWD were present in different countries, notably with a higher prevalence in Scandinavian countries (2.4–3.12 per million) [15]. The highest prevalence of type 3 VWD was, however, observed by Berliner *et al.* [16] in Arabs, in whom consanguinity is rather frequent, with an estimated prevalence of 5.3 per million.

No data are available about the prevalence of type 2 VWD, while the prevalence of severe type 1 (e.g. VWF level <10 U/dL) could be higher than previously believed. For example, VWD Vicenza (R1205H), an increasingly frequently recognized mutation across several countries, has been identified at our center in 98 patients from a resident population of 807 000 inhabitants, leading to a rough estimation of 12 cases/100 000 inhabitants, somewhat greater than the prevalence of hemophilia A. This estimate appears reliable since all the patients and relatives undergo extended family studies to identify early potential patients who will require specific treatment or prophylaxis for invasive procedures. These estimates could be biased by the presence of a founder effect; nevertheless this situation could occur with other mutations in other countries.

Prevalence of intermediate von Willebrand disease (group B)

Like for severe VWD, prevalence estimates for intermediate VWD are available only from hospital-based cohorts: these are

Table 49.2 Prevalence of referred von Willebrand disease. Modified from [18]. Reproduced with permission of Elsevier.

Area	Population (million)	Patients reported	Corrected prevalence, per million
Scandinavia	21.5	4749	239
Rest of Europe	441	6514	23
Australasia	16	599	42
North America	237	2263	22
Israel	3.5	106	60.4
Far East	286	1673	8.1
South America	133	600	3.7
South Africa	24	80	7.4

calculated as the number of patients registered at a single specialized center, divided by the total population served by the center. The first data published with this methodology date to 1984, when Nilsson estimated that there were about 530 known cases (230 families) of VWD in Sweden, corresponding to a prevalence of seven VWD patients per 100 000 inhabitants, the same figure as for hemophilia in that country [17]. This study, however, also included patients with type 3. In 1991, Bloom and Giddins [18] carried out an international survey of the prevalence of acquired immune deficiency syndrome (AIDS) in VWD, trying to indirectly estimate the prevalence of VWD. A questionnaire was dispatched to the hemophilia center directors of 59 countries and information was received from 63% of the centers (37 countries) concerning 16 664 identified patients, of whom 7534 were treated. The prevalence estimate was consequently very heterogeneous in the various countries, ranging from 3.7 to 239 cases per million inhabitants (Table 49.2). Whatever the limitations of this approach, the prevalence of patients with intermediate VWD requiring specific treatment has been estimated to range from 40 to 100 cases per million [17–20], a figure often quoted as a reliable estimation [21].

Prevalence of mild von Willebrand disease

Four population-based studies are available (Table 49.3). Rodeghiero *et al.* [2,22] evaluated 1218 schoolchildren aged 11–14 years in a well-defined territory of northern Italy. Diagnosis of VWD was considered "probable" in the following children: those with low VWF levels (VWF:RCo below an ABO-adjusted reference range) belonging to a family with more than two members, including or not the subject under investigation, and those with a bleeding history consisting of two or more symptoms. A definite diagnosis was assigned if, in addition to these criteria, at least one other family member on the hemorrhagic side had a low VWF level. Ten children (four with probable and six with definite VWD) were classified as affected (0.82%). This figure could range from 7 (0.57%) to 14 (1.15%) taking into account the 90% confidence interval for the lower limit of the normal range. It turned out that all these children

Table 49.3 Estimates of prevalence of von Willebrand disease (VWD).

VWD severity	Study	Methodology	Population	Prevalence
Severe	Weiss et al. [14]	Mail survey to 354 hematology departments	USA, Canada, 17 European countries, Iran, Israel	1.38–1.51 per million
	Mannucci et al. [15]	Patients identified through a questionnaire; plasma VWF assay and recruitment of patients with VWF:Ag <1% by IRMA	Western European countries plus Israel	0.1–3.12 per million
	Berliner et al. [16]	Investigation of patients followed at a single center	Cases followed in Israel	5.3 per million among Arabs
Intermediate	Nilsson [17]	Cases registered at specialized centers in Sweden	230 Swedish families (530 patients) with VWD already known	70 cases per million inhabitants (about 15% severe type 3)
Mild	Rodeghiero et al. [2]	Anamnesis + VWF:RCo. Family study	Caucasian children	0.82% (8200 per million)
	Rodeghiero et al. [22]	As above + VWF:Ag instead of VWF:RCo	As above	0.7%
	Miller et al. [24]	VWF:RCo	Adult blood donors	1.6% (0.2% bleeder)
	Meriane et al. [25]	Anamnesis + VWF:RCo. Family study	Arabic–Turkish adult students	1.23%
	Werner et al. [23]	Anamnesis + VWF:RCo. Family study	Caucasian–black children	1.3% (1.15% Caucasian, 1.81% black)

IRMA, immunoradiometric assay; VWF, von Willebrand factor.

had at least one bleeding symptom. This translates into a prevalence of 0.57–1.15%, or 5700–11 500 per million. Interestingly, in about half of the diagnosed families from this investigation, linkage was not subsequently confirmed [12].

In 1993, Werner et al. [23] published the results of a similar investigation carried out in 600 American schoolchildren aged 12–18 years undergoing well-child or school physical examinations at the pediatric ambulatory clinics of the hospitals located in Virginia, Ohio, and Mississippi. The criteria were seemingly less restrictive and included all three of at least one bleeding symptom, a family member with at least one bleeding symptom, and low VWF. The overall prevalence was estimated at 1.3%, with no racial difference (1.15% among white and 1.8% among black people). These data have been confirmed in two additional studies, not reported as full papers. Miller et al. [24], in 1987, found a prevalence of VWD of 1.6% in adult blood donors from New York, with a prevalence of symptomatic subjects with low VWF:RCo was 0.2%. In an additional study, Meriane et al. [25] studied the prevalence in Arabic–Turkish adult subjects. The figure was 1.23%, again with no racial differences. In all these studies the same functional test (VWF:RCo) and separate normal ranges according to blood groups were used, thus providing uniformity to the results. Although these figures appear high, it should be emphasized that the prevalence is probably even higher since the sensitivity of the functional test is about 50%. This assumption stems from the demonstration by Miller et al. [26] that among the obligatory carriers for type 1 disease, only 42% had abnormal VWF activity on their initial test. As previously mentioned, most of these cases will resist a Bayesian approach as sufficiently proved VWD cases, in keeping with their lack of linkage with a VWF allele [12]. Of note, in a murine model a phenotype mimicking VWD was produced by a mutation in the glycosyltransferase (GALgt2) gene [27] and the occurrence of similar mutations in human "VWD" cannot presently be ruled out.

Prevalence of a mutant *VWF* gene

While it is appreciated that a mild VWF deficiency is rather frequent in the general population, an estimate of the prevalence of mutant(s) *VWF* gene possibly causing disease is unknown. The main difficulty in such an estimation relies on the fact that while some heterozygous mutations are highly penetrant and fully expressing (e.g. R1205H, C1130F, R1374H/C, etc.) giving a severe reduction of VWF levels and a clear-cut bleeding tendency, others do not. Type 3 VWD carriers are usually asymptomatic but they carry a mutation which in compound heterozygous or homozygous state produces a relevant bleeding tendency. For example, in the Veneto Region through family studies we have identified at least 120 subjects with C2362F heterozygous mutation; individuals with a single gene dose do not have any bleeding while the phenotype in two homozygous patients and in several other compound heterozygous individuals with null alleles is severe. These patients are truly recessive, although their features do not completely match with the usual classification of type 3, further adding to the complexity of the genetic basis of VWD.

Thus, mutations in the *VWF* gene appear to be rather frequent in the general population, producing through their functional diversity the full range of different VWD phenotypes.

Table 49.4 Frequency of von Willebrand disease types in different series of patients.

Authors	Number of patients	Type 1 (%)	Type 2 (%)	Type 3 (%)
Tuddenham *et al.* [28]	134	75	19	6
Lenk *et al.* [29]	111	76	12	12
Nilsson [17]	106 families	70	10	20
Hoyer *et al.* [30]	116	71	23	6
Awidi [31]	65	59	29.5	11.5
Berliner *et al.* [16]	60	62	9	29
Overall	592	70	17	13

Frequency of von Willebrand disease subtypes

The relative frequency of subtypes of VWD has been estimated only from the series of single institutions. These are obviously flawed since they are based on severe and intermediate VWD patients (group A and B patients) only, indicative of a reporting bias. On epidemiologic grounds, the prevalence of mild VWD (group C patients), which is almost invariably due to type 1 VWD, appears to be 100–1000 times higher than that of the group A and B patients. Consequently, type 1 VWD in the population should be at least 100-fold more common than the other subtypes. Nevertheless, in referred patients there is a rather homogeneous distribution of VWD subtypes (Table 49.4) [16,17,28–31]. Overall, the data could be summarized for a relative percentage frequency of 70, 17, and 13 respectively for type 1, 2, and 3 VWD in the 592 patients considered in these studies. These data are quite in accordance with an extensive recent survey carried out by Federici *et al.* [32] among Italian hemophilia centers reporting a relative percentage frequency of 73, 21, and 6, respectively, for type 1, 2, and 3 VWD.

This general view has recently been challenged by the demonstration that several subtle abnormalities of multimeric pattern can be observed in patients previously diagnosed as type 1 VWD by using well-standardized laboratory methods [33]. However, from a practical point of view, these minor abnormalities do not prevent a complete biologic response to desmopressin, which is a good criterion for considering these patients to have a true quantitative deficiency of VWF [34].

Prevalence of von Willebrand disease in developing countries

Limited investigations have been carried out in developing countries, based on voluntary reporting in mail questionnaire-based surveys through national or regional hemophilia centers [21]. In general, major underreporting is evident compared with the expected prevalence. In a more recent unpublished survey, the ratio between severe hemophilia A (taken as a normalizing prevalence) and that of VWD in the same region was investigated, showing an underreporting rate of more than 60%

of cases of VWD. Surprisingly, the distribution of severity in reported cases is apparently not much different from that reported in developed countries, indicating the lack of a regional or national strategy for the detection of more severe cases [35]. Sadly, unlike in economically more developed countries, deaths secondary to hemorrhage in VWD patients are still reported from these countries, despite cryoprecipitate and VWF/factor VIII concentrates being generally available.

Practical implications

Type 3 VWD is a rare disorder, with a prevalence similar to that of other severe, homozygous coagulopathies, but the prevalence of the other severe cases could be more prevalent. Intermediate VWD prevalence is probably similar to the cumulative prevalence of hemophilia A and B. The prevalence of mild VWD is still uncertain, but a reasonable estimate is possibly one case between 1000 and 10 000 subjects. About 1% of the normal population could satisfy quite conservative epidemiologic criteria sufficient to diagnose VWD in *ad-hoc* cross-sectional investigations. This rather high prevalence figure must be interpreted with caution, as many of these subjects will experience only minor or trivial bleedings during their lifetime and will probably never be referred for medical assistance. It is therefore of paramount importance to distinguish between a diagnosis satisfying only minimal criteria and a clinically meaningful diagnosis. The first type of diagnosis is relevant for the epidemiologist but could be dangerous to the patients and his/her family in terms of generated anxiety and social burden; by contrast, the second one is certainly more useful for the patient and the physician alike [36,37]. We will discuss here two initiatives to clarify this issue using an epidemiologic approach.

Presurgical screening

A prevalence of 1/500 subjects of a hemorrhagic disease may certainly be alarming for a surgeon facing an elective mucous surgery (e.g. tonsillectomy) who is keen to avoid any hemorrhagic risk. However, despite such a high prevalence in the population, presurgical screening is probably not cost-effective for two reasons: First, all available phenotypic laboratory tests have their specificity based on the "reference limit" concept, which means that the specificity is usually set at 97.5%. Even assuming a sensitivity of 100% for a laboratory test (a very optimistic estimate indeed), for every 1000 subjects screened, the test would identify 25 subjects as affected, of whom 23 would be false positives and only two would have mild VWD. Second, the chance of patients with mild VWD bleeding significantly after surgery may be less than 50%, which means that more than 1000 subjects would need to be screened to avoid surgical bleeding related to mild VWD, at the cost of excluding all the false positives.

Diagnosis based on mild bleeding symptoms

Similarly, pursuing the diagnosis of mild VWD in a subject without a convincing personal or familial bleeding history poses the problems mentioned for presurgical screening and for cross-sectional epidemiologic surveys. As an example, we could examine the case of a woman investigated for VWD because of menorrhagia. Menorrhagia is found in 29–44% of otherwise healthy women [38,39] compared with 50–60% of VWD females [39]. Is screening for VWD advisable for all patients referred for menorrhagia? Consider a town with a population of 20 000 fertile women (Figure 49.2). Based on the prevalence of 0.5% of VWD and the above-mentioned figures, based on the frequency of menorrhagia in women with type 1 VWD [40] and in normal women [5], the ratio of VWD:normal in women with menorrhagia is 45:2985 in a population of 20 000 fertile women. By using the same laboratory test with a sensitivity of 100% and a specificity of 97.5% in all women complaining of menorrhagia, we can identify all the 45 women with VWD, but also 75 false positively "labeled" women. This represents a positive predictive value of only 37.5%.

Therefore, although it is recognized that menorrhagia could be the sole presenting symptom of a hemorrhagic disorder [41] and that in women with menorrhagia there is a high prevalence of women with VWD [42], a generalized screening is not advised. This is even more true if one considers that only a limited benefit is expected from a specific diagnosis in most women.

A clinically useful diagnosis

The two above-mentioned instances share a common feature: a laboratory diagnosis is made on the basis of a personal history with few symptoms (e.g. menorrhagia) or no symptoms at all (screening). In a recent multicenter survey, we demonstrated that the pretest probability (likelihood ratio) of VWD is significantly increased only when a clinically relevant history of bleeding is present (at least two hemorrhagic symptoms in the proband or a bleeding score ≥ 3 in males and ≥ 5 in females) [5]. Moreover, at least two (but preferably three) family members should be present in a family to reasonably suspect VWD in cases with mild VWF reduction or dubious bleeding symptoms [13]. Therefore, every laboratory assessment should be undertaken only in subjects presenting with significant bleeding symptoms or having two first-degree relatives with hemorrhagic symptoms or a VWF level $\leq 40 \, IU/dL$. Most importantly,

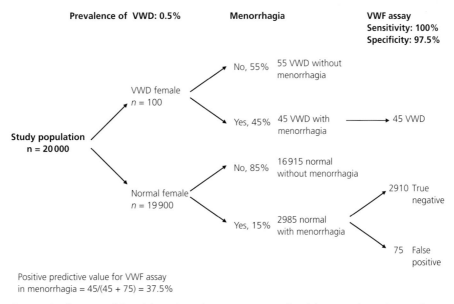

Figure 49.2 Positive predictive value for von Willebrand factor (VWF) assay in women referred for menorrhagia. See text for assumptions. Study population $n = 20\,000$.

subjects and families identified by these criteria are also those who are more likely to benefit from an appropriate therapy (e.g. desmopressin treatment or prophylaxis).

These epidemiologic data further reaffirm the concept that physicians should always base their diagnoses on sound clinical criteria that will translate their specific diagnosis into a beneficial way to treat or prevent the consequences of this still intriguing disorder [36].

Acknowledgment

We wish to thank Dr Alberto Tosetto for his helpful suggestions and for his invaluable contribution to the development of the epidemiologic simulations.

References

1 von Willebrand EA. Hereditär pseudohemofili. *Finska Läkarsällskapets Handl* 1926; **67**: 7–112.

2 Rodeghiero F, Castaman G, Dini E. Epidemiological investigation of the prevalence of von Willebrand's disease. *Blood* 1987; **69**: 454–9.

3 Higham JM, O'Brien PM, Shaw RW. Assessment of menstrual blood loss using a pictorial chart. *Br J Obstet Gynaecol* 1990; **97**: 734–9.

4 Friberg B, Orno AK, Lindgren A, Lethagen S. Bleeding disorders among young women: a population-based prevalence study. *Acta Obstet Gynecol Scand* 2006; **85**: 200–6.

5 Rodeghiero F, Castaman G, Tosetto A, *et al*. The discriminant power of bleeding history for the diagnosis of von Willebrand disease type 1: an international, multicenter study. *J Thromb Haemost* 2005; **3**: 2619–26.

6 Hedlund-Treutiger I, Revel-Vilk S, Blanchette VS, Curtin JA, Lillicrap D, Rand ML. Reliability and reproducibility of classification of children as "bleeders" versus "non-bleeders" using a questionnaire for significant mucocutaneous bleeding. *J Pediatr Hematol Oncol* 2004; **26**: 488–91.

7 Sadler JE, Budde U, Eikenboom JC, *et al.*, and the Working Party on von Willebrand Disease Classification. Update on the pathophysiology and classification of von Willebrand disease: a report of the Subcommittee on von Willebrand Factor. *J Thromb Haemost* 2006; **4**: 2103–14.

8 Castaman G, Federici AB, Rodeghiero F, Mannucci PM. Von Willebrand's disease in the year 2003: towards the complete identification of gene defects for correct diagnosis and treatment. *Haematologica* 2003; **88**: 94–108.

9 Goodeve A, Eikenboom J, Castaman G, *et al*. Phenotype and genotype of a cohort of families historically diagnosed with type 1 von Willebrand disease in the European study, Molecular and Clinical Markers for the Diagnosis and Management of Type 1 von Willebrand Disease (MCMDM-1VWD). *Blood* 2007; **109**: 112–21.

10 Eikenboom J, Van Marion V, Putter H, *et al*. Linkage analysis in families diagnosed with type 1 von Willebrand disease in the European study, molecular and clinical markers for the diagnosis and management of type 1 VWD. *J Thromb Haemost* 2006; **4**: 774–82.

11 James PD, Paterson AD, Notley C, *et al.*, and the Association of Hemophilia Clinic Directors of Canada. Genetic linkage and association analysis in type 1 von Willebrand disease: results from the Canadian type 1 VWD study. *J Thromb Haemost* 2006; **4**: 783–92.

12 Castaman G, Eikenboom JCJ, Bertina R, Rodeghiero F. Inconsistency of association between type 1 von Willebrand disease phenotype and genotype in families identified in an epidemiologic investigation. *Thromb Haemost* 1999; **82**: 1065–70.

13 Tosetto A, Castaman G, Rodeghiero F. Evidence-based diagnosis of type 1 von Willebrand disease: a Bayes theorem approach. *Blood* 2008; **111**: 3998–4003.

14 Weiss HJ, Ball AP, Mannucci PM. Incidence of severe von Willebrand's disease. *N Engl J Med* 1982; **307**: 127.

15 Mannucci PM, Bloom AL, Larrieu MJ, Nilsson IM, West RR. Atherosclerosis and von Willebrand factor. I. Prevalence of severe von Willebrand's disease in Western Europe and Israel. *Br J Haematol* 1984; **57**: 163–9.

16 Berliner SA, Seligsohn U, Zivelin A, Zwang E, Sofferman G. A relatively high frequency of severe (type III) von Willebrand's disease in Israel. *Br J Haematol* 1986; **62**: 535–43.

17 Nilsson IM. Von Willebrand disease from 1926 to 1983. *Scand J Haematol* 1984; **33**(Suppl. 40): 21–43.

18 Bloom AL, Giddins JC. HIV infection and AIDS in von Willebrand's disease. An international survey including data on the prevalence of clinical von Willebrand's disease. In: Lusher JM, Kessler CM (eds.) *Hemophilia and von Willebrand's Disease in 1990s*. Amsterdam: Elsevier Science Publishers, 1991: 405–11.

19 Bloom AL. The von Willebrand syndrome. *Semin Hematol* 1980; **17**: 215–27.

20 Bachman F. Diagnostic approach to mild bleeding disorders. *Semin Hematol* 1980; **17**: 292–312.

21 Sadler JE, Mannucci PM, Berntorp E, *et al*. Impact, diagnosis and treatment of von Willebrand disease. *Thromb Haemost* 2000; **84**: 160–74.

22 Rodeghiero F, Castaman G, Tosetto A. von Willebrand factor antigen is less sensitive than ristocetin cofactor for the diagnosis of type I von Willebrand disease—results based on a epidemiological investigation. *Thromb Haemost* 1990; **64**: 349–52.

23 Werner EJ, Broxson EH, Tucker EL, *et al*. Prevalence of von Willebrand disease in children: A multiethnic study. *J Pediatr* 1993; **123**: 893–8.

24 Miller CH, Lenzi R, Breen C. Prevalence of von Willebrand's disease among U.S. adults. *Blood* 1987; **70**(Suppl. 1): 377 (Abstract).

25 Meriane F, Sultan Y, Arabi H, *et al*. Incidence of a low von Willebrand factor activity in a population of Algerian students. *Blood* 1991; **78**(Suppl. 1): 484 (Abstract).

26 Miller CH, Graham JB, Goldin LR, Elston RC. Genetics of classic von Willebrand's disease. I. Phenotypic variation within families. *Blood* 1979; **54**: 117–36.

27 Nichols WC, Cooney KA, Mohlke KL, *et al*. von Willebrand disease in the RIIIS/J inbred mouse strain as a model for von Willebrand disease. *Blood* 1994; **83**: 3225–8.

28 Tuddenham EGD. von Willebrand factor and its disorders: an overview of recent molecular studies. *Blood Rev* 1989; **3**: 251–62.

29 Lenk H, Nilsson IM, Holmberg L, Weissbach G. Frequency of different types of von Willebrand's disease. *Acta Med Scand* 1988; **224**: 275–80.

VWF:PB

Direct platelet-binding assays are used to confirm the diagnosis of type 2B VWD. In this assay, fixed platelets are incubated with plasma and low-dose ristocetin (typically <0.6 mg/mL). A neutral antibody is used to detect VWF that binds spontaneously to the normal platelets [38]. This test will confirm that the gain-of-function defect is due to plasma VWF, and exclude the possibility of platelet-type, pseudo-VWD.

VWF:F8B

In type 2N VWD, the defect is in the ability of VWF to bind FVIII. FVIII-binding assays are also ELISA based, and utilize an antibody to isolate plasma VWF from the patient [28,39]. Recombinant FVIII is added, its presence detected by antibody or activity assays, and compared to the amount of VWF:Ag. The ratio of FVIII to VWF will be decreased in type 2N VWD, in contrast to normal individuals or those with mild hemophilia A, where normal VWF-FVIII binding is present. In addition, type 2N VWD patients typically have a heightened FVIII response to deamino-D-arginine vasopressin (DDAVP) administration, but a shortened FVIII survival due to the lack of normal FVIII-VWF binding. This assay may help to distinguish 2N VWD from mild FVIII deficiency [40].

VWFpp

The VWF propolypeptide, VWFpp, is secreted from cells in equimolar concentration to mature VWF [41]. Some VWD patients have increased clearance of VWF from the circulation, and these patients are characterized by high propeptide levels and a short half-life of VWF following administration of desmopressin. An abnormal VWFpp/VWF:Ag ratio therefore is consistent with increased clearance, with a proposed classification of VWD 1C [32]. This category would also include the well-recognized Vicenza variant [42]. VWFpp levels may be helpful in distinguishing patients with clearance defects from those with suboptimal VWF expression. In those with accelerated clearance of VWF, FVIII levels are also reduced through this accelerated clearance [32]. VWFpp is also decreased in type 2A and type 2B VWD [43].

VWF gene sequencing

Genetic testing is also becoming more widely available. DNA analysis of *VWF* is challenging due to the large size of the VWF protein and complexity of the genomic DNA, with 52 exons and approximately 8.4 kb of coding sequence [44]. Type 2 and type 3 VWD are more likely to be associated with gene defects, while type 1 VWD patients, especially those with VWF:Ag > 20 IU/dL, most often do not have an associated mutation in the *VWF* gene, especially if normal multimers are present [45,46]. The majority of type 2A, 2B, and 2M mutations are located in exon 28, although some type 2A mutations have been found in other regions, including exons 11–16, 26, 51, and 52. While type 2N defects are most often seen in exon 18,

mutations affecting FVIII binding have also been reported in exons 17–27. Type 1 defects are scattered throughout the gene. The mutations and polymorphisms in the *VWF* gene are detailed in an online database (https://grenada.lumc.nl/LOVD2/VWF/home.php?select_db=VWF). There are numerous naturally occurring polymorphisms as well, making it difficult to use gene sequencing for the definitive diagnosis of type 1 VWD patients. Some sequence variations that have been previously reported as *VWF* mutations are more likely benign variants, found at increased frequency in certain ethnic populations [47]. Those type 1 patients who do not have a documented mutation may have a splice site mutation, promoter defect or a defect in a related gene that causes low VWF levels (e.g. blood type). The possibility also exists that such patients simply have low VWF levels and do not truly have hereditary VWD.

Diagnosis

If there is clinical suspicion for the diagnosis of VWD, specific VWF testing should be performed as there are no reliable screening tests. Recommended initial testing includes VWF:Ag, VWF:RCo, FVIII:C, and multimer analysis [1]. A discrepancy between VWF:Ag and VWF:RCo should prompt further testing. A testing algorithm for the work-up of a potential VWD patient is shown in Figure 50.1. If FVIII is low, consideration of type 2N should occur, in which case VWF:F8B or DNA sequencing of the commonly affected exons may be helpful. Thrombocytopenia is frequently (although not always) seen with type 2B, and may prompt LD-RIPA, VWF:PB, and/or exon 28 sequencing. DNA sequencing may also be helpful in type 2A or type 2M VWD diagnosis. Expected results of VWD laboratory testing for the various VWD subtypes are shown in Figure 50.2.

Limitations of the currently available testing include the high variability present in the VWF:RCo and the need for more physiologic assays of VWF function. VWF *in vivo* is active under conditions of high shear forces, yet none of the readily available diagnostic tests specifically evaluate VWF under shear conditions. Also, laboratory testing provides an incomplete picture without adding in bleeding symptoms and family history. Recent efforts to generate predictive models have incorporated laboratory data and bleeding symptoms from family members as part of the work-up for VWD [48]. Although family testing is not an obligatory part of the VWD work-up, it may provide additional diagnostic information. The laboratory results should always be correlated with clinical symptoms for the most accurate diagnosis of VWD and optimal patient care. In patients with low VWF levels who do not meet the criteria for diagnosis of VWD, treatment may depend on symptoms and clinical history, consistent with the concept of low VWF levels as a risk factor for bleeding.

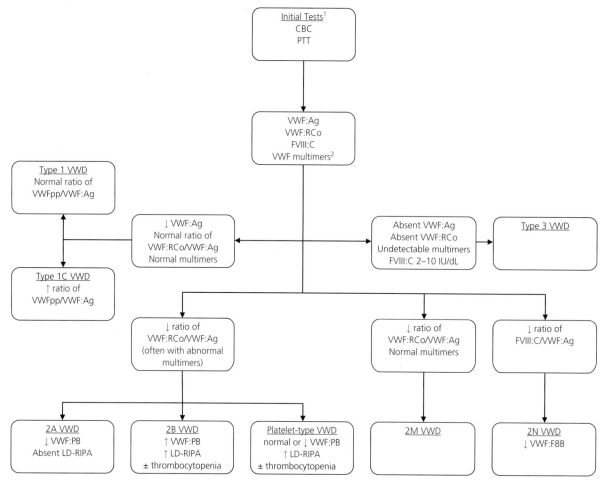

Figure 50.1 Laboratory testing algorithm for von Willebrand disease (VWD). [1]Additional screening tests may be indicated depending on symptoms and other diagnoses under consideration. [2]Particularly if ↓ VWF:Ag or ↓ VWF:RCo/VWF:Ag. CBC, complete blood count; FVIII, factor VIII; LD-RIPA, low-dose ristocetin-induced platelet aggregation; PTT, partial thromboplastin time; VWF, von Willebrand factor. (See Table 50.1 for other definitions.)

	Normal	Type 1	Type 1C (Vicenza)	Type 3	Type 2A	Type 2B	Type 2N	Type 2M	PT-VWD
VWF:Ag	N	↓	↓↓	absent	↓	↓	N or ↓	↓ or N	↓
VWF:RCo	N	↓	↓↓	absent	↓↓↓	↓↓	N or ↓	↓↓	↓↓
FVIII:C	N	N or ↓	↓	2–10 IU/dL	N or ↓	N or ↓	↓↓	N	N or ↓
VWFpp/VWF:Ag ratio	N	N	↑↑	absent	N or ↑	↑	N	N	↑
RIPA	N	often N	↓	absent	↓	often N	N	N or ↓	often N
LD-RIPA	absent	absent	absent	absent	absent	↑↑↑	absent	absent	↑↑↑
PFA*	N	N or ↑	↑	↑↑↑	↑	↑	N	↑	↑
BT*	N	N or ↑	↑	↑↑↑	↑	↑	N	↑	↑
Platelet count	N	N	N	N	N	↓ or N	N	N	↓
VWF multimers	N	N but ↓	N but ↓	absent	abnormal	abnormal	N but ↓	N but ↓	abnormal

Figure 50.2 Expected results of von Willebrand disease (VWD) laboratory testing. BT, bleeding time; FVIII, factor VIII; LD-RIPA, low-dose ristocetin-induced platelet aggregation; N, normal; N but ↓, normal but decreased in intensity; PT-VWD, platelet-type VWD; VWF, von Willebrand factor; ↓,↓↓,↓↓↓, relative decrease; ↑,↑↑,↑↑↑, relative increase; *not routinely recommended. (See Table 50.1 for other definitions.) Used by permission of R.R. Montgomery.

References

1 Nichols WL, Hultin MB, James AH, *et al*. Von Willebrand disease (VWD): evidence-based diagnosis and management guidelines, the National Heart, Lung, and Blood Institute (NHLBI) expert panel report (USA). *Haemophilia* 2008; **14**: 171–232.

2 Rodeghiero F, Castaman G, Tosetto A, *et al*. The discriminant power of bleeding history for the diagnosis of type 1 von Willebrand disease: An international, multicenter study. *J Thromb Haemost* 2005; **3**: 2619–26.

3 Federici AB, Mannucci PM, Castaman G, *et al*. Clinical and molecular predictors of thrombocytopenia and risk of bleeding in patients with von Willebrand disease type 2B: A cohort study of 67 patients. *Blood* 2009; **113**: 526–34.

4 Nilsson IM, Magnusson S, Borchgrevink C. The Duke and Ivy methods for determination of the bleeding time. *Thromb Diath Haemorrh* 1963; **10**: 223–34.

5 Dean JA, Blanchette VS, Carcao MD, *et al*. Von Willebrand disease in a pediatric-based population—comparison of type 1 diagnostic criteria and use of the PFA-100 and a von Willebrand factor/collagen-binding assay. *Thromb Haemost* 2000; **84**: 401–9.

6 Quiroga T, Goycoolea M, Munoz B, *et al*. Template bleeding time and PFA-100 have low sensitivity to screen patients with hereditary mucocutaneous hemorrhages: Comparative study in 148 patients. *J Thromb Haemost* 2004; **2**: 892–8.

7 Kundu SK, Heilmann EJ, Sio R, Garcia C, Davidson RM, Ostgaard RA. Description of an in vitro platelet function analyzer, PFA-100. *Semin Thromb Hemost* 1995; **21**: 106–12.

8 Fressinaud E, Veyradier A, Truchaud F, *et al*. Screening for von Willebrand disease with a new analyzer using high shear stress: A study of 60 cases. *Blood* 1998; **91**: 1325–31.

9 Castaman G, Tosetto A, Goodeve A, *et al*. The impact of bleeding history, von Willebrand factor and PFA-100((R)) on the diagnosis of type 1 von Willebrand disease: Results from the European study MCMDM-1VWD. *Br J Haematol* 2010; **151**: 245–51.

10 Hubbard AR, Hamill M, Beeharry M, Bevan SA, Heath AB, and the SSC Sub-Committees on Factor VIII/Factor IX and von Willebrand Factor of ISTH. Value assignment of the WHO 6th International Standard for Blood Coagulation Factor VIII and von Willebrand Factor in Plasma (07/316). *J Thromb Haemost* 2011; **9**: 2100–2.

11 Ingerslev J. A sensitive ELISA for von Willebrand factor (vWf:Ag). *Scand J Clin Lab Invest* 1987; **47**: 143–9.

12 Castaman G, Tosetto A, Cappelletti A, *et al*. Validation of a rapid test (VWF-LIA) for the quantitative determination of von Willebrand factor antigen in type 1 von Willebrand disease diagnosis within the European multicenter study MCMDM-1VWD. *Thromb Res* 2010; **126**: 227–31.

13 Sadler JE. Von Willebrand disease type 1: A diagnosis in search of a disease. *Blood* 2003; **101**: 2089–93.

14 Gill JC, Endres-Brooks J, Bauer PJ, Marks WJ Jr, Montgomery RR. The effect of ABO blood group on the diagnosis of von Willebrand disease. *Blood* 1987; **69**: 1691–5.

15 Miller CH, Haff E, Platt SJ, Rawlins P, Drews CD, Dilley AB, Evatt B. Measurement of von Willebrand factor activity: Relative effects of ABO blood type and race. *J Thromb Haemost* 2003; **1**: 2191–7.

16 Pottinger BE, Read RC, Paleolog EM, Higgins PG, Pearson JD. Von Willebrand factor is an acute phase reactant in man. *Thromb Res* 1989; **53**: 387–94.

17 Jenkins PV, O'Donnell JS. ABO blood group determines plasma von Willebrand factor levels: A biologic function after all? *Transfusion* 2006; **46**: 1836–44.

18 Howard MA, Sawers RJ, Firkin BG. Ristocetin: A means of differentiating von Willebrand's disease into two groups. *Blood* 1973; **41**: 687–90.

19 Kitchen S, Jennings I, Woods TA, Kitchen DP, Walker ID, Preston FE. Laboratory tests for measurement of von Willebrand factor show poor agreement among different centers: Results from the United Kingdom national external quality assessment scheme for blood coagulation. *Semin Thromb Hemost* 2006; **32**: 492–8.

20 Meijer P, Haverkate F. An external quality assessment program for von Willebrand factor laboratory analysis: An overview from the European Concerted Action on Thrombosis and Disabilities Foundation. *Semin Thromb Hemost* 2006; **32**: 485–91.

21 Murdock PJ, Woodhams BJ, Matthews KB, Pasi KJ, Goodall AH. Von Willebrand factor activity detected in a monoclonal antibody-based ELISA: An alternative to the ristocetin cofactor platelet agglutination assay for diagnostic use. *Thromb Haemost* 1997; **78**: 1272–7.

22 Federici AB, Canciani MT, Forza I, *et al*. A sensitive ristocetin co-factor activity assay with recombinant glycoprotein ibalpha for the diagnosis of patients with low von Willebrand factor levels. *Haematologica* 2004; **89**: 77–85.

23 Chen D, Daigh CA, Hendricksen JI, *et al*. A highly-sensitive plasma von Willebrand factor ristocetin cofactor (VWF:RCo) activity assay by flow cytometry. *J Thromb Haemost* 2008; **6**: 323–30.

24 Favaloro EJ, Bonar R, Chapman K, Meiring M, Funk Adcock D. Differential sensitivity of von Willebrand factor (VWF) 'activity' assays to large and small VWF molecular weight forms: A cross-laboratory study comparing ristocetin cofactor, collagen-binding and mAb-based assays. *J Thromb Haemost* 2012; **10**: 1043–54.

25 Hulstein JJ, de Groot PG, Silence K, Veyradier A, Fijnheer R, Lenting PJ. A novel nanobody that detects the gain-of-function phenotype of von Willebrand factor in ADAMTS13 deficiency and von Willebrand disease type 2B. *Blood* 2005; **106**: 3035–42.

26 Flood VH, Gill JC, Morateck PA, *et al*. Gain-of-function GPIb ELISA assay for VWF activity in the Zimmerman program for the molecular and clinical biology of VWD. *Blood* 2011; **117**: e67–74.

27 Flood VH, Gill JC, Morateck PA, *et al*. Common VWF exon 28 polymorphisms in African Americans affecting the VWF activity assay by ristocetin cofactor. *Blood* 2010; **116**: 280–6.

28 Mazurier C, Meyer D. Factor VIII binding assay of von Willebrand factor and the diagnosis of type 2N von Willebrand disease—results of an international survey. On behalf of the subcommittee on von Willebrand factor of the Scientific and Standardization Committee of the ISTH. *Thromb Haemost* 1996; **76**: 270–4.

29 Ruggeri ZM, Zimmerman TS. Variant von Willebrand's disease: Characterization of two subtypes by analysis of multimeric composition of factor VIII/von Willebrand factor in plasma and platelets. *J Clin Invest* 1980; **65**: 1318–25.

30 Budde U, Pieconka A, Will K, Schneppenheim R. Laboratory testing for von Willebrand disease: Contribution of multimer analysis to diagnosis and classification. *Semin Thromb Hemost* 2006; **32**: 514–21.

31 Gill JC, Wilson AD, Endres-Brooks J, Montgomery RR. Loss of the largest von Willebrand factor multimers from the plasma of patients with congenital cardiac defects. *Blood* 1986; **67**: 758–61.

32 Haberichter SL, Balistreri M, Christopherson P, *et al.* Assay of the von Willebrand factor (VWF) propeptide to identify patients with type 1 von Willebrand disease with decreased VWF survival. *Blood* 2006; **108**: 3344–51.

33 Brown JE, Bosak JO. An ELISA test for the binding of von Willebrand antigen to collagen. *Thromb Res* 1986; **43**: 303–11.

34 Favaloro EJ. Collagen binding assay for von Willebrand factor (VWF:CBA): Detection of von Willebrands disease (VWD), and discrimination of VWD subtypes, depends on collagen source. *Thromb Haemost* 2000; **83**: 127–35.

35 Ribba AS, Loisel I, Lavergne JM, *et al.* Ser968Thr mutation within the A3 domain of von Willebrand factor (VWF) in two related patients leads to a defective binding of VWF to collagen. *Thromb Haemost* 2001; **86**: 848–54.

36 Flood VH, Lederman CA, Wren JS, *et al.* Absent collagen binding in a VWF A3 domain mutant: Utility of the VWF:CB in diagnosis of VWD. *J Thromb Haemost* 2010; **8**: 1431–3.

37 Flood VH, Gill JC, Christopherson PA, *et al.* Critical von Willebrand factor A1 domain residues influence type VI collagen binding. *J Thromb Haemost* 2012; **10**: 1417–24.

38 Scott JP, Montgomery RR. The rapid differentiation of type IIb von Willebrand's disease from platelet-type (pseudo-) von Willebrand's disease by the "neutral" monoclonal antibody binding assay. *Am J Clin Pathol* 1991; **96**: 723–8.

39 Montgomery RR, Hathaway WE, Johnson J, Jacobson L, Muntean W. A variant of von Willebrand's disease with abnormal expression of factor VIII procoagulant activity. *Blood* 1982; **60**: 201–7.

40 Mazurier C, Gaucher C, Jorieux S, Goudemand M. Biological effect of desmopressin in eight patients with type 2N ('Normandy') von Willebrand disease. collaborative group. *Br J Haematol* 1994; **88**: 849–54.

41 Borchiellini A, Fijnvandraat K, ten Cate JW, *et al.* Quantitative analysis of von Willebrand factor propeptide release in vivo: Effect of experimental endotoxemia and administration of 1-deamino-8-D-arginine vasopressin in humans. *Blood* 1996; **88**: 2951–8.

42 Mannucci PM, Lombardi R, Castaman G, *et al.* Von Willebrand disease "Vicenza" with larger-than-normal (supranormal) von Willebrand factor multimers. *Blood* 1988; **71**: 65–70.

43 McCarroll DR, Ruggeri ZM, Montgomery RR. Correlation between circulating levels of von Willebrand's antigen II and von Willebrand factor: Discrimination between type I and type II von Willebrand's disease. *J Lab Clin Med* 1984; **103**: 704–11.

44 Mancuso DJ, Tuley EA, Westfield LA, *et al.* Structure of the gene for human von Willebrand factor. *J Biol Chem* 1989; **264**: 19514–27.

45 Goodeve A, Eikenboom J, Castaman G, *et al.* Phenotype and genotype of a cohort of families historically diagnosed with type 1 von Willebrand disease in the European study, molecular and clinical markers for the diagnosis and management of type 1 von Willebrand disease (MCMDM-1VWD). *Blood* 2007; **109**: 112–21.

46 James PD, Notley C, Hegadorn C, *et al.* The mutational spectrum of type 1 von Willebrand disease: Results from a Canadian cohort study. *Blood* 2007; **109**: 145–54.

47 Bellissimo DB, Christopherson PA, Flood VH, *et al.* VWF mutations and new sequence variations identified in healthy controls are more frequent in the African-American population. *Blood* 2012; **119**: 2135–40.

48 Tosetto A, Castaman G, Rodeghiero F. Evidence-based diagnosis of type 1 von Willebrand disease: A Bayes theorem approach. *Blood* 2008; **111**: 3998–4003.

CHAPTER 51

Classification and clinical aspects of von Willebrand disease

Augusto B. Federici
University of Milan, Milan, Italy

Introduction

von Willebrand disease (VWD), the most common inherited bleeding disorder, is due to quantitative and/or qualitative defects of von Willebrand factor (VWF), the adhesive glycoprotein synthesized by endothelial cells and megakaryocytes that mediates platelet adhesion/aggregation and stabilizes factor VIII (FVIII) in the circulation [1]. In VWD, bleeding events are thus caused in VWD not only by the impaired platelet adhesion usually measured in plasma as ristocetin cofactor activity (VWF:RCo) but also by reduced FVIII levels associated with VWF defects. The pathophysiology, diagnosis, and classification of VWD are complex, but characterization of VWD patients is always important for providing correct management. VWD is inherited by autosomal dominant or recessive patterns, but women with milder VWD forms are apparently more symptomatic [1].

Prevalence and classification in the von Willebrand disease registries

In population-based studies, the prevalence of VWD is very high (0.6–1.3%) [2,3], but the clinical relevance of many of these cases is uncertain. However, if we consider patients referred for clinical manifestations of bleeding at hemophilia centers, the actual prevalence is 0.005–0.01%, thus two orders of magnitude lower [4–8].

The most updated classification of VWD has proposed six different types: VWD1, VWD3, VWD2A, VWD2B, VWD2M, and VWD2N [1]. A partial quantitative defect marks VWD1, whereas VWD3 is characterized by the nearly total absence of VWF in plasma and platelets. VWD1 is easily distinguished from VWD3 by milder VWF deficiency (usually in the range of 10–40 U/dL), an autosomal dominant pattern of inheritance, and the presence of a milder bleeding tendency [1]. In the past,

VWD1 was reported to be the most frequent form of VWD, accounting for approximately 70–75% of cases. A study based on the reappraisal of diagnoses of VWD1 after 10 years (1998–2008) in 1234 patients followed by 16 Italian centers has established that VWD1 represents only 779/1234 (63%) [9], because many cases previously diagnosed as VWD1 were rediagnosed as VWD2A or VWD2M. The percentages of type distribution reported in the two VWD cohorts, the specific VWD registry with 1234 followed by 16 centers [9] and those of the more general registry on Hemophilia and Allied Disorders of the Italian Association of Hemophilia Centers (AICE) with 2420 cases followed by 48 centers [10], are shown in Table 51.1. The percentages of VWD2A, VWD2B, VWD2N, and VWD3 are similar while the difference refers to VWD1 (18 vs 6%) and VWD2M (63 vs 73%).

This change in classification was made because of discrepant VWF measurements (ratio of VWF:RCo to VWF:Ag < 0.6) upon retesting based on more sensitive VWF:RCo assays [11]. The presence of qualitative defects of VWF in previously diagnosed VWD1 has also been reported in 154 families evaluated prospectively by the European study [12]. The main demographic, clinical, and laboratory data are summarized in Table 51.2. Women are more frequent in mild forms of VWD1, VWD2B, and VWD2M while male/female ratio is equal in VWD3 and VWD2A. The median age is 20–32 years, with extremely wide range (1–96 years). The levels of VWF activities are always below the normal range observed in healthy individuals: however, the VWF:RCo level varies from very low (<10 U/dL), to moderate (10–30 U/dL), and mild (31–56 U/dL) within each VWD type.

With regard to qualitative defects of VWF, four types are identified, reflecting different pathophysiologic mechanisms [9]. VWD2A is marked by the absence of high-molecular-weight VWF multimers in plasma and VWD2B is identified by increased affinity of VWF for its platelet receptor, the glycoprotein Ib α (GpIbα). Characterization of qualitatively abnormal

Textbook of Hemophilia, Third Edition. Edited by Christine A. Lee, Erik E. Berntorp and W. Keith Hoots.
© 2014 John Wiley & Sons, Ltd. Published 2014 by John Wiley & Sons, Ltd.

Table 51.1 Italian hemophilia centers and patients included in the Italian national registry on von Willebrand disease (VWD) RENAWI versus those reported annually in the Registry on Hemophilia and Allied Disorders of the AICE [9,10]. The case number (%) of VWD1 and VWD2 are underlined in the table to indicate significant changes observed in RENAWI versus AICE data.

Numbers of participating hemophilia centers	16	48
Patients enrolled in the registry in January 2005	1529	2420
Patients not included in the registry:	295	Not applicable
Included by more than one center	35	Verified
Did not meet criteria for VWD diagnosis	246	Analyses not tested
Lost at the follow-up or died	14	Verified
Classification of total VWD included:	1234	2420
VWD1	779 (63%)	1,773 (73%)[a]
VWD2A	87 (7%)	208 (9%)
VWD2B	73 (6%)	113 (5%)
VWD2M	219 (18%)	164 (6%)[a]
VWD2N	10 (1%)	40 (2%)
VWD3	66 (5%)	122 (5%)

[a]The case number (%) of VWD1 and VWD2 are underlined in the table to indicate significant changes observed in RENAWI versus AICE data. This is mainly due to the more sensitive enzyme-linked immunosorbent assay (ELISA)-VWF:RCo and multimeric analyses used in the RENAWI allowing to better identify VWD2M versus previously diagnosed VWD1 according to these additional tests.

variants with decreased platelet-dependent function and a normal multimeric structure defines VWD2M. The VWD2N phenotype displays a full array of multimers, the defect being in the N-terminal region of the *VWF* where the binding domain for FVIII is located. This type is distinguishable from mild hemophilia A only by the abnormal binding of FVIII to VWF (VWF:FVIIIB).

Criteria for diagnosis

Three main criteria are required for the correct diagnoses of VWD: (1) positive bleeding history since childhood; (2) reduced VWF activity in plasma; and (3) history of bleeding in the family with autosomal dominant or recessive inheritance.

Positive bleeding history since childhood

Clinical manifestations of VWD are excessive mucocutaneous bleeding and prolonged oozing after surgical procedures. In women, menorrhagia may be the only clinical manifestation. Soft-tissue and joint bleeding are rare, except in patients with VWD3 and other VWD types who are characterized by severe deficiencies of FVIII. The clinical expression of the disease is usually mild in most patients with VWD1, whereas severity is typically greater in VWD2A and particularly in VWD3. Generally, the severity of bleeding correlates with the degree of reduction of VWF:RCo and FVIII. To date, only a few detailed

Table 51.2 Demographic, clinical and lab data expressed in median (*range*) of the patients enrolled into the Italian national registry on von Willebrand disease (RENAWI).

	VWD1	VWD2A	VWD2B	VWD2M	VWD2N	VWD3	All VWD
Case number	779	87	73	219	10	66	1234
(%)	(63)	(7)	(6)	(18)	(1)	(5)	(100)
Family number	279	31	22	67	5	47	451
Gender M/F	311/468	45/42	29/44	101/118	5/5	32/34	523/711
(% female)	(60%)	(48%)	(60%)	(54%)	(50%)	(51%)	(58%)
Median age	35	34	33	37	20	28	32
(range)	(2–87)	(3–77)	(5–87)	(4–96)	(4–54)	(1–72)	(1–96)
Bleeding time	7	21	14	10	7	35	15
(min)	(2.50–35)	(6–35)	(4–35)	(3–35)	(5–13)	(15–35)	(2.50–35)
RIPA	1.30	2.00	0.60	1.60	1.10	3.50	1.50
(mg/mL)	(1.10–3.50)	(1.40–3.50)	(0.30–0.80)	(1.30–3.50)	(1.10–1.20)		(0.30–3.50)
VWF:RCo	37	6	20	7	37	<3	18
(U/dL)	(5–56)	(2–68)	(6–79)	(3–50)	(26–100)		(<3–100)
VWF:Ag	40	36	48	24	33	<1	28
(U/dL)	(5–60)	(6–140)	(16–180)	(3–120)	(26–98)		(<1–180)
VWF:RCo/Ag	0.92	0.23	0.46	0.50	1.00	n.c.	0.61
(ratio)	(0.60–1.60)	(0.10–0.60)	(0.10–1.00)	(0.10–0.60)	(0.90–1.30)		(0.10–1.60)
FVIII:C	52	46	50	35	20	6	35
(U/dL)	(2–187)	(12–140)	(16–140)	(2–144)	(6–33)	(1–22)	(1–140)
FVIII/VWF:Ag	1.65	1.23	1.27	1.40	0.46	n.c.	1.28
(ratio)	(0.80–2.00)	(0.60–2.00)	(0.40–2.00)	(0.60–2.00)	(0.20–0.60)		(0.20–2.00)

Bleeding time >30 min was calculated as 35; RIPA >3 mg/mL was calculated as 3.5; VWF:RCo <3 and VWF:Ag < 1 U/dL was considered as 1 U/dL to calculate ratios.
n.c., not calculated; RIPA, ristocetin-induced platelet aggregation; VWD, von Willebrand disease; VWF, von Willebrand factor.

Table 51.3 Number of patients (%) who showed one of the different bleeding symptoms.

	VWD1	VWD2A	VWD2B	VWD2M	VWD2N	VWD3	All VWD
Case number	779	87	73	219	10	66	1234
(%)	(63)	(7)	(6)	(18)	(1)	(5)	(100)
Epistaxis	412	61	49	123	4	51	699
	(53)	(70)	(67)	(56)	(40)	(77)	(57)
Menorrhagia[a]	374	25	26	105	2	22	654
	(48)	(40)	(59)	(58)	(40)	(65)	(53)
Postdental extraction	327	37	27	92	3	27	456
	(42)	(43)	(37)	(42)	(30)	(41)	(37)
Bleeding from minor wounds	273	31	37	81	3	36	469
	(35)	(36)	(51)	(37)	(30)	(55)	(38)
Gum bleeding	210	38	31	70	0	38	394
	(27)	(44)	(42)	(32)	(–)	(58)	(32)
Postsurgical bleeding	280	42	35	98	2	30	494
	(36)	(48)	(48)	(45)	(20)	(45)	(40)
Gastrointestinal bleeding	31	15	7	18	0	13	87
	(4)	(17)	(10)	(8)	(–)	(20)	(7)
Hematomas	93	12	12	13	4	31	161
	(12)	(14)	(16)	(6)	(40)	(47)	(13)
Joint bleeding	15	7	12	13	1	27	78
	(2)	(8)	(16)	(6)	(10)	(41)	(6)
Hematuria	16	5	3	7	1	8	40
	(2)	(6)	(4)	(3)	(10)	(12)	(3)
Cerebral bleeding	5	2	0	1	0	6	14
	(0.60)	(2)	(–)	(0.60)	(–)	(9)	(1)

[a]Women only; underlined values indicate similar percentages among von Willebrand factor (VWF) types.

descriptions of symptoms are available [5,13,14]. Table 51.3 shows a more updated relative frequency of bleedings among the VWD types collected in the Italian Registry on VWD (RENAWI-1).

Several attempts were recently made to evaluate sensitivity and specificity of categorized bleeding symptoms to predict a VWD diagnosis, especially among mild cases thought to be VWD1 (VWF:RCo levels of 20–40 U/dL). A questionnaire-based screening tool designed to identify patients with bleeding disorders has been proposed since 1995 [15]: additional tools specifically devoted to VWD were also designed 10 years later [16,17]. The bleeding score (BS) calculated after exposing patients to the detailed questionnaire proposed by Tosetto et al. [18] was used to quantify symptoms for the confirmation of diagnosis in a large cohort of European VWD type 1 [12]: such BS with some modifications was also applied in VWD studies by others [19]. The list of symptoms considered in the detailed questionnaire, together with their severity degree calculated from –1 to 4, is summarized in Table 51.4. BS together with baseline VWF levels and family history have been proposed as more evidence-based criteria for VWD1 diagnosis [20] to better define "possible" type 1 VWD [21–23]. Indeed, a few attempts to assess the determinant of bleeding in VWD have been made for the last 5 years, but only in a limited number of cases with certain VWD types. The risk of bleeding assessed by BS appears to be greater in VWD2B than in VWD1 with increased VWF

clearance [24,25]. More recently, a head-to-head comparison between VWD2A and VWD2M using BS did result in higher risk of bleeding in VWD2A because of the higher frequency of gastrointestinal bleeds [26].

Reduced von Willebrand factor activity in plasma

The diagnosis of VWD may require several laboratory tests to be repeated on different occasions. These tests are usually performed on patients with suspected bleeding disorders. Table 51.5 provides the list of clinical and laboratory tests useful for VWD diagnosis. The bleeding time (BT), the original in-vivo test used for diagnosing VWD, is not always prolonged and may be normal in patients with mild VWD, such as those with VWD1 and normal platelet VWF content [1]. Hence, it is not particularly useful for diagnosis. Evaluation of closure time (CT) with the platelet function analyzer (PFA-100) gives rapid and simple measures of VWF-dependent platelet function at high shear stress: it can be performed in whole blood and therefore can be employed instead of BT in children or when BT is not feasible. This system is sensitive and reproducible for VWD screening, but CT is normal in VWD2N and cannot be modified in VWD3 after the administration of VWF/FVIII concentrates [27]. Based on these observations, BT and CT were not included in the flow chart to be used in the differential diagnosis of VWD types as previously proposed [28]: an updated version of this flow chart is shown in Figure 51.1.

Table 51.4 Bleeding score used to evaluate patient bleeding history. Adapted from [18].

Symptom	Score −1	0	1	2	3	4
Epistaxis	—	No or trivial (<5)	>5 or more than 10	Consultation only	Packing or cauterization or antifibrinolytic	Blood transfusion or replacement therapy or desmopressin
Cutaneous	—	No or trivial (<1 cm)	>1 cm and no trauma	Consultation only	—	—
Bleeding from minor wounds	—	No or trivial (<5)	>5 or more than 5	Consultation only	Surgical hemostasis	Blood transfusion or replacement therapy or desmopressin
Oral cavity	—	No	Referred at least one	Consultation only	Surgical hemostasis or antifibrinolytic	Blood transfusion or replacement therapy or desmopressin
Gastrointestinal bleeding	—	No	Associated with ulcer, portal hypertension, hemorrhoids, angiodysplasia	Spontaneous	Surgical hemostasis, blood transfusion, replacement therapy, desmopressin, antifibrinolytics	—
Tooth extraction	No bleeding in at least 2 extractions	None done or no bleeding in 1 extraction	Referred in <25% of all procedures	Referred in >25% of all procedures, no intervention	Resuturing or packing	Blood transfusion or replacement therapy or desmopressin
Surgery	No bleeding in at least 2 surgeries	None done or no bleeding in 1 surgery	Referred in <25% of all surgeries	Referred in >25% of all procedures, no intervention	Surgical hemostasis or antifibrinolytic	Blood transfusion or replacement therapy or desmopressin
Menorrhagia	—	No	Consultation only	Antifibrinolytics, pill use	Dilatation & currettage, iron therapy	Blood transfusion or replacement therapy or desmopressin or hysterectomy
Postpartum hemorrhage	No bleeding in at least 2 deliveries	None done or no bleeding in 1 delivery	Consultation only	Dilatation & currettage, iron therapy, antifibrinolytics	Blood transfusion or replacement therapy or desmopressin	Hysterectomy
Muscle hematomas	—	Never	Post trauma no therapy	Spontaneous, no therapy	Spontaneous or traumatic, requiring desmopressin or replacement therapy	Spontaneous or traumatic, requiring surgical intervention or blood transfusion
Hemarthrosis	—	Never	Post trauma no therapy	Spontaneous, no therapy	Spontaneous or traumatic, requiring desmopressin or replacement therapy	Spontaneous or traumatic, requiring surgical intervention or blood transfusion

Table 52.1 Schedule for the test dose of desmopressin to assess responsiveness in patients with von Willebrand disease (and mild hemophilia). If the subcutaneous or intranasal routes are preferred for desmopressin administration, the same schedule should be followed.

Step 1	Infuse over 30 min 0.3 μg/kg of desmopressin in 100 mL saline in newly diagnosed patients or in those who must undergo an elective treatment
Step 2	Obtain citrated blood samples at 60 min after starting desmopressin (postinfusion peak) and at 4 h (to assess the rate of factor clearance)
Step 3	Measure factor VIII coagulant activity and ristocetin cofactor or collagen-binding activity in plasma

Table 52.2 Target levels of factor VIII (FVIII) and von Willebrand factor recommended in patients with von Willebrand disease for clinical situations.

Clinical situation	Target
Major surgery	Peak FVIII levels[a] of 100% and trough daily levels of at least 50% until healing is complete (usually 5–10 days)
Minor surgery	Peak FVIII levels of 60% and trough daily levels of at least 30% until healing is complete (usually 2–4 days)
Dental extractions	Peak FVIII levels of 60% (single dose)
Spontaneous bleeding episodes	Peak FVIII levels higher than 50% until bleeding stops (usually 2–4 days)
Delivery and puerperium[a]	Peak FVIII levels higher than 80% and trough levels of at least 30% (usually for 3–4 days)

[a]For those who prefer to monitor and measure von Willebrand factor, the same target levels of ristocetin cofactor or collagen-binding activity are recommended.

Responses to desmopressin can also be predicted to some extent from knowledge of the different subtypes of VWD. Type 1, the most frequent phenotype accounting for 60–80% of cases and due to the quantitative deficiency of VWF and FVIII, is the most responsive to desmopressin [7–10]. There is some variability in the response to desmopressin among patients with type 1 VWD. For instance, those who carry gene mutations in the D–D3 domains of the *VWF* gene have the greatest relative response, whereas partially or nonresponsive patients have mutations more frequently in the A1–A3 domains. In practise, the predictive usefulness of genotyping is limited and the test dose recommended above is of greater practical value [11].

Type 2, accounting for 20–30% of cases and due to dysfunctional VWF proteins synthesized in normal amounts, is generally poorly responsive to desmopressin, because the compound triggers the secretion into plasma of a dysfunctional moiety [7,8,12]. Exceptions to this general rule are some cases with the subtypes 2N, in whom low FVIII levels increase postinfusion [8,13]. Type 3 VWD, the most severe form accounting for 2–5% of cases, is almost invariably unresponsive to desmopressin, because these patients lack secretable VWF.

Desmopressin is sometimes clinically useful for patients with the acquired von Willebrand syndrome, which occurs in association with lymphoproliferative, cardiovascular, and myeloproliferative disorders. Management of bleeding episodes in these patients is based on the choice between desmopressin, FVIII/VWF concentrates, and high-dose intravenous immunoglobulins, but no single drug is effective for all [14]. In a large series of 186 cases infused with desmopressin to control bleeding episodes, this treatment was clinically effective in 20% of cases. The variability of the clinical response to desmopressin was explained by the variably short half-life of endogenous FVIII and VWF released by the compound [15].

A limit of DDAVP is a progressive decrease in the degree of factor rise observed in patients with VWD (and mild hemophilia) who are repeatedly treated [16]. In general, treatment with desmopressin can be usefully repeated at least 3–4 times. The only way to ascertain whether and when tachyphylaxis develops is to measure FVIII and VWF levels in plasma after each desmopressin infusion. Depending on the peak factor levels attained postinfusion and on trough levels, the clinician can decide whether or not treatment can be safely stopped because rebleeding is unlikely to occur or whether it is necessary to resort to the infusion of plasma fractions.

The obvious advantages of desmopressin are the absent risk of the transmission of bloodborne infections and its relatively low cost. For this reason, desmopressin is the treatment of choice in responsive patients with VWD (and mild hemophilia). Desmopressin is listed by the World Health Organization among essential drugs. However, not all countries have implemented the WHO recommendations, and in many of them desmopressin is not available or licenced only for the other main clinical indications of the compound, i.e. diabetes insipidus and nocturnal enuresis.

Monitoring treatment

The purpose of monitoring desmopressin treatment with laboratory testing is to establish whether or not the degree of correction over time of FVIII and VWF defects is adequate to control bleeding, spontaneous or postoperative (Table 52.2). For minor bleeding episodes and invasive procedures such as dental extractions, monitoring is usually not necessary because the hemostatic response is quite predictable if the dosages recommended above are used. For more severe bleeding episodes and major surgery monitoring is usually necessary to establish, as outlined above, whether or not the occurrence of tachyphylaxis has rendered the patient unresponsive.

Assays for FVIII are the tests of choice for monitoring treatment in patients with VWD. VWF measurements, such as the ristocetin cofactor and collagen-binding assays, can also be used, but they are less standardized than FVIII assays. Moreover, there is much less experience than for FVIII on peaks and troughs of VWF levels needed to reach and maintain hemostasis

(Table 52.2). If one chooses to monitor patients with VWF assays, the same peak and trough levels recommended for FVIII are tentatively recommended (Table 52.2).

It is usually not necessary to monitor the skin bleeding time, not only because this test is difficult to standardize and poorly reproducible, but mainly because it is a poor predictor of hemostasis during soft-tissue and postoperative bleeding. There is evidence, for instance, that surgical hemostasis is reached and maintained by desmopressin and by plasma fractions even if the skin bleeding time is prolonged, provided sufficient levels of plasma FVIII are reached. It is also unnecessary to evaluate the post-treatment multimeric pattern of VWF, whereas knowledge of this pattern is necessary to establish the phenotype of VWD and thus to decide the optimal treatment with desmopressin or plasma fractions.

Side-effects of desmopressin

Transient headache, facial flushing, and mild tachycardia are relatively frequent side-effects, usually well tolerated by patients. The antidiuretic effect is not perceived clinically in patients with a normal capacity to excrete water, if the drug is given at the recommended time intervals (every 12–24 h) and fluid intake is not excessive. Regular laboratory monitoring of osmolality and electrolytes is not necessary, but body weighing is a recommendable simple and inexpensive precautionary measure. Severe symptoms due to water intoxication such as cerebral edema and seizures are seldom reported, more often in infants and young children [17], but sometimes also in adults. There are reports of arterial thrombosis during treatment [18,19], so that the drug should be avoided in patients with overt cardiovascular disease. Desmopressin can be safely used in women during the first months of pregnancy, because it is devoid of oxytocic properties [20].

Adjuvant treatments

Treatment with desmopressin for mucous membrane bleeding is usually given in association with antifibrinolytic amino acids. Epsilon aminocaproic acid and tranexamic acid are synthetic compounds that inhibit fibrinolysis by saturating the binding sites on plasminogen thereby impeding plasmin formation. Epsilon aminocaproic acid can be administered orally, intravenously, or topically at doses of 60 mg/kg every 6 h, tranexamic acid by the same routes at doses of 15 mg/kg every 8 h. In general, the effectiveness of these compounds in the treatment of bleeding disorders is explained by the role of local hyperfibrinolysis in the onset and maintenance of bleeding in such mucosal tracts as the nasopharynx, the gastrointestinal, and the genitourinary tracts. Sometimes in these situations, antifibrinolytic drugs are sufficient to stop bleeding without the need to recur to desmopressin or plasma products. More often, they are given as adjuvants, because they help to reduce the total amount of coagulation factors or desmopressin by stabilizing the formed fibrin clots. A typical example is dental surgery, in which these drugs can also be used locally, as mouthwashes. We recommend the use of antifibrinolytic amino acids together with desmopressin for the aforementioned reasons. Even though desmopressin induces a brisk, short-term increase of tissue plasminogen activator, there is no evidence that this potential antihemostatic effect affects the efficacious control of bleeding in treated patients.

Conclusion

The therapeutic use of desmopressin in VWD (and mild hemophilia) has now withstood the experience of nearly 40 years. There is no doubt that the use of this compound in the late 1970s to early 1980s at a time when plasma concentrates were not virus inactivated has spared many patients with mild hemophilia and VWD from bloodborne infections and the related consequences [21], felt as particularly dramatic in patients with mild bleeding disorders who need treatment much less frequently than those with severe disease. The advent of virus-inactivated plasma concentrates and the availability of recombinant factors have currently rendered less crucial the safety afforded by a synthetic drug as desmopressin. Hence its main appeal is its relatively low cost, particularly for developing countries. It is baffling that, despite its early inclusion in the WHO recommended list of essential drugs, desmopressin is not licenced nor available in many developing countries.

References

1 Sadler JE. Biochemistry and genetics of von Willebrand factor. *Ann Rev Biochem* 1998; **67**: 395–424.

2 Kaufmann JE, Oksche A, Wollheim CB, Gunther G, Rosenthal W, Vischer UM. Vasopressin induced von Willebrand factor secretion from endothelial cells involves V2 receptors and cAMP. *J Clin Invest* 2000; **106**: 107–16.

3 Mannucci PM, Aberg M, Nilsson IM, Robertson B. Mechanism of plasminogen activator and factor VIII increase after vasoactive drugs. *Br J Haematol* 1975; **30**: 81–93.

4 Mannucci PM, Canciani MT, Rota L, Donovan BS. Response of factor VIII/von Willebrand factor to DDAVP in healthy subjects and patients with haemophilia A and von Willebrand disease. *Br J Haematol* 1981; **47**: 283–93.

5 Rodeghiero F, Castaman G, Mannucci PM. Prospective multicenter study on subcutaneous concentrated desmopressin for home treatment of patients with von Willebrand disease and mild or moderate hemophilia A. *Thromb Haemost* 1996; **76**: 692–6.

6 Mannucci PM, Ruggeri ZM, Pareti FI, Capitanio AM. Deamino-8-D-arginine vasopressin: a new pharmacological approach to the management of haemophilia and von Willebrand disease. *Lancet* 1977; **1**: 869–72.

7 Revel-Vilk S, Schmugge M, Carcao MD, Blanchette P, Rand ML, Blanchette VS. Desmopressin (DDAVP) responsiveness in children with von Willebrand disease. *J Pediatr Hematol Oncol* 2003; **25**: 874–9.

8 Federici AB, Mazurier C, Berntorp E, *et al.* Biological response to desmopressin in patients with severe type 1 and type 2 von Willebrand disease. Results of a Multicenter European Study. *Blood* 2004; **103**: 2032–8.

9 Rodeghiero F, Castaman G, Di Bona E, Ruggeri M. Consistency of responses to repeated DDAVP infusions in patients with von Willebrand's disease and hemophilia A. *Blood* 1989; **74**: 1997–2000.

10 Mannucci PM, Lombardi R, Bader R, *et al.* Heterogeneity of type I von Willebrand disease: evidence for a subgroup with an abnormal von Willebrand factor. *Blood* 1985; **66**: 796–802.

11 Castaman G, Lethagen S, Federici AB, *et al.* Response to desmopressin is influenced by the genotype and phenotype in type 1 von Willebrand disease (VWD): results from the European Study MCMDM-1VWD. *Blood* 2008; **111**: 3531–9.

12 Ruggeri ZM, Mannucci PM, Lombardi R, Federici AB, Zimmerman TS. Multimeric composition of factor VIII/von Willebrand factor following administration of DDAVP: implications for pathophysiology and therapy of von Willebrand's disease subtypes. *Blood* 1982; **59**: 1272–8.

13 Mazurier C, Gaucher C, Jorieux S, Goudemand M, and the Collaborative Group. Biological effect of desmopressin in eight patients with type 2 N ("Normandy") von Willebrand disease. *Br J Haematol* 1994; **88**: 849–54.

14 Federici AB, Rand JH, Bucciarelli P, *et al.*, and the Subcommittee on von Willebrand Factor. Acquired von Willebrand syndrome: data from an international registry. *Thromb Haemost* 2000; **84**: 345–9.

15 Federici AB, Stabile F, Castaman G, Canciani MT, Mannucci PM. Treatment of acquired von Willebrand syndrome in patients with monoclonal gammopathy of uncertain significance: comparison of three different therapeutic approaches. *Blood* 1998; **92**: 2707–11

16 Mannucci PM, Bettega D, Cattaneo M. Patterns of development of tachyphylaxis in patients with hemophilia and von Willebrand disease after repeated doses of desmopressin (DDAVP). *Br J Haematol* 1992; **82**: 87–93.

17 Smith TJ, Gill JC, Ambroso DR, Hathaway WE. Hyponatremia and seizures in young children given DDAVP. *Am J Hematol* 1989; **31**: 199–202.

18 Bond L, Bevin D. Myocardial infarction in a patient with hemophilia A treated with DDAVP. *N Engl J Med* 1988; **318**: 121 (letter).

19 Byrnes JJ, Larcada A, Moake JL. Thrombosis following desmopressin for uremic bleeding. *Am J Hematol* 1988; **28**: 63–5.

20 Mannucci PM. Use of desmopressin (DDAVP) during early pregnancy in factor VIII-deficient women. *Blood* 2005; **105**: 3382.

21 Mannucci PM, Ghirardini A. Desmopressin: twenty years after. *Thromb Haemost* 1997; **78**: 958.

CHAPTER 53

Treatment of von Willebrand disease: therapeutic concentrates

Erik E. Berntorp
Skåne University Hospital, Malmö, Sweden

Introduction

Treatment with von Willebrand factor (VWF) containing factor VIII (FVIII) concentrates is indicated in some cases of type 1 von Willebrand disease (VWD), a majority of type 2 and all type 3 VWD where hemophilia-like bleeding due to their FVIII deficiency occurs, and in acute situations where replacement with FVIII and VWF is a prerequisite for achieving hemostasis. As increased levels of VWF prolong and more or less restore FVIII level, it may be feasible to use purified VWF concentrates given well ahead of, for example, elective surgery. There are several types of licenced VWF/FVIII containing concentrates. In this chapter, treatment effects and adverse advents with concentrates are discussed.

Concentrates

Plasma-derived, viral-inactivated concentrates used for correction of the hemostatic defect in VWD vary among brands in their composition and quantitative levels of content of VWF relative to FVIII levels. Budde *et al.* [1] reported a comparative study of 12 different concentrates. They found that Haemate (CSL Behring) had the highest content of high-molecular-weight multimers (HMWM) and highest specific activity of VWF:Ag, VWF:RCo, and VWF:CB per FVIII molecule. Lethagen *et al.* [2] in a study of six concentrates reported similar findings. Mannucci and Franchini [3] published the characteristics of eight VWF/FVIII concentrates tested in prospective clinical trials. Concordant with the two previous studies, they found that Haemate-P had the highest VWF:RCo/FVIII ratio, closely followed by Biostate with ratios of 2–2.5. The other concentrates had ratios around 1. In Table 53.1, published characteristics of selected VWF/FVIII concentrates are given. A broad variation of content and quality of VWF and FVIII can be seen. The ratio of VWF:RCo/FVIII is

by far highest in Facteur Willebrand (a predecessor of Wilfact/Wilfactin) implying a very high content of VWF compared to FVIII. In addition, the content of HMWM varied with Haemate-P and Facteur Willebrand showing the highest values, 82–94%, of the content in normal human plasma. Definition of HMWM is not universal, and the function of different multimeric sizes has not yet been satisfactorily clarified. A recombinant VWF concentrate has been developed devoid of FVIII [4] and is currently in clinical trials. The role of this product in the management of VWD remains to be seen.

It can be concluded that treating physicians must be aware of the large differences among VWF concentrates and the potential clinical implications. Concentrates lacking HMWM are probably less efficient for mucosal bleeding. FVIII is most important for surgical bleeding. A low FVIII content may be preferable, except in cases of acute surgery, provided that dosing is prescribed according to content of VWF:RCo levels. In Europe, dosing is usually guided by the FVIII content in concentrates whereas in North America the content of VWF:RCo is used for dose calculation. The latter option is probably the most relevant as quantitative and/or qualitative changes of VWF is the basis of the disorder.

Clinical studies with von Willebrand factor/factor VIII concentrates

A systematic review of concentrate treatment of hemophilia A and B and VWD was performed under the auspices of the Swedish Council on Health Technology Assessment (SBU) to evaluate the knowledge of and evidence underpinning concentrate treatment of these diseases [5,6]. A literature search was performed for the years 1985 to 2010. The inclusion criteria for the VWD section were patients with VWD who do not respond satisfactorily to desmopressin.

Textbook of Hemophilia, Third Edition. Edited by Christine A. Lee, Erik E. Berntorp and W. Keith Hoots.
© 2014 John Wiley & Sons, Ltd. Published 2014 by John Wiley & Sons, Ltd.

Table 53.1 von Willebrand factor/factor XIII (VWF/FVIII) concentrates. Ratios of FVIII:C/VWF:RCo and content of high-molecular-weight VWF multimers (HMWM). Data from [1–3].

Concentrate	Manufacturer	VWF:RCo/ FVIII:C ratio	Content of HMWM in % of normal human plasma
Haemate-P	CSL Behring	2.04–2.88	91–94
Wilate	Octapharma	0.9	na
Alphanate	Grifols	0.82–0.91	29
Fandhi	Grifols	1.04–1.29	32
Biostate	CSL Bioplasma	2	na
Koate DVI	Talecris	1.1–1.2	61
Immunate	Baxter	0.17–1.1	4–15
Factor 8Y	BioProducts Laboratory	0.81–1.87	32
Facteur Willebrand	LFB	50	82

Types of studies searched included randomized and controlled studies, cohort and case–control studies, registry studies, and case series. Overviews such as national guidelines and/or systematic literature reviews were also accepted. Pharmacokinetic studies were not included. The number of patients required was 20 or more. The search resulted in 18 articles that met the inclusion criteria, including four articles that presented overviews. Fourteen studies presented original research, of which six were prospective and eight are retrospective. The study populations included between 21 and 100 patients. The severe and painful symptoms caused by acute bleeds in VWD (at times life threatening), and the good clinical effects observed from treatment render placebo-controlled studies unethical. Consequently, the scientific evidence for the studies was low. Investigations included in the report and a few more recent studies will be described below.

Prospective studies

Mannucci et al. [7] studied the VWF/FVIII concentrate Alphanate in a multicenter cohort study. Of the 81 patients, 32 had type 3 VWD. Dosing was 40–50 IU/kg VWF:RCo for bleeding and 60–75 IU for surgery. Less bleeding than expected was observed during surgery and the median number of infusions for stopping bleeding events was one for type 1 and 2A and three for type 3 VWD. Two adverse events were recorded, i.e. one thrombophlebitis and one deep venous thrombosis in connection with surgery

Cox Gill [8] reported a study of 41 patients, 12 of whom were type 3 VWD. Fifty-three acute bleeding episodes were treated with Haemate at an initial dose of 67 IU/kg VWF:RCo and usually for 3 days. In 98% of the cases, the effects were found to be excellent/good.

Similar to the preceding study, Thompson et al. [9] reported a multicenter study including treatment of 39 surgical patients with Haemate. Initial doses were 60–80 IU/kg VWF:RCo with a somewhat lower dose on subsequent days for up to 7 days. In all cases, the hemostatic effect was reported to be excellent/good.

Borel-Derlon et al. [10] conducted a study with Wilfactin in 50 patients, including 18 with type 3 VWD. For spontaneous bleeds, a median dose per infusion of 41.8 units VWF:RCo per kilogram of body weight was given, and the mean number of infusions was three. Effects were reported to be excellent/good in 88% and 89% at 6 and 24 h post-treatment, respectively. In elective surgery, only Wilfactin was administered, starting 12–24 h prior to the procedure, but in emergency surgery FVIII was also given for a rapid effect on FVIII plasma levels. The median dose of Wilfactin was 45.5 units (range 11.1–100), treatment was 3 days (range 1–57), and the median number of infusions 3.0 (range 1–65). Neither thromboembolic complications, nor the development of antibodies, were observed.

Lethagen et al. [11] reported results from a study of 29 patients, in which 27 underwent elective surgery under the protection of Haemate. Eight patients had type 3 VWD. Sixteen procedures were classified as major surgery. The preoperative median dose was 62.4 IU/kg VWF:RCo, and the maintenance dose was lower—a median of 19.4 IU/kg. On the first postoperative day, 92.6% had excellent effects and 7.4% good effects. One patient, reportedly having multiple risk factors, was affected by a pulmonary embolism.

Berntorp and Windyga [12] presented 44 patients treated with Wilate for acute bleeding or as long-term prophylaxis. In 1095 bleeding episodes treated, the effects were rated as excellent/good in 96% of cases. Median dose was 26 units FVIII:C (about 23 U VWF:RCo) per kilogram of body weight, and treatment averaged 2 days. The dose for gastrointestinal bleeding was higher, 44 units, and the treatment time was longer, 4 days. Nineteen patients received prophylactic treatment over a long period (average 14.8 months) at a mean dose of 27.4 units FVIII:C and an interval of 1.9 infusions per week. The bleeding frequency decreased significantly during prophylaxis, and no serious side-effects were observed.

In the study by Windyga and von Depka-Prondzinski [13], data for VWD patients receiving Wilate for perioperative management were presented. A total of 57 surgical procedures were performed (major: n = 27; minor n = 30) in 32 patients. The majority of patients (n = 19, 59.4%) had type 3 VWD, nine (28.1%) had type 2 VWD, and four (12.5%) had type 1 VWD. During major surgery, median daily FVIII dose and mean total number of infusions were 25 IU/kg FVIII (VWF:RCo ∼ 23 IU) and 11.0, respectively. Corresponding values for minor surgery were 35 IU/kg (VWF:RCo ∼ 32 IU) and 1.5. Efficacy was excellent or good in 51/53 (96%) procedures and no significant side-effects were observed.

Gill et al. [14] evaluated the safety, efficacy, and optimal dosing of Humate-P in subjects with VWD undergoing elective surgery. Dosing was based on VWF:RCo and FVIII pharmacokinetic assessments performed before surgery. Overall, effective hemostasis was achieved in 32/35 subjects. Median VWF/FVIII concentrate loading doses ranged from 42.6 IU/kg VWF:RCo (oral surgery) to 61.2 IU/kg VWF:RCo (major surgery), with a median of 10 (range, 2–55) doses administered per subject. Adverse events considered possibly treatment related ($n = 6$) were generally mild and of short duration.

Castaman et al. [15] assessed the efficacy, safety, and ease of use of a new volume-reduced (VR) formulation of Haemate-P. Of the 121 patients enrolled, 25.6% had type 3 VWD and greater than 40% had severe disease. All patients were followed for 2 years, a total of 521 visits. On-demand treatment was given to 61.9% of patients, secondary long-term prophylaxis to 25.6%, and prophylaxis for surgery, dental, or invasive procedures to 45.5%. The response to treatment was rated as good to excellent in 93–99% of interventions. The new formulation was well tolerated.

Dunkley et al. [16] evaluated the efficacy and safety of Biostate when used for nonsurgical bleeds, surgical procedures, and prophylactic therapy. Twenty-three patients (seven type 1, nine type 2, and seven type 3; 12 male, 11 female) were treated. Dosing was based on pretreatment FVIII:C and/or VWF:RCo plasma levels and a predetermined dosing guide. Hemostatic efficacy was rated as excellent or good for all major and minor surgery events, long-term prophylaxis, and for four of the six assessable nonsurgical bleeding events. The median overall exposure to Biostate across all groups was 8 days, greater in the prophylactic group (range 53–197) compared with major surgery (3–24), minor surgery (1–8), and nonsurgical bleeds (1–10).

Retrospective studies

Goudemand et al. [17] reported a cohort study of 75 patients comprising a spectrum of different types of VWD. The majority of patients ($n = 42$) had type 1 VWD. Fourteen bleeding episodes and 54 surgical procedures (31 minor and 23 major) were treated with Wilfactin. Initial doses were approximately 50 IU/kg VWF:RCo. Epistaxis and gingival bleeding was generally stopped after one infusion. No bleeding complications were seen during surgery.

Nitu-Whalley et al. [18] reported a study of 65 patients who underwent 103 surgical procedures, in which 38 patients (68 surgical procedures) were treated with concentrate, namely BPL 8Y or Haemate. The initial dose was approximately 50 IU FVIII/kg. Hemostatic effects were reported to be excellent in 82% of the procedures, while the remainder were equally distributed between moderate and poor effects.

Federici et al. [19] conducted a review of 22 patients treated with Fandhi for surgery or acute bleeding. Hemostatic effects were excellent to good in 92% of the treatment cases. The median dose of FVIII was 51 IU/kg given within the initial days of major surgery.

Franchini et al. [20] presented a study including 26 patients treated with Haemate for 43 procedures, 14 of which were major surgery. Initial doses in major surgery averaged 61.2 units VWF:RCo per kilogram of body weight with a range of 47.5–81.1 units. The mean daily dose administered was 39.3 units (range 25–52.5), and the number of treatment days was 9.7 (range 5–23). In all cases, the effects were judged to be excellent/good. No side-effects were observed.

Federici et al. [21] reported a study with Haemate conducted in 10 centers. It included 100 patients, of whom 37 had type 3 VWD. Fifty-nine patients were treated for 280 apparently spontaneous bleeds, with 1003 infusions at a daily median dose of 72 units/kg (range 27–135) VWF:RCo. In 95% of the cases, the effects were excellent/good. Fifty-six patients underwent a variety of procedures, 17 of which were major. The daily median dose for all types of procedures was 80 units/kg (range 27–146). Effects were rated as excellent/good in 97% of the cases. Seventeen patients received long-term prophylaxis to prevent bleeds in joints or the gastrointestinal tract and were dosed 2–3 times per week. Effects were excellent/good in 100% of cases. No side-effects were observed.

Rivard et al. [22] reported the results of a surgical study that included 39 patients, nine with type 3 VWD. The patients were treated with Alphanate in 61 procedures, 12 of which were major surgery. The maximum dose administered was 80 units VWF:RCo per kilogram of body weight, with a total perioperative dose of 34 229 units for major surgery. Excellent/good effects were observed in 95.1% of the procedures on day 1 and 91.8% on the following day. No serious side-effects were observed.

Viswabandya et al. [23] reported experiences with Koate DVI in a surgery study. Ten of the 21 patients underwent 10 major procedures. The mean dose was 35 units FVIII per kilogram of body weight as an initial dose followed by 10–20 units/kg daily for 7 days. In minor surgery, the doses were approximately half that for major surgery, and treatment time was 2 days. Adequate hemostasis was observed in all cases.

Howman et al. [24] retrospectively assessed the efficacy and safety of Biostate in 43 children with VWD who received treatment for surgery, nonsurgical bleeds, or continuous prophylaxis. Excellent/good hemostatic efficacy was observed in 90% of surgical procedures ($n = 42$) with a mean daily FVIII dose of 47 IU/kg FVIII:C and a median treatment duration of 3 days. Excellent/good hemostatic efficacy was achieved in 94% of nonsurgical bleeding events ($n = 72$) with a mean FVIII dose of 45 IU/kg FVIII:C per day and a median treatment duration of 1 day. One case of nausea, possibly related to product administration, was reported.

Prophylaxis

In several of the studies mentioned, small cohorts of patients treated with secondary prophylaxis for varying time periods with excellent results have been reported.

A few studies have focused on prophylaxis with larger cohorts and longer periods of follow-up. The studies, cited below, are retrospective. Prospective studies are underway but results are not yet available [25,26].

Berntorp and Petrini [27] presented experiences in prophylactic treatment for VWD in a cohort including 35 patients, of which 28 had type 3 VWD. In children, the indications for prophylaxis were bleeding in the nose or mouth and, in older children, joint bleeds as well. Bleeding in joints dominated among adults, but gastrointestinal bleeds and profuse menstruation were also common indications. Before the mid-1980s, AHF-Kabi (fraction I-0, produced by Kabi, no longer available) was used, and thereafter Haemate. The doses were 24 units FVIII/kg (range 12–50 units), given 1–3 times per week. Of the adult patients, 63% were treated with prophylaxis for at least 10 years, and 89% of the 18 children for at least 5 years. The results showed that the number of bleeds decreased substantially and significantly during prophylaxis, and in many patients bleeding ceased.

The Von Willebrand Disease Prophylaxis Network (VWDPN) was formed to investigate the role of prophylaxis in VWD [28]. Sixty-one subjects from 20 centers in 10 countries were enrolled. Data for 59 were used in the analysis. The median age at onset of prophylaxis was 22.4 years. Type 3 VWD accounted for the largest number ($n = 34$, 57.6%). Differences in bleeding rates within individuals during prophylaxis compared with before prophylaxis were significant for the total group ($P < 0.0001$), and for those with primary bleeding indications of epistaxis ($P = 0.0005$), joint bleeding ($P = 0.002$), and gastrointestinal bleeding ($P = 0.001$). The effect of prophylaxis was similar among those aged <18 years and those ≥18. One person developed an inhibitor during treatment.

Halimeh et al. [29] reported results on secondary prophylactic VWF replacement therapy applied in 32 patients (children, $n = 13$; adolescents, $n = 7$; adults, $n = 12$) with VWD (type 1, $n = 4$; type 2, $n = 15$; type 3, $n = 13$]. Eight patients were treated with Humate-P and 24 with Wilate. The median dose vWF:RCo was 40 IU/kg (range 20–47). Twenty-three patients were given substitution therapy twice weekly, seven patients three times a week, and two children four times per week. Within a 12-month period hemoglobin concentrations returned to normal values. The median duration of prophylaxis was 3 years. Recurrent bleeding episodes stopped in 31/32 patients, whereas inhibitors developed in one.

Information from guidelines and reviews

Several guidelines are available which give recommendations about treatment with concentrates. Pasi et al. [30] reported the British UK Haemophilia Centre Doctors' Organization (UKHCDO) recommendations and guidelines for the care management of VWD. Nichols et al. [31] presented guidelines

from the US National Heart, Lung, and Blood Institute (NHLBI). Federici et al. [32] reported guidelines from the Italian Association of Hemophilia Centres (AICE).

Discussion and recommendations

The ratio between VWF and FVIII varies among products and is generally in the range of 1–2.5. Infusion with these concentrates provides an immediate rise in VWF and FVIII which is beneficial when treating acute bleeds and acute surgery. A secondary rise in FVIII levels occurs with some concentrates after 12–24 h; in others, a parallel decay over time for VWF and FVIII [33] has been reported. However, infusion of virtually pure VWF will also restore FVIII levels due to binding and stabilization of endogenous FVIII. This takes 12–24 h and in connection with treatment of acute bleeds and surgery infusion of exogenous FVIII is sometimes needed.

Studies presented are retrospective or prospective cohort studies without controls, and they represent a low grade of evidence. However, the effects of concentrate are generally reported to be very good and cause few side-effects. Rarely, venous thromboembolism have been reported in VWD [34], but it is important to be aware that infusion of VWF and FVIII may result in supranormal levels of FVIII. Thromboprophylaxis cannot therefore be recommended if patients are treated appropriately.

Prophylactic treatment of VWD is sometimes considered indicated particularly for type 3. Available evidence indicates high clinical efficacy.

Guidelines for dosing are available but need to be highly individualized taking into account the product used, the type of bleeding, or prevention of bleeding and type of VWD. Use of pharmacokinetic evaluation prior to surgery has not been particularly successful [35]. Dosing should be done according to VWF:RCo, but FVIII plasma levels also need to be monitored during major surgery and bleeding. The initial dose for major events should be around 50 IU/kg giving a rise in plasma level to approximately 100% (baseline not taken into account) and repeated after 12 h, then every 24 h until hemostasis is secured. Dosing for minor events may be half of that used for major events, and additional doses must be determined individually. For regular prophylaxis, 20–50 IU/kg 1–3 times per week may be recommended, with a more intensive schedule for gastrointestinal bleeding tendency.

References

1 Budde U, Metzner HJ, Muller HG. Comparative analysis and classification of von Willebrand factor/factor VIII concentrates: impact on treatment of patients with von Willebrand disease. *Semin Thromb Hemost* 2006; **32**(6): 626–35.

2 Lethagen S, Carlson M, Hillarp A. A comparative in vitro evaluation of six von Willebrand factor concentrates. *Haemophilia* 2004; **10**(3): 243–9.

3 Mannucci P, Franchini M. The use of plasma-derived concentrates. In: Federici AB, Lee CA, Berntorp E, Lillicrap D, Montgomery A (eds.) *Von Willebrand Disease Basic and Clinical Aspects*. Oxford: Wiley-Blackwell, 2011: 200–6.

4 Turecek PL, Schrenk G, Rottensteiner H, *et al*. Structure and function of a recombinant von Willebrand factor drug candidate. *Semin Thromb Hemost* 2010; **36**(5): 510–21.

5 Swedish Council on Health Technology Assessment (www.sbu.se/en/). Treatment of hemophilia and von Willebrand disease.

6 Berntorp E, Astermark J, Baghaei F, *et al*. Treatment of haemophilia A and B and von Willebrand's disease: summary and conclusions of a systematic review as part of a Swedish health-technology assessment. *Haemophilia* 2011; **18**(2): 158–65.

7 Mannucci PM, Chediak J, Hanna W, *et al*. Treatment of von Willebrand disease with a high-purity factor VIII/von Willebrand factor concentrate: a prospective, multicenter study. *Blood* 2002; **99**(2): 450–6.

8 Cox Gill J. Diagnosis and treatment of von Willebrand disease. *Hematol/Oncol Clin N Am* 2004; **18**: 1277–99.

9 Thompson AR, Gill JC, Ewenstein BM, Mueller-Velten G, Schwartz BA, Humate PSG. Successful treatment for patients with von Willebrand disease undergoing urgent surgery using factor VIII/VWF concentrate (Humate-P). *Haemophilia* 2004; **10**(1): 42–51.

10 Borel-Derlon A, Federici AB, Roussel-Robert V, *et al*. Treatment of severe von Willebrand disease with a high-purity von Willebrand factor concentrate (Wilfactin): a prospective study of 50 patients. *J Thromb Haemost* 2007; **5**(6): 1115–24.

11 Lethagen S, Kyrle PA, Castaman G, Haertel S, Mannucci PM. von Willebrand factor/factor VIII concentrate (Haemate-P) dosing based on pharmacokinetics: a prospective multicenter trial in elective surgery. *J Thromb Haemost* 2007; **5**(7): 1420–30.

12 Berntorp E, Windyga J. Treatment and prevention of acute bleedings in von Willebrand disease—efficacy and safety of Wilate, a new generation von Willebrand factor/factor VIII concentrate. *Haemophilia* 2009; **15**(1): 122–30.

13 Windyga J, von Depka-Prondzinski M, European Wilate Study G. Efficacy and safety of a new generation von Willebrand factor/factor VIII concentrate (Wilate(R)) in the management of perioperative haemostasis in von Willebrand disease patients undergoing surgery. *Thromb Haemost* 2011; **105**(6): 1072–9.

14 Gill JC, Shapiro A, Valentino LA, *et al*. von Willebrand factor/factor VIII concentrate (Humate-P) for management of elective surgery in adults and children with von Willebrand disease. *Haemophilia* 2011; **17**(6): 895–905.

15 Castaman G, Coppola A, Zanon E, *et al*. Efficacy and safety during formulation switch of a pasteurized VWF/FVIII concentrate: results from an Italian prospective observational study in patients with von Willebrand disease. *Haemophilia* 2012; **19**(1): 82–8.

16 Dunkley S, Baker RI, Pidcock M, *et al*. Clinical efficacy and safety of the factor VIII/von Willebrand factor concentrate BIOSTATE in patients with von Willebrand's disease: a prospective multi-centre study. *Haemophilia* 2010; **16**(4): 615–24.

17 Goudemand J, Negrier C, Ounnoughene N, Sultan Y. Clinical management of patients with von Willebrand's disease with a VHP vWF concentrate: the French experience. *Haemophilia* 1998; **4** (Suppl. 3): 48–52.

18 Nitu-Whalley IC, Griffioen A, Harrington C, Lee CA. Retrospective review of the management of elective surgery with desmopressin and clotting factor concentrates in patients with von Willebrand disease. *Am J Hematol* 2001; **66**(4): 280–4.

19 Federici AB, Baudo F, Caracciolo C, *et al*. Clinical efficacy of highly purified, doubly virus-inactivated factor VIII/von Willebrand factor concentrate (Fanhdi) in the treatment of von Willebrand disease: a retrospective clinical study. *Haemophilia* 2002; **8**(6):761–7.

20 Franchini M, Rossetti G, Tagliaferri A, *et al*. Efficacy and safety of factor VIII/von Willebrand's factor concentrate (Haemate-P) in preventing bleeding during surgery or invasive procedures in patients with von Willebrand disease. *Haematologica* 2003; **88**(11): 1279–83.

21 Federici AB, Castaman G, Franchini M, *et al*. Clinical use of Haemate-P in inherited von Willebrand's disease: a cohort study on 100 Italian patients. *Haematologica* 2007; **92**(7): 944–51.

22 Rivard GE, Aledort L. Alphanate Surgical I. Efficacy of factor VIII/von Willebrand factor concentrate Alphanate in preventing excessive bleeding during surgery in subjects with von Willebrand disease. *Haemophilia* 2008; **14**(2): 271–5.

23 Viswabandya A, Mathews V, George B, *et al*. Successful surgical haemostasis in patients with von Willebrand disease with Koate DVI. *Haemophilia* 2008; **14**(4): 763–7.

24 Howman R, Barnes C, Curtin J, *et al*. The clinical efficacy and safety of the FVIII/VWF concentrate, BIOSTATE(R), in children with von Willebrand disorder: a multi-centre retrospective review. *Haemophilia* 2011; **17**(3): 463–9.

25 Federici AB. Highly purified VWF/FVIII concentrates in the treatment and prophylaxis of von Willebrand disease: the PRO.WILL Study. *Haemophilia* 2007; **13**(Suppl.): 15–24.

26 Berntorp E, Abshire T. The von Willebrand disease prophylaxis network: exploring a treatment concept. *J Thromb Haemost* 2006; **4**(11): 2511–12.

27 Berntorp E, Petrini P. Long-term prophylaxis in von Willebrand disease. *Blood Coag Fibrinol* 2005; **16**(Suppl. 1): S23–6.

28 Abshire TC, Federici AB, Alvarez MT, *et al*. Prophylaxis in severe forms of von Willebrand's disease: results from the von Willebrand Disease Prophylaxis Network (VWD PN). *Haemophilia* 2012; Jan **19**(1): 76–81.

29 Halimeh S, Krumpel A, Rott H, *et al*. Long-term secondary prophylaxis in children, adolescents and young adults with von Willebrand disease. Results of a cohort study. *Thromb Haemost* 2011; **105**(4): 597–604.

30 Pasi KJ, Collins PW, Keeling DM, *et al*. Management of von Willebrand disease: a guideline from the UK Haemophilia Centre Doctors' Organization. *Haemophilia* 2004; **10**(3): 218–31.

31 Nichols WL, Hultin MB, James AH, *et al*. von Willebrand disease (VWD): evidence-based diagnosis and management guidelines, the National Heart, Lung, and Blood Institute (NHLBI) Expert Panel report (USA). *Haemophilia* 2008; **14**(2): 171–232.

32 Federici AB, Castaman G, Mannucci PM, and the Italian Association of Hemophilia C. Guidelines for the diagnosis and management of von Willebrand disease in Italy. *Haemophilia* 2002; **8**(5): 607–21.

33 Kessler CM, Friedman K, Schwartz BA, Gill JC, Powell JS. The pharmacokinetic diversity of two von Willebrand factor

(VWF)/factor VIII (FVIII) concentrates in subjects with congenital von Willebrand disease. Results from a prospective, randomised crossover study. *Thromb Haemost* 2011; **106**(2): 279–88.

34 Coppola A, Franchini M, Makris M, Santagostino E, Di Minno G, Mannucci PM. Thrombotic adverse events to coagulation factor concentrates for treatment of patients with haemophilia and von

Willebrand disease: a systematic review of prospective studies. *Haemophilia* 2012; **18**(3): e173–87.

35 Di Paola J, Lethagen S, Gill J, *et al.* Presurgical pharmacokinetic analysis of a von Willebrand factor/factor VIII (VWF/FVIII) concentrate in patients with von Willebrand's disease (VWD) has limited value in dosing for surgery. *Haemophilia* 2011; **17**(5): 752–8.

PART XVI

Rare bleeding disorders

CHAPTER 54

Factor II

Jan Astermark
Skåne University Hospital, Malmö, Sweden

Introduction

Factor II (FII; prothrombin) deficiency is a rare bleeding disorder that in the homozygous severe form is associated with high mortality. Milder deficiencies, however, may actually be underdiagnosed, since routine laboratory screening tests are often only slightly affected and many patients do not experience bleeding symptoms requiring medical care. This chapter provides an overview of the structure and function of prothrombin and some clinical perspectives on the various deficiency states.

Biosynthesis

Prothrombin is synthesized as a preproprotein in hepatocytes and encoded by a gene on chromosome 11 (11p11-q12) of 21 kb containing 14 exons and 13 intervening sequences [1]. The prepeptide directs the synthesized protein to the endoplasmic reticulum and is then removed prior to the process of post-translational modification. The mature molecule is a plasma glycoprotein and zymogen of a serine protease requiring vitamin K for normal biosynthesis [2]. The common feature of all vitamin K-dependent proteases is an N-terminal noncatalytic module containing γ-carboxyglutamic acid (Gla) residues, but, unlike the procoagulant factor VII (FVII), factor IX (FIX), and factor X (FX), prothrombin consists not of epidermal growth factor (EGF)-like modules but of two kringle domains separated from the Gla module by a disulfide loop. The propeptide serves as an anchor for the γ-carboxylase, and is cleaved off before secretion [3]. The catalytic serine protease part contains the active site and is located at the C-terminal end of the molecule.

Structure and function

The binding of calcium to the Gla module is fundamental for proper folding of the vitamin K-dependent enzymes and for the accumulation of the factors on a negatively charged phospholipid membrane at concentrations high enough to promote fibrin formation [4,5]. The Gla residues have also been associated with normal intracellular transportation. The function of the kringles, named after a pastry because of their pretzel-like form, is to some extent unclear, although the second kringle seems to be involved in the binding of activated factor Va (FVa) and thrombin. Thrombin is the active form of prothrombin. It is formed by the cleavage of two peptide bonds by the prothrombinase complex composed of FXa, FVa, and calcium on a phospholipid surface (Figure 54.1). In contrast to the other activated vitamin K-dependent coagulation factors, thrombin contains none of the noncatalytic modules and therefore has no phospholipid-binding capacity, but dissociates from the prothrombinase complex by diffusion. Thrombin exerts several pro- and anticoagulant effects. It triggers platelet aggregation and promotes coagulation by activating regulatory pathways and generating fibrin monomers by cleavage of a peptide bond in each of the α- and β-subunits of fibrinogen [6].

Prothrombin deficiency

Congenital prothrombin deficiency was first described by Quick in 1947 and further explored in subsequent reports [7,8]. The condition is inherited as an autosomal recessive trait with a prevalence of the presumed homozygous form in the general population of about 1 : 2 000 000 [9–12]. The prevalence, however, varies between ethnic groups and is strongly influenced by the rate of consanguinity. Based on the immunoreactive component in plasma and the functional activity, two different phenotypic deficiencies have been described. In type 1 deficiency, or hypoprothrombinemia, the levels of antigen and functional activity are decreased to a similar extent, whereas in type 2 deficiency, or dysprothrombinemia, the enzyme itself is synthesized and present in plasma at a more or less normal level, but the coagulant activity is low. Mutations found in patients with hypo- and dysprothrombinemia have been reviewed and are summarized

Textbook of Hemophilia, Third Edition. Edited by Christine A. Lee, Erik E. Berntorp and W. Keith Hoots.
© 2014 John Wiley & Sons, Ltd. Published 2014 by John Wiley & Sons, Ltd.

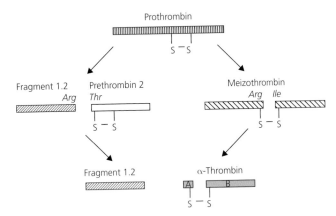

Figure 54.1 Schematic overview of the pathways for prothrombin activation. α-Thrombin is formed by the cleavage of two peptide bonds in prothrombin (Arg271-Thr272) and (Arg320-Ile321). Depending on which bond is cleaved first, fragment 1.2 and prethrombin 2 or meizothrombin is formed as an intermediate product. The activation by the prothrombinase complex is thought to mainly proceed through the formation of meizothrombin.

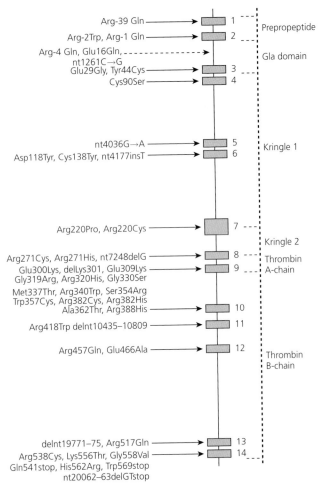

Figure 54.2 Mutations in the prothrombin gene associated with prothrombin deficiency projected on the corresponding exons and protein domains. Modified from [10].

in Figure 54.2 [9,11,13–20]. The mutations associated with dysprothrombinemia are mainly missense mutations, most of which interfere with the FXa-binding site and the active site in the serine protease domain. In patients with hypoprothrombinemia, nonsense and small deletions have also been found, but the mechanisms by which these defects affect function largely remain to be settled. Compound heterozygosity for dys- and hypoprothrombinemia has been described [21]. In addition, combined defects with the other vitamin K-dependent coagulation factors FVII, FIX, and FX, and protein C and S, have been found with variable clinical manifestations and in some cases associated with skeletal abnormalities [22–26]. The molecular defects in these cases are thought to reside in the gene of the γ-glutamyl carboxylase [27,28].

Acquired prothrombin deficiency is usually associated with neutralizing anticoagulants, the lupus anticoagulant-hypoprothrombinemia syndrome (LA-HPS), in patients with systemic lupus erythematosus (SLE), or following viral infections [29–32]. However, non-neutralizing antibodies accelerating the clearance of prothrombin have also been described [33,34].

Laboratory diagnosis

Specific tests are usually required to identify prothrombin deficiency. Screening tests such as prothrombin time (PT) and activated partial thromboplastin time (aPTT) are variably prolonged and in milder cases often more or less normal, suggesting that milder cases could be underdiagnosed. Several specific diagnostic tools are available, some of which are based on viper venoms [9]. The most widely used test is a one-stage assay using thromboplastin as the activating agent. The test is reliable for

screening purposes. In patients with homozygous type 1 prothrombin deficiency activity is usually less than 10% of normal, whereas subjects heterozygous for the same deficiency usually have values between 40% and 60%. Type 1 deficient patients generally have similar results regardless of the diagnostic method used, whereas the results for patients with type 2 deficiency may be inconsistent from method to method. Immunologic methods are required to fully characterize the deficient state in terms of true hypo- or dysprothrombinemia.

Clinical manifestations

The most typical manifestation of the disease, common to most rare bleeding disorders, is the occurrence of excessive bleeding at the time of minor invasive procedures, but a range of bleeding symptoms have been reported [11,35,36]. Heterozygous patients are usually asymptomatic, but homozygosity with activity levels less than 10% of normal may be associated with severe bleeding

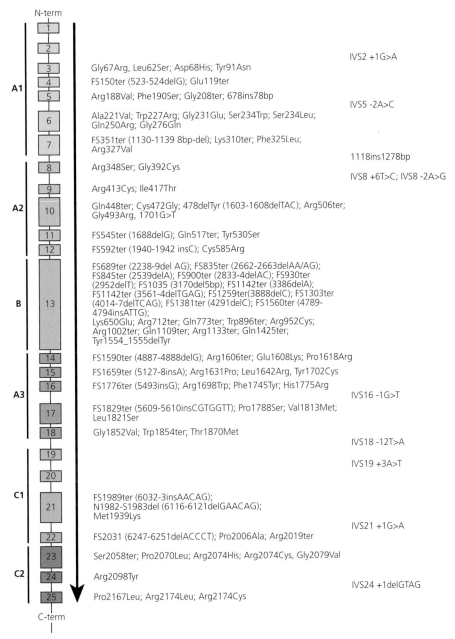

Figure 55.1 Mutations in the *F5* gene, projected on the exons encoding the domains of the protein. Exons and introns are represented by boxes and lines, respectively, and are not drawn to scale. Arrow indicates gross deletion. The FV domain structure is also indicated.

Clinical manifestations

Generally, bleeding symptoms develop during the first 6 years of life, and even bleeding from the umbilical stump has been reported [34]. Heterozygotes are usually asymptomatic or experience only mild bleeding. Frequent symptoms are epistaxis and menorrhagia, which occur in approximately 50% of patients, as well as postoperative and oral cavity hemorrhages [2]. Other less common symptoms include hemarthroses and hematomas, whereas life-threatening bleeding episodes in the gastrointestinal tract and in the central nervous system are rare [34].

The FV activity level has limited correlation with the severity of bleeding. Overall, patients with lower levels are more likely to have bleeding episodes than those with higher levels. Patients who come to medical attention are typically symptomatic homozygotes or compound heterozygotes with FV activity levels less than 5%, although some patients who are compound heterozygotes with levels that ranged from 24% to 68% had no bleeding symptoms [32,35].

Recently, the relationship between coagulation factor activity level and bleeding severity in patients with RBDs has been evaluated by a cross-sectional study using data from 489 patients registered in the EN-RBD. Among them, 60 patients affected with FV deficiency showed a poor association between coagulant activity level and bleeding severity. This could be explained by the FV deficiency association with reduced plasma levels of total and free tissue factor pathway inhibitor antigen, which decreases the FV requirement for minimal thrombin generation in FV-deficient plasma to <1 U/dL [36]. Moreover, in four patients with congenital FV deficiency and undetectable plasma FV, residual platelet FV was shown to support enough thrombin generation to rescue patients from fatal hemorrhage [37].

Treatment

The choice of dosages and modalities of treatment of bleeding episodes is based on the type of bleeding, on FV levels of affected individuals, and on FV plasma half-life (36 h). Replacement therapy of FV can be administered only through fresh frozen plasma (FFP), preferably virus inactivated, since FV concentrates are not available and FV is not present in cryoprecipitate or prothrombin complex concentrates [38]. FV levels should be raised to at least 25 IU/dL [36] by using 15–20 mL/kg FFP [2]. The initial dose should be 15–20 mL/kg followed by smaller amounts, such as 5 mL/kg every 12 h, adjusting the dosage on the basis of FV levels, prothrombin time (PT), and partial thromboplastin time (PTT). Studies of FV recovery recommend maintaining a level of 20–25% of FV activity for surgery or in cases of severe bleeding [38]. Surgical procedures should be addressed by administering FFP once a day to achieve minimum levels of FV of 25 IU/dL until wound healing is established [38]. A single report by Mathias *et al.* described the use of recombinant activated factor VII (rFVIIa) in combination with FFP and platelets to be successful in the management of 13 invasive procedures in three children with severe FV deficiency [39].

It has been suggested that in cases of severe bleeding not controlled with FFP replacement, or in cases of inhibitor development, platelet transfusions may be considered. A case of severe FV deficiency associated with multiple episodes of intracranial bleeding at birth was reported, where the inhibitor development owing to FFP infusion was solved by additional administration of platelets [40]. Platelets provide a concentrated supply of FV (approximately 20% of total circulating FV). Therefore, following α-granule release upon platelet activation, FV can presumably bind immediately to surface receptors optimizing prothrombinase complex activity [38].

Development of alloantibodies to FV in FFP is a potential complication of hereditary FV deficiency [38]. Following FFP replacement therapy, the occurrence of inhibitors, especially transient ones of low level, may not be uncommon and can be neutralized using large amounts of FFP [38]. However, as in the treatment of surgical cases, there are concerns over fluid overload in this situation, and close cardiovascular monitoring is advised. Intravenous immunoglobulin also may be effective in

eradicating the FV inhibitor [41]. Platelet infusions have been reported to be effective in acquired FV deficiency [42], but it was reported to be effective in stabilizing a subdural hematoma also in a patient with hereditary FV deficiency, complicated by inhibitors [40].

Menorrhagia is a common bleeding symptom in women with severe FV deficiency. Management of this symptom usually includes medical treatment such as antifibrinolytics, desmopressin (deamino-D-arginine vasopressin or DDAVP), oral contraceptives, levonorgestrel intrauterine device placement, replacement therapy, and/or surgical treatments, such as endometrial ablation and hysterectomy [43]. No data are available on the management of pregnancy; however, the administration of FFP to maintain a FV level above 15 IU/dL is recommended as soon as the patient is in established labor, and to maintain minimum hemostatic FV levels until after delivery [38]. Management of women with FV deficiency requires additional monitoring of the hemostatic parameters and awareness of the increased risk of bleeding with any surgical interventions [43].

Combined deficiency of factor V and factor VIII

Combined deficiency of FV and FVIII (F5F8D, OMIM 227300) is an autosomal recessive bleeding disorder characterized by concomitantly low levels (usually between 5% and 20%) of the two coagulation factors. F5F8D is completely separate from FV deficiency and FVIII deficiency. The latter two are transmitted with different patterns of inheritance (autosomal recessive for FV, X-linked for FVIII) and involve proteins encoded by two different genes (*F5* gene and *F8* gene). F5F8D was first described by Oeri *et al.* in 1954 [44]; however, the molecular mechanism of the association of the combined factor deficiency was not understood until late 1990s, when Nichols *et al.* [45,46] discovered that the cause of the deficiency was associated with null mutations in the *ERGIC-53* gene, now called *LMAN1* gene (lectin mannose binding protein). *LMAN1* encodes an endoplasmic reticulum (ER)–Golgi intermediate compartment (ERGIC) marker protein; mutations in *LMAN1* were found in ~70% of affected patients but 30% of this population had no detectable mutation in *LMAN1*. In 2003, Zhang *et al.* [47] identified a second locus associated with the deficiency in about 15% of affected families with no mutation in *LMAN1*: the *MCFD2* (multiple coagulation factor deficiency 2) gene encoding for a cofactor for LMAN1 [46]. Even if a debate was carried out on the possible existence of other loci involved in the intracellular transport of FV and FVIII and associated with the disease, until now previous biochemical studies have failed to identify additional components of the LMAN1–MCFD2 receptor complex [48], supporting the idea that F5F8D might be limited to the *LMAN1* and *MCFD2* genes [49].

Congenital F5F8D is estimated to be extremely rare (1/1 000 000) in the general population [4]. However, this disorder was reported to be particularly prevalent among Middle Eastern Jewish and non-Jewish Iranians, where the incidence was estimated to reach ~1/100 000 [50], probably due, at least in part, to the high incidence of consanguineous marriages in these populations [51]; nonetheless, other cases were also reported from different countries of the world: Europe, Asia, Africa, and America [51].

The worldwide prevalence of F5F8D patients, as indicated by the last WFH 2010 global survey and the EN-RBD project seem to be ~3% of the total number of patients affected with RBDs, indicating that F5F8D is one of the rarest coagulation disorders. Nonetheless, F5F8D may be significantly underdiagnosed because of the often mild bleeding symptoms.

LMAN1 and MCFD2 proteins

LMAN1 is a 53-kDa type 1 transmembrane nonglycosylated protein with homology to leguminous lectin proteins [52]. It displays different oligomerization states—monomer, dimer, and hexamer—which have been implicated in its exit/retention within the ER, and it is thought to bind correctly folded glycosylated cargo proteins, including FV and FVIII in the ER, recruiting the cargo for package into coat protein complex II (COPII)-coated vesicles and to transport them first to the ERGIC and then to the Golgi [53]. Indeed, LMAN1 resides in the early secretory pathway, with highest concentration in the ERGIC compartment. LMAN1 consists of a luminal, a transmembrane and a short cytoplasmatic domain for a total of 513 residues. The luminal domain can be divided into two subdomains, an N-terminal carbohydrate recognition domain (CRD) (residues 31–285) and a membrane-proximal α-helical coiled domain, the stalk domain (residues 290–460). The CRD is responsible for the calcium ion-dependent binding of the protein to mannose-rich glycans. The stalk domain, which is predicted to be a coiled-coil structure, contains two cysteines thought to mediate oligomerization of the protein through disulfide interactions [54,55] while the cytoplasmic tail binds to the COPII component of vesicle coats, allowing efficient ER export; it also includes a retrieval sequence to bring the transporter back to the ER after release of its cargo in the ERGIC [56]. Efficient transport of coagulation FV and FVIII along the secretory pathway requires the integrity of their heavily glycosylated B domains and a functional LMAN1 protein, and an interaction between FVIII and LMAN1 has been demonstrated [48,57]. LMAN1 has thus been implicated to act as a sorting receptor, mediating transport of certain glycoproteins from the ER to Golgi. In support of such an important function, homologs of LMAN1 have been identified in levels of the animal kingdom ranging from *Caenorhabditis elegans* to man and display a high degree of sequence identity [58].

MCFD2 is a small (146 residues) soluble protein of 16 kDa with a signal sequence-mediating translocation into the ER and two calmodulin-like EF-hand motifs that may bind Ca^{2+} ions in the C-terminal region. MCFD2 forms a Ca^{2+}-dependent 1:1 stoichiometric complex with LMAN1, which works as a cargo receptor for efficient ER–Golgi transfer of coagulation FV and FVIII during their secretion [45]. While, to date, several proteins have been identified as cargo of LMAN1 (FV, FVIII, cathepsin C, cathepsin Z, nicastrin, and α1-antitrypsin) [59–62], MCFD2 is only known to be required for transport of the blood coagulation factors, suggesting a possible role for MCFD2 as a specific recruitment factor for this subset of LMAN1 cargo proteins [63]. Interestingly, an MCFD2 mutant which fails to coimmunoprecipitate with LMAN1 has been shown to retain the ability to interact with FVIII, implying that the interaction between MCFD2 and the coagulation factors may be independent of MCFD2/LMAN1 binding [48]. Unlike LMAN1, MCFD2 does not include the Phe–Phe (FF) motif required for COPII binding or the Lys–Lys (KK) motif which functions as an ER retrieval signal, suggesting that correct localization of MCFD2 is reliant on its interaction with LMAN1 [47]. In 2010, Nishio *et al.* [64] determined the three-dimensional structure of the complex between MCFD2 and the CRD of LMAN1 They proposed a model of functional coordination between the two proteins: MCFD2 is converted into the active form upon complex formation with LMAN1 thereby enabling capture of the polypeptide segments of FV and FVIII. The coagulation factors bind the LMAN1 oligomer in the ER, but become released upon arrival to acidic post-ER compartments because the sugar binding of ERGIC-53 is pH dependent [64]. In the same year Zheng *et al.*, using a systematic mutagenesis analysis, tested the effects of LMAN1 mutations on the interactions with both MCFD2 and FV/FVIII; they found that the CRD of LMAN1 contains separate binding sites for MCFD2 and FV/FVIII, and that the oligomerization of LMAN1 is required for MCFD2 binding and the ER exit, but dispensable for FV/FVIII binding [65]. In a second study, the same authors demonstrated that the EF hands of MCFD2 contain separate binding sites required for LMAN1–MCFD2 receptor complex formation and for the interaction between MCFD2 and FV and FVIII [66].

Genes structure and mutations

LMAN1 is encoded by a gene of approximately 29 kb located on chromosome 18q21 and containing 13 exons [67]. MCFD2 is encoded by a gene of approximately 19 kb located on chromosome 2p21 and containing 4 exons [47]. To date, more than 50 mutations in *LMAN1* and *MCFD2* genes have been described (http://www.isth.org/?MutationsRareBleedin) (Figures 55.2 and 55.3). Almost 70% of the identified mutations were on the *LMAN1*, either nonsense or frameshift mutations whose truncated protein products would be predicted to lack the normal LMAN1 function. In contrast, both null mutations and missense mutations have been identified in *MCFD2*.

Mutations in *LMAN1* and *MCFD2* are associated with indistinguishable phenotypes [47]. However, a selective delay in

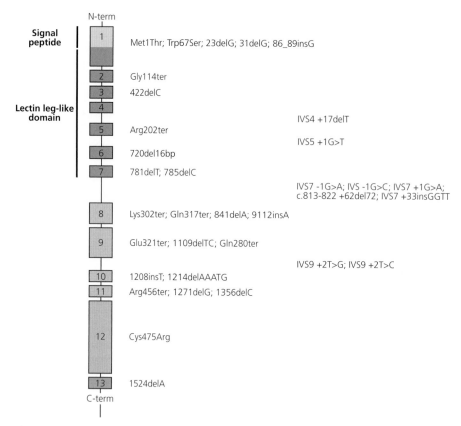

Figure 55.2 Mutation in the *LMAN1* gene, projected on the exons encoding the domains of the protein. Exons and introns are represented by boxes and lines, respectively, and are not drawn to scale.

secretion of the protein procathepsin C has been observed in HeLa cells overexpressing a dominant negative form of LMAN1 [60]. These results were confirmed by Nyfeler *et al.*, showing that LMAN1 also interacts with the two lysosomal glycoproteins cathepsin Z and cathepsin C; in contrast, MCFD2 is not needed for the binding of them to LMAN1 [63]. Zhang *et al.* [68] performed a genotype–phenotype analysis to evaluate whether mutations in different genes are associated with differences in the FV and FVIII plasma levels: they found that the mean FV and FVIII levels in patients with *MCFD2* mutations were significantly lower than the corresponding levels in patients with *LMAN1* mutations. These data suggest that MCFD2 may play a primary role in the export of FV and FVIII from the ER, with the impact of LMAN1 being mediated indirectly through its interaction with MCFD2 [68].

Some of the identified mutations, in both the *LMAN1* and *MCFD2* genes have been reported in more than one family. *LMAN1* mutations, such as c.86_89insG, IVS9+2T>C, IVS7-1G>A, Met1Thr, Arg202ter, and Lys302ter, have been observed in more than four patients [46,69,70–73]. Similarly, the c.149+5G>A and Ile136Thr mutations in *MCFD2* have also been commonly reported [68,73–75]. Moreover, some of the mutations identified on the *LMAN1* were found only in certain populations, suggesting a founder effect: the

IVS9+2T>C splicing mutation prevalent in Jews originating from the island of Djerba in Tunisia [66] and the c.86_89insG unique to Middle Eastern Jews [46]. Another notable mutation is the missense mutation Met1Thr that truncates the initiation codon of LMAN1 and which has only been reported in families of Italian origin. In-vitro expression studies of *LMAN1* and *MCFD2* gene mutations and characterization of the activity of the corresponding recombinant proteins in the secretion of coagulation FV and FVIII proved to be of help in describing the mechanism of the deficiency. Five out of the six identified *MCFD2* missense mutations (Asp81Tyr, Asp89Ala, Asp122Val, Asp129Glu, and Ile136Thr) result in an amino acid substitution at a highly conserved amino acid residue. All these mutations are in one of the two EF-hand domains. They were expressed in COS-1 transfected cells [47,53,68,76], and have been shown to disrupt LMAN1 binding. All the other identified mutations were demonstrated to be associated with the deficiency through analysis performed on Epstein–Barr virus (EBV)-transformed lymphoblasts of the patients that showed the presence or absence of the mutated protein [47,49,70].

Clinical manifestations

F5F8D is characterized by concomitantly low levels (usually between 5% and 20%) of FV and FVIII, both as coagulant activ-

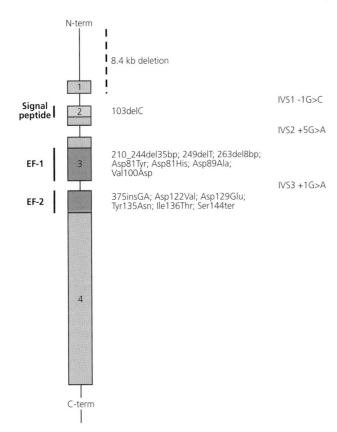

Figure 55.3 Mutation in the *MCFD2* gene, projected on the exons encoding the domains of the protein. Exons and introns are represented by boxes and lines, respectively, and are not drawn to scale.

ity and antigen. F5F8D is associated with a mild to moderate bleeding tendency and the concomitant presence of two coagulation defects does not enhance the hemorrhagic tendency that was observed in each defect separately [4,50,69,77,78]. Mild bleeding symptoms such as easy bruising, epistaxis, and gum bleeding are not uncommon in affected individuals. Other common bleedings include soft-tissue hematomas [4,78]; bleeding after surgery, dental extraction and trauma; and menorrhagia and postpartum hemorrhage in affected women [50,78]. Excessive bleeding after circumcision was also reported in a high number of male patients [77,78]. In F5F8D patients, circulating levels of FV and FVIII are usually sufficient to prevent more severe spontaneous bleeding episodes [38,50,78]. More severe symptoms, such as gastrointestinal and central nervous system bleedings were rarely reported: in a study of 27 Iranian patients, only one with FV and FVIII level of 8 and 7%, respectively, had a central nervous system bleed, while two patients with FV and FVIII level <10% had gastrointestinal bleeding [78].

Treatment

In F5F8D, bleeding episodes are usually treated on demand and do not require regular prophylaxis [36]. Treatment of bleeding episodes is generally chosen according to the nature of the bleed and the FV and FVIII levels of affected individuals. Both

FV and FVIII sources are needed and their respective plasma half-lives (FV: 36h; FVIII: 10–14h) have to be taken into consideration.

As there are no FV concentrates available and FV is not present in cryoprecipitate or prothrombin complex concentrates, replacement of FV could be achieved only through the use of FFP, preferably with virus-inactivated plasma. For FVIII replacement, a large number of products are available, including FFP, plasma-derived concentrates, or recombinant FVIII (rFVIII) (different generations).

Factor V replacement
See section on factor V deficiency.

Factor VIII replacement
Factor VIII levels should be raised to at least 30–50 IU/dL for the treatment of minor bleeding episodes and to at least 50–70 IU/dL for more severe bleeds. The synthetic hormone DDAVP as well as antifibrinolytics or combined hormonal contraceptives, can be successfully used for minor bleeding episodes [38]. For severe bleedings, rFVIII concentrate is the treatment of choice. Surgical procedures should be addressed by administering FVIII 30 min before surgery and then every 12 h to maintain FVIII levels above 50 IU/dL [38].

Prenatal diagnosis

In developing countries, where management is still largely inadequate, patients with rare bleeding disorders rarely live beyond childhood. Thus, molecular characterization, carrier detection, and prenatal diagnosis remain key steps for genetic counseling and education. In neonates born with these rare conditions, there is a need for an emergent contingency planning for on-demand replacement therapy in the event of neonatal hemorrhages. As for FV deficiency, though life-threatening episodes at birth are rare, the use of prenatal diagnosis can be advisable only in those families with severe clinical history, presenting affected members. Patients with F5F8D have a mild to moderate bleeding tendency; hence, prenatal diagnosis is not currently performed and not recommended.

Only recently a FV concentrate has been developed for clinical use in deficient patients and preclinical studies are currently being performed for the orphan drug designation application to European Medicine Agency (EMA) and Food and Drug Administration (FDA), in order to make it available on the market as soon as possible.

Acknowledgments

We are grateful to the Fondazione Italo Monzino, Milan, Italy, for its continued support for studies in rare coagulation disorders.

References

1 Dahlback B. Blood coagulation. *Lancet* 2000; **355**: 1627–32.

2 Peyvandi F, Duga S, Akhavan S, *et al.* Rare coagulation deficiencies. *Haemophilia* 2002; **8**: 308–21.

3 Chiu HC, Whitaker E, Colman RW. Heterogeneity of human factor V deficiency. Evidence for the existence of an antigen-positive variant. *J Clin Invest* 1983; **72**: 493–503.

4 Mannucci PM, Duga S, Peyvandi F. Recessively inherited coagulation disorders. *Blood* 2004; **104**: 1243–52.

5 Kingsley CS. Familial factor V deficiency: the pattern of heredity. *Q J Med* 1954; **23**: 323–9.

6 Jenny RJ, Pittman DD, Toole JJ, *et al.* Complete cDNA and derived amino acid sequence of human factor V. *Proc Natl Acad Sci USA* 1987; **84**: 4846–50.

7 Cripe LD, Moore KD, Kane WH. Structure of the gene for human coagulation factor V. *Biochemistry* 1992; **31**: 3777–85.

8 Janeway CM, Rivard GE, Tracy PB, *et al.* Factor V Quebec revisited. *Blood* 1996; **87**: 3571–8.

9 Streiff MB, Ness PM. Acquired FV inhibitors: a needless iatrogenic complication of bovine thrombin exposure. *Transfusion* 2002; **42**: 18–26

10 Zhang B, Spreafico M, Zheng C, *et al.* Genotype–phenotype correlation in combined deficiency of factor V and factor VIII. *Blood* 2008; **111**: 5592–600.

11 Camire RM, Pollak ES, Kaushansky K, Tracy PB. Secretable human platelet-derived factor V originates from the plasma pool. *Blood* 1998; **92**: 3035–41.

12 Suehiro Y, Veljkovic DK, Fuller N, *et al.* Endocytosis and storage of plasma factor V by human megakaryocytes. *Thromb Haemost* 2005; **94**: 585–92.

13 Kane WH, Davie EW. Blood coagulation factor V and VIII: structural and functional similarities and their relationship to hemorrhagic and thrombotic disorders. *Blood* 1988; **71**: 539–55.

14 Ortel TL, Takahashi N, Putnam FW. Structural model of human ceruloplasmin based on internal triplication, hydrophilic/hydrophobic character, and secondary structure of domains. *Proc Nat Acad Sci USA* 1984; **81**: 4761–5.

15 Baumgartner S, Hofmann K, Chiquet-Ehrismann R, *et al.* The discoidin domain family revisited: new members from prokaryotes and a homology-based fold prediction. *Protein Sci* 1998; **7**: 1626–31.

16 Macedo-Ribeiro S, Bode W, Huber R, *et al.* Crystal structures of the membrane-binding C2 domain of human coagulation factor V. *Nature* 1999; **402**: 434–9.

17 Adams TE, Hockin MF, Mann KG, *et al.* The crystal structure of activated protein C inactivated bovine factor Va: implications for cofactor function. *Proc Natl Acad Sci USA* 2004; **101**: 8918–23.

18 Stoilova-McPhie S, Parmenter CD, Segers K, *et al.* Defining the structure of membrane-bound human blood coagulation factor Va. *J Thromb Haemost* 2008; **6**: 76–82.

19 Lee CJ, Lin P, Chandrasekaran V, *et al.* Proposed structural models of human factor Va and prothrombinase. *J Thromb Haemost* 2008; **6**: 83–9.

20 Foster WB, Nesheim ME, Mann KG. The factor Xa-catalyzed activation of factor V. *J Biol Chem* 1983; **258**: 13970–7.

21 Huang JN, Koerper MA. Factor V deficiency: a concise review. *Haemophilia* 2008; **14**: 1164–9.

22 Kalafatis M, Rand MD, Mann KG. The mechanism of inactivation of human factor V and human factor Va by activated protein C. *J Biol Chem* 1994; **269**: 31869–80.

23 Cui J, O'Shea KS, Purkayastha A, *et al.* Fatal haemorrhage and incomplete block to embryogenesis in mice lacking coagulation factor V. *Nature* 1996; **384**: 66–8.

24 Yang TL, Cui J, Taylor JM, *et al.* Rescue of fatal neonatal hemorrhage in factor V deficient mice by low transgene expression. *Thromb Haemost* 2000; **83**: 70–7.

25 Tuddenham EGD, Cooper DN. *The Molecular Genetics of Hemostasis and its Inherited Disorders.* Oxford: Oxford University Press, 1994.

26 Dall'osso C, Guella I, Duga S, *et al.* Molecular characterization of three novel splicing mutations causing factor V deficiency and analysis of the F5 gene splicing pattern. *Haematologica* 2008; **93**: 1505–13.

27 Frischmeyer PA, Dietz HC. Nonsense-mediated mRNA decay in health and disease. *Hum Mol Genet* 1999; **10**: 1893–900.

28 Guasch JF, Cannegieter S, Reitsma PH, *et al.* Severe coagulation factor V deficiency caused by a 4 bp deletion in the factor V gene. *Br J Haematol* 1998; **101**: 32–9.

29 Castoldi E, Lunghi B, Mingozzi F, *et al.* A missense mutation (Y1702C) in the coagulation factor V gene is a frequent cause of factor V deficiency in the Italian population. *Haematologica* 2001; **86**: 629–33.

30 Scanavini D, Girelli D, Lunghi B, *et al.* Modulation of factor V levels in plasma by polymorphisms in the C2 domain. *Arterioscler Thromb Vasc Biol* 2004; **24**: 200–6.

31 Yamazaki T, Nicolaes GA, Sorensen KW, *et al.* Molecular basis of quantitative factor V deficiency associated with factor V R2 haplotype. *Blood* 2002; **100**: 2515–21.

32 Murray JM, Rand MD, Egan JO, *et al.* Factor V New Brunswick: Ala221-to-Val substitution results in reduced cofactor activity. *Blood* 1995; **86**: 1820–7.

33 Steen M, Miteva M, Villoutreix BO, *et al.* Factor V New Brunswick: Ala221Val associated with FV deficiency reproduced in vitro and functionally characterized. *Blood* 2003; **102**: 1316–22.

34 Lak M, Sharifian R, Peyvandi F, *et al.* Symptoms of inherited factor V deficiency in 25 Iranian patients. *Br J Haematol* 1998; **103**: 1067–9.

35 Kingsley CS. Familial factor V deficiency: the pattern of heredity. *Q J Med* 1954; **23**: 323–9.

36 Peyvandi F, Palla R, Menegatti M, *et al.* Coagulation factor activity and clinical bleeding severity in rare bleeding disorders: results from the European network of rare bleeding disorders. *J Thromb Haemost* 2012; **10**: 615–21.

37 Duckers C, Simioni P, Spiezia L, *et al.* Residual platelet factor V ensures thrombin generation in patients with severe congenital factor V deficiency and mild bleeding symptoms. *Blood* 2010; **115**: 879–86.

38 Bolton-Maggs PH, Perry DJ, Chalmers EA, *et al.* The rare coagulation disorders—review with guidelines for management from the United Kingdom Haemophilia Centre Doctors' Organisation. *Haemophilia* 2004; **10**: 593–628.

39 Mathias M, Tunstall O, Khair K, Liesner R. Management of surgical procedures in children with severe FV deficiency: experience of 13 surgeries. *Haemophilia* 2013; **19**: 256–8.

40 Salooja N, Martin P, Khair K, *et al.* Severe factor V deficiency and neonatal intracranial haemorrhage: a case report. *Haemophilia* 2000; **6**: 44–6.

41 Tarantino MD, Ross MP, Daniels TM, *et al.* Modulation of an acquired coagulation factor V inhibitor with intravenous immune globulin. *J Pediatr Hematol Oncol* 1997; **19**: 226–31.

42 Chediak J, Ashenhurst JB, *et al.* Successful management of bleeding in a patient with factor V inhibitor by platelet transfusions. *Blood* 1980; **56**: 835–41.

43 Lee CA, Chi C, Pavord SR, *et al.* The obstetric and gynaecological management of women with inherited bleeding disorders—review with guidelines produced by a taskforce of UK Haemophilia Centre Doctors Organization. *Haemophilia* 2006; **12**: 301–36.

44 Oeri J, Matter M, Isenschmid H, *et al.* Congenital factor V deficiency (parahemophilia) with true hemophilia in two brothers. *Bibl Paediatr* 1954; **58**: 575–88.

45 Nichols WC, Seligsohn U, Zivelin A, *et al.* Linkage of combined factors V and VIII deficiency to chromosome 18q by homozygosity mapping. *J Clin Invest* 1997; **99**: 596–601.

46 Nichols WC, Seligsohn U, Zivelin A, *et al.* Mutations in the ER–Golgi intermediate compartment protein ERGIC-53 cause combined deficiency of coagulation factors V and VIII. *Cell* 1998; **93**: 61–70.

47 Zhang B, Cunningham MA, Nichols WC, *et al.* Bleeding due to disruption of a cargo-specific ER-to-Golgi transport complex. *Nat Genet* 2003; **34**: 220–5.

48 Zhang B, Kaufman RJ, Ginsburg D. LMAN1 and MCFD2 form a cargo receptor complex and interact with coagulation factor VIII in the early secretory pathway. *J Biol Chem* 2005; **280**: 25881–6.

49 Zhang B, McGee B, Yamaoka JS, *et al.* Combined deficiency of factor V and factor VIII is due to mutations in either LMAN1 or MCFD2. *Blood* 2006; **107**: 903–7.

50 Seligsohn U, Zivelin A, Zwang E. Combined factor V and factor VIII deficiency among non-Ashkenazi Jews. *N Engl J Med* 1982; **307**: 1191–5.

51 Spreafico M, Peyvandi F. Combined FV and FVIII deficiency. *Haemophilia* 2008; **14**: 1201–8.

52 Itin C, Roche AC, Monsigny M, *et al.* ERGIC-53 is a functional mannose-selective and calcium-dependent human homologue of leguminous lectins. *J Cell Biol* 1996; **107**: 483–93.

53 Guy JE, Wigren E, Svärd M, *et al.* New insights into multiple coagulation factor deficiency from the solution structure of human MCFD2. *J Mol Biol* 2008; **381**: 941–55.

54 Lahtinen U, Svensson K, Pettersson RF. Mapping of structural determinants for the oligomerization of p58, a lectin-like protein of the intermediate compartment and cis-Golgi. *Eur J Biochem* 1999; **260**: 392–7.

55 Nufer F, Kappeler S, Guldbrandsen S, *et al.* ER export of ERGIC-53 is controlled by cooperation of targeting determinants in all three of its domains. *J Cell Sci* 2003; **116**: 4429–40.

56 Tisdale EJ, Plutner H, Matteson J, *et al.* p53/58 binds COPI and is required for selective transport through the early secretory pathway. *J Cell Biol* 1997; **137**: 581–93.

57 Cunningham MA, Pipe SW, Zhang B, *et al.* LMAN1 is a molecular chaperone for the secretion of coagulation factor VIII. *J Thromb Haemost* 2003; **1**: 2360–7.

58 Wen C, Greenwald I. p24 proteins and quality control of LIN-12 and GLP-1 trafficking in Caenorhabditis elegans. *J Cell Biol* 1999; **145**: 1165–75.

59 Appenzeller C, Andersson H, Kappeler F, *et al.* The lectin ERGIC-53 is a cargo transport receptor for glycoproteins. *Nat Cell Biol* 1999; **1**: 330–4.

60 Vollenweider F, Kappeler F, Itin C, *et al.* Mistargeting of the lectin ERGIC-53 to the endoplasmic reticulum of HeLa cells impairs the secretion of a lysosomal enzyme. *J Cell Biol* 1998; **142**: 377–89.

61 Nyfeler B, Reiterer V, Wendeler MW, *et al.* Identification of ERGIC-53 as an intracellular transport receptor of alpha1-antitrypsin. *J Cell Biol* 2008; **180**: 705–12.

62 Morais VA, Brito C, Pijak DS, *et al.* N-glycosylation of human nicastrin is required for interaction with the lectins from the secretory pathway calnexin and ERGIC-53. *Biochim Biophys Acta* 2006; **1762**: 802–10.

63 Nyfeler B, Zhang B, Ginsburg D, *et al.* Cargo selectivity of the ERGIC-53/MCFD2 transport receptor complex. *Traffic* 2006; **7**: 1473–81.

64 Nishio M, Kamiya Y, Mizushima T, *et al.* Structural basis for the cooperative interplay between the two causative gene products of combined factor V and factor VIII deficiency. *Proc Natl Acad Sci USA* 2010; **107**: 4034–9.

65 Zheng C, Liu H, Yuan S, Zhou J, Zhang B. Molecular basis of LMAN1 in coordinating LMAN1-MCFD2 cargo receptor formation and ER-to-Golgi transport of FV/FVIII. *Blood* 2010; **116**: 5698–706.

66 Zheng C, Liu H, Zhou J, Zhang B. EF-hand domains of MCFD2 mediate interactions with both LMAN1 and coagulation factor V or VIII. *Blood* 2010; **115**: 1081–7.

67 Neerman-Arbez M, Antonarakis SE, Blouin JL, *et al.* The locus for combined factor V–factor VIII deficiency (F5F8D) maps to 18q21, between D18S849 and D18S1103. *Am J Hum Genet* 1997; **61**: 143–50.

68 Zhang B, Spreafico M, Zheng C, *et al.* Genotype–phenotype correlation in combined deficiency of factor V and factor VIII. *Blood* 2008; **111**: 5592–600.

69 Segal A, Zivelin A, Rosenberg N, *et al.* A mutation in LMAN1 (ERGIC-53) causing combined factor V and factor VIII deficiency is prevalent in Jews originating from the island of Djerba in Tunisia. *Blood Coag Fibrinol* 2004; **15**: 99–102.

70 Neerman-Arbez M, Johnson KM, Morris MA, *et al.* Molecular analysis of the ERGIC-53 gene in 35 families with combined factor V-factor VIII deficiency. *Blood* 1999; **93**: 2253–60.

71 Nichols WC, Valeri HT, Wheatley MA, *et al.* ERGIC-53 gene structure and mutation analysis in 19 combined factors V and VIII deficiency families. *Blood* 1999; **93**: 2261–6.

72 D'Ambrosio R, Santacroce R, Di Perna P, *et al.* A new case of combined factor V and factor VIII deficiency further suggests that the LMAN1 M1T mutation is a frequent cause in Italian patients. *Blood Coagul Fibrinol* 2007; **18**: 203–4.

73 Dansako H, Ishimaru F, Takai Y, *et al.* Molecular characterization of the *ERGIC-53* gene in two Japanese patients with combined factor V–factor VIII deficiency. *Ann Hematol* 2001; **80**: 292–4.

74 Jayandharan G, Spreafico M, Viswabandya A, *et al.* Mutations in the MCFD2 gene are predominant among patients with hereditary combined FV and FVIII deficiency (F5F8D) in India. *Haemophilia* 2007; **13**: 413–19.

75 Mohanty D, Ghosh K, Shetty S, *et al.* Mutations in the *MCFD2* gene and a novel mutation in the *LMAN1* gene in Indian families with combined deficiency of factor V and VIII. *Am J Hematol* 2005; **79**: 262–6.

76 Gifford JL, Walsh MP, Vogel HJ. Structures and metal-ion-binding properties of the Ca^{2+}-binding helix-loop-helix EF-hand motifs. *Biochem J* 2007; **405**: 199–221.

77 Mansouritorgabeh H, Rezaieyazdi Z, Pourfathollah AA, *et al.* Haemorrhagic symptoms in patients with combined factors V and VIII deficiency in north-eastern Iran. *Haemophilia* 2004; **10**: 271–5.

78 Peyvandi F, Tuddenham EG, Akhtari AM, *et al.* Bleeding symptoms in 27 Iranian patients with the combined deficiency of factor V and factor VIII. *Br J Haematol* 1998; **100**: 773–6.

A recent review reported 60 patients with amyloidosis and isolated FX deficiency (FX:C $\leq$ 50%) of which six were classified as severe (FX:C < 10%), 15 as moderate (FX:C 10–25%), and 39 as mild (FX:C 26–50%). These 60 individuals underwent 112 invasive procedures, 19 of whom (17%) received treatment with one or more hemostatic agents. There were complications in 14 (13%) procedures (bleeding 12, thrombosis 1, and death 1). Baseline FX levels were not predictive of the bleeding risk and bleeding complications were relatively infrequent, particularly in patients with mild or moderate FX deficiency undergoing nonvascular procedures.

- Miscellaneous causes: acquired FX inhibitors are rare but have been reported in patients with leprosy, in association with *Mycoplasma pneumonia* chest and in some cases with no preceding or concomitant illness. FX deficiency has been reported in patients with myeloma (without amyloidosis), following exposure to the fungicide methylbromide, in association with various tumors, in acute myeloid leukemia treated with amsacrine, and in severe burns patients.

Treatment of factor X deficiency

Inherited FX is a rare disorder and management of this disorder can be difficult. Evidence-based guidelines are lacking. The UK Haemophilia Centre Doctors' Organisation (UKHCDO) have published guidelines on the management of FX deficiency (and other rare inherited bleeding disorders) based upon a literature review and personal experience [24]. Current therapeutic options to manage patients with FX deficiency include fibrinolytic inhibitors such as ε-aminocaproic acid (EACA) and tranexamic acid, solvent detergent treated fresh frozen plasma (FFP), and prothrombin complex concentrates (PCCs). A plasma-derived FX concentrate is currently undergoing clinical study in both adults and children (Bio Products Laboratory, UK). Recombinant VIIa (rVIIa) has been used successfully to treat acquired FX deficiency secondary to amyloidosis [25].

The need for replacement therapy is guided by the particular hemorrhagic episode. The biological half-life of FX is 20–40 h [26] so an adequate level can be achieved with repeated infusions. Factor levels of 10–20 U/dL are generally sufficient for hemostasis, even in the immediate postoperative period [27] although some data suggest that levels of 5 IU/dL may be sufficient for adequate hemostasis [28] and the thrombogram would suggest that levels of >10 U/dL are sufficient to restore thrombin generation to normal [19,29].

Tranexamic acid
Tranexamic acid, a fibrinolytic inhibitor, may be of value in the management of patients with FX deficiency. For oral bleeding, 10 mL of a 5% solution of tranexamic acid as a mouthwash every 8 h has shown efficacy. However, this is not commercially available, and therefore will need to be formulated by the hospital pharmacy. In women with menorrhagia, tranexamic acid 15 mg/kg 8 hourly (in practise 1 g 6–8 hourly) may be effective when taken for the duration of the menstrual period.

Fibrin glue
Fibrin glue can be effective in facilitating local hemostasis.

Fresh frozen plasma
Fresh frozen plasma has been successfully used to manage patients with FX deficiency. A dose of 20 mL/kg followed by 3–6 mL/kg twice daily is recommended, aiming to keep X:C trough levels above 10–20 U/dL [29]. This frequently requires large volumes of FFP and problems with fluid overload may be encountered. A virally inactivated FFP should be used.

Prothrombin complex concentrates
In many centres, PCCs are used to manage patients with FX deficiency particularly severe FX deficiency. The calculated required dosage for treatment is based on the empirical finding that 1 IU of FX per kilogram of body weight raises the FX level by 1.5%.

Historically, PCCs have been used with caution in patients with concomitant liver disease, large hematomas, major trauma, in the neonate, or in individuals with antithrombin deficiency because of concerns that they may precipitate a thrombosis. However, the risks associated with PCCs are small and appear to be less so with the newer formulations of PCCs [30]. Tranexamic acid is generally avoided with PCCs because of the risk of thrombosis. The half-life of FX is 20–40 h and daily treatment is not usually required. However, in cases where replacement therapy is given, levels should be monitored on a daily basis. In children, the biologic half-life of FX may be shortened and fall-off studies may be required to establish an appropriate dosing regimen [28].

Recombinant factor VIIa
Recombinant FVIIa (rFVIIa) has been used to treat amyloid-associated FX deficiency [25] but the data on its use in patients with inherited FX deficiency are limited.

Factor X concentrates
Factor X P Behring
This is a freeze-dried human FIX–FX concentrate that is used in the management of patients with FX deficiency [31]. When reconstituted it contains (nominally) 600–1200 IU human coagulation FX and 600 IU human coagulation FIX per vial.

Factor X concentrate
A single plasma-derived FX concentrate (Bio Products Laboratory) is currently in clinical trial for patients with FX deficiency and this may prove to be useful in individuals with FX deficiency requiring treatment.

Management of an acute bleed in patients with severe factor X deficiency

At present and until an FX concentrate becomes licensed, PCCs are the treatment of choice to manage patients with severe FX deficiency who present with an acute bleeding problem. The aim in such cases is to treat with a PCC to raise the endogenous FX levels to 20–30 U/dL on the basis that this dose is sufficient to prevent bleeding during surgery. Daily treatment may be required depending upon the severity of the bleeding problem.

Management of surgery in patients with severe factor X deficiency

Surgery in individuals with severe FX deficiency (FX:C < 1 IU/dL) has been successfully performed following infusion of either FFP or PCCs. In the case of FFP, a level of 35 U/dL was achieved prior to surgery and FX levels were maintained above 20 U/dL in the postoperative period with no bleeding reported [27]. An FX level of 20 U/dL appears to be sufficient for efficient hemostasis. However, a recent report has shown that lower FX levels, in the region of 5 U/dL achieves adequate hemostasis [28]. Similarly, data using the thrombogram suggests that FX levels of >10 U/dL may be effective [19].

Factor X prophylaxis

Prophylaxis in patients with severe FX deficiency using PCCs has been reported [28,32–36]. In data from Iran in 10 patients with severe FX deficiency (FX:C < 1 U/dL) in whom prophylaxis was instituted using an FX–FIX concentrate (Factor X P Behring) at a dose of 20 IU/kg once weekly, all patients were followed up for a period of 12 months [31]. One patient had an anaphylactic reaction to the treatment and this was stopped; the remaining patients had no bleeding symptoms and all were reported to have a FX:C > 1 U/dL.

Pharmacokinetic studies can be invaluable when prophylaxis is being considered to guide the frequency/dose of administration with the aim of keeping the FX:C > 1 U/dL.

Management of severe factor X deficiency in pregnancy

Factor X levels increase during pregnancy (in women with normal FX levels at the start of pregnancy) [13] but women with severe FX deficiency and a history of adverse outcome in pregnancy may benefit from aggressive replacement therapy [37,38].

Management of the neonate with severe factor X deficiency

In families in whom both parents are known to have FX deficiency, pregnancy and delivery should be managed in such a way as to minimize the potential risk of bleeding in both mother and baby. This requires close liaison with the obstetric unit including obstetric anesthetists: a management plan should be prepared for the delivery and subsequent investigation of the neonate. An FX assay should be performed prior to delivery. At birth, a cord blood sample should be taken for FX assay.

Cranial ultrasound should be undertaken in severely affected neonates because of the increased risk of intracranial hemorrhage. Prophylaxis during the neonatal period may be necessary in severely affected neonates.

Management of moderate factor X deficiency (FX:C > 2 U/dL)

Patients with FX levels greater than 10 U/dL or a lower level and no significant bleeding history (despite hemostatic challenges) require no replacement therapy. However, the nature of the surgery and any bleeding history in relation to previous hemostatic challenges must be considered.

Liver transplantation for factor X deficiency

Liver transplantation in one case of FX deficiency has been reported and was associated with subsequent normalization of FX levels and no bleeding problems [39].

References

1 Telfer TP, Denson KW, Wright DR. A new coagulation defect. *Br J Haematol* 1956; **2**(3): 308–16.

2 Hougie C, Barrow EM, Graham JB. The Stuart factor: a hitherto unrecognized blood coagulation factor. *Bibl Haematol* 1958; **7**: 336–40.

3 Wright IS. The nomenclature of blood clotting factors. *Thromb Diathesis Haemorrh* 1962; **7**: 381–8.

4 Scambler PJ, Williamson R. The structural gene for human coagulation factor X is located on chromosome 13q34. *Cytogen Cell Genet* 1985; **39**(3): 231–3.

5 Davidson CJ, Hirt RP, Lal K, et al. Molecular evolution of the vertebrate blood coagulation network. *Thromb Haemost* 2003; **89**(3): 420–8.

6 Degen SJ, Davie EW. The prothrombin gene and serine proteinase evolution. *Ann N York Acad Sci* 1986; **485**: 66–72.

7 Patthy L. Evolution of the proteases of blood coagulation and fibrinolysis by assembly from modules. *Cell* 1985; **41**(3): 657–63.

8 Fung MR, Hay CW, MacGillivray RT. Characterization of an almost full-length cDNA coding for human blood coagulation factor X. *Proc Natl Acad Sci USA* 1985; **82**(11): 3591–5.

9 Peyvandi F, Menegatti M, Santagostino E, *et al.* Gene mutations and three-dimensional structural analysis in 13 families with severe factor X deficiency. *Br J Haematol* 2002; **117**(3): 685–92.

10 Philippou H, Adami A, Boisclair MD, Lane DA. An ELISA for factor X activation peptide: application to the investigation of thrombogenesis in cardiopulmonary bypass. *Br J Haematol* 1995; **90**(2): 432–7.

11 Wei Z, Yan Y, Carrell RW, Zhou A. Crystal structure of protein Z-dependent inhibitor complex shows how protein Z functions as a cofactor in the membrane inhibition of factor X. *Blood* 2009; **114**(17): 3662–7.

12 Epstein DJ, Bergum PW, Bajaj SP, Rapaport SI. Radioimmunoassays for protein C and factor X. Plasma antigen levels in abnormal hemostatic states. *Am J Clin Pathol* 1984; **82**(5): 573–81.

13 Condie RG. A serial study of coagulation factors XII, XI and X in plasma in normal pregnancy and in pregnancy complicated by pre-eclampsia. *Br J Obstet Gynaecol* 1976; **83**(8): 636–9.

14 Williams MD, Chalmers EA, Gibson BE. The investigation and management of neonatal haemostasis and thrombosis. *Br J Haematol* 2002; **119**(2): 295–309.

15 Girolami A, Vettore S, Scarparo P, Lombardi AM. Persistent validity of a classification of congenital factor X defects based on clotting, chromogenic and immunological assays even in the molecular biology era. *Haemophilia* 2011; **17**(1): 17–20.

16 Peyvandi F, Mannucci PM, Lak M, *et al.* Congenital factor X deficiency: spectrum of bleeding symptoms in 32 Iranian patients. *Br J Haematol* 1998; **102**(2): 626–8.

17 Herrmann FH, Auerswald G, Ruiz-Saez A, *et al.* Factor X deficiency: clinical manifestation of 102 subjects from Europe and Latin America with mutations in the factor 10 gene. *Haemophilia* 2006; **12**(5): 479–89.

18 Acharya SS, Coughlin A, Dimichele DM. Rare Bleeding Disorder Registry: deficiencies of factors II, V, VII, X, XIII, fibrinogen and dysfibrinogenemias. *J Thromb Haemost* 2004; **2**(2): 248–56.

19 Al Dieri R, Peyvandi F, Santagostino E, *et al.* The thrombogram in rare inherited coagulation disorders: its relation to clinical bleeding. *Thromb Haemost* 2002; **88**(4): 576–82.

20 Dewerchin M, Liang Z, Moons L, *et al.* Blood coagulation factor X deficiency causes partial embryonic lethality and fatal neonatal bleeding in mice. *Thromb Haemost* 2000; **83**(2): 185–90.

21 Tai SJ, Herzog RW, Margaritis P, *et al.* A viable mouse model of factor X deficiency provides evidence for maternal transfer of factor X. *J Thromb Haemost* 2008; **6**(2): 339–45.

22 Zivelin A, Seligsohn U. Mutations causing rare bleeding disorders, 2011. Available at: http://www.isth.org/?MutationsRareBleedin

23 Korsan-Bengtsen K, Hjort PF, Ygge J. Acquired factor X deficiency in a patient with amyloidosis. *Thromb Diathesis Haemorrh* 1962; **7**: 558–66.

24 Bolton-Maggs PH, Perry DJ, Chalmers EA, *et al.* The rare coagulation disorders–review with guidelines for management from the United Kingdom Haemophilia Centre Doctors' Organisation. *Haemophilia* 2004; **10**(5): 593–628.

25 Boggio L, Green D. Recombinant human factor VIIa in the management of amyloid-associated factor X deficiency. *Br J Haematol* 2001; **112**(4): 1074–5.

26 Roberts HR, Lechler E, Webster WP, Penick GD. Survival of transfused factor x in patients with Stuart disease. *Thromb Diathesis Haemorrh* 1965; **13**: 305–13.

27 Knight RD, Barr CF, Alving BM. Replacement therapy for congenital Factor X deficiency. *Transfusion* 1985; **25**(1): 78-80.

28 McMahon C, Smith J, Goonan C, Byrne M, Smith OP. The role of primary prophylactic factor replacement therapy in children with severe factor X deficiency. *Br J Haematol* 2002; **119**(3): 789–91.

29 Anwar M, Hamdani SN, Ayyub M, Ali W. Factor X deficiency in North Pakistan. Journal of Ayub Medical College, Abbottabad. *J Ayub Med Coll Abbottabad* 2004; **16**(3): 1–4.

30 Franchini M, Lippi G. Prothrombin complex concentrates: an update. *Blood Transf* 2010; **8**(3): 149–54.

31 Karimi M, Menegatti M, Afrasiabi A, Sarikhani S, Peyvandi F. Phenotype and genotype report on homozygous and heterozygous patients with congenital factor X deficiency. *Haematologica* 2008; **93**(6): 934–8.

32 Auerswald G. Prophylaxis in rare coagulation disorders—factor X deficiency. *Thromb Res* 2006; **118** (Suppl. 1): S29–31.

33 Karimi M, Vafafar A, Haghpanah S, *et al.* Efficacy of prophylaxis and genotype-phenotype correlation in patients with severe Factor X deficiency in Iran. *Haemophilia* 2012; **18**(2): 211–15.

34 Kouides PA, Kulzer L. Prophylactic treatment of severe factor X deficiency with prothrombin complex concentrate. *Haemophilia* 2001; **7**(2): 220–3.

35 Todd T, Perry DJ. A review of long-term prophylaxis in the rare inherited coagulation factor deficiencies. *Haemophilia* 2010; **16**(4): 569–83.

36 Todd T, Perry DJ, Hayman E, Lawrence K, Gattens M, Baglin T. Severe factor X deficiency due to a homozygous mutation (Cys364Arg) that disrupts a disulphide bond in the catalytic domain. *Haemophilia* 2006; **12**(6): 621–4.

37 Kumar M, Mehta P. Congenital coagulopathies and pregnancy: report of four pregnancies in a factor X-deficient woman. *Am J Hematol* 1994; **46**(3): 241–4.

38 Romagnolo C, Burati S, Ciaffoni S, *et al.* Severe factor X deficiency in pregnancy: case report and review of the literature. *Haemophilia* 2004; **10**(5): 665–8.

39 Bang SH, Oh SH, Kim KM, *et al.* Successful liver transplantation for a child with life-threatening recurrent bleeding episodes due to congenital factor X deficiency: a case report. *Transpl Proc* 2012; **44**(2): 583–4.

CHAPTER 58

Factor XI deficiency

Paula H.B. Bolton-Maggs[1] and Uri Seligsohn[2]
[1] Serious Hazards of Transfusion Haemovigilance Scheme, Manchester Blood Centre, and University of Manchester, Manchester, UK
[2] Sheba Medical Center and Sackler Faculty of Medicine, Tel Aviv University, Tel Hashomer, Israel

History

Factor XI (FXI) deficiency was first described in 1953 by Rosenthal *et al.* [1] as a new type of hemophilia, later termed hemophilia C. Its presence in two sisters and their maternal uncle was interpreted as an indication that the mode of inheritance was autosomal dominant. However, a seminal study in 1961 clearly established that transmission of the disorder was autosomal [2], and distinguished between patients with major FXI deficiency, with an activity of <20 U/dL, and patients with minor deficiency with an activity of 30–60 U/dL. This study, as well as a later study [3], also delineated that FXI deficiency was particularly common in Jews.

In the classic "waterfall" or "cascade" scheme of coagulation, designed in 1964, FXI was assigned a role in the initial "contact phase" of the intrinsic system. It was shown that negatively charged surfaces trigger activation of factor XII (FXII), later found to occur in the presence of prekallikrein (PK) and high-molecular-weight kininogen (HK), and that FXIIa, in turn, activates FXI. FXIa then activates factor IX (FIX) in the presence of Ca^{2+} ions, which leads through additional reactions to the generation of thrombin. Yet this sequence of reactions was difficult to reconcile with the clinical observations which indicated that patients with severe deficiencies of FXII, PK, or HK had no bleeding tendency, whereas patients with FXI deficiency exhibited a significant bleeding tendency, particularly following trauma. In 1991, two groups of researchers showed that FXI was activated by thrombin, thereby bypassing the initial contact reactions [4,5]. Although this was challenged by the suggestion that thrombin activation was caused in these experiments by contact activation [6], further work confirmed the role of thrombin activation of FXI, and in addition demonstrated that it required a normal thrombin-binding site, and normal FXI catalytic activity [7]. These experiments coincide with a renewed interest in the contact system and further understanding of the roles of FXI and FXII in hemostasis and thrombosis which are discussed below.

Biochemical features and function of factor XI

Factor XI is a 160-kDa glycoprotein that consists of two identical polypeptide subunits of 80 kDa linked by a disulfide bond. Each subunit contains 607 amino acids organized in a heavy chain with four tandem repeats of 90 or 91 amino acids, designated "apple domains," and a light chain in which a serine protease domain is located. The first apple domain contains the binding sites for HK, with which FXI circulates as a complex, and for prothrombin. Apple 3 contains the binding sites for platelets and FIX, and apple 4 harbors the binding site for FXII and is important for the dimerization of the subunits [8–10]. Analysis of the crystal structure [9] has shown that these four apple domains form a disc-like structure around the catalytic domain and has increased our understanding of the relationship between the dimers. Activation of FXI is associated with a conformational change which exposes sites recognizing FIX on the third apple domain, particularly Arg184 which is critical for FIX activation. This may be a switch holding FXI in its inactive form.

The gene encoding for FXI (GenBank M18295) consists of 15 exons and 14 introns and is located on chromosome 4q34–35 close to the gene for PK [11]. FXI is synthesized in the liver. The physiologic activator of FXI is thrombin, which converts zymogen FXI to a serine protease (FXIa) by cleavage of the Arg369–Ile370 bond, giving rise to a 47-kDa heavy chain and a 33-kDa light chain. This reaction is greatly accelerated when FXI is bound to activated platelets in the presence of prothrombin and Ca^{2+} ions or HK and Zn^{2+} ions [12]. Recent work shows that polyphosphates are key in FXI activation by thrombin [13]. Polyphosphates are released from activated platelets, and provide a template for the assembly of the contact factors including FXI, FXII, PK, and HK, and thereby act as a cofactor, accelerating thrombin activation of FXI. Polyphosphates are ubiquitous in nature and their roles have been recently reviewed [13]. Function is related to the

Textbook of Hemophilia, Third Edition. Edited by Christine A. Lee, Erik E. Berntorp and W. Keith Hoots.
© 2014 John Wiley & Sons, Ltd. Published 2014 by John Wiley & Sons, Ltd.

length: very long-chain molecules (as are found in bacteria) are 1000 times more potent in coagulation activation than those released from platelets. Polyphosphates also accelerate the thrombin burst by promoting factor V (FV) activation by FXa and thrombin, and abrogate tissue factor pathway inhibitor (TFPI) which would normally inhibit FXa. It is suggested that one of the FXI subunits binds to the platelet membrane while the other subunit binds to FIX [8], thereby enabling efficient activation of FXI by thrombin and then activation of FIX by FXIa. FXIa initially cleaves FIX at the Arg146–Ala147 bond in the presence of Ca^{2+} ions and subsequently an Arg180–Val181 bond yielding fully activated FIXa and an activation peptide. FIXa then activates FX in the presence of factor VIIIa, negatively charged phospholipids and Ca^{2+} ions, and FXa in turn converts prothrombin to thrombin in the presence of FVa, negatively charged phospholipids, and Ca^{2+} ions.

FXI activated by thrombin is essential for sustained thrombin generation, which is particularly important after clot formation. It also diminishes fibrinolysis as thrombin activates procarboxypeptidase B, also termed thrombin-activatable fibrinolysis inhibitor (TAFI). Activated TAFI removes terminal lysine residues from fibrin, the binding sites of plasminogen and tissue plasminogen activator thereby inhibiting fibrinolysis [14]. FXI can thus be regarded as a procoagulant and an indirect inhibitor of fibrinolysis. This conclusion is supported by the clinical observation that patients with severe FXI deficiency are specifically prone to bleeding when trauma is inflicted at sites where there is enhanced fibrinolytic activity [14]. FXIa is inhibited by antithrombin in the presence of heparin, protease nexin II, C_1-inhibitor, and protein C inhibitor.

The physiologic role of the contact system is better understood as a result of recent research, particularly animal experiments (reviewed in [15]). These confirm Ratnoff's "seamless web of host defence reactions" by demonstrating the interaction of coagulation, fibrinolysis, and inflammatory pathways [16]. Mice with absent FIX, FXI, or FXII on a background of low tissue factor illustrate the different functions of these factors. Mice with low TF have a bleeding disorder, and when either combined with absent FXI or FIX die *in utero* from bleeding. In contrast, those with low TF and absent FXII are viable, but have a bleeding disorder. Earlier data suggested that at high TF concentrations, fibrin formation is independent of FXI, but with decreasing TF concentration, the contribution of FXI becomes more important [17]. These experiments are particularly interesting as they suggest that the risk of bleeding with FXI deficiency may vary with TF availability. The role of the contact pathway in infection [18] is supported by further observations in animals. For example, FXI deficient mice survive longer than wild-type mice in a peritoneal sepsis model [19] and inhibition of FXI by a monoclonal antibody attenuates development of disseminated intravascular coagulation in a mouse model of sepsis [20].

Inheritance and functional defect

Factor XI deficiency is inherited as an autosomal disorder. Homozygotes or compound heterozygotes have a FXI activity of less than 15 U/dL and heterozygotes have an activity range of 25–70 U/dL or are within normal limits. Vertical transmission of severe FXI deficiency or apparent dominance has been observed in Ashkenazi Jewish families but stems from matings between homozygotes and heterozygotes in this population, in which the prevalence of mutant genes and affected individuals is high [3]. In the vast majority of patients with FXI deficiency, FXI activity is concordant with antigenicity [21]. Only a few patients have so far been described with dysfunctional FXI (i.e. 100 U/dL antigenicity and <1 U/dL activity) [22].

Mutations

Three mutations in the *FXI* gene, termed types I, II, and III, were first described in 1989 in six Ashkenazi Jews who had severe FXI deficiency [23]. Type I mutation is a G to A change at the splice junction of the last intron of the gene, type II mutation is a G to T change in exon 5 leading to Glu117stop, and type III mutation is a T to C change in exon 9, giving rise to Phe283Leu substitution. Homozygotes for type II mutation have a mean FXI activity of 1.2 U/dL, homozygotes for type III mutation have a mean FXI activity of 9.7 U/dL, and compound heterozygotes for types II and III mutations have a mean activity of 3.3 U/dL [24]. Types II and III mutations are the predominant mutations causing FXI deficiency in Ashkenazi Jews [24,25]. Table 58.1 demonstrates that in 414 unrelated Jewish patients of various ethnic origins with severe FXI deficiency, 53.9% of the alleles harbored type II mutation, 43.8% type III mutation, 1.2% type I mutation, and 1.1% other mutations. Databases listing more than 200 published mutations are available (http://isth.org/?MutationsRareBleedin under Registries/Databases/Mutations Causing Rare Bleeding Disorders; www.hgmd.org and www.factorxi.com). Most mutations responsible for FXI deficiency are missense mutations displaying equal reduction in

Table 58.1 Molecular analysis in 414 unrelated Jewish patients with severe factor XI deficiency.

Mutant allele	*n*	%
Type II: Glu117Ter	446	53.9
Type III: Phe283Leu	363	43.8
Type I: IVS 14+1 (Ggt→Gat)	10	1.21
Type IV: 14bp deletion (IVS 14/exon 15)	2	0.24
Gly555Glu	2	0.24
Tyr427Cys	1	0.12
Glu323Lys	1	0.12
nt73del14bp	1	0.12
Unknown	2	0.24
Total	**828**	**100**

both activity and antigen. Ten mutations are reported with discrepant activity and antigen (www.factorxi.org). Expression of several missense mutations revealed impaired secretion of FXI from transfected cells [26,27]. For one of these mutations, the type III mutation (Phe283Leu) in apple 4, the impaired secretion was related to defective dimerization [26].

Prevalence and ethnic distribution

The highest prevalence of FXI deficiency has been observed in Ashkenazi Jews [3]. Among 531 control individuals of Ashkenazi Jewish origin, the allele frequency of type II and type III mutations was 0.0217 and 0.0254, respectively [28]. Thus, 9.1% of subjects belonging to this ethnic group are predicted to be carriers of either mutation and 1/450 individuals (0.22%) is expected to have severe FXI deficiency. The Iraqi Jews, who represent the ancient gene pool of Jews from Babylonian times 2500 years ago, have only the type II mutation. Among 507 subjects, an allele frequency of 0.0167 was found, predicting heterozygosity in 1/30 individuals and homozygosity in 1/3600 individuals in the general Iraqi Jewish community [28].

Interestingly, among 382 Arabs, type II mutation was detected with an allele frequency of 0.0065. A study of intragenic polymorphisms in patients with severe FXI deficiency from all the three ethnic groups (Ashkenazi Jews, Arabs, and Iraqi Jews) enabled haplotype analysis, which disclosed distinct founder effects for the type II and type III mutations [28] (Figure 58.1). Based on the distribution of allelic variants at a microsatellite marker flanking the *FXI* gene (D4S171), the type II mutation was estimated to have occurred more than 120 generations ago, while the type III mutation was of a more recent origin [29] (Figure 58.2). Another cluster of patients with FXI deficiency was observed in Basques residing in south-western France, and a recent study revealed that the predominant mutation in this population is Cys38Arg, with an allele frequency of 0.005 [30]. Another cluster of FXI-deficient patients harboring a C128X mutation was described in Caucasians living or originating in the UK [31]. Haplotype analysis for this mutation was consistent with a founder effect.

Factor XI deficiency has also been reported sporadically in other patients of English, African-American, German, Indian, Italian, Korean, Japanese, Chinese, Portuguese, Swedish, Yugoslav, Arab, and Iranian origin.

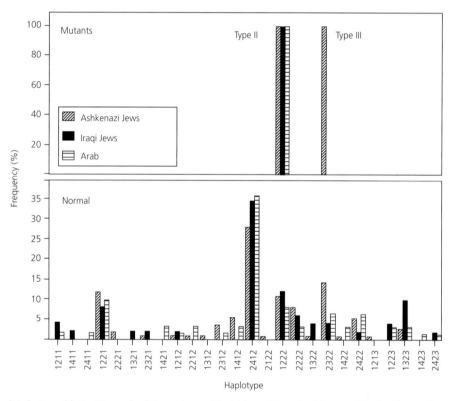

Figure 58.1 Frequency distribution of factor XI gene haplotypes observed in Ashkenazi Jews, Iraqi Jews, and Arabs. The numbers on the abscissa denote, from bottom to top, the allele numbers of polymorphisms in introns A, B, E, and M. For example, the haplotype designated 1-2-1-1 comprises allele 1 of intron A polymorphism, allele 2 of intron B polymorphism, allele 1 of intron E polymorphism, and allele 1 of intron M polymorphism. The lower and upper panels represent normal chromosomes and chromosomes bearing type II or type III mutations, respectively. Note that all chromosomes carrying the type II mutation are characterized by the same 1-2-2-2 haplotype that is observed in 8–12% of normal chromosomes. The chromosomes bearing the type III mutation are confined to Ashkenazi Jews, all characterized by haplotype 2-3-2-2. From [28]. Copyright of the American Society of Hematology, used with permission.

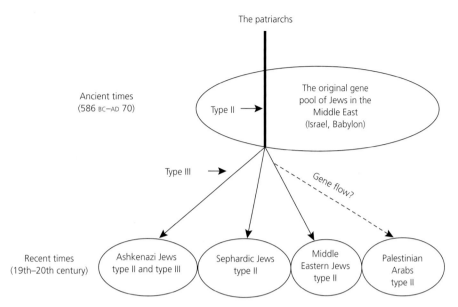

Figure 58.2 A simplified scheme showing the common origin of the three major segments of contemporary Jews and explaining the current distribution of the type II and type III mutations. The predicted time when type II and type III mutations occurred in the factor XI gene are indicated by horizontal arrows. We speculate that gene flow has been responsible for the transfer of type II mutation from Middle Eastern Jews to Palestinian Arabs after the settlement of Arabs in Israel in the seventh century AD. From [28]. Copyright of the American Society of Hematology, used with permission.

Bleeding manifestations in patients with severe deficiency

Spontaneous bleeding manifestations are rare in patients with severe FXI deficiency. The common presentation is an injury-related bleeding tendency, particularly at sites where tissues contain activators of the fibrinolytic system, such as the oral cavity, nose, tonsils, and urinary tract [24,32,33]. Bleeding is less common at other sites of trauma, such as encountered during orthopedic surgery, appendicectomy, circumcision, or cuts in the skin. Postpartum hemorrhage occurs in only 20–30% of affected women [33,34]. Some patients with a very low level of FXI may not bleed at all following trauma [2], while in others the bleeding tendency varies in the same patient over time even when provoked by similar hemostatic challenges [24,32,33]. Bleeding can be brisk at the time of injury and persists unless treated, or can begin several hours following trauma.

Bleeding manifestations in heterozygotes

Some heterozygotes exhibit abnormal bleeding. In one study, bleeding was observed in 9/94 (9.6%) of patients who underwent surgical procedures, including tooth extractions, tonsillectomy, and nasal operation [2]. In another study, no bleeding was observed following urologic surgery unless FXI activity was 25 U/dL or less [35]. In contrast, two studies from the UK and one from Iran [33,36,37] described injury-related bleeding in 48–60% of cases, as well as spontaneous bleeding

manifestations. An assessment of the risk of bleeding in a large cohort of patients with severe and partial FXI deficiency yielded an odds ratio of 13 [confidence interval (CI) 3.8–45] for patients with severe FXI deficiency and an odds ratio of 2.6 (CI 0.8–9.0) for patients with partial deficiency [38]. Analysis of data from an international rare bleeding disorders registry found no relationship between the FXI level and bleeding risk [39]. These discrepancies may relate to the observation that the plasma FXI level may not be the best measure of the role of FXI in coagulation. For example, the activated partial thromboplastin time (APTT) can be normal in patients with a mutation which disrupts platelet binding of FXI, yet exhibit bleeding. Thrombin generation under low TF conditions may correlate better with bleeding risk, and new methods are needed to permit investigation of the role of platelet polyphosphates. It can be concluded that patients with partial FXI deficiency may exhibit a bleeding tendency but the risk is lower than in patients with severe FXI deficiency. Whatever the cause of the discrepancy among the studies, patients with partial FXI deficiency who have a bleeding history should be carefully examined for additional inherited disorders of hemostasis such as platelet dysfunction or von Willebrand disease (VWD), and for acquired hemostatic defects.

Thrombosis

The effect of FXI in promoting coagulation and inhibiting fibrinolysis could hypothetically predict that in patients with severe FXI deficiency, thrombosis would occur infrequently. However, unlike patients with severe hemophilia A or hemophilia B, in whom the incidence of acute myocardial infarction is significantly reduced, patients with severe FXI deficiency are not protected against such events. In a study of 96 adult patients with severe FXI deficiency, 16 (17%) had an acute myocardial infarction, which occurred at median ages of 64.5 and 58 years in women and men, respectively [40]. The observed incidence of acute myocardial infarction in this cohort was not statistically different from the expected incidence in the general population. As anticipated, one or more of the conventional atherosclerotic risk factors was detected in 13 of the 16 patients who had an acute myocardial infarction (81%), whereas, among patients with severe FXI deficiency who had not experienced an acute myocardial infarction, the presence of these risk factors was significantly lower. In contrast, a reduced incidence of ischemic stroke has been observed in severe FXI deficiency. A cohort of 115 patients over 45 years of age with severe FXI deficiency (level <15 U/dL) was compared with an Israeli health survey of 9509 people. After correction for the common risk factors, the expected incidence of stroke was 8.56 but only one was observed [41]. Another recent study in Israel addressed the question whether severe FXI deficiency protects against deep vein thrombosis. The incidence of venous thrombosis in 219 unrelated patients aged 20–94 years was compared to the incidence in a large population-based study. The calculated expected number of patients with deep vein thrombosis in the FXI deficient cohort was 4.68, whereas the observed number was 0 ($P < 0.019$). Collectively, these observations suggest that severe FXI deficiency is protective against deep vein thrombosis and ischemic stroke but not against myocardial infarction [42].

Animal experiments have shown an important role of FXI and FXII in thrombosis and are consistent with the human data [43]. Gene knock-outs for FXII or FXI demonstrate protection against both arterial and venous thrombosis in various experimental systems yet do not cause injury-related bleeding despite prolonged coagulation tests [15]. These observations suggest that FXI or FXII inhibition could be developed as a new antithrombotic strategy and several animal studies support this approach [44]. Since FXII is pivotal in activation of other pathways involving the kinin system, fibrinolysis, and complement, it may not be desirable to block its action. FXII roles are reviewed by Renne *et al.* [45]. Several options for inhibition of FXI are under investigation including monoclonal antibodies, small molecules [44], and a specific domain of the FXI inhibitor protease nexin 2 [46] Another novel strategy is development of antisense oligonucleotides which interfere with hepatic FXI RNA, thereby reducing FXI production. This has already yielded good results in mice, preventing thrombosis without increasing bleeding [47]. Reducing FXI level by 80% in monkeys with this technique was not accompanied by bleeding [48]. These developments are promising a new approach to anticoagulation which may have a better safety profile than current agents.

Development of inhibitors

Inhibitors to FXI have been described in patients with severe FXI deficiency. Fortunately, bleeding manifestations in such patients are not aggravated following inhibitor formation, but trauma or surgery presents a substantial hemostatic challenge. In a study of 118 unrelated patients with severe FXI deficiency, seven were found to harbor an inhibitor [49]. All seven patients had received plasma replacement therapy prior to the development of the inhibitor and all were homozygous for the type II null allele, which is associated with extremely low levels of FXI. Of 84 patients with other genotypes, i.e. type III homozygotes or type II and type III compound heterozygotes (of whom 43 had received plasma), none was found to have an inhibitor to FXI. Patients with these genotypes have measurable levels of FXI in the range 2–15 U/dL. These observations suggest that only homozygotes or compound heterozygotes for two null alleles are prone to the development of an inhibitor following exposure to exogenous FXI. This study also revealed that the seven patients who developed an inhibitor were among 21 homozygotes for the type II mutation who had received plasma, which suggests that 33% of patients with almost no FXI have a predilection for development of an inhibitor. The antibodies isolated from patients with an inhibitor display various effects, i.e. impaired FXI activation by thrombin or by FXIIa, inhibition of binding of FXI to HK, and diminished activation of FIX by FXIa [49].

Diagnosis

Excessive bleeding following injury, such as tooth extraction, tonsillectomy, nose surgery, and urologic procedures, or an incidental finding of a prolonged APTT are the common modes of presentation of FXI deficiency. Excessive menstrual bleeding is also a recognized presentation. All patients with severe FXI deficiency (activity of <15 U/dL) exhibit an APTT value that is more than two standard deviations above the normal mean [50]. Heterozygotes may have a slightly prolonged APTT or values within the normal range but this is dependent upon the APTT reagent. Similarly, FXI levels overlap with normal levels. [3,33,36]. Therefore, for diagnosis of partial FXI deficiency in suspected heterozygotes, only genotyping for the responsible mutation can be diagnostic.

Because severe FXI deficiency can remain asymptomatic until injury is inflicted, it is desirable for all Ashkenazi Jews in need of surgery (particularly at sites of enhanced fibrinolysis) to undergo screening tests including APTT. If a prolonged APTT is obtained, FXI activity can be measured by an APTT-based assay.

Therapy

Spontaneous bleeding is rare in patients with severe FXI deficiency, and when it occurs it is usually mild and terminates without therapy. Sometimes, spontaneous bleeding follows the inadvertent use of antiplatelet agents and discontinuation of their use solves the problem. Deliveries are infrequently complicated by excessive bleeding in patients with severe FXI deficiency and thus on-demand, rather than preventive, blood product therapy can be advocated [34]. Oral antifibrinolytic drugs are useful both for menorrhagia and for bleeding after childbirth when it occurs.

Surgery or trauma can be associated with excessive and prolonged bleeding unless treated properly. Consequently, careful evaluation of patients with severe FXI deficiency prior to surgery is indispensable, as well as meticulous planning of the procedure and the postsurgical course. The following are some considerations and guidelines:

1 The surgical procedure should be absolutely indicated.
2 Previous bleeding episodes and their severity should be taken into account.
3 A test for an inhibitor to FXI should be performed and its presence ruled out.
4 The prothrombin time and platelet count should be normal.
5 Use of antiplatelet drugs should be discontinued 1 week before surgery.
6 Both site and type of surgery are significantly related to the risk of bleeding and, hence, planning of surgery should be tailored accordingly. Examples include: (i) patients in need of tooth extraction can be treated by tranexamic acid alone; (ii) for prostatectomy and other lower urinary tract surgery, both blood component therapy and local flushing by saline containing tranexamic acid can be used; (iii) for nasal surgery and tonsillectomy, replacement therapy and parenteral tranexamic acid administration are advisable; and (iv) for major surgery, plasma or FXI concentrate infusions should be targeted at trough FXI levels of 45 U/dL for approximately 10 days; for minor surgery a trough level of 30 U/dL during approximately 5 days is usually sufficient.
7 Assessment of the cardiovascular status of the patient is essential for two reasons: (i) when use of fresh frozen plasma is planned, the patient's incapacity to tolerate volume overload can be a serious impediment; and (ii) compromised cardiovascular function confers a risk of thrombosis when FXI concentrate is used.
8 Replacement therapy should be started prior to surgery and carefully monitored thereafter by assays of FXI activity.
9 Use of fibrin glue during surgery can significantly contribute to successful hemostasis.

Replacement therapy is usually by fresh frozen plasma. The main disadvantages of this mode of therapy are potential transmission of infectious agents, allergic reactions, and volume overload. Treatment of fresh frozen plasma by solvent/detergent or by pasteurization has increased its safety, with preservation of FXI activity [51].

Two concentrates of FXI have been produced, one in the UK and the other in France, and both were found to be safe with regard to transmission of infectious agents. However, approximately 10% of patients who were treated by these products developed arterial thrombosis or venous thromboembolism which was fatal in several cases. Since almost all patients who developed these unfortunate complications were elderly and had pre-existing cardiovascular disease [51], these products should be avoided in such patients or used with extreme caution. Caution should also be exercised in patients with prothrombotic states such as pregnancy and malignant disorders. Notwithstanding these limitations, FXI concentrates have been successfully used in many patients. Studies have shown a 90% recovery of FXI after infusion of these concentrates and a half-life of 46–52 h. The relatively small volume that needs to be infused, the excellent *in-vivo* recovery of FXI, and the extended half-life of FXI substantially facilitate therapy.

For several types of minor surgery, such as tooth extractions and skin biopsy, there is no need for replacement therapy. In 19 patients with severe FXI deficiency who have had a history of bleeding following tooth extractions or trauma, tooth extractions were uneventfully performed under treatment with tranexamic acid alone started 12 h prior to surgery and continued until 7 days after surgery [52]. Fibrin glue can also be used in such cases and in patients undergoing resection of skin lesions.

The approach to patients with partial FXI deficiency who need surgery varies among centers. Excessive bleeding following surgery in some patients with FXI levels of approximately 50 U/dL is used to support the view that such patients need replacement therapy during surgery [36]. Other observations of patients who underwent uneventful prostatectomy with a level of 30 U/dL support the view that replacement therapy is unnecessary during most surgical procedures in patients with partial FXI deficiency [35]. Notwithstanding these inconsistencies, a reasonable practice in patients with partial FXI deficiency can be:

1 Obtain a detailed history of bleeding.
2 If a clear history of a bleeding tendency is obtained, perform a thorough investigation of other potential inherited or acquired hemostatic disorders; abnormal results should be taken into account in the planning of surgery.
3 Use tranexamic acid and/or fibrin glue when there is a bleeding history or when high-risk surgery such as prostatectomy is planned.
4 Use replacement therapy in patients with an unequivocal bleeding tendency (after ruling out other hemostatic defects) aiming at a trough FXI level of 45 U/dL for 5 days after surgery.

Surgery in patients who have developed an inhibitor to FXI presents a great challenge. When the titer of the inhibitor is very low, use of a FXI concentrate can suffice, but an anamnestic reaction is to be expected. A one-time low dose of recombinant factor VIIa given during surgery and prolonged therapy by tranexamic acid have been successfully used in three such patients who underwent major surgery [53].

References

1 Rosenthal R, Dreskin O, Rosenthal N. New hemophilia-like disease caused by deficiency of a third plasma thromboplastin factor. *Proc Soc Exp Biol Med* 1953; **82**: 171–4.

2 Rapaport SI, Proctor RR, Patch NJ, Yettra M. The role of inheritance of PTA deficiency: evidence for the existence of major PTA deficiency and minor PTA deficiency. *Blood* 1961; **18**: 149–65.

3 Seligsohn U. High gene frequency of factor XI (PTA) deficiency in Ashkenazi Jews. *Blood* 1978; **516**; 1223–8.

4 Gailani D, Broze GJ. Factor XI activation in a revised model of blood coagulation. *Science* 1991; **253**: 909–12.

5 Naito K, Fujikawa K. Activation of human blood coagulation factor XI independent of factor XII. Factor XI is activated by thrombin and factor XIa in the presence of negatively charged surfaces. *J Biol Chem* 1991; **266**: 7353–8.

6 Pedicord DL, Seiffert D, Blat Y. Feedback activation of factor XI by thrombin does not occur in plasma. *Proc Natl Acad Sci USA* 2007; **104**: 12855–60.

7 Kravtsov DV, Matafonov A, Tucker EI, *et al.* Factor XI contributes to thrombin generation in the absence of factor XII. *Blood* 2009; **114**: 452–8.

8 Gailani D, Ho D, Sun MF, *et al.* Model for a factor IX activation complex on blood platelets: dimeric conformation of factor XIa is essential. *Blood* 2001; **97**: 3117–22.

9 Papagrigoriou E, McEwan PA, Walsh PN, Emsley J. Crystal structure of the factor XI zymogen reveals a pathway for transactivation. *Nature Struct Mol Biol* 2006; **13**: 557–8.

10 Emsley J, McEwan PA, Gailani D. Structure and function of factor XI. *Blood* 2010; **115**: 2569–77.

11 Kato A, Asakai R, Davie EW, Aoki N. Factor XI gene (F11) is located on the distal end of the long arm of human chromosome 4. *Cytogenet Cell Genet* 1989; **52**: 77–8.

12 Baglia FA, Badellino KO, Li CQ, *et al.* Factor XI binding to the platelet glycoprotein Ib–IX–V complex promotes factor XI activation by thrombin. *J Biol Chem* 2002; **277**: 1662–8.

13 Morrissey JH, Choi SH, Smith SA. Polyphosphate: an ancient molecule that links platelets, coagulation, and inflammation. *Blood* 2012; **119**: 5972–9.

14 Bouma BN, Marx PF, Mosnier LO, Meijers JC. Thrombin-activatable fibrinolysis inhibitor (TAFI, plasma procarboxypeptidase B, procarboxypeptidase R, procarboxypeptidase U). *Thromb Res* 2001; **101**: 329–54.

15 Muller F, Gailani D, Renne T. Factor XI and XII as antithrombotic targets. *Curr Opin Hematol* 2011; **18**: 349–55.

16 Ratnoff OD. Some relationships among hemostasis, fibrinolytic phenomena, immunity, and the inflammatory response. *Adv Immunol* 1969; **10**: 145–227.

17 von dem Borne PA, Cox LM, Bouma BN. Factor XI enhances fibrin generation and inhibits fibrinolysis in a coagulation model initiated by surface-coated tissue factor. *Blood Coag Fibrinol* 2006; **17**: 251–7.

18 Frick IM, Bjorck L, Herwald H. The dual role of the contact system in bacterial infectious disease. *Thromb Haemost* 2007; **98**: 497–502.

19 Tucker EI, Gailani D, Hurst S. Survival advantage of coagulation factor XI-deficient mice during peritoneal sepsis. *J Infect Dis* 2008; **198**: 271–4.

20 Tucker EI, Verbout NG, Leung PY, *et al.* Inhibition of factor XI activation attenuates inflammation and coagulopathy while improving the survival of mouse polymicrobial sepsis. *Blood* 2012; **119**: 4762–8.

21 Saito H, Ratnoff OD, Bouma BN, Seligshon U. Failure to detect variant (CRM) plasma thromboplastin antecedent (factor XI) molecules in hereditary plasma thromboplastin antecedent deficiency: a study of 125 patients in several ethnic backgrounds. *J Lab Clin Med* 1985; **106**: 718–22.

22 Zivelin A, Ogawa T, Bulvik S, *et al.* Severe factor XI deficiency caused by a Gly555 to Glu mutation (factor XI- Glu555): a cross-reactive material positive variant defective in factor XI activation. *J Thromb Haemost* 2004; **2**: 1782–9.

23 Asakai R, Chung DW, Ratnoff OD, Davie EW. Factor XI (plasma thromboplastin antecedent) deficiency in Ashkenazi Jews is a bleeding disorder that can result from three types of point mutations. *Proc Natl Acad Sci USA* 1989; **8**: 7667–71.

24 Asakai R, Chung DW, Davie EW, Seligsohn U. Factor XI deficiency in Ashkenazi Jews in Israel. *N Engl J Med* 1991; **3253**: 153–8.

25 Hancock JF, Wieland K, Pugh RE, *et al.* A molecular genetic study of factor XI deficiency. *Blood* 1991; **77**: 1942–8.

26 Meijers JC, Mulvihill ER, Davie EW, Chung DW. Apple four in human blood coagulation factor XI mediates dimer formation. *Biochemistry* 1992; **31**: 4680–4.

27 Pugh RE, McVey JH, Truddenham EG, Hancock JF. Six point mutations that cause factor XI deficiency. *Blood* 1995; **85**: 1509–16.

28 Peretz H, Mulai A, Usher S, *et al.* The two common mutations causing factor XI deficiency in Jews stem from distinct founders: one of ancient Middle Eastern origin and another of more recent European origin. *Blood* 1997; **90**: 2654–9.

29 Goldstein DB, Reich DE, Bradman N, *et al.* Age estimates of two common mutations causing factor XI deficiency: recent genetic drift is not necessary for elevated disease incidence among Ashkenazi Jews. *Am J Hum Genet* 1999; **64**: 1071–5.

30 Zivelin A, Bauduer F, Ducout L, *et al.* Factor XI deficiency in French Basques is caused predominantly by an ancestral Cys38Arg mutation in the factor XI gene. *Blood* 2002; **99**: 2448–54.

31 Bolton-Maggs PHB, Peretz H, Butler R, *et al.* A common ancestral mutation (C128X) occurring in 11 non-Jewish families from the UK with factor XI deficiency. *J Thromb Haemost* 2004; **2**: 918–24.

32 Salomon O, Steinberg DM, Seligsohn U. Variable bleeding manifestations characterize different types of surgery in patients with severe factor XI deficiency enabling parsimonious use of replacement therapy. *Haemophilia* 2006; **12**: 490–3.

33 Bolton-Maggs PH, Patterson DA, Wensley RT, Tuddenham EG. Definition of the bleeding tendency in factor XI-deficient kindreds—a clinical and laboratory study. *Thromb Haemost* 1995; **73**: 194–202.

34 Salomon O, Steinberg DM, Tamarin I, *et al.* Plasma replacement therapy during labor is not mandatory for women with sever factor XI deficiency. *Blood coagul Fibrinolysis* 2005; **16**: 37–41.

35 Sidi A, Seligsohn U, Jonas P, Many M. Factor XI deficiency: detection and management during urological surgery. *J Urol* 1978; **119**: 528–30.

36 Bolton-Maggs PH, Young Wan-Yin B, McCraw AH, *et al.* Inheritance and bleeding in factor XI deficiency. *Br J Haematol* 1988; **69**: 521–8.

37 Peyvandi F, Lak M, Mannucci PM. Factor XI deficiency in Iranians: its clinical manifestations in comparison with those of classic hemophilia. *Haematologica* 2002; **87**: 512–14.

38 Brenner B, Laor A, Lupo H, *et al.* Bleeding predictors in factor-XI-deficient patients. *Blood Coag Fibrinol* 1997; **8**: 511–15.

39 Peyvandi F, Palla R, Menegatti M, *et al.* Coagulation factor activity and clinical bleeding severity in rare bleeding disorders: results from the European Network of Rare Bleeding Disorders. *J Thromb Haemost* 2012; **10**: 615–21.

40 Salomon O, Steinberg DM, Dardik R, *et al.* Inherited factor XI deficiency confers no protection against acute myocardial infarction. *J Thromb Haemost* 2003; **1**: 658–61.

41 Salomon O, Steinberg DM, Koren-Morag N, *et al.* Reduced incidence of ischemic stroke in patients with severe factor XI deficiency. *Blood* 2008; **111**: 4113–17.

42 Salomon O, Steinberg DM, Zucker M, *et al.* Patients with severe factor XI deficiency have a reduced incidence of deep-vein thrombosis. *Thromb Haemost* 2011; **105**: 269–73.

43 Renne T, Oschatz C, Seifert S, *et al.* Factor XI deficiency in animal models. *J Thromb Haemost* 2009; **7**(Suppl. 1): 79–83.

44 Schumacher WA, Luettgen JM, Quan ML, *et al.* Inhibition of factor XIa as a new approach to anticoagulation. *Arterioscler Thromb Vasc Biol* 2010; **30**: 388–92.

45 Renne T, Schmaier AH, Nickel KF, *et al.* In vivo roles of factor XII. *Blood* 2012; **120**: 4296–303.

46 Wu W, Li H, Navaneetham, D, *et al.* The kunitz protease inhibitor domain of protease nexin-2 inhibits factor XIa and murine carotid artery and middle cerebral artery thrombosis. *Blood* 2012; **120**: 671–7.

47 Zhang H, Lowenberg EC, Crosby JR, *et al.* Inhibition of the intrinsic coagulation pathway factor XI by antisense oligonucleotides: a novel antithrombotic strategy with lowered bleeding risk. *Blood* 2010; **116**: 4684–92.

48 Younis HS, Crosby J, Huh JI, *et al.* Antisense inhibition of coagulation factor XI prolongs APTT without increased bleeding risk in cynomolgus monkeys. *Blood* 2012; **119**: 2401–8.

49 Salomon O, Zivelin A, Livnat T, *et al.* Prevalence, causes, and characterization of factor XI inhibitors in patients with inherited factor XI deficiency. *Blood* 2003; **101**: 4783–8.

50 Seligsohn U, Modan M. Definition of the population at risk of bleeding due to factor XI deficiency in Ashkenazic Jews and the value of activated partial thromboplastin time in its detection. *Isr J Med Sci* 1981; **17**: 413–15.

51 Bolton-Maggs PHB. Factor XI deficiency and its management. *Haemophilia* 2000; **6**: 100–9.

52 Berliner S, Horowitz I, Martinowitz U, *et al.* Dental surgery in patients with severe factor XI deficiency without plasma replacement. *Blood Coag Fibrinol* 1992; **3**: 465–8.

53 Livnat T, Tamarin I, Mor Y, *et al.* Recombinant activated factor VII and tranexamic acid are hemostatically effective during major surgery in factor XI-deficient patients with inhibitor antibodies. *Thromb Haemost* 2009; **102**: 487–92.

CHAPTER 59

Factor XIII deficiency

Diane Nugent and Loan Hsieh

Division of Hematology, Children's Hospital of Orange County and Center for Inherited Blood Disorders, California, USA

Introduction

Factor XIII (FXIII) is a transglutaminase enzyme that was first discovered as a clotting protein in the coagulation cascade. However, recent literature describes multiple roles for this factor, including the ability to cross-link proteins in the plasma, vascular matrix, endothelial cells, platelets, and monocytes. In addition to maintaining normal hemostasis, FXIII plays a role in atherosclerosis, wound healing, inflammation, and pregnancy [1–3].

Factor XIII circulates in plasma as a tetramer protein (FXIII-A_2B_2) held together by noncovalent bonds. FXIII has a molecular weight of 325 kDa with two catalytic A-subunits (FXIII-A_2) of 83 kDa and two noncatalytic B-subunits or carrier subunits (FXIII-B_2) of 79 kDa [4–6]. Table 59.1 shows the International Society of Thrombosis Hemostasis (ISTH) recommended nomenclature for the various forms of FXIII used for research publications [7].

Intracellular FXIII-A_2 exists as a homodimer and can be found in platelets, monocytes, tissue macrophages, and placenta. Nearly half of the total amount of FXIII in whole blood can be found in association with circulating platelets [1–3,8]. Intracellular FXIII-A_2 is released during hemostasis and binds to FXIII-B_2 to form the tetramer complex (FXIII-A_2B_2), which functions to stabilize the fibrin clot. Platelet FXIII can also enhance clot formation by cross-linking platelets to clotting proteins such as von Willebrand factor, factor V, and fibrinogen [9,10]. FXIII-A contains the activation site of the enzyme and is synthesized by hematopoietic cells such as monocytes and megakaryocytes with some production from hepatocytes as well [11–13]. Intracellular platelet FXIIIA has also been found to play a role in lamellipodia formation and spreading on a fibrinogen-coated surface [14].

Approximately 50% of total FXIII-B can be found in plasma as a free form with the remainder existing in the heterotetrameric form (FXIII-A_2B_2) bound to FXIII-A_2 [1–4,15]. The main role of FXIII-B is to protect FXIII-A_2 from proteolytic degradation and inactivation, thereby extending the time FXIII-A_2 remains in circulation. Another critical role of FXIII-B is the localization of FXIII to the polymerizing fibrin chains to facilitate cross-linking. FXIII-B is primarily produced in the liver [12,16]. Plasma FXIII-B specifically binds to the γ' chain of fibrinogen type 2 [17]. Fibrinogen acts as a carrier for FXIII in plasma and helps to downregulate potential cross-linking activity [1–6,18].

Structure/function

Factor XIII plays an important role in hemostasis by catalyzing the cross-linking of fibrin as well as enhancing fibrin interaction with a variety of integrins within the platelet membrane and matrix proteins throughout thrombus formation. In aggregate, these biologic processes strengthen and stabilize the blood clot [2,4] (Figure 59.1). Both plasma and platelet FXIII-A originate from the same gene, making them functionally indistinguishable. Intracellular FXIII represents nearly 50% of total FXIII activity in the body [8]. Platelet FXIII-A is present in large concentrations in circulating platelets and appears to play an important role in the cytoskeletal remodeling associated with the activation of platelets [14,19,20]. As early as 1982, Cohen *et al.* observed that FXIII-deficient plasma did not support platelet fibrin association and retraction in humans [21]. This observation has now been validated in the FXIII knock-out mouse where clot retraction is entirely lost [22]. Following activation with calpain, intracellular FXIII-A2 has been shown to enhance platelet adhesion and clot retraction via FXIII–fibrin–GPIIb/IIIa cross-linking with myosin fibrils [20]. Plasma FXIII also has been shown to bind specifically to fibrinogen linked to the GPIIb/IIIa receptor in thrombin-activated platelets. Several excellent recent reviews are recommended for those wishing to delve deeper into the expanding role of both intracellular and extracellular FXIII in platelet function and clot retraction [1–3,23].

Textbook of Hemophilia, Third Edition. Edited by Christine A. Lee, Erik E. Berntorp and W. Keith Hoots.

© 2014 John Wiley & Sons, Ltd. Published 2014 by John Wiley & Sons, Ltd.

In the past decade, more information has been gleaned from X-ray crystallography where the FXIII-A-subunit is shown to contain an activation peptide, a β-sandwich, a catalytic core, and barrel 1 and barrel 2 domains [9]. The activation peptide, composed of 37 amino acids, restricts the access of the substrate to the active site cysteine. Activated FXIII (FXIIIa) binds to fibrin through the α-C-domain enhancing dissociation of the FXIII-subunits [9]. The B-subunit is composed of 10 repeated Sushi or glycoprotein 1 domains [24]. Each Sushi domain has two disulfide bridges that sustain its tertiary structure. The B-subunit binds to fibrinogen 2 γ-chain and helps regulate cross-linking activity [9,24]. Souri *et al.* studied the function of FXIII-B by expressing recombinant FXIII-B protein in baculovirus [25]. These studies revealed specific roles for the individual Sushi components: the first Sushi domain was involved in the binding of FXIII-B to FXIII-A, whereas the fourth and ninth Sushi domains were responsible for the FXIII-B homodimer assembly. The study also confirmed that rFXIII-B in the heterotetramer form (FXIII-A_2B_2) protected FXIII-A from proteolytic digestion [25].

Activation of FXIII begins with thrombin cleavage of A-subunits and requires a critical mass of fibrin polymers.

Table 59.1 Factor XIII nomenclature.

Plasma FXIII	FXIII-A_2B_2
Cellular FXIII	FXIII-A_2
A-subunit of FXIII	FXIII-A (monomer)
A-subunit of FXIII	FXIII-A_2 (dimer)
B-subunit of FXIII	FXIII-B (monomer)
B-subunit of FXIII	FXIII-B_2 (dimer)
Inactive intermediate after thrombin cleavage	FXIIIa′
Thrombin + Ca^{2+}-activated FXIII	FXIIIa*

Thrombin mediates cleavage of the activation peptides (AP-FXIII) of FXIII-A from the N-terminus at position 37 [26–28]. In the presence of Ca^{2+} and fibrin, the B-subunits dissociate from the A-subunits causing a conformational change exposing the active site [29] (Figure 59.2). This active site contains a cysteine residue (Cys311) which is found within the sequence Tyr–Gly–Gln–Cys–Trp. Activated FXIII-A_2 (FXIII-A_2*) will then cross-link fibrin through ε-amino(γ-glutamyl) lysine isopeptide bond [30,31]. The B-subunits dissociate while the majority of A-subunits remain bound to fibrin [30]. Thrombin catalyzes formation of γ-glutamyl-ε lysl bonds between fibrin monomers, resulting in a fibrin meshwork that is insoluble in mild acids and urea. Activated FXIII cross-links fibrin polymers present at very low concentrations, before a clot is visible [32]. FXIIIa can also cross-link fibrinogen but at a much slower rate [33,34]. The activation rate of intracellular factor XIII by thrombin is more rapid than plasma FXIII thrombin conversion to XIIIa. Studies have shown a lag time between the first steps of plasma FXIII activation: thrombin cleavage and exposure of the active site [35–37]. This delay corresponds to the amount of time needed for the B-subunit to dissociate from activated plasma FXIII. In contrast to plasma FXIII activation, platelet FXIII activation depends on high levels of intracellular Ca^{2+} triggering the protein to undergo a nonproteolytic conformation change to its active form.

In addition to binding fibrin(ogen), FXIII cross-links numerous substrates involved in hemostasis and antifibrinolysis [9,33]. FXIII incorporates antifibrinolytic proteins such as $α_2$-antiplasmin, plasminogen activator inhibitor 2 (PAI-2), and thrombin activatable fibrinolysis inhibitor (TAFI) into fibrin [9,35]. The main substrate for FXIII is fibrin, with only the α- and γ-chains participating in cross-linking activity [1]. There

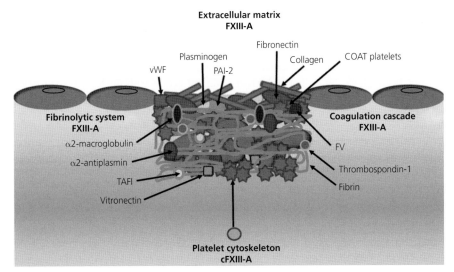

Figure 59.1 Role of cross-linking in thrombus consolidation and extracellular matrix attachment. COAT, collagen- and thrombin-activated (platelets); FV, factor V; FXIII, factor XIII; PAI-2, plasminogen activator inhibitor-2; TAFI, thrombin-activatable fibrinolysis inhibitor; vWF, von Willebrand factor. From [2]. Reproduced with permission of Portland Press Limited. (See also Plate 59.1.)

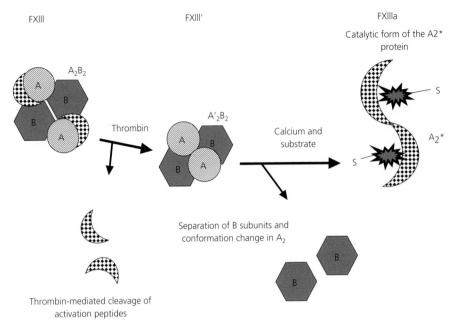

Figure 59.2 Activation of plasma factor XIII (FXIII) heterotetramer.

are several other proteins that FXIII cross-links: von Willebrand factor, factor V, vitronectin, vinculin, myosin, and actin [1–3]. Plasma FXIII binds to glycoprotein IIb/IIIa on platelets and α (v)β3 integrin on endothelial cells [38,39]. FXIII also plays an important function in wound healing and tissue repair by binding proteins fibronectin and collagen [2–4,40]. The cross-linking of these proteins to fibrin enhances migration and proliferation of fibroblasts, which in turn stabilizes the extracellular matrix formed at the site of tissue injury [2,4,9,40].

Molecular genetics

Since the first molecular mutation of FXIII deficiency was published in 1992, there have now been over 70 mutations reported [41,42]. The majority of the mutations for FXIII-A are due to missense or nonsense mutations (Table 59.2). For a current listing of all subunit A or B mutations reported, please see the Human Gene Mutation Database at the Institute of Medical Genetics in Cardiff website (http://www.hgmd.cf.ac.uk) and the Factor XIII Registry Database website (http://www.f13-database.de).

The vast majority of FXIII-deficient patients have mutations in the *F13A* gene, with more than 60 different types of mutations reported. Most of the mutations code for a single amino acid change (missense mutation), resulting in irregular folding and instability of the altered protein. Other types of mutations such as nonsense mutations, frame-shift mutations, and intronic mutations at splice sites leading to incorrect post-transcriptional processing of the mRNA have also been reported. Splice-site mutations have been reported to occur in introns 3, 5, 7, 8, 10,

11, and 14 [43]. To date, only four mutations have been described for the *F13B* gene, leading to the rarer form of the disease.

The FXIII-A gene (*F13A*) has been localized to chromosome 6p24–p25, spanning more than 160 kb, and has 15 exons separated by 14 introns encoding 731 amino acids (Figure 59.3). The FXIII-B gene (*F13B*) is located on chromosome 1q32–q32.1 and spans 28 kb in size with 12 exons interrupted by 11 introns encoding 641 amino acids [44,45] (Figure 59.4).

In addition to the numerous mutations reported in the *FXIII-A* gene, there are five common coding polymorphisms that have been identified: Val34Leu, Tyr204Phe, Pro564Leu, Val650Ile, and Glu651Gln. The most common single nucleotide polymorphism (SNP) is Val34Leu, occurring with an allele frequency of about 0.35 to 0.30 in the Caucasian population [46–48]. The nucleotide change from G to T does not result in FXIII deficiency, but does alter the function of the protein. Tyr204Phe variant occurs with the lowest frequency, at 0.01–0.03, and has been associated with an increased risk for recurrent miscarriages [49].

The Val34Leu variant has been most studied, with the amino acid substitution occurring in the activation peptide sequence, three amino acids upstream from the thrombin cleavage site. Studies show that activation of the Leu34 variant FXIII by thrombin proceeds more rapidly than the wild-type Val 34 [50]. Fibrin clots formed in the presence of Leu34 FXIII have thinner fibers, smaller pores, and altered permeation characteristics when compared with fibrin clots formed in the presence of Val34 variant [51]. Several studies support the protective role Val34Leu plays in myocardial infarctions and venous thrombosis [52–54]; however, there are reports of no association with or increased risk of thrombosis [55–58]. There is a correlation

Table 59.2 Factor XIII-A missense/nonsense mutations. Adapted from http://www.f13-database.de/%28ghloq2yn111bja55r0kqnhev%29/content .aspx?menu=1,6,21

Exon	Nucleotide change	Amino acid change	References
3	c.183C > A	Asn60Lys	Anwar *et al.* (1995)
3	c.232C > T	Arg77Cys	Duan *et al.* (2002)
3	c.233G > A	Arg77His	Peyvandi *et al.* (2004)
3	c.306G > A	Glu102Lys	Anwar (2002)
4	c.479T > G	Met159Arg	Schroeder *et al.* (2006)
4	c.514C > T	Arg171Stop	Standen & Bowen (1993)
5	c.631G > A	Gly210Arg	Vysokovsky *et al.* (2004)
5	c.646G > A	Gly215Arg	Schroeder *et al.* (2006)
6	c.707T > G	Leu235Arg	Birben *et al.* (2003)
6	c.728T > C	Met242Thr	Mikkola *et al.* (1994)
6	c.758G > T	Arg252Ile	Mikkola *et al.* (1996)
6	c.781C > T	Arg260Cys	Ichinose (1998)
6	c.782G > T	Arg260Leu	Vysokovsky *et al.* (2004)
6	c.782G > A	Arg260His	Kangsadalampai (1999)
6	c.788G > A	Gly262Glu	Onland *et al.* (2005)
7	c.851A > G	Tyr283Cys	Souri *et al.* (2001)
7	c.888C > G	Ser295Arg	Anwar *et al.* (2000)
7	c.949G > T	Val316Phe	Onland *et al.* 2005
7	c.956C > T	Ala318Val	Vysokovsky *et al.* (2004)
8	c.980G > A	Arg326Gln	Mikkola *et al.* (1996)
8	c.978C > T	Arg326Stop	Anwar (2005)
8	c.1064T > C	Leu354Pro	Anwar *et al.* (2001)
9	c.1128G > T	Trp375Cys	Schroeder *et al.* (2006)
9	c.1149G > T	Arg382Ser	Peyvandi *et al.* (2003)
9	c.1183C > T	Ala394Val	Izumi (1998)
9	c.1196C > A	Thr398Asn	Vysokovsky *et al.* (2004)
9	c.1201C > T	Gln400Stop	Kangsadalampai *et al.* (1996)
10	c.1226G > A	Arg408Gln	Anwar *et al.* 1995
10	c.1241C > T	Ser413Leu	Niya *et al.* (1999)
10	c.1241C > G	Ser413Trp	Duan *et al.* (2003)
10	c.1243G > T	Val414Phe	Aslam (1997)
10	c.1216G > A	Gly420Ser	Kangsadalampai *et al.* (2000)
11	c.1325C > A	Tyr441Stop	Anwar (1995)
11	c.1504G > A	Gly501Arg	Board (1993)
12	c.1496T > C	Leu498Pro	Mikkola *et al.* (1996)
12	c.1626C > G	Asn541Lys	Birben *et al.* (2002)
12	c.1687G > A	Gly562Arg	Takahashi *et al.* (1998)
14	c.1982T > C	Leu660Pro	Inbal *et al.* (1997)
14	c.1984C > T	Arg661Stop	Mikkola *et al.* (1994)
14	c.2003T > C	Leu667Pro	Aslam (1995)
15	c.2074G > A	Trp691Stop	Anwar (2005)
15	c.2150A > G	His716Arg	Schroeder *et al.* (2006)

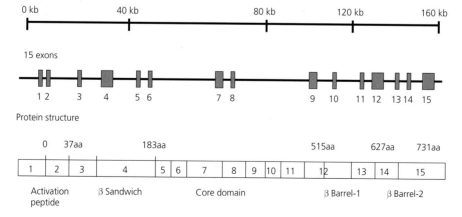

Figure 59.3 Factor XIII-A gene (*F13A*) and protein structure. *F13A* gene on chromosome 6 at bands p24–25: length 160 kb.

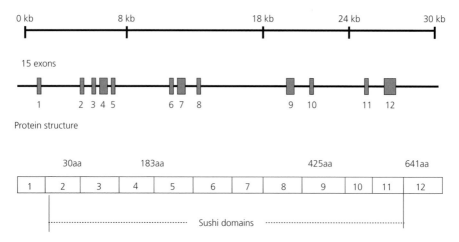

Figure 59.4 Factor XIII-B gene (*F13B*) and protein structure. The *F13B* gene is located on the long arm of chromosome 1 (q32–32.1). The 10 FXIII-B-subunit tandem repeats (known as Sushi domains) are encoded by a single exon 2–11.

between geographic area and the Leu34 allele prevalence contributing to a difference in arterial thrombosis rates among different populations.

Two polymorphisms, Tyr204Phe and Pro564Leu, have been associated with an increased risk of hemorrhagic stroke in young women [59]. The other two polymorphisms, Glu651Gln and Val650Ile, have been studied the least.

As these examples of gene variants influencing phenotype suggest, there is a high level of heterogeneity observed in the clinical presentation among patients with FXIII deficiency. This heterogeneity represents the gamut of molecular variation of the *FXIII* gene: rare mutations to common polymorphisms.

Clinical presentation

Factor XIII deficiency is a rare bleeding disorder with an incidence of 1/1–3 million individuals [60,61]. The inheritance pattern of FXIII deficiency is autosomal recessive, with the expected higher incidence among populations with consanguinity. Clinical manifestations of FXIII deficiency include severe bleeding in the joints or soft tissue, spontaneous intracranial hemorrhage, poor wound healing, and spontaneous abortions. The factor XIII international registry data, recorded from 1993 to 2005, showed over half of the patients (57%) presented with subcutaneous bleeding, followed closely by delayed umbilical cord bleeding (56%), a characteristic finding in these patients [60,61].

Patients with congenital homozygous FXIII deficiency present with severe bleeding symptoms and plasma FXIII levels of <1%. The incidence of intracranial hemorrhage has been reported to be 25–35%. This high incidence of life-threatening bleeding complications in FXIII-deficient patients distinguishes it from other types of bleeding disorders such as hemophilia A or B. This potentially fatal bleeding complication is the major reason the treatment plan for these patients is so aggressive.

Postoperative bleeding 24–48 h later is commonly seen in FXIII-deficient patients because of normal clot formation, but early fibrinolysis because of weak cross-linking of fibrin. Ecchymoses and mucosal bleeding represent the more mild bleeding symptoms observed in these patients [60].

Homozygous congenital FXIII deficiency can be due to defects in either *FXIII-A* genes (also known as type 2 defect) or *FXIII-B* genes (type 1 defect). The majority of patients with FXIII deficiency are lacking FXIII-A, leading to a greater tendency to bleed compared with patients missing FXIII-B. This clinical difference can be attributed to the preservation of intracellular FXIII-A in the case of B-subunit deficiency. Patients lacking FXIII-B will still have normal levels of FXIII-A in platelets to help stabilize clot formation [61].

FXIII-A$_2$, produced in the placenta, plays an important role in early pregnancy. Low levels of maternal FXIII-A$_2$ can lead to poor formation of cytotrophoblastic shell and placental detachment. FXIII-A$_2$ is not critical for fertilization or early implantation but is necessary to minimize decidual bleeding starting at 5 weeks' gestation [62,63]. Impaired placental adhesion along with a tendency for hemorrhage in FXIII-deficient women likely lead to the increased risk of miscarriages and recurrent fetal loss reported.

Factor XIII cross-linking plays an important role in innate immunity. Inflammation, sepsis, and clotting are being shown to have shared activation pathways and regulatory mechanisms. Various hypotheses regarding the evolution of coagulation and the complement system focus on our need to both recognize and curtail the spread of infection [64,65]. In two landmark articles, it has been shown that mannose-binding lectin-associated serine protease (MASP)-1 of the *complement* system cleaves fibrinogen and activates FXIII of the *coagulation* system [66,67]. The MASP-1catalyzed deposition and polymerization of fibrin on the microorganisms outer surface aids in sequestering infection. Indeed, human FXIII has been shown to completely encapsulate bacteria quite effectively [68]. Much work has also focused on the role of FXIII in the monocyte, which when transformed into a macrophage, is key to host defense in innate immunity. Adany et al. recently reported that monocytes activated by interleukin-4 are converted to M2 cells with a striking increase in the expression of intracellular FXIII-A [69,70]. When this occurs, phagocytosis of opsonized red cells or complement coated yeast ensues when cells are derived from normal individuals, while this activity is completely absent when cells are derived from patients with FXIII deficiency [70]. Excellent reviews of this and neutrophil–FXIII interactions can be found in the following articles [3,4,23,40].

Diagnosis

Since most clinical FXIII assays focus on the cross-linking that occurs late in the clotting cascade after fibrin has already been formed, its activity is not reflected in routine coagulation assays. Standard screening tests, such as prothrombin time, activated partial thromboplastin time, fibrinogen level, platelet count, and bleeding time, are all normal in patients with FXIII deficiency. Clot formation is normal with FXIII deficiency, but the quality of the clot is weak because of lack of fibrin cross-linking. As in the early studies of FXIII deficiency, this can be seen in thromboelastography with a decrease in clot size and early lysis, but clearly this is not specific and may not be used in definitive diagnosis [61,71,72]. Best practise currently includes quantitative FXIII enzyme activity, and where available, determination of the FXIII antigens, both A- and B-subunits.

The majority of hospitals will perform a clot solubility test as rapid qualitative screen for FXIII, but this test is easily affected by other factors, such as an elevated fibrinogen, and thus may be falsely normal. Importantly, the clot solubility test is only sensitive at extremely low levels of FXIII and will be normal if levels are above 1–3% [72]. Therefore, additional quantitative testing can be accomplished using commercially available enzyme assays used to quantitate FXIII activity based on monitoring the amount of ammonia (NH_3) released. There are a number of assays currently available and the majority of clinical laboratories have modified these commercial kits to be sensitive down to levels of 1% activity [71,72]. An enzyme-linked immunoadsorbent assay (ELISA) can measure FXIII tetramer or FXIII subunit (A or B) antigens by specific antibodies, respectively. Knowing the subunit deficiency will become an increasingly important distinction, as the use of recombinant FXIIIa for prophylaxis would not be indicated in the very rare FXIII B-subunit deficiency.

Treatment

Once the diagnosis of FXIII deficiency is confirmed, prophylactic therapy with FXIII replacement is critical to prevent severe disability or even death because of bleeding complications. As in other forms of hemophilia, blood product has now been replaced with safer heat-treated plasma concentrate (Corifact, CSL-Behring) and most recently recombinant FXIII-A2 (NovoNordisk). However, if these products are not available, FXIII replacement can be accomplished with cryoprecipitate or fresh frozen plasma. Cryoprecipitate can be given in doses of one bag per 10–20 kg every 3–4 weeks. Fresh frozen plasma can be administered at 10 mL/kg every 4–6 weeks. Blood products are not optimal for long-term treatment due to the high rate of sensitization to plasma proteins and potential for transmission of infectious agents. Because of the long half-life of endogenous FXIII (ranging from 7 to 13 days), dosing frequency can be spaced out to 4–6 weeks for most FXIII-containing products. Any given patient may vary in FXIII half-life, therefore dosing for prophylaxis should be based on levels obtained at a minimum of 1 day, 14 days, and 28 days postinfusion initially, and then obtain nadir levels for 2–3 months to be sure that the patient is within a safe range throughout the month.

Successful treatment with FXIII concentrate was demonstrated by a striking decrease in bleeding frequency and confirmed by restoration of normal thromboelastography [73,74]. Based in this and subsequent studies this plasma-derived product (Corifact, CSL) was approved in the USA and Europe in 2010 [75]. Recombinant FXIII-A$_2$ (Novo Nordisk; Bagsvaerd, Denmark) is already commercially available in Europe, and is anticipated to receive US approval in 2014. This investigational drug is a homodimer (rFXIII-A$_2$) that binds to endogenous plasma FXIII-B-subunits to form plasma FXIII-A$_2$B$_2$. Lovejoy et al. and Inbal et al. showed that rFXIII-A2 demonstrated normal pharmacokinetics, and subsequent phase 3 trials confirmed efficacy as an alternative therapy for FXIII A-subunit-deficient patients [76,77].

Perinatal management of FXIII-deficient women varies according to the weeks of gestation. In general, coagulation factor levels tend to increase during gestation, with the exception of FXIII-A activity, which decreases during pregnancy. Since decidual bleeding begins early in gestation (week 5–6), FXIII replacement is critical to maintaining pregnancy. However, FXIII-A is not necessary for fertilization or early implantation. The half-life of FXIII-A concentrate ranges from 7 to 13 days during the nongestational period but progressively decreases to as low as 1.8 days in late pregnancy (32 weeks' gestation) [78–80]. Plasma levels of FXIII-A need to be sustained above 10% to prevent spontaneous abortion [81–83]. Recommended therapy for pregnancy at this time is with plasma-derived FXIII concentrate at a dosing every 14 days in early pregnancy and increasing to every 7 days later in pregnancy to maintain levels of at least 20–30% activity [78–83]. During labor, an additional dose is recommended to reach minimum plasma FXIII levels of 50% to avoid bleeding complications [80].

Data regarding the use of either product for surgical or dental procedures is limited, and currently only the heat-treated plasma-derived concentrate (Corifact) has US Food and Drug Administration (FDA) approval for use during surgery. As in the case of perinatal management, FXIII activity of 50% or greater would be recommended for surgical procedures. [84].

Prognosis

The risk for intracranial hemorrhage increases the morbidity and mortality of patients with FXIII deficiency. However, the prognosis is excellent with the current availability of plasma-derived products such as cryoprecipitate, fresh frozen plasma, or FXIII concentrate. As seen in large registries, lifelong therapy would be necessary to prevent bleeding complications, miscarriage, and especially life-threatening intracranial hemorrhage.

References

1 Lorand L, Losowsky MS, Miloszewski KJ. Human factor XIII: fibrin-stabilizing factor. *Prog Hemost Thromb* 1980; **5**: 245–90.

2 Richardson VR, Cordell P, Standeven KF, Carter AM. Substrates of Factor XIII-A: roles in thrombosis and wound healing. *Clin Sci (Lond)* 2013; **124**: 123–37.

3 Schroeder V, Kohler HP. New developments in the area of factor XIII. *J Thromb Haemost* 2013; **11**: 234–44.

4 Muszbek L, Bereczky Z, Bagoly Z, Komáromi I, Katona É. Factor XIII: a coagulation factor with multiple plasmatic and cellular functions. *Physiol Rev* 2011; **91**: 931–72.

5 Komáromi I, Bagoly Z, Muszbek L. Factor XIII: novel structural and functional aspects. *J Thromb Haemost* 2011; **9**: 9–20.

6 Ashcroft AE, Grant PJ, Ariens RAS. A study of human coagulation factor XIII-subunit by electrospray ionization mass spectrometry. *Rapid Commun Mass Spectrom* 2000; **14**: 1607–11.

7 Muszbek L, Ariens RA, Ichinose A, on behalf of the ISTH SSC Subcommittee on Factor XIII. Factor XIII: recommended terms and abbreviations. *J Thromb Haemost* 2007; **5**: 181–3.

8 McDonagh J, McDonagh RP Jr, Delage JM, *et al.* Factor XIII in human plasma and platelets. *J Clin Invest* 1969; **48**: 940–6.

9 Muszbek L, Adany R, Mikkola H. Novel aspect of blood coagulation Factor XIII. I. Structure, distribution, activation, and function. *Crit Rev Clin Lab Sci* 1996; **33**: 357–421.

10 Nagy B Jr, Simon Z, Bagoly Z, *et al.* Binding of plasma factor XIII to thrombin-receptor activated human platelets. *Thromb Haemost* 2009; **102**: 83–9.

11 Henricksson P, Becker S, Lynch G, *et al.* Identification of intracellular factor XIII in human monocytes and macrophages. *J Clin Invest* 1985; **76**: 528–34.

12 Wolpl A, Lattke H, Board PG, *et al.* Coagulation factor XIII A and B subunits in bone marrow and liver transplantation. *Transplantation* 1987; **43**: 151–3.

13 Poon MC, Russell JA, Low S, *et al.* Hematopoietic origin of factor XIII A subunits in platelets, monocytes, and plasma. Evidence from bone marrow transplantation studies. *J Clin Invest* 1989; **84**: 787–92.

14 Jayo A, Conde I, Lastres P, *et al.* New insights into the expression and role of platelet factor XIII-A. *J Thromb Haemost* 2009; **7**: 1184–91.

15 Yorifuji H, Anderson K, Lynch GW, *et al.* B protein of factor XIII: differentiation between free B and complexed B. *Blood* 1988; **72**: 1645–50.

16 Nagy JA, Henriksson P, McDonagh J. Biosynthesis of factor XIII B subunit by human hepatoma cell lines. *Blood* 1986; **68**: 1272–9.

17 Siebenlist KR, Meh DA, Mosesson MW. Plasma factor XIII binds specifically to fibrinogen molecules containing gamma chains. *Biochemistry* 1996; **35**: 10448–53.

18 Mosesson MW. Fibrinogen gamma chain functions. *J Thromb Haemost* 2003; **1**: 231–8.

19 Adany R, Bardos H. Factor XIII subunit A as an intracellular transglutaminase. *Cell Mol Life Sci* 2003; **60**: 1049–60.

20 Magwenzi SG, Ajjan RA, Standeven KF, Parapia LA, Naseem KM. Factor XIII supports platelet activation and enhances thrombus formation by matrix proteins under flow conditions. *J Thromb Haemost* 2011; **9**: 820–33.

21 Cohen I, Gerrard JM, White JG. Ultrastructure of clots during isometric contraction. *J Cell Biol* 1982; **93**: 775–87.

22 Kasahara K, Souri M, Kaneda M, Miki T, Yamamoto N, Ichinose A. Impaired clot retraction in factor XIII A subunit-deficient mice. *Blood* 2010;**115**: 1277–9.

23 Ichinose A. Factor XIII is a key molecule at the intersection of coagulation and fibrinolysis as well as inflammation and infection control. *Int J Hematol* 2012; **95**: 362–70.

24 Ichinose A, McMullen BA, Fjuikawa K, *et al.* Amino acid sequence of the B subunit of human factor XIII, a protein composed of ten repetitive segments. *Biochemistry* 1986; **25**: 4633–8.

25 Souri M, Kaetsu H, Ichinose A. Sushi domains in the B subunit of factor XIII responsible for oligomer assembly. *Biochemistry* 2008; **47**: 8656–64.

26 Mikuni, Y, Iwanga S, Konishi KA. Peptide released from plasma fibrin stabilizing factor in the conversion to the active enzyme by thrombin. *Biochem Biophys Res Commun* 1973; **54**: 1393–402.

27 Nakamura S, Iwanga S, Suzuki T, *et al.* Amino acid sequence of the peptide released from bovine factor XIII following activation by thrombin. *Biochem Biophys Res Commun* 1974; **58**: 250–6.

28 Takgai T, Doolittle RF. Amino acid sequence studies on factor XIII and the peptide released during its activation by thrombin. *Biochemistry* 1974; **13**: 750–6.

29 Lorand L, Konishi K. Activation of the fibrin stabilizing factor of plasma by thrombin. *Arch Biochem Biophys* 1964; **105**: 58–67.

30 Pisano JJ, Finlayson JS, Peyton MP. Crosslink in fibrin polymerized by factor XIII:e-(gamma-glutamyl) lysine. *Science* 1968; **160**: 892–3.

31 Matacic S, Loewy AG. The identification of isopeptide crosslink in insoluble fibrin. *Biochem Biophys Res Com* 1968; **30**: 356–62.

32 Ariens RAS, Lai TS, Weisel JW, *et al.* Role of factor XIII in fibrin clot formation and effects of genetic polymorphisms. *Blood* 2002; **100**: 743–54.

33 Greenberg CS, Miraglia CC, Rickles FR, *et al.* Cleavage of blood coagulation factor XIII and fibrinogen by thrombin during in vitro clotting. *J Clin Invest* 1985; **75**: 1463–70.

34 Kanaide H, Shainoff JR. Cross-linking of fibrinogen and fibrin by fibrin-stabilizing factor (factor XIIIa). *J Lab Clin Med* 1975; **85**: 574–97.

35 Mosesson MW, Siebenlist KR, Hainfeld JF, *et al.* The covalent structure of factor XIIIa crosslinked fibrinogen fibrils. *J Str Biol* 1995; **115**: 88–101.

36 Greenberg GS, Achyuthan KE, Fenton JW. Factor XIIIa formation promoted by complexing of alpha-thrombin, fibrin, and plasma factor XIII. *Blood* 1987; **69**: 867–71.

37 Lorand L. Factor XIII: Structure, activation, and interactions with fibrinogen and fibrin. *Ann NY Acad Sci* 2001; **936**: 291–311.

38 Cox AD, Devine DV. Factor XIIIa binding to activated platelets is mediated through activation of glycoprotein IIb-IIIa. *Blood* 1994; **83**: 1006–16.

39 Dardik R, Shenkman B, Tamarin I, *et al.* Factor XIII mediates adhesion of platelets to endothelial cells through alpha(v) beta(3) and glycoprotein IIb/IIIa integrins. *Thromb Res* 2002; **105**: 317–23.

40 Bagoly Z, Katona E, Muszbek L. Factor XIII and inflammatory cells. *Thromb Res* 2012; **129**(Suppl. 2): S77–81.

41 Kamura T, Okamura T, Murakawa M, *et al.* Deficiency of coagulation factor XIII A subunit caused by the dinucleotide deletion at the 5' end of exon III. *J Clin Invest* 1992; **90**: 315–19.

42 Board P, Coggan M, Miloszewski K. Identification of a point mutation in factor XIII A subunit deficiency. *Blood* 1992; **80**: 937–41.

43 Schroeder V, Durrer D, Mell E, *et al.* Congenital factor XIII deficiency in Switzerland. *Swiss Med Wkly* 2007; **137**: 272–8.

44 Bottenus RE, Ichinose A, Davie EW. Nucleotide sequence of the gene for the b subunit of human factor XIII. *Biochemistry* 1990; **29**: 11195–209.

45 Webb GC, Coggan M, Ichinose A, *et al.* Localization of the coagulation factor XIIIB subunit gene (F13B) to chromosome bands 1q31–32.1 and restriction fragment length polymorphism at the locus. *Hum Genet* 1989; **81**: 157–60.

46 Kohler HP, Stickland MH, Ossei-Gerning N, *et al.* Association of a common polymorphism in the factor XIII gene with myocardial infraction. *Thromb Haemost* 1998; **79**: 8–13.

47 McCormack LJ, Kain K, Catto AJ, *et al.* Prevalence of FXIII V34L in populations with different cardiovascular risk. *Thromb Haemost* 1998; **80**: 601–3.

48 Attie-Castro FA, Zago MA, Lavinha J, *et al.* Ethnic heterogeneity of the factor XIII Val34Leu polymorphism. *Thromb Haemost* 2000; **84**: 601–3.

49 Anwar R, Gallivan L, Edmonds SD, *et al.* Genotype/phenotype correlations for coagulation factor XIII: specific normal polymorphisms are associated with high or low factor XIII specific activity. *Blood* 1999; **93**: 897–905.

50 Wartiovaara U, Mikkola H, Szoke G, *et al.* Effect of Val34Leu polymorphism on the activation of the coagulation factor XIII-A. *Thromb Haemost* 2000; **84**: 595–600.

51 Ariens RAS, Philippou H, Nagaswami C, *et al.* The factor XIII V34L polymorphism accelerates thrombin activation of factor XIII and affects cross-linked fibrin structure. *Blood* 2000; **96**: 988–95.

52 Hancer VS, Diz-Kucukkaya R, Bilge AK, *et al.* The association between factor XIII Val34Leu polymorphism and early myocardial infarction. *Circ J* 2006; **70**: 239–42.

53 Wells PS, Anderson JL, Scarvelis DK, *et al.* Factor XIII Val34Leu variant is protective against venous thromboembolism: a HuGE review and meta-analysis. *Am J Epidemiol* 2006; **164**: 101–9.

54 Catto AJ, Kohler HP, Coore J, *et al.* Association of a common polymorphism in the factor XIII gene with venous thrombosis. *Blood* 1999; **93**: 906–8.

55 Franco RF, Reitsma PH, Lourenco D, *et al.* Factor XIII Val34Leu is a genetic factor involved in the etiology of venous thrombosis. *Thromb Haemost* 1999; **81**: 676–9.

56 Aleksic N, Ahn C, Wang YW, *et al.* Factor XIII Val34Leu polymorphism does not predict risk of coronary heart disease: The Atherosclerosis Risk in Communities (ARIC) study. *Arterioscler Thromb Vasc Biol* 2002; **22**: 348–52.

57 Balogh I, Szoke G, Karpati L, *et al.* Val34Leu polymorphism of plasma factor XIII: biochemistry and epidemiology in familial thrombophilia. *Blood* 2000; **96**: 2479–86.

58 Margaglione M, Bossone A, Brancaccio V, *et al.* Factor XIII Val-34Leu polymorphism and risk of deep vein thrombosis. *Thromb Haemost* 2000; **84**: 1118–19.

59 Reiner AP, Schwartz SM, Frank MB, *et al.* Polymorphisms of coagulation factor XIII subunit A and risk of nonfatal hemorrhagic stroke in young white women. *Stroke* 2001; **32**: 2580–6.

60 Peyvandi F, Palla R, Menegatti M, *et al.*, and the European Network of Rare Bleeding Disorders Group. Coagulation factor activity and clinical bleeding severity in rare bleeding disorders: results from the European Network of Rare Bleeding Disorders. *J Thromb Haemost* 2012; **10**: 615–21.

61 Kohler HP, Ichinose A, Seitz R, Ariens RA, Muszbek L, and the Factor XIII and Fibrinogen SSC Subcommittee of the ISTH. Diagnosis and classification of factor XIII deficiencies. *J Thromb Haemost* 2011; **9**: 1404–6.

62 Asahina T, Kobayashi T, Takeuchi K, *et al.* Congenital blood coagulation factor XIII deficiency and successful deliveries: a review of the literature. *Obstet Gynecol Surv* 2007; **62**: 255–60.

63 Ajjan RA, Standeven KF, Parapia LA, Naseem KM. Factor XIII supports platelet activation and enhances thrombus formation by matrix proteins underflow conditions. *J Thromb Haemost* 2011; **9**: 820–33.

64 Ding JL, Li P, Ho B. The Sushi peptides: structural characterization and mode of action against Gram-negative bacteria. *Cell Mol Life Sci* 2008; **65**: 1202–19.

65 Loof TG, Mörgelin M, Johansson L, *et al.* Coagulation, an ancestral serine protease cascade, exerts a novel function in early immune defense. *Blood* 2011; **118**: 2589–98.

66 Krarup A, Gulla KC, Gal P, Hajela K, Sim RB. The action of MBL-associated serine protease 1 (MASP1) on factor XIII and fibrinogen. *Biochim Biophys Acta* 2008; **1784**: 1294–300.

67 Gulla KC, Gupta K, Krarup A, Gal P, *et al.* Activation of mannan-binding lectin associated serine proteases leads to generation of a fibrin clot. *Immunology* 2010; **129**: 482–95.

68 Wang Z, Wilhelmsson C, Hyrsl P, *et al.* Pathogen entrapment by transglutaminase—a conserved early innate immune mechanism. *PLoS Path* 2010; **6**: e1000763.

69 Torocsik D, Szeles L, Paragh G Jr, *et al.* Factor XIII-A is involved in the regulation of gene expression in alternatively activated human macrophages. *Thromb Haemost* 2010; **104**: 709–17.

70 Sarvary A, Szucs S, Balogh I, *et al.* Possible role of factor XIII subunit A in Fc gamma and complement receptor-mediated phagocytosis. *Cell Immunol* 2004; **228**: 81–90.

71 Katona É, Pénzes K, Molnár É, Muszbek L. Measurement of factor XIII activity in plasma. *Clin Chem Lab Med* 2012; **50**: 1191–202.

72 Lawrie AS, Green L, Mackie IJ, Liesner R, Machin SJ, Peyvandi F. Factor XIII—an under diagnosed deficiency—are we using the right assays? *J Thromb Haemost* 2010; **8**: 2478–82.

73 Lusher J, Pipe SW, Alexander S, Nugent D. Prophylactic therapy with Fibrogammin P is associated with a decreased incidence of bleeding episodes: a retrospective study. *Haemophilia* 2010; **16**(2): 316–21.

74 Dreyfus M, Barrois D, Borg JY, *et al.* and the Groupe d'Etudes Francophone du FXIII. Successful long-term replacement therapy with FXIII concentrate (Fibrogammin(*) P) for severe congenital factor XIII deficiency: a prospective multicentre study. *J Thromb Haemost* 2011; **9**(6): 1264–6.

75 Nugent D. Corifact™/Fibrogammin® P in the prophylactic treatment of hereditary factor XIII deficiency: results of a prospective, multi-center, open-label study. *Thromb Res* 2012; **130**(Suppl. 2): S12–14.

76 Lovejoy AE, Reynolds TC, Visich JE, *et al.* Safety and pharmacokinetics of recombinant factor XIII-A2 administration in patients with congenital factor XIII deficiency. *Blood* 2006; **108**: 57–62.

77 Inbal A, Oldenburg J, Carcao M, Rosholm A, Tehranchi R, Nugent D. Recombinant factor XIII: a safe and novel treatment for congenital factor XIII deficiency. *Blood* 2012; **119**: 5111–17.

78 Kadir R, Chi C, Bolton-Maggs P. Pregnancy and rare bleeding disorders. *Haemophilia* 2009; **15**: 990–1005.

79 Naderi M, Eshghi P, Cohan N, Miri-Moghaddam E, Yaghmaee M, Karimi M. Successful delivery in patients with FXIII deficiency receiving prophylaxis: report of 17 cases in Iran. *Haemophilia* 2012; **18**: 773–6.

80 Peyvandi F, Bidlingmaier C, Garagiola I. Management of pregnancy and delivery in women with inherited bleeding disorders. *Semin Fetal Neonatal Med* 2011; **16**: 311–17.

81 Asahina T, Kobayshi T, Okada Y. Studies on the role of adhesive proteins in maintaining pregnancy. *Horm Res* 1998; **50**(Suppl. 2): 37–45.

82 Ichinose A, Asahina T, Kobayashi T. Congenital blood coagulation factor XIII deficiency and perinatal management. *Curr Drug Targets* 2005; **6**: 541–9.

83 Asahina T, Kobayashi T, Takeuchi K, *et al.* Congenital blood coagulation factor XIII deficiency and successful deliveries: a review of the literature. *Obstet Gynecol Surv* 2007; **62**: 255–60.

84 Ivaskevicius V, Seitz R, Kohler HP *et al.* and the Study Group. International registry on factor XIII deficiency: a basis formed mostly on European data. *Thromb Haemost* 2007; **97**: 914–21.

CHAPTER 60

Fibrinogen deficiency

Michael Laffan

Imperial College and Hammersmith Hospital, London, UK

Introduction

Fibrinogen is a soluble 340-kDa dimeric plasma glycoprotein. Its principal importance lies in its conversion into the insoluble fibrin clot by the action of thrombin. However, it also has important interactions with other adhesion molecules, platelets, endothelial cells, and cells involved in the inflammatory response. Where appropriate the nomenclature used here follows published guidelines [1].

Fibrinogen structure

Each half of the fibrinogen molecule is composed of three polypeptide chains designated Aα, Bβ, and γ. The properties of each chain are listed in Table 60.1. The aminoterminals of the three pairs of polypeptide chains are held together by disulfide bridges (two γ–γ and one α–α) to form the globular E region (Figure 60.1). All of the total 58 cysteine residues in each six-chained molecule are incorporated into 29 inter- and intrachain disulfide bridges. From the central E region, the two sets of three chains extend out in an antiparallel fashion in a coiled-coil to the D region which is comprised of the somewhat separate globular carboxytermini of the γ- and β-chains. From this region the α-chain extends back in a structure called the αC region with its carboxyterminus resting adjacent to the E region (Figure 60.1).

A variant γ-chain denoted γ' is produced by a variation in mRNA splicing which results in the replacement of aa residues 408–411 by a novel 20 aa residues terminating at residue 427. In the process, a platelet-binding site is lost and high-affinity binding sites for FXIII and thrombin gained. The γ' variant constitutes approximately 10% of plasma fibrinogen. A less common (<2%) α-chain variant "αE" is also produced by splice variation and has an additional 236 carboxyterminal amino acids.

Genetics and regulation of synthesis

The sequences of the three fibrinogen chains exhibit a high degree of homology suggesting that they have arisen by duplication events. This conclusion is supported by similarities in the intron-exon structure of the three genes fibrinogen A (*FGA*), *FGB*, and *FGG*, and their genomic position in a contiguous cluster on chromosome 4q31.3, with *FGB* in the opposite transcriptional orientation to *FGA* and *FGG*. Transcription of the three genes is highly coordinated, but at the protein level, production of Bβ-chain seems to be the limiting factor in humans. Studies from liver transplant patients indicate that the liver is the only major site of fibrinogen synthesis in humans, producing 1.7–5.0 g/day; sufficient to replace metabolized/utilized fibrinogen in the steady-state condition. The plasma half-life is 3–5 days. Synthesis of fibrinogen is upregulated by interleukin-6 (IL-6) as part of the acute phase reaction but IL-1β and transforming growth factor (TGF)-β have an opposing effect. Several polymorphisms of the fibrinogen genes have been described and most interest has focused on the −455G/A dimorphism in the *FGB* gene. This is estimated to account for 1–5% of the population variation in fibrinogen levels. The presence of the A allele was associated with a 0.15 g/L rise in fibrinogen level [2]. Other studies have only detected this effect in smokers or those with coronary artery disease, suggesting an environmentally influenced dynamic expression of the allele.

Plasma fibrinogen is a heterogeneous pool resulting from differential splicing of mRNA transcripts (Table 60.1) and from partial cleavage in plasma by thrombin and plasmin. Fibrinogen is also found in platelets but this is derived from α_{IIb}-β_3 (glycoprotein IIb-IIIa)-mediated endocytosis of plasma fibrinogen which is then stored in α-granules, rather than synthesis by megakaryocytes. Thus fibrinogen mRNA is not detected in megakaryocytes [3] and platelet fibrinogen is absent in severe forms of Glanzmann's thrombasthenia.

Textbook of Hemophilia, Third Edition. Edited by Christine A. Lee, Erik E. Berntorp and W. Keith Hoots.
© 2014 John Wiley & Sons, Ltd. Published 2014 by John Wiley & Sons, Ltd.

Table 60.1 Characteristics of the fibrinogen chains.

Chain	Aα	Bβ	γ
aa residues	610	461	411
Molecular weight	66500	52000	46500
Variants (% total)	AαE +296aa (2%)	–	γ′+408–427 (10%)
Thrombin cleavage	R16-17G	R14-15G	–
Cys residues	8	11	10
Factor XIII cross-link residues	Gln: 221,237,328,366	none	Gln: 398,399
(Gln acceptor, Lys donor)	Lys:208, 219, 224, 418, 427, 429, 446, 448, 508, 539, 556, 580, 583, 601, 606.		Lys: 406
Glycosylation sites	(αE) Asn 667	Asn 364	Asn 52
$\alpha_{IIb}\beta_3$ binding RGDF motif	95–98	–	–
$\alpha_{IIb}\beta_3$ binding RGDS motif	572–575	–	–
$\alpha_{IIb}\beta_3$ binding dodecapeptide	–	–	400–411
$\alpha_{IIb}\beta_3$ and $\alpha_5\beta_1$ binding site	–	–	370–383
$\alpha_v\beta_3$ on endothelial cells	–	–	346–358

RGDF, arginine-glycine-aspartic acid-phenylalanine; RGDS, arginine-glycine-aspartic acid-serine.

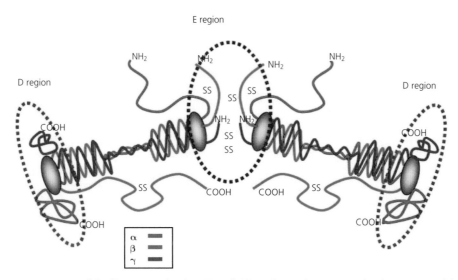

Figure 60.1 A schematic representation of the fibrinogen molecule. NH2 and COOH denote the amino- and carboxytermini of the α-chain (red), β-chain (green), and γ-chain (blue) respectively. The free carboxyterminal of the α-chain is referred to as Cα. The variant γ′-chain extends from the carboxyterminus of the γ-chain (not shown). SS identifies disulfide bonds. The E region is located in the central region of the molecule and is roughly composed of amino acids 1–49 of the α-chain, 1–80 of the β-chain, and 1–23 of the γ-chain. The E region is flanked by two D regions roughly composed of amino acids 111–197 of the α-chain, 134–461 of the β-chain, and 88–406 of the γ-chain. From [44]. Reproduced with permission of John Wiley and Sons. (See also Plate 60.1.)

Fibrin clot formation

Conversion of fibrinogen into the insoluble fibrin clot can be considered to take place in three stages as follows:

1 Thrombin cleavage of fibrinopeptides A and B.
2 Assembly of insoluble fibrin monomers into protofibrils and fibers.
3 Cross-linking by FXIII.

The initiating event in fibrin formation is the cleavage of the Aα Arg16-Gly17 bond by thrombin, releasing fibrinopeptide A (FpA) from desA fibrin. This exposes an "A" site (knob) in the E region which can then bind to a pre-existing "a" site (hole) on the γ-chain of another molecule's D region. Thus begins a staggered assembly of half overlapping fibrin monomers which extends to form a double-stranded protofibril (Figure 60.2). At this stage, FXIII activation by thrombin has already occurred and cross-linking has begun.

Cleavage of Fibrinopeptide B (FpB) follows that of FpA; however, this sequential release of FpA and then FpB reflects the differing affinity of thrombin for these two substrates rather than a change in conformation after FpA release. Fibrin polymerization facilitates FpB cleavage but it remains incomplete with only 33% of the potential FpB being released. FpB release exposes a "B" site in the E region which binds to a

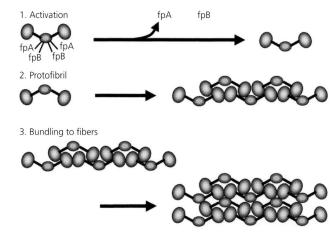

1. Activation   fpA   fpB

fpA   fpA
fpB   fpB

2. Protofibril

3. Bundling to fibers

Figure 60.2 A schematic representation of the conversion of fibrinogen to a fibrin clot by thrombin. Thrombin cleavage of fibrinopeptide A (amino acids 1–16 of the α-chain) followed by cleavage of fibrinopeptide B (amino acids 1–14 of the β-chain) leads to formation of fibrin monomers. Fibrin monomers then self-assemble in a half-staggered linear overlap to form protofibrils. Protofibril formation is governed by the interaction of the thrombin exposed "a" site on the E region with "A" site on the D region. The protofibrils are then bundled into fibrin fibers through interaction of the "b" site on the E region with the "B" site located on the D region. From [44]. Reproduced with permission of John Wiley and Sons. (See also Plate 60.2.)

corresponding "b" hole on the carboxyterminus of a β-chain in an adjacent molecule. This facilitates lateral assembly of thick fibers. FpB cleavage also releases the Cα region from its non-covalent association with the E region freeing it to participate in lateral interactions with other Cα regions [4]. Nonetheless, FpA release appears sufficient for the entire process of clot formation; although it is enhanced by FpB removal and mutations of the FpB cleavage site result in prolonged clotting times and reduced functional fibrinogen assay results. FpB cleavage alone (e.g. by Venzyme [5]) is not sufficient to induce fibrin clot formation under normal conditions.

Lateral association of fibrils leads to formation of thick fiber bundles. Convergence of two or three double-stranded fibrils results in tetra- and trimolecular branch points, effectively joining the nascent fibers and producing a complex three-dimensional network [6].

Formation of fibrin also accelerates the formation of activated FXIII. In plasma, fibrinogen functions as a carrier protein for the A2B2 FXIII tetramer which appears to bind specifically to the γ'-chains. Fibrin polymer formation accelerates FXIII cleavage but the A-chain is not active until the activation peptide has been released and it has dissociated from the B-chain. One or both of these dissociation events are facilitated by binding of activated FXIII to the γ' region of fibrin. The active A-chain released then binds to fibrin in the Aα 242–424 region and leaves behind a vacant thrombin-binding site. Thus fibrin formed from γ' containing fibrinogen is more extensively cross-linked and higher γ' levels are a risk factor for coronary heart

disease [7]. Platelet FXIII comprises the A-chains only and is not dependent on fibrin for activation.

Factor XIII-mediated cross-linking begins by joining D regions in an end-to-end or longitudinal fashion via reciprocal γGln398-γLys406 links. Side-to-side links between γ-chains then follow. Cross-linking between α-chains occurs more slowly but at multiple sites (Table 60.1). "α"-chain cross-linking is important in blocking plasmin access to the coiled-coil regions linking D and E regions and thus preventing break down of the fibrin clot. Finally, some cross-linking between α- and γ-chains takes place.

At the same time fibrin formation exposes binding sites for tissue plasminogen activator (tPA) and plasminogen. High-affinity sites for both tPA and plasminogen are exposed in the Aα392–610 segment (Cα) and lower affinity sites on Aα 148–160 and γ 312–324 (D region). Adjacent binding of tPa and plasminogen greatly reduces the Km and increases the V_{max} for the activation reaction [8]. The plasmin thus activated then cleaves fibrin, exposing further carboxyterminal lysine residues of Cα, allowing more plasminogen and tPA to bind, accelerating and targeting the fibrinolytic system. This process is now known to be in competition with the activity of TAFI (thrombin activatable fibrinolysis inhibitor) which selectively removes these lysine residues and thus limits fibrinolysis. FXIII also cross-links antiplasmin to Lys303 in the α-chain whilst retaining its antiplasmin activity. It has recently been shown that this occurs extensively in plasma so that approximately 1.2–1.8 mol of antiplasmin are bound per mole of fibrinogen [9]. Recent work has shown that cross-linking of antiplasmin to fibrin is more important than fibrin–fibrin cross-linking in conferring resistance to fibrinolysis [10].

Fibrinogen interaction with other cells

In addition to its self-associating properties, fibrin also has other important interactions. At least four integrin-binding motifs have been identified in fibrinogen not all of which contain the classic RGD (arginine-glycine-aspartic acid) sequence (Table 60.1). The γ-terminal sequence is involved in platelet adherence and aggregation whereas the two α-chain RGD sequences are important in promoting clot retraction [11]. These sequences mediate binding to platelet $α_{IIb}β_3$ to effect platelet retraction but also to leukocyte $α_Mβ_2$ and to endothelial cell $α_Vβ_3$. Mice with fibrinogen lacking the terminal γ-chain sequence had a severe bleeding tendency [11]. Fibrinogen binding to endothelial cell integrins is mediated by the Aα RGD sequence at 572–574 [12] and by the γchain 346–358 [13]. However, fibrin-specific binding to endothelial cells is mediated by the β15–42 region exposed by thrombin cleavage. Fibrin or fibrin peptide interaction with endothelial cells results in numerous changes including release of Weibel–Palade bodies, prostacyclin and tPA release and monolayer disruption. Finally, fibrinogen is important in mediating adherence and migration of activated monocytes and neutrophils through endothelium.

Fibrinogen is also able to bind several cytokines, in particular vascular endothelial growth factor, fibroblast growth factor (FGF)-2, and IL-1β. This is postulated to concentrate the factors at the site of vascular injury and promote wound healing. Loss of this function may contribute to the phenotype seen in afibrinogenemic mice and humans [14].

Measuring fibrinogen

An international standard for fibrinogen assays has been prepared [15]. The normal plasma concentration of fibrinogen is approximately 1.7–4.0 g/L when measured by clotting assays and slightly higher (2.5–6.0 g/L) by immunoassay. The ability to detect abnormalities of fibrinogen depends critically on the assay methods used and guidelines for fibrinogen assays have been published in the UK [16]. A deficiency or abnormality of fibrinogen may be first suspected from prolongation of clotting times. In afibrinogenemia all the clotting times will be prolonged but in less marked deficiency or the presence of a dysfibrinogenemia, it may only be the thrombin time which is prolonged.

Although the international reference method for fibrinogen measurement has traditionally been by the total clottable fibrinogen method, this is not practical for routine laboratory use. In hospital practice, fibrinogen is usually assayed by a functional (clotting) assay; either that of Clauss or estimated from plasma turbidity in the prothrombin time (derived fibrinogen: PT-Fg). In the Clauss assay, a high concentration of thrombin is used to clot a diluted aliquot of patient plasma. Typically, one volume of a 100 NIH u/mL thrombin solution is added to two volumes of plasma to give a final concentration of approximately 33 NIH u/mL. The clotting time is then compared with a standard curve prepared using dilutions of a reference plasma. When automated, the assay is quite reproducible (CV 3–9%) and the combination of dilution and high thrombin concentration makes it relatively insensitive to the effect of heparin. It is, however, sensitive to high concentrations of fibrin(ogen) degradation products and some kits contain agents to overcome these effects. The PT-Fg can give misleading results and is not recommended. Fibrinogen can also be assayed using immunologic techniques, but this requires the use of monoclonal antibodies to avoid interference from degraded and partially degraded fibrinogen fragments. The performance of different fibrinogen assays has been reviewed [17].

When a low fibrinogen is determined by clotting assay then the presence of a dys- or hypofibrinogen can be resolved by performing a physicochemical or immunologic assay. In practice, a simple (gravimetric) clot weight determination is usually sufficient to demonstrate the discrepancy between function and protein characteristic of a dysfibrinogenemia.

Table 60.2 Relative frequency of bleeding symptoms in 55 patients with afibrinogenemia compared with 100 patients with severe hemophilia A (factor VIII 1%). From [18]. Reproduced with permission of John Wiley and Sons.

Symptom	In afibrinogenemia	In hemophilia A
Umbilical cord bleeding	45/55 (85%)	0
Central nervous system bleeding	3/55 (10%)	4/100 (4%)
Hemarthrosis	30/55 (54%)	86/100 (86%)
Muscle hematoma	40/55 (72%)	93/100 (93%)
Gastrointestinal bleeding	0	10/100 (10%)
Urinary tract bleeding	0	12/100 (12%)
Epistaxis	40/55 (72%)	50/100 (50%)
Menorrhagia	14/20 (70%)	Not applicable
Oral cavity bleeding	40/55 (72%)	55/100 (55%)
Postoperative bleeding	23/55 (40%)	36/100 (36%)
Thrombotic symptoms	2/55 (4%)	0

Afibrinogenemia

The complete absence of fibrinogen, *afibrinogenemia*, is accompanied by a clinical syndrome that is surprisingly mild and generally less severe than hemophilia (Table 60.2) [18]. An early and characteristic feature is umbilical cord bleeding: present in 85% of cases [18]. Thereafter muscle bleeds and hemarthroses are relatively frequent but rarely result in disability. Unlike hemophilia, epistaxis is also common (72%) and spontaneous splenic rupture is reported. Bleeding is sometimes followed by poor wound healing [18]. In mice rendered afibrinogenemic by disruption of the *FGA* gene, all three chains are absent from plasma and a similar phenotype is seen: bleeding begins shortly after birth in approximately 30% but is not usually severe and the mice survive into maturity [19]. The European Network of Rare Bleeding Disorders found that grade III bleeding (i.e. spontaneous major bleeding) was present in patients whose fibrinogen level was undetectable and that a level of 1 g/L was required to remain asymptomatic. [20].

In affected women, menorrhagia is common and recurrent early abortion is seen, presumed to reflect poor implantation as also observed in the fibrinogen-deficient mice. Afibrinogenemic mice are still capable of developing atheromatous plaques although murine plaques are not as complex as those in humans.

Remarkably, spontaneous thrombosis (venous and arterial) has been reported in patients with afibrinogenemia. A plausible explanation is that an increase in free thrombin results from the loss of the thrombin-binding capacity of fibrin and that this results in excessive platelet activation.

Genetics and molecular biology

Inheritance of afibrinogenemia is autosomal recessive and the disorder is thus more common in populations favoring consanguineous marriages. The estimated frequency in Europe is $1/10^6$. Obligate heterozygotes have plasma fibrinogen levels of approximately half normal but are asymptomatic. The majority of cases appear to arise from mutations in the *FGA* gene; in particular a recurrent 11 kb deletion probably results from a nonhomologous recombination mediated by 7-bp direct repeats. Haplotype analysis suggests that the mutation has arisen independently on several occasions. Indeed the majority of null mutations are in the *FGA* gene and the most common recurrent mutation occurs at the donor splice site of *FGA* intron 4 [21]. A number of other truncating mutations in *FGA* as well as *FGB* and *FGG* are also described (reviewed in [22]). Failure to produce any of the individual peptide chains results in a virtually complete absence of the mature protein. A small number of missense mutations also cause afibrinogenemia as a result of intracellular retention of the abnormal protein.

Therapy

Guidelines for treatment and literature reviews have been published [23,24] based largely on case reports and small case series. The basis of therapy is replacement of fibrinogen. Historically, the principal source of fibrinogen has been cryoprecipitate which contains approximately 1.5 g fibrinogen per unit. Plasma-derived virally inactivated concentrates are now available and are the recommended choice but are not uniformly licenced. When concentrate is not available, UK-BCSH (British Committee for Standards in Haematology) guidelines recommend virally inactivated plasma over cryoprecipitate if volume is not a limiting factor [25]. Methylene blue treatment of plasma is reported to result in a 40% loss of fibrinogen but fibrinogen content of solvent/detergent-treated plasma is normal. The half-life of infused fibrinogen concentrate was similar in two studies at approximately 3–5 days. However, the recovery showed considerable variation: in the study by Negrier *et al.*, a dose of 0.06 g/kg produced a rise of 1.39 g/L; whereas the data from Kreuz *et al.* suggest a similar dose would produce a rise of 0.84 g/L [26,27].

A level of 1 g/L is regarded as sufficiently hemostatic to arrest bleeding (20–40 mg/kg of fibrinogen concentrate) [23]. Bleeding problems may be sufficient to warrant prophylactic treatment and the long half-life of fibrinogen allows prophylactic infusions of fibrinogen concentrate or cryoprecipitate to be given weekly. In one report, a dose of 100 mg/kg/week was sufficient to maintain a trough level of 0.5 g/L which prevented recurrence of hemorrhage [28]. A trough level of 0.5 g/L is recommended for primary prophylaxis [23]; however, in this context, even lower levels may be effective in preventing bleeding and 2–4 weekly infusions have been reported as successful [29]. A survey of hematologists reported a considerable diversity of practise: prophylactic doses ranged from 18 to 120 mg/kg (median 53 mg/kg) and most patients (59%) were treated weekly (remainder 2–4 weekly). However, the survey also revealed that prophylaxis completely prevented bleeds in only nine of 19 patients [30]. Replacement therapy is not usually complicated by the development of antifibrinogen antibodies but these have been reported [31]. Menorrhagia may be controlled by use of the combined oral contraceptive pill and adjunctive therapy with tranexamic acid has also been suggested.

Prophylactic therapy appears necessary for successful completion of pregnancy: fibrinogen replacement must be begun before 5 weeks gestation to prevent abortion and maintained at >1.0 g/L throughout the pregnancy. Fibrinogen consumption increases markedly as gestation progresses and the amount and frequency of fibrinogen infusion must be increased accordingly [32]. A level of >1.5 g/L is recommended for delivery [33].

Hypofibrinogenemia may be used to describe patients with incomplete deficiency of fibrinogen and a corresponding intermediate phenotype. Some of these will be heterozygotes for null mutations and are generally asymptomatic.

Dysfibrinogenemia

Dysfibrinogens are usually inherited in an autosomal dominant fashion but a few cases are found as recessives with asymptomatic heterozygotes. Dysfibrinogen generally arises from missense mutations in any of the three *FG* genes, but small deletions or insertions may also be responsible and the clinical phenotype is correspondingly diverse. A database of mutations responsible is available at http://www.geht.org/databaseang/fibrinogen/. The diagnosis is suspected from prolonged coagulation times, especially the thrombin time, with low fibrinogen by functional assay. Prolongation of the Reptilase time may also be useful. Determination of a discrepantly high fibrinogen protein concentration confirms the presence of a dysfibrinogen. Rare examples where the clotting times are shortened or where the functional and immunologic assays are concordant have been described.

The majority of dysfibrinogens are found incidentally and have no associated phenotype [34] (55%), whereas 20% are associated with thrombosis and 25% with hemorrhage. A few cases have been reported with both hemorrhagic and thrombotic problems (e.g. Marburg, Bethesda III, and Baltimore I). It is not possible to predict the phenotype from the standard laboratory tests and so sequencing of the gene has been recommended to allow comparison with other published cases.

Dysfibrinogens associated with thrombosis

Although usually detected as a result of a prolonged thrombin clotting time, a dysfibrinogen is reported in approximately 0.8% of patients with thrombosis: rarer than the anticoagulant deficiencies but unlike them associated with both venous and arterial events, although venous are more common. The rarity of each individual dysfibrinogen makes it difficult to be certain there is a causal relationship underlying the association but a survey conducted by the International Society on Thrombosis and Haemostasis (ISTH) in 1995 [35] concluded it was genuine: an increased incidence of thrombosis was found in affected relatives of the dysfibrinogenemia proband but not in the 88 unaffected relatives. As with other thrombophilic traits, women affected with dysfibrinogenemia appear to suffer an increased rate of pregnancy complications [35]. It is postulated that dysfibrinogens may increase the risk of thrombosis either by producing clots that are more resistant to fibrinolysis or by failing to sequester normal amounts of thrombin resulting in increased amounts of the free enzyme. Several mutations at or close to the thrombin cleavage sites have been reported in association with thrombosis (i.e. Marburg, Malmo, New York, and Naples), presumably via the latter mechanism [36]. The best described association with thrombosis is that of fibrinogen Dusart Arg554Cys (also called Paris V and Chapel Hill III) as it has occurred several times [37]. The new Cys residue crosslinks with albumin resulting in formation of thin but plasmin-resistant fibrin fibers [38]. Similar phenomena have been reported in other dysfibrinogens with free thiol groups. In one case, that of fibrinogen Oslo I [39], the dysfibrinogen was associated with thrombosis, shortened clotting times and enhancing platelet activation. Morris *et al.* reported a surprisingly high incidence of dysfibrinogenemia in patients with chronic thromboembolic pulmonary hypertension and showed that they all conferred resistance to fibrinolysis [40].

Dysfibrinogens associated with bleeding

Some dysfibrinogens, particularly those with fibrinogen levels <1 g/L are associated with an increased frequency of bleeding. The mechanisms are diverse, for example fibrinogen Bremen (Gly17Val), results in delayed polymerization and symptomatic bleeding as a result of impaired interaction of the "A" and "a" sites [41]. Many other examples can be found in the database. The symptoms are usually mild and may be associated with wound dehiscence. For those patients with a history of bleeding associated with a dysfibrinogen or hypofibrinogen, tranexamic acid or replacement therapy may be needed as for afibrinogenemia.

Other syndromes associated with dysfibrinogens

Several mutations in the Aa-chain gene have been found to cause hereditary renal amyloidosis (R554L, E526V and 4904delG and 4897delT which both lead to premature termination at codon 548). The fibrinogen behaves normally from a coagulation point of view and cannot be detected by this means. The role of fibrinogen was originally revealed by sequence analysis of the amyloid deposits [42]. Some dysfibrinogens result in misfolded chains which are retained in the endoplasmic reticulum resulting in hepatic storage disease [43].

Acquired dysfibrinogenemia

An acquired abnormality of fibrinogen typically arises in association with liver disease, especially hepatocellular carcinoma, due to an increased number of sialic acid residues. The thrombin time is prolonged but the Clauss fibrinogen assay is normal or more frequently elevated. This is not associated with any bleeding tendency and can be ignored. A similar abnormality of fibrinogen is seen in neonates reflecting hepatic immaturity. Occasionally, laboratory results simulating the presence of a dysfibrinogenemia may be produced by a paraprotein or autoantibody interfering with fibrin polymerization. Although the fibrinogen may in fact be normal, this can nonetheless result in a hemorrhagic tendency.

References

1 Medved L, Weisel JW. Fibrinogen, factor XSoSSCoISoT, haemostasis. Recommendations for nomenclature on fibrinogen and fibrin. *J Thromb Haemost* 2009; **7**: 355–9.

2 Tybjaerg-Hansen A, Agerholm-Larsen B, Humphries SE, Abildgaard S, Schnohr P, Nordestgaard BG. A common mutation (G-455-> A) in the beta-fibrinogen promoter is an independent predictor of plasma fibrinogen, but not of ischemic heart disease. A study of 9,127 individuals based on the Copenhagen City Heart Study. *J Clin Invest* 1997; **99**: 3034–9.

3 Rox JM, Muller J, Potzsch B. Absence of fibrinogen alpha-, beta- and gamma-chain mRNA in human platelets. *Br J Haematol* 2005; **130**: 647–8.

4 Gorkun OV, Veklich YI, Medved LV, Henschen AH, Weisel JW. Role of the alpha C domains of fibrin in clot formation. *Biochemistry* 1994; **33**: 6986–97.

5 Shainoff JR, Dardik BN. Fibrinopeptide B in fibrin assembly and metabolism: physiologic significance in delayed release of the peptide. *Ann NY Acad Sci* 1983; **408**: 254–68.

6 Mosesson MW. Fibrinogen and fibrin polymerization: appraisal of the binding events that accompany fibrin generation and fibrin clot assembly. *Blood Coag Fibrinol* 1997; **8**: 257–67.

7 Lovely RS, Falls LA, Al-Mondhiry HA, *et al.* Association of gammaA/gamma' fibrinogen levels and coronary artery disease. *Thromb Haemost* 2002; **88**: 26–31.

8 Medved L, Nieuwenhuizen W. Molecular mechanisms of initiation of fibrinolysis by fibrin. *Thromb Haemost* 2003; **89**: 409–19.

9 Mosesson MW, Siebenlist KR, Hernandez I, Lee KN, Christiansen VJ, McKee PA. Evidence that alpha2-antiplasmin becomes covalently ligated to plasma fibrinogen in the circulation: a new role for plasma factor XIII in fibrinolysis regulation. *J Thromb Haemost* 2008; **6**: 1565–70.

10 Fraser SR, Booth NA, Mutch NJ. The antifibrinolytic function of factor XIII is exclusively expressed through alpha2-antiplasmin cross-linking. *Blood* 2011; **117**: 6371–4.

11 Holmback K, Danton MJ, Suh TT, Daugherty CC, Degen JL. Impaired platelet aggregation and sustained bleeding in mice lacking the fibrinogen motif bound by integrin alpha IIb beta 3. *EMBO J.* 1996; **15**: 5760–71.

12 Suehiro K, Gailit J, Plow EF. Fibrinogen is a ligand for integrin alpha5beta1 on endothelial cells. *J Biol Chem* 1997; **272**: 5360–6.

13 Yokoyama K, Erickson HP, Ikeda Y, Takada Y. Identification of amino acid sequences in fibrinogen gamma -chain and tenascin C C-terminal domains critical for binding to integrin alpha vbeta 3. *J Biol Chem* 2000; **275**: 16891–8.

14 Peng H, Sahni A, Fay P, *et al.* Identification of a binding site on human FGF-2 for fibrinogen. *Blood* 2004; **103**: 2114–20.

15 Whitton CM, Sands D, Hubbard AR, Gaffney PJ. A collaborative study to establish the 2nd International Standard for Fibrinogen, Plasma. *Thromb Haemost* 2000; **84**: 258–62.

16 Mackie IJ, Kitchen S, Machin SJ, Lowe GD. Haemostasis, Thrombosis Task Force of the British Committee for Standards in Haemostasis Guidelines on fibrinogen assays. *Br J Haematol* 2003; **121**: 396–404.

17 Mackie J, Lawrie AS, Kitchen S, *et al.* A performance evaluation of commercial fibrinogen reference preparations and assays for Clauss and PT-derived fibrinogen. *Thromb Haemost* 2002; **87**: 997–1005.

18 Lak M, Keihani M, Elahi F, Peyvandi F, Mannucci PM. Bleeding and thrombosis in 55 patients with inherited afibrinogenaemia. *Br J Haematol* 1999; **107**: 204–6.

19 Suh TT, Holmback K, Jensen NJ, *et al.* Resolution of spontaneous bleeding events but failure of pregnancy in fibrinogen-deficient mice. *Genes Devel* 1995; **9**: 2020–33.

20 Peyvandi F, Palla R, Menegatti M, *et al.* Coagulation factor activity and clinical bleeding severity in rare bleeding disorders: results from the European Network of Rare Bleeding Disorders. *J Thromb Haemost* 2012; **10**: 615–21.

21 Neerman-Arbez M. The molecular basis of inherited afibrinogenaemia. *Thromb Haemost* 2001; **86**: 154–63.

22 Vu D, Neerman-Arbez M. Molecular mechanisms accounting for fibrinogen deficiency: from large deletions to intracellular retention of misfolded proteins. *J Thromb Haemost* 2007; **5**(Suppl. 1): 125–31.

23 Bolton-Maggs PHB, Perry DJ, Chalmers EA, *et al.* The rare coagulation disorders–review with guidelines for management from the United Kingdom Haemophilia Centre Doctors' Organisation. *Haemophilia* 2004; **10**: 593–628.

24 Bornikova L, Peyvandi F, Allen G, Bernstein J, Manco-Johnson MJ. Fibrinogen replacement therapy for congenital fibrinogen deficiency. *J Thromb Haemost* 2011; **9**: 1687–704.

25 Keeling D, Tait C, Makris M. Guideline on the selection and use of therapeutic products to treat haemophilia and other hereditary bleeding disorders. A United Kingdom Haemophilia Center Doctors' Organisation (UKHCDO) guideline approved by the British Committee for Standards in Haematology. *Haemophilia* 2008; **14**: 671–84.

26 Kreuz W, Meili E, Peter-Salonen K, *et al.* Pharmacokinetic properties of a pasteurised fibrinogen concentrate. *Transfus Apheresis Sci* 2005; **32**: 239–46.

27 Negrier C, Rothschild C, Goudemand J, *et al.* Pharmacokinetics and pharmacodynamics of a new highly secured fibrinogen concentrate. *J Thromb Haemost* 2008; **6**: 1494–9.

28 Parameswaran R, Dickinson JP, de Lord S, Keeling DM, Colvin BT. Spontaneous intracranial bleeding in two patients with congenital afibrinogenaemia and the role of replacement therapy. *Haemophilia* 2000; **6**: 705–8.

29 Neerman-Arbez M, Honsberger A, Antonarakis SE, Morris MA. Deletion of the fibrinogen [correction of fibrogen] alpha-chain gene (FGA) causes congenital afibrogenemia. [Erratum: *J Clin Invest* 1999; **103**(5): 759]. *J Clin Invest* 1999; **103**: 215–18.

30 Peyvandi F, Haertel S, Knaub S, Mannucci PM. Incidence of bleeding symptoms in 100 patients with inherited afibrinogenemia or hypofibrinogenemia. *J Thromb Haemost* 2006; **4**: 1634–7.

31 Ra'anani P, Levi Y, Varon D, Gitel S, Martinowitz U. Congenital afibrinogenemia with bleeding, bone cysts and antibodies to fibrinogen. *Harefuah* 1991; **121**: 291–3.

32 Mensah PK, Oppenheimer C, Watson C, Pavord S. Congenital afibrinogenaemia in pregnancy. *Haemophilia* 2011; **17**: 167–8.

33 Kobayashi T, Kanayama N, Tokunaga N, Asahina T, Terao T. Prenatal and peripartum management of congenital afibrinogenaemia. *Br J Haematol* 2000; **109**: 364–6.

34 Shapiro SE, Phillips E, Manning RA, *et al.* Clinical phenotype, laboratory features and genotype of 35 patients with heritable dysfibrinogenaemia. *Br J Haematol* 2012; **15**: 12085.

35 Haverkate F, Samama M. Familial dysfibrinogenemia and thrombophilia. Report on a study of the SSC Subcommittee on Fibrinogen. *Thromb Haemost* 1995; **73**: 151–61.

36 Koopman J, Haverkate F, Lord ST, Grimbergen J, Mannucci PM. Molecular basis of fibrinogen Naples associated with defective thrombin binding and thrombophilia. Homozygous substitution of B beta 68 Ala-Thr. *J Clin Invest* 1992; **90**: 238–44.

37 Wada Y, Lord ST. A correlation between thrombotic disease and a specific fibrinogen abnormality (A alpha 554 Arg ->Cys) in two unrelated kindred, Dusart and Chapel Hill III. *Blood* 1994; **84**: 3709–14.

38 Koopman J, Haverkate F, Grimbergen J, *et al.* Molecular basis for fibrinogen Dusart (A alpha 554 Arg-->Cys) and its association with abnormal fibrin polymerization and thrombophilia. *J Clin Invest* 1993; **91**: 1637–43.

39 Egeberg O. Inherited fibrinogen abnormality causing thrombophilia. *Thromb Diathes Haemorrhag* 1967; **17**: 176–87.

40 Morris TA, Marsh JJ, Chiles PG, *et al.* High prevalence of dysfibrinogenemia among patients with chronic thromboembolic pulmonary hypertension. *Blood* 2009; **114**: 1929–36.

41 Wada Y, Niwa K, Maekawa H, *et al.* A new type of congenital dysfibrinogen, fibrinogen Bremen, with an A alpha Gly-17 to Val substitution associated with hemorrhagic diathesis and delayed wound healing. *Thromb Haemost* 1993; **70**: 397–403.

42 Hamidi Asl L, Liepnieks JJ, Uemichi T, *et al.* Renal amyloidosis with a frame shift mutation in fibrinogen aalpha-chain gene producing a novel amyloid protein. *Blood* 1997; **90**: 4799–805.

43 Brennan SO, Davis RL, Conard K, Savo A, Furuya KN. Novel fibrinogen mutation gamma314Thr->Pro (fibrinogen AI duPont) associated with hepatic fibrinogen storage disease and hypofibrinogenaemia. *Liver Int* 2010; **30**: 1541–7.

44 Roberts HR, Stinchcombe TE, Gabriel DA. The dysfibrinogenaemias. *Br J Haematol* 2001; **114**: 249–57.

CHAPTER 61

Miscellaneous rare bleeding disorders

Frederico Xavier and Amy D. Shapiro
Indiana Hemophilia and Thrombosis Center, Indiana, USA

Introduction

The primary function of the coagulation system is to maintain hemostasis, prevent uncontrolled clot propagation, and assist in the restoration of normal vascular architecture. Hemostasis involves a series of complex physiologic processes related to prevention of blood loss and the maintenance of both vascular integrity and blood fluidity. Upon vascular injury, coagulation is activated through a cascade of proteolytic reactions culminating in the generation of thrombin (factor IIa) and fibrin mesh (clot) formation (Figure 61.1). Finely orchestrated interactions between the vascular endothelium, platelets/von Willebrand factor, and procoagulant proteins are crucial to the formation of a clot at the site of vessel wall injury. Coagulation is downregulated through naturally occurring anticoagulants and normal architecture is restored through the fibrinolytic system; natural anticoagulants control thrombin generation by direct inhibition or inactivation of procoagulants while the fibrinolytic system restores normal architecture through gradual clot dissolution after appropriate healing has occurred. Thus, qualitative and quantitative defects of platelets, vessel wall, coagulation and fibrinolytic systems may result in a bleeding diathesis. Bleeding disorders owing to congenital deficiencies of coagulation proteins including factors V, VII, VIII, combined V and VIII, IX, X, XI, and XIII, and prothrombin, fibrinogen, and von Willebrand factor are discussed in other chapters.

This chapter will briefly review the fibrinolytic system and bleeding diathesis associated with congenital deficiencies of plasminogen activator inhibitor 1 (PAI-1), α2-plasmin inhibitor, and familial deficiency of vitamin K-dependent clotting factors (VKCFD).

Overview of fibrinolytic system

The fibrinolytic system is complex and regulates hemostasis thorough clot lysis and degradation of extracellular matrix [1].

This system contains a pivotal inactive proenzyme, plasminogen, that is converted into an active enzyme, plasmin, to degrade fibrin into soluble degradation products (Figure 61.1) [2]. Dissolution of fibrin is integral to wound healing and to maintain and restore vascular integrity.

Plasminogen is converted into plasmin by two immunologically distinct physiologic plasminogen activators (serine proteases): tissue-type plasminogen activator (t-PA) and urokinase-type plasminogen activator (uPA). Inhibition of fibrinolysis occurs at the levels of plasminogen activators by serine protease inhibitors (serpines), via specific plasminogen activator inhibitors (PAI-1 and PAI-2) and at the level of plasmin, mainly through α2-antiplasmin (α2-AP; Figure 61.1). Tissue-type plasminogen activator-mediated plasminogen activation is primary to the dissolution of fibrin in the circulation while uPA binds to a specific cellular receptor (uPAR) resulting in enhanced activation of cell-bound plasminogen. In normal plasma, tPA activity is extremely low and the majority of tPA is in complex with PAI-l. Regulation and control of the fibrinolytic system is mediated through synthetic control and release of plasminogen activators and plasminogen activator inhibitors, primarily from endothelial cells. Hyperfibrinolysis, owing to excessive synthesis or insufficient downregulation of plasmin, is associated with a bleeding diathesis. To date, deficiencies of two fibrinolytic proteins, PAI-1 and α2-AP, have been documented to be associated with a congenital bleeding diathesis.

Congenital plasminogen activator inhibitor 1 deficiency

Role of plasminogen activator inhibitor 1 in fibrinolysis

This is a single-chain glycoprotein with a molecular weight of approximately 50 kDa consisting of 379 amino acids preceded by a signal peptide of 23 amino acids. PAI-1 controls the proteolytic action of plasmin through inhibition of plasminogen

Textbook of Hemophilia, Third Edition. Edited by Christine A. Lee, Erik E. Berntorp and W. Keith Hoots.
© 2014 John Wiley & Sons, Ltd. Published 2014 by John Wiley & Sons, Ltd.

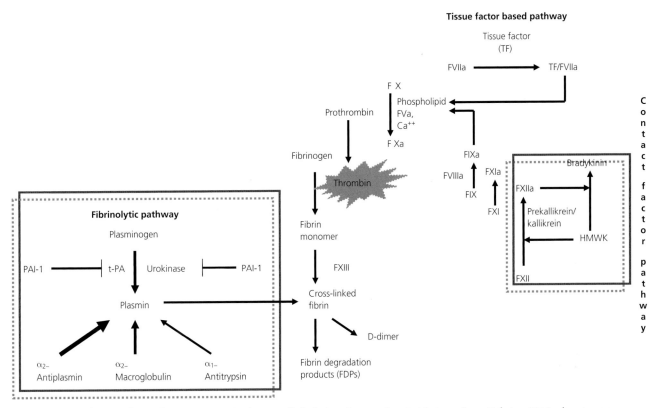

Figure 61.1 Coagulation pathways depicting interaction between fibrinolytic pathway and contact factor pathway. F, factor; PAI-1, plasminogen activator inhibitor 1; t-PA, tissue plasminogen activator.

activators, tPA and uPA. The *PAI-1* gene has been mapped at 7q22.1 locus (OMIM #173360) and consists of nine exons and eight introns distributed over 12.2 kb of DNA [3]. Its expression is induced by insulin, transforming growth factor beta, and endotoxin. PAI-1 is synthesized and secreted from endothelial cells, megakaryocytes, hepatocytes, and adipocytes [4]. Platelet PAI-1 is present in α-granules, mostly in an inactive form [5]. In healthy individuals, there exist highly variable plasma antigenic levels of PAI-1 ranging from 6 to 85 ng/mL (geometric mean, 24 ng/mL) [6]. PAI-1 exhibits a circadian variability with a peak plasma concentration in the morning and troughs achieved in the late afternoon and evening [7]. This variability may be regulated through proteins CLOCK:ARNTL1 and CLOCK:ARNTL2 which bind to the *SERPINE1* promoter and upregulate its expression [8,9]. These proteins are contained in *ARNTL* locus of the chromosome 11p15.2.

Plasminogen activator inhibitor 1 is a relatively unstable molecule with both a latent and active conformational form. PAI-1 spontaneously inactivates under physiologic conditions with an *in-vitro* half-life of 1–2 h. Binding of PAI-I to vitronectin, a cellular adhesion molecule from the extracellular matrix, stabilizes the active conformation, prolonging its half-life [10]. In humans, PAI-1 is present in human plasma, platelet α-granules, the placenta, and the extracellular matrix. Presently, the origin of plasma PAI-1 has not been completely elucidated, but most

likely originates from endothelial cells and/or hepatocytes. Synthesis and secretion of PAI-1 can be modulated by various chemical mediators including hormones, growth factors, endotoxin, cytokines, and phorbol esters. PAI-1 belongs to the family of serine protease inhibitors (serpin) and inhibits both single-chain and two-chain tPA, and only single-chain uPA through formation of a 1:1 stoichiometric complex through its reactive peptide bond, Arg346–Met347 [11]. The majority of tPA in plasma is in complex with PAI-1; the level of active PAI-1 in the blood is an important regulator of the concentration, half-life, and circadian variation of active tPA.

In addition to its central role in fibrinolysis, PAI-1 is involved in multiple other physiologic pathways and may be related to the pathogenesis of obesity, insulin resistance, and type 2 diabetes. A role for PAI-1 has also been implicated in tumor angiogenesis, bone remodeling, asthma, rheumatoid arthritis, glomerulonephritis, and sepsis [12]. Ongoing research is currently investigating the true role of PAI-1 as a risk factor for cardiovascular disease [9].

Clinical presentation

Plasminogen activator inhibitor 1 deficiency may result from either a quantitative (decreased or absent protein) [13,14] or qualitative defect (detectable protein with reduced or absent functional activity) [15,16]. In quantitative PAI-1 deficiency, affected patients carry one (heterozygote) or two (double het-erozygous or homozygote) alleles with a mutation, resulting in partial or total antigenic deficiency of PAI-1. It is important to note that heterozygous PAI-1 deficiency is not associated with a clinical bleeding diathesis even when the individual experi-ences significant hemostatic challenge including trauma or surgery. Both partial and total PAI-1 deficiencies are extremely rare disorders; the prevalence of this condition in the general population is not established. In large part, an inability to estab-lish true prevalence rates results from lack of accurate sensitive diagnostic of PAI-1 activity assays.

Plasminogen activator inhibitor 1 deficiency is inherited in an autosomal recessive inheritance pattern. Fay et al. [13] reported an Amish pedigree of 19 individuals who carried a homozygous null mutation in the PAI-1 gene with resultant quantitative PAI-1 deficiency. Affected patients had a two base pair (TA) insertion at 3' end of exon 4 in the PAI-1 gene result-ing in a frame-shift in exon 4 with early truncation of the PAI-1 protein and a corresponding absence of PAI-1 antigen in both platelets and plasma. Interestingly, isolated deficiency of plasma PAI-1 with normal platelet PAI-1 has been reported, question-ing the role of PAI-1 in the platelet compartment [13]. There is some suggestion that platelet PAI-1 may be protective against premature clot lysis early in coagulation but subsequently may not be available when delayed bleeding occurs [10]. Thus, it is thought that the local concentrations of PAI-1 and the dynamic time course are important in hemostatic control. Other anecdo-tal mutations include the missense mutation G to A transition at nucleotide position 4497 in exon 2 causing replacement of alanine 15 to threonine (Ala15Thr mutation) described in 34-year-old man heterozygous for the mutation [17].

The literature on PAI-1 deficiency is limited; a few reports provide the most complete information available on the clinical phenotype of PAI-1 deficiency [18]. Complete PAI-1 deficiency was first described in an Amish girl and later in seven individu-als from the same family. The spectrum of bleeding episodes ranged from intracranial hemorrhage and hemarthrosis after injury or mild trauma, delayed surgical bleeding, severe menor-rhagia, and frequent bruising. A well-described case was reported in an elderly male presenting with delayed bleeding diathesis after transurethral prostatic resection [16]. Similar to those with a quantitative PAI-1 deficiency, this patient had a lifelong history of delayed postoperative bleeding and bleeding after trauma [16]. His euglobulin clot lysis assay revealed a shortened clot lysis time (50 min with normal exhibiting no lysis at 2 h) which partially corrected (1 h 45 min) after addition of an antifibrinolytic medication (ε-aminocaproic acid). Extensive evaluation for a deficiency in the fibrinolytic pathway confirmed what appeared to be a functional deficiency of PAI-1 despite a normal PAI-1 antigen. In addition, Minowa et al. (1999) reported four members of a family with early-onset bleeding symptoms (e.g. easy bruising, prolonged bleeding after tooth extractions or trauma, and abnormal uterine bleeding) with the diagnosis being established through documented decreased

Table 61.1 General principles of supportive care in patients with miscellaneous rare bleeding disorders.

General measures
- Avoidance of trauma, contact sports, fastidious dental care, use of MedicAlert bracelet
- Safety checks for infants and toddlers at home

Local measures
- Local bleeding: local pressure, application of ice
- Dental bleeding: local application of fibrin sealants
- Epistaxis: local pressure, ice, nasal packing, application of gel foam, topical thrombin, cauterization, rhinoplasty, or arterial embolization
- Gingival bleeding: regular dental care, topical antifibrinolytic agents

Specific therapies
- Dental bleeding: topical fibrin glue/thrombin, use of DDAVP and antifibrinolytic drugs, dental splints to prevent blood loss accompanying the loss of deciduous teeth
- Menorrhagia: hormone suppression, antifibrinolytics and consider DDAVP
- Iron-deficiency anemia secondary to blood loss: iron supplementation
- Surgery/child birth: involvement of hematology service, type and cross for blood transfusions, use of hemostatic agents such as DDAVP, antifibrinolytics, replacement of deficient coagulation proteins through fresh frozen plasma, use of platelets in platelet function disorders
- Surveillance for alloantibody formation and virus transmission if patient exposed to blood products
- Life-threatening bleeding: consider using recombinant factor VIIa in addition to other supportive measures

PAI-1 activity [19]. Zhang et al. (2005) reported a Chinese man with significant bleeding symptoms after trauma or surgery without spontaneous bleeds. His diagnosis was confirmed using genetic analysis which identified a heterozygous mutation in the SERPINE1 gene inherited from his father. In this report, a second mutation was not identified [17]. A list of the signs and symptoms of PAI-1 deficiency is described in the Table 61.1.

Despite the occurrence of some life-threatening bleeding events, the clinical phenotype is characterized as a moderate bleeding disorder with hemorrhagic manifestations restricted to injury or surgery in homozygous affected individuals; no bleed-ing manifestations were observed in heterozygotes [18]. The clinical manifestations in homozygous individuals are consist-ent with excessive fibrinolysis, resulting in early destruction and detachment of the normal fibrin clot prior to adequate wound healing. In general, bleeding is expected to be most pronounced after trauma/surgical procedures especially involving the oral and urogenital areas owing to the increased fibrinolytic activity in saliva and urine, respectively.

Diagnosis and management

Accurate diagnosis of PAI-1 deficiency is pivotal for effective management with fibrinolytic inhibitors, thereby decreasing the need for blood product support and/or risk of uncontrolled hemorrhage [13,19]. Typically, hyperfibrinolytic bleeding is characterized by normal platelet function tests and screening coagulation tests. The euglobulin clot lysis assay and whole blood clotting assays [20], such as the thromboelastogram, may be helpful to indicate a diagnosis of hyperfibrinolytic states, but are largely insufficient to confirm PAI-1 deficiency whose diagnosis is based on the measurement of antigenic [enzyme-linked immunoadsorbent assay (ELISA)] and functional (chromogenic test) PAI-1 assays. The major limitation of the currently available activity assay is its inability to differentiate low normal levels from a deficiency state. Currently, reported variability of the PAI-1 levels within the normal population include at the lower ranges a PAI-1 activity level of zero, confounding the clinician's ability to diagnosis a deficiency state. Owing to these limitations of activity assays, unless a genetic alteration leads to complete absence of the protein as in the cases reported by Fay *et al.* [13], the diagnosis of PAI-1 deficiency remains problematic and is oftentimes deduced or assumed rather than proven. Genetic analysis could be helpful, yet is also not widely available outside specific research laboratories. Accredited laboratories in Europe can be determined through country-specific rare bleeding disorder societies as listed at www.orpha.net (the portal for rare diseases and orphan drugs).

As many bleeding episodes in patients with PAI-1 deficiency result from injury or invasive interventions, the use of appropriate precautions for bleed prevention are critical to prevent life-threatening haemorrhage. Supportive care may be required to ameliorate bleeding (Table 61.1). Importantly, bleeding episodes are effectively managed with antifibrinolytic agents including oral or intravenous tranexamic acid or ε-aminocaproic acid; treatment duration is dependent upon the severity of the bleeding episode or intervention (Table 61.2). Persistent excessive menorrhagia may be managed with hormonal suppression and long-term prophylactic antifibrinolytic therapy if necessary. Severe bleeding events, including intracranial hemorrhage with or without hematoma evacuation, have been successfully managed with intravenous fibrinolytic inhibitors; use of fresh frozen plasma (dose 10–15 mL/kg) may be utilized to acutely increase PAI-1 activity at initiation of therapy prior to achievement of steady-state levels of antifibrinolytics. The need for on-going treatment with fresh frozen plasma is dependent on the individual patient's circumstances and response to therapy.

Table 61.2 Commonly used hemostatic agents to control bleeding in patients with plasminogen activator inhibitor 1 (PAI-1) deficiency and α1-antiplasmin deficiency.

	Aminocaproic acid	Tranexamic acid	rFVIIa
Mechanism of action	Inhibitor of plasminogen activation	Competitive inhibitor of plasminogen activation; noncompetitive plasmin inhibition at higher concentrations	When complexed with tissue factor, NovoSeven can activate FX to FXa, as well as FIX to FIXa. FXa, in complex with other factors, then converts prothrombin to thrombin, which leads to the formation of a hemostatic plug by converting fibrinogen to fibrin and thereby inducing local hemostasis
Dosage forms	500 mg and 1 g tablets; 250 mg/mL syrup; 250 mg/mL injection in 20 cc and 100 cc vials	500 mg tablets (not available in the USA); 100 mg/mL injection	Intravenous form available as single-use vials of 1.2 mg, 2.4 mg, and 4.8 mg
Oral dosage	3 g every 6 h or 10 g orally followed by 5 g every 6 h	25 mg/kg three to four times/day; absorption not affected by food	No oral dosage form available
Pediatric dosage	200 mg/kg as loading dose orally followed by 100 mg/kg every 6 h. Alternatively, 50–100 mg/kg/dose	Limited data in children to date; dosing instructions for adults may be used	15–30 mcg/kg bolus every 2–3 h for minor bleeds; 30–120 mcg/kg bolus every 2–3 h for significant bleeds
Monitoring parameters	Laboratory monitoring evaluation usually not performed	Laboratory monitoring evaluation usually not performed; higher concentrations may prolong thrombin time	Laboratory monitoring evaluation not performed
Contraindications (absolute and relative)	DIC (disseminated intravascular coagulation); upper urinary tract bleeding; history of thrombosis or thrombophilia	Defective vision; subarachnoid hemorrhage; renal compromise: dose adjustment required; history of thrombosis or thrombophilia	Known hypersensitivity to any component of the drug; known hypersensitivity to mouse, hamster, or bovine proteins; history of thrombosis or thrombophilia
Adverse events	Urinary obstruction if used for upper gastrointestinal tract bleeding	Visual changes with prolonged treatment	Potential risk of thrombosis
Use in pregnancy[a]	Category C	Category B	Category C
Drug interactions	Concomitant use with oral contraceptives or estrogens may potentiate a hypercoagulable state	Concomitant use with oral contraceptives or estrogens may potentiate a hypercoagulable state	None known

[a] US Food and Drug Administration (FDA) safety category of a drug for use in pregnancy. Category B indicates that the drug is potentially safe in animal studies but there is a lack of adequate clinical data in humans, while category C indicates that animal studies have demonstrated adverse effects in fetus but there are no clinical data in humans.

In Indiana, at least two female siblings in the Amish community with homozygous complete PAI-1 deficiency have controlled menstrual flow and achieved successful pregnancies with the use of antifibrinolytic agents (unpublished observations, Indiana Hemophilia and Thrombosis Center). The pregnancies were complicated with intermittent bleeding in the antenatal period and preterm labor, although the newborns were healthy.

To date, there are no reports of the development of inhibitory antibodies against exogenously administered PAI-1 in complete congenital PAI-1 deficiency. Owing to the significant limitations in the diagnosis of PAI-1 deficiency, a clinical trial of antifibrinolytic agents should be considered when a high index of suspicion is present for PAI-1 deficiency and after all other known bleeding disorders have been excluded. Currently, antenatal diagnosis of PAI-1 deficiency is not available.

α2-Plasmin inhibitor deficiency

Role of α2-plasmin inhibitor in fibrinolysis

α2-Plasmin inhibitor deficiency, also known as α2-antiplasmin, is a single-chain glycoprotein consisting of 452 amino acids with a molecular weight of 70 kDa [21] synthesized in the liver and stored in platelet α-granules. The primary function of α2-PI is inhibition of the proteolytic action of plasmin through direct inhibition of plasmin(ogen). Inhibition of fibrin-bound plasmin is more efficient. The gene for α2-PI is located at 17p13.3 (OMIM# 262850) and contains 10 exons and nine introns and spans over 16 kb of DNA. In humans, α2-PI is synthesized primarily in the liver. High levels of α2-PI mRNA have been observed in proximal convoluted tubules, smooth muscles, placenta, and the central nervous system; the clinical significance of these findings is not well elucidated. The mature α2-PI protein belongs to the serine protease inhibitor (Serpin) family and consists of NH_2-terminal Met (Met-form) [22]. In the circulation, the mature protein loses its 12 aminoterminal residues and is converted to the NH_2-terminal Asn (Asn-form) [23]. The Asn-form is present in plasma as 60–70% of the total α2-PI [22]. The reactive site, reacting with the active center of plasmin, consists of Arg376–Met377, based upon the amino acid numbering of the Met-form [21]. α2-PI has a strong affinity for plasmin(ogen) and noncovalently binds to the lysine-binding site (LBS) of plasminogen leading to inhibition of plasmin(ogen) [24]. LBSs are sites at which fibrin is also noncovalently bound. Therefore, α2-PI competitively inhibits the binding of plasminogen to fibrin [25]. In addition to inhibition of plasmin, α2-PI inhibits plasmin(ogen) binding to fibrin. The inhibition of plasmin at the clot level involves covalent binding (cross-linking) of α2-PI with the α-chains of fibrin that are catalyzed by factor XIII. The plasma concentration of α2-PI is 0.7 ± 0.06 mg/L. α2-PI is also present in platelet α-granules at low concentrations and constitutes only 0.05% of α2-PI present in whole blood [26]. Its half-life is 2.6 days, whereas the half-life is 0.5 days for the plasmin–α2-PI complex [27].

Clinical presentation

Owing to the rarity of this disorder, an accurate prevalence is not clearly established. Based on the results of both functional and immunologic assays, two types of deficiency states have been reported: type I (quantitative) [28,29], defined by similar decrease in both antigen and activity, and type II (qualitative), in which a discrepancy between the activity and antigen is found with a lowered activity compared with a normal antigen. The mode of inheritance is autosomal recessive.

The first well-described case report of α2-PI deficiency was in 1979 by Koie et al. [28]. Similar to PAI-1 deficiency, the bleeding manifestations are characterized by post-traumatic or surgical bleeding, and are attributed to premature hemostatic plug dissolution prior to complete vessel repair. Reported bleeding episodes range from moderate to severe and often present in childhood. Reported hemorrhagic episodes include umbilical stump bleeding, prolonged bleeding from wounds, epistaxis, gingival bleeding, hematuria, subcutaneous and intramuscular hematomas, hemothorax, central nervous system hemorrhage, and hemarthroses. An unusual bleeding site, intramedullary hematoma in the diaphyses of the long bones, has been reported in patients with α2-PI deficiency [30,31]. Radiography indicates homogenous hyperlucent lesions with well-defined margins without marginal sclerosis that may be difficult to distinguish from cystic fibrous dysplasia, Langerhans cell histiocytosis, or metastatic neuroblastoma. Accurate diagnosis of these intramedullary hematomas may be confirmed with magnetic resonance imaging revealing homogeneous hyperintense signals in the medulla and a hypointense signal surrounding the lesion. The fact that the spectrum of severity exhibited by homozygous or compound heterozygous affected individuals varies from severe to moderate may relate to the variability of genetic defects and their specific impact on enzymatic function and other, as yet unidentified, factors.

In general, compound heterozygous and homozygous affected individuals experience a significant bleeding tendency while clinical bleeding in heterozygotes (one abnormal allele) is a matter of controversy. The majority of heterozygous individuals are discovered through family studies of compound heterozygous/homozygous individuals, and have not experienced a bleeding tendency. However, there remain a few case reports that describe bleeding manifestations in what appears to be heterozygous individuals [32,33]. Bleeding events in heterozygotes have been reported in association with trauma, including surgery or dental extraction, and have occurred in children [32] and in adults [33]. There is a suggestion that the bleeding tendency may increase with age [34]. Intramedullary hematomas have not been reported in heterozygotes.

Three different mutations have been described: SERPINF2, GLU137DEL; SERPINF2, 1-BP insertion, 1438C; and SERPINF2, VAL384MET. The first mutation ever described was reported by

Miura *et al.* in 1989 [35,36]. The authors described homozygosity for a nucleotide deletion in exon 7 that resulted in deletion of glu137. This mutation transcribes a mutant protein the majority of which remains intracellular as an endoglycosidase causing a block in intracellular trafficking from the endoplasmic reticulum to the Golgi apparatus. The family studied contained three consanguineous marriages and had lived for generations on Okinawa. The proband had less than 1 μg/mL of protein; heterozygous family members, including both parents, exhibited about 50% of the normal concentration as measured immunologically or functionally. This mutation was designated α2-plasmin inhibitor Okinawa. A second mutation was described by Yoshioka *et al.* (1982) in a Japanese family [29]. This mutation was designated α2-plasmin inhibitor Nara and is characterized by single cytidine nucleotide insertion at nucleotide 1438 in the exon coding for the C-terminal region (exon 10). This frameshift mutation led to replacement of the C-terminal 12 amino acid residues of the normal inhibitor with 178 amino acid residues entirely unrelated to the normal amino acid sequence. Lind and Thorsen described the third mutation in 1999 [37]. The authors reported heterozygosity for a G-to-A transition in the PLI gene resulting in a val384-to-met mutation in a woman and two of her children who displayed a bleeding tendency. The mother experienced a traumatic breast hematoma and peripostoperative bleeding. An affected daughter required a blood transfusion after a normal delivery, and a son had prolonged bleeding after a dental extraction. The plasma plasmin inhibitor activities were reduced to 49–66% of normal [37].

Diagnosis and management

Diagnosis of α2-PI requires a high index of suspicion as screening coagulation assays and platelet function tests are normal even in those severely affected with α2-PI deficiency. The euglobulin clot lysis time and whole-blood clotting assays may be useful tin pointing towards a hyperfibrinolytic state; functional and immunologic α2-PI assays are required for diagnosis.

Supportive care and antifibrinolytic medications, including ε-aminocaproic acid and tranexamic acid, are the mainstay of treatment (Table 61.2). Fresh frozen plasma may be used as an alternative or as adjunct to antifibrinolytic therapy in specific situations when an acute increase of the clotting factor is required. Based on the observation of Yoshioka *et al.* [29], infusion of FFP (17.5 mL/kg) increased the plasma concentration of α2-PI antigen and activity to 15.6% and 19%, respectively. The half-life of infused α2-PI antigen and activity was 35.5 and 21 h, respectively [29]. It is important to emphasize that treatment with fresh frozen plasma may be ineffective in individuals with a reduced concentration of factor XIII (FXIII) activity as α2-PI induced inhibition of fibrin-bound plasmin is catalyzed by FXIII [38]. Treatment of intramedullary hematomas may require curettage with local application of hemostatic agents, such as fibrin glues, along with systemic antifibrinolytic therapy.

Vitamin K

Vitamin K is a family of molecules (phylloquinone, menaquinone, and the synthetic menadione) that share a common functional methylated naphthoquinone ring. The first mention of vitamin K in the literature was in 1929 by Henrik Dam who observed that removing a fat-soluble compound ("Koagulation Vitamin") from the diet of chickens resulted in a bleeding diathesis [39]. The members of this family of molecules differ in their pharmacokinetics (e.g. intestinal absorption, distribution, metabolism, and excretion) due to the lipophilicity profile of the side chains and the food matrices where they are found [40,41]. Among this family of molecules, phylloquinone is the most abundant in our diet and is found in green vegetables. Human colonic intestinal flora also produces vitamin K and requires bile salts for its absorption. Circulating levels of vitamin K in healthy adults range between 200 and 800 pg/mL after an overnight fasting period [42]. In nonfasting individuals, vitamin K levels may vary based upon dietary consumption. A commercially available form of vitamin K is phylloquinone.

In mammals, vitamin K is a required cofactor for γ-glutamylcarboxylase critical to the carboxylation of glutamate residues into γ-carboxyglutamate (Gla) in liver microsomes [43,44]. Vitamin K deficiency may be established through the detection of undercarboxylated forms of Gla proteins, designated proteins induced by vitamin K absence (PIVKAs).

The Gla portion of the vitamin K-dependent proteins (factors II, VII, IX, and X, and protein C, S, and Z) is primarily involved in facilitating the binding of the protein to negatively charged phospholipids on the surface membrane of activated platelets thereby promoting thrombin formation. The Gla residues form calcium-binding groups and the binding of calcium ions results in conformational changes of the coagulation factors leading to the internalization of the Gla–Ca^{2+} complex and exposure of the phospholipid-binding domain that allows binding to activated platelets [45,46] .

Familial deficiency of vitamin K-dependent clotting factors

Hereditary combined deficiency of factor II, factor VII (FVII), factor IX, and factor X, is a rare autosomal recessive bleeding disorder that is estimated to occur at a frequency of 1/2 000 000 births [47]. This disorder also involves the naturally occurring anticoagulants (e.g. proteins C and S), as well as vitamin K-dependent bone proteins resulting in a vulnerability to osteopenia and skeletal defects in affected individuals [48–50]. The diagnosis should be considered only after other more common causes of vitamin K deficiency are ruled out including liver disease, vitamin K antagonist (e.g. warfarin or anticoagulant rodenticides) overdose, malabsorption (e.g. inflammatory bowel disease or celiac disease), use of anticonvulsants, or prolonged therapy with antibiotics. The etiology of VKCFD is due to a defective step in the carboxylation of the vitamin K-dependent factors due to mutations (point mutations) in genes responsible for encoding two enzymes involved in this process: γ-glutamyl carboxylase (GGCX) and the vitamin K epoxide reductase (VKORC). Mutations in GGCX (two kindreds) and functional deficiency of the VKOR (three kindreds) have been described [51,52]. The only deletion mutation (14 bp) was described in a kindred in intron 1 of GGCX by Thomas and Stirling in 2003 [53].

Familial deficiency of vitamin K-dependent clotting factors has been reported in less than 30 families worldwide; carriers are usually asymptomatic. The rarity of the disorder may be explained by the risk of fetal lethality with complete deficiency as is supported by observations in the GGCX knock-out mouse [54].

Clinical presentation

Vitamin K-dependent clotting factor deficiency was first described in 1966 in a 3-month-old female with multiple episodes of spontaneous bleeding and easy bruising [55]. Affected individuals may exhibit a severe bleeding phenotype including intracranial hemorrhage early in life identical to hemorrhagic disease of the newborn observed prior to institution of vitamin K prophylaxis. Some cases may be associated with dysmorphic features similar to warfarin embryopathy, developmental delay, skeletal defects, osteoporosis, and a high incidence of miscarriage [48–50]. The severity of symptoms may be impacted by diet, gastrointestinal microflora, and mutational genetic penetrance. Anecdotal reports of affected patients with cases of thrombosis due to associated proteins C and S deficiencies are reported [56].

Diagnosis and management

After excluding other causes of vitamin K deficiency, genotyping of VKORC and GGCX are available and recommended. The vitamin K assay, if available, may be useful. Final diagnosis requires genetic confirmation. Screening laboratory tests reveal a prolonged prothrombin time (PT) and activated partial thromboplastin time (aPTT).

Administration of large doses of vitamin K remains the current standard of care; however, bleeding symptoms may still occur. Administration of an oral dose of 10 mg twice or three times weekly commonly avoids frequent mucocutaneous bleeding [47]. Alternatively, if not tolerated orally, the same dose of vitamin K may be regularly administered via the intravenous route at intervals based upon the PT-INR values. Despite the generally acknowledged efficacy of vitamin K, a fixed therapeutic schedule does not exist. Sequential transfusions of prothrombin-complex concentrates (PCCs) would be the treatment of choice during bleeding events. Standardized treatment for VKCFD is not available and current management are derived from the reversal of vitamin K antagonists, with a suggested dose of 500 IU given intravenously (8.8 IU/kg) for an INR below 5. PCCs may be divided in two categories based on their coagulation factor composition. All PCCs contain factors II, IX, and X (three-factor PCC) while some contain higher levels of FVII (four-factor PCC). Four-factor PCC (Octaplex, Beriplex P/N) is a relatively newer product and may not be widely available. Some studies suggest that the four-factor PCC is more effective in the reversal of vitamin-K antagonist effects as evidenced by normalization of the INR, due to a higher FVII content [57]. The risk of thrombosis must be considered when using PCCs due to their containing activated forms of coagulation factors although these doses are significantly below those used in hemophilia patients complicated by inhibitors [47]. If PCCs are not available, fresh frozen plasma may be used at 15–20 mL/kg. Another alternative is the use of recombinant activated FVII (rFVIIa), but certain features, including its containing a single vitamin K-dependent coagulation factor, the short in-vivo half-life, and the increased clearance rate in young children, influence its use. The recommended dose of rFVIIa is 35–90 µg/kg every 4–6 h; however, much lower doses have been used successfully 15–30 µg/kg every 4–6 h in patients with FVII deficiency [58]. As rFVIIa and vitamin K have associated differing expected peak action (4 h and 24 h, respectively), their combined use with a simultaneous infusion at the doses mentioned above may result in a sustained normalization of clotting times required in episodes of major or life-threatening hemorrhagic episodes and/or more complex surgical procedures [47].

Conclusion

Miscellaneous rare bleeding disorders comprise a group of heterogeneous disorders that present with a wide variety of clinical bleeding symptoms ranging from mucocutaneous bleeding, bleeding after hemostatic challenge such as surgery, menorrhagia, bleeding with pregnancy, labor, and delivery, to catastrophic life-threatening haemorrhage. Diagnosis of these disorders requires skilled clinical evaluation, with a detailed family history, and knowledge of the disorders and their associated presentation and sequelae, and use of specific tests to substantiate the diagnosis. Quite often, immediate and accurate laboratory diagnosis may not be possible due to limitations in test availability or insensitivity of currently available assays as exemplified PAI-1 activity assays. Therefore, a high index of suspicion is required to establish these diagnoses and provide optimal medical care. Therapeutic interventions should be administered after careful consideration of the risk–benefit ratio and not necessarily to treat an abnormal laboratory result. In the majority of cases, judicious use of hemostatic agents including antifibrinolytic therapies, fresh frozen plasma, PCCs, or rFVIIa dependent on the deficiency state, control bleeding symptoms. On rare occasions when catastrophic or refractory haemorrhage is encountered, blood component support may be required. Therapeutic interventions are tailored to the specific deficiency. For example, antifibrinolytics are utilized as primary hemostatic agents in PAI-1 and α2-PI deficiency. Patients affected with rare disorders should, whenever possible, be reported to national and/or international registries to accumulate the much needed information to better define their incidence, clinical manifestations, define optimal treatment algorithms, long-term safety and efficacy of hemostatic interventions, and long-term disease associated and treatment outcomes.

Resources

- Global Bleeding Disorder Community: www.wfh.org
- Rare Coagulation Disorder Resource Room: www.rarecoagulationdisorders.org and International Registry of Rare Bleeding Disorder database: http://rbdd.org
- Online Mendelian Inheritance in Man: www.omim.org

References

1 Collen D, Lijnen HR. Basic and clinical aspects of fibrinolysis and thrombolysis. *Blood* 1991; **78**: 3114–24.

2 Rijken DC. Plasminogen activators and plasminogen activator inhibitors: biochemical aspects. *Baillieres Clin Haematol* 1995; **8**: 291–312.

3 Ny T, *et al.* Cloning and sequence of a cDNA coding for the human beta-migrating endothelial-cell-type plasminogen activator inhibitor. *Proc Natl Acad Sci USA* 1986; **83**: 6776–80.

4 Dellas C, Loskutoff DJ. Historical analysis of PAI-1 from its discovery to its potential role in cell motility and disease. *Thromb Haemost* 2005; **93**: 631–40.

5 Booth NA, *et al.* Plasminogen activator inhibitor (PAI-1) in plasma and platelets. *Br J Haematol* 1988; **70**: 327–33.

6 Alessi MC, *et al.* Correlations between t-PA and PAI-1 antigen and activity and t-PA/PAI-1 complexes in plasma of control subjects and of patients with increased t-PA or PAI-1 levels. *Thromb Res* 1990; **60**: 509–16.

7 Rydzewski A, *et al.* Diurnal variation in serum remnant-like lipoproteins, platelet aggregation and fibrinolysis in healthy volunteers. *Haemostasis* 1997; **27**: 305–14.

8 Schoenhard JA, *et al.* Regulation of the PAI-1 promoter by circadian clock components: differential activation by BMAL1 and BMAL2. *J Mol Cell Cardiol* 2003; **35**: 473–81.

9 Huang J, *et al.* Genome-wide association study for circulating levels of PAI-1 provides novel insights into its regulation. *Blood* 2012; **120**: 4873–81.

10 Wiman B, *et al.* Plasminogen activator inhibitor 1 (PAI) is bound to vitronectin in plasma. *FEBS Lett* 1988; **242**: 125–8.

11 Lindahl TL, Ohlsson PI, Wiman B. The mechanism of the reaction between human plasminogen-activator inhibitor 1 and tissue plasminogen activator. *Biochem J* 1990; **265**: 109–13.

12 Lijnen HR, *et al.* On the role of plasminogen activator inhibitor-1 in adipose tissue development and insulin resistance in mice. *J Thromb Haemost* 2005; **3**: 1174–9.

13 Fay WP, *et al.* Human plasminogen activator inhibitor-1 (PAI-1) deficiency: characterization of a large kindred with a null mutation in the PAI-1 gene. *Blood* 1997; **90**: 204–8.

14 Lee MH, *et al.* Deficiency of plasma plasminogen activator inhibitor 1 results in hyperfibrinolytic bleeding. *Blood* 1993; **81**: 2357–62.

15 Pannekoek H, *et al.* Functional display of human plasminogen-activator inhibitor 1 (PAI-1) on phages: novel perspectives for structure-function analysis by error-prone DNA synthesis. *Gene* 1993; **128**: 135–40.

16 Schleef RR, *et al.* Bleeding diathesis due to decreased functional activity of type 1 plasminogen activator inhibitor. *J Clin Invest* 1989; **83**: 1747–52.

17 Zhang ZY, *et al.* A case of deficiency of plasma plasminogen activator inhibitor-1 related to Ala15Thr mutation in its signal peptide. *Blood Coag Fibrinol* 2005; **16**: 79–84.

18 Mehta R, Shapiro AD. Plasminogen activator inhibitor type 1 deficiency. *Haemophilia* 2008; **14**: 1255–60.

19 Minowa H, *et al.* Four cases of bleeding diathesis in children due to congenital plasminogen activator inhibitor-1 deficiency. *Haemostasis* 1999; **29**: 286–91.

20 Rijken DC, *et al.* Development of a new test for the global fibrinolytic capacity in whole blood. *J Thromb Haemost* 2008; **6**: 151–7.

21 Holmes WE, *et al.* Primary structure of human alpha 2-antiplasmin, a serine protease inhibitor (serpin). *J Biol Chem* 1987; **262**: 1659–64.

22 Bangert K, *et al.* Different N-terminal forms of alpha 2-plasmin inhibitor in human plasma. *Biochem J* 1993; **291**(Pt 2): 623–5.

23 Koyama T, *et al.* Different NH2-terminal form with 12 additional residues of alpha 2-plasmin inhibitor from human plasma and culture media of Hep G2 cells. *Biochem Biophys Res Commun* 1994; **200**: 417–22.

24 Wiman B, Lijnen HR, Collen D. On the specific interaction between the lysine-binding sites in plasmin and complementary sites in alpha2-antiplasmin and in fibrinogen. *Biochim Biophys Acta* 1979; **579**: 142–54.

25 Moroi M, Aoki N. Inhibition of plasminogen binding to fibrin by alpha2-plasmin inhibitor. *Thromb Res* 1977; **10**: 851–6.

26 Mui PT, James HL, Ganguly, P. Isolation and properties of a low molecular weight antiplasmin of human blood platelets and serum. *Br J Haematol* 1975; **29**: 627–37.

27 Collen D, Wiman B. Turnover of antiplasmin, the fast-acting plasmin inhibitor of plasma. *Blood* 1979; **53**: 313–24.

28 Koie K, *et al.* Alpha2-plasmin-inhibitor deficiency (Miyasato disease). *Lancet* 1978; **2**: 1334–6.

29 Yoshioka A, *et al.* Congenital deficiency of alpha 2-plasmin inhibitor in three sisters. *Haemostasis* 1982; **11**: 176–84.

30 Devaussuzenet VM, *et al.* A case of intramedullary haematoma associated with congenital alpha2-plasmin inhibitor deficiency. *Pediatr Radiol* 1998; **28**: 978–80.

31 Takahashi Y, *et al.* Intramedullary multiple hematomas in siblings with congenital alpha-2-plasmin inhibitor deficiency: orthopedic surgery with protection by tranexamic acid. *Haemostasis* 1991; **21**: 321–7.

32 Griffin GC, *et al.* Alpha 2-antiplasmin deficiency. An overlooked cause of hemorrhage. *Am J Pediatr Hematol Oncol* 1993; **15**: 328–30.

33 Kordich L, *et al.* Severe hemorrhagic tendency in heterozygous alpha 2-antiplasmin deficiency. *Thromb Res* 1985; **40**: 645–51.

34 Ikematsu S, Fukutake K, Aoki N. Heterozygote for plasmin inhibitor deficiency developing hemorrhagic tendency with advancing age. *Thromb Res* 1996; **82**: 129–16.

35 Miura O, *et al.* Molecular basis for congenital deficiency of alpha 2-plasmin inhibitor. A frameshift mutation leading to elongation of the deduced amino acid sequence. *J Clin Invest* 1989; **83**: 1598–604.

36 Miura O, Sugahara Y, Aoki N. Hereditary alpha 2-plasmin inhibitor deficiency caused by a transport-deficient mutation (alpha 2-PI-Okinawa). Deletion of Glu137 by a trinucleotide deletion blocks intracellular transport. *J Biol Chem* 1989; **264**: 18213–19.

37 Lind B, Thorsen S. A novel missense mutation in the human plasmin inhibitor (alpha2-antiplasmin) gene associated with a bleeding tendency. *Br J Haematol* 1999; **107**: 317–22.

38 Kluft C, *et al.* A familial hemorrhagic diathesis in a Dutch family: an inherited deficiency of alpha 2-antiplasmin. *Blood* 1982; **59**: 1169–80.

39 Dam H. Cholesterinstoffwechsel in Hühnereiern und Hühnehen. *Biochem Z* 1929; **215**: 475.

40 Reedstrom CK, Suttie WJ. Comparative distribution, metabolism, and utilization of phylloquinone and menaquinone-9 in rat liver. *Proc Soc Exp Biol Med* 1995; **209**: 403–9.

41 Will BH, Suttie JW. Comparative metabolism of phylloquinone and menaquinone-9 in rat liver. *J Nutr* 1992; **122**: 953–8.

42 Vermeer C, Schurgers LJ. A comprehensive review of vitamin K and vitamin K antagonists. *Hematol Oncol Clin North Am* 2000; **14**: 339–53.

43 Suttie JW. Vitamin K-dependent carboxylase. *Annu Rev Biochem* 1985; **54**: 459–77.

44 Furie BBA, Bouchard A, Furie BC. Vitamin K-dependent biosynthesis of gamma-carboxyglutamic acid. *Blood* 1999; **93**: 1798–808.

45 Soriano-Garcia M, *et al.* Structure of Ca2+ prothrombin fragment 1 including the conformation of the Gla domain. *Biochemistry* 1989; **28**: 6805–10.

46 Li L, *et al.* Refinement of the NMR solution structure of the gamma-carboxyglutamic acid domain of coagulation factor IX using molecular dynamics simulation with initial Ca2+ positions determined by a genetic algorithm. *Biochemistry* 1997; **36**: 2132–8.

47 Napolitano M, Mariani G, Lapecorella M. Hereditary combined deficiency of the vitamin K-dependent clotting factors. *Orphanet J Rare Dis* 2010; **5**: 21.

48 Darghouth D, *et al.* Compound heterozygosity of novel missense mutations in the gamma-glutamyl-carboxylase gene causes hereditary combined vitamin K-dependent coagulation factor deficiency. *Blood* 2006; **108**: 1925–31.

49 Pauli RM, *et al.* Association of congenital deficiency of multiple vitamin K-dependent coagulation factors and the phenotype of the warfarin embryopathy: clues to the mechanism of teratogenicity of coumarin derivatives. *Am J Hum Genet* 1987; **41**: 566–83.

50 Boneh A, Bar-Ziv J. Hereditary deficiency of vitamin K-dependent coagulation factors with skeletal abnormalities. *Am J Med Genet* 1996; **65**: 241–3.

51 Soute BA, *et al.* Congenital deficiency of all vitamin K-dependent blood coagulation factors due to a defective vitamin K-dependent carboxylase in Devon Rex cats. *Thromb Haemost* 1992; **68**: 521–5.

52 Oldenburg J, *et al.* Congenital deficiency of vitamin K dependent coagulation factors in two families presents as a genetic defect of the vitamin K-epoxide-reductase-complex. *Thromb Haemost* 2000; **84**: 937–41.

53 Thomas A, Stirling D. Four factor deficiency. *Blood Coag Fibrinol* 2003; **14** (Suppl. 1): S55–7.

54 Zhang B, Ginsburg D. Familial multiple coagulation factor deficiencies: new biologic insight from rare genetic bleeding disorders. *J Thromb Haemost* 2004; **2**: 1564–72.

55 McMillan CW, Roberts HR. Congenital combined deficiency of coagulation factors II, VII, IX and X. Report of a case. *N Engl J Med* 1966; **274**: 1313–15.

56 Weston BW, Monahan PE. Familial deficiency of vitamin K-dependent clotting factors. *Haemophilia* 2008; **14**: 1209–13.

57 Voils SA, Baird B. Systematic review: 3-factor versus 4-factor prothrombin complex concentrate for warfarin reversal: does it matter? *Thromb Res* 2012; **130**(6): 833–40.

58 Mariani G, *et al.* Invasive procedures and minor surgery in factor VII deficiency. *Haemophilia* 2012; **18**: e63–5.

Emergency medicine

CHAPTER 62

Emergency management of hemophilia

W. Keith Hoots

National Heart, Lung, and Blood Institute, National Institutes of Health, Maryland, USA

Introduction

Patients with hemophilia A or B of all severities are at increased bleeding risk following injury of any origin. Even when prophylaxis is being employed to reduce or eliminate hemarthroses in patients with severe or moderately severe hemophilia, a significant portion of an individual hemophilic patient's daily living is occurring with subphysiologic plasma levels of his missing clotting factor. Should he incur a major injury during these periods of nonoptimal levels of factor VIII (FVIII) or factor IX (IX), he is at increased risk for life- or limb-threatening bleeding, at a minimum analogous to that of a patient with mild hemophilia having a comparable injury. Hence, therapeutic strategies for treating life- or limb-threatening injuries follow common principles regardless of severity or whether the patient has hemophilia A or B. This chapter reviews these therapies for injuries to vital organs and provides a guidance concerning key therapeutic issues such as duration of clotting factor replacement and other acute care management strategies.

Central nervous system bleeding

The most frequently encountered life-threatening event among the hemophilia population is intracranial hemorrhage (ICH). Supporting this conclusion is a recent report concerning inhibitor mortality reduction among patients with high-titer inhibitors reported from the UK Haemophilia Centre Doctors' Organisation database during the last decade of the 20th century compared with death rates for the aggregate hemophilia population during the prior two decades [1]. Trauma is the inciting event for severe central nervous system (CNS) hemorrhage (intracranial or paraspinal) in hemophilia patients most commonly. However, it is well recognized that slowly evolving hemorrhages or hematomas that begin as inconsequential can be followed by recurrent bleeding in the area of the initial bleeding leading to a much greater neurologic impairment. Therefore,

a bleed thought to have occurred spontaneously may well reflect this scenario rather than a *de-novo* event [2,3]. Stated another way, spontaneous CNS bleeding in hemophilia, even among patients with a severe phenotype, appears to be rare. Exceptions may indicate the presence of an anatomic lesion, such as an arteriovenous malformation or aneurysm. Besides trauma, other predisposing risk factors for ICH include human immunodeficiency virus (HIV) infection accompanied by immune suppression, the presence of an inhibitor, and age <5 years or >51 years [3]. All severities of hemophilia are at increased risk for CNS hemorrhage compared with the normal population and even patients with >5% FVIII or FIX have an increased risk approaching 50% of those with severe disease.

Proper assessment of CNS bleeding cannot be achieved without proper imaging technology. This reality is not unique to CNS hemorrhage; however, the capacity to adequately and assiduously image the brain, spinal cord, and other anatomy associated with the CNS (e.g. the optic nerve) is essential for rapid diagnosis and appropriate intervention. The proper application of these imaging techniques is beyond the scope of this chapter. Constantine *et al.* have recently provided a comprehensive review of hemophilia-specific imaging including that for CNS-associated bleeding [4].

Intracranial hemorrhage

Compression from an increasing volume of blood inside the calvarium or spinal canal can rapidly induce a compression injury of the vulnerable neurons and glial cells. Depending on the location of the bleed, even small volumes of blood can induce such injury because of markedly constrained expansion capacity in these anatomic sites. Therefore, from a therapeutic standpoint, it is critical that a physiologic hemostatic potential through infusion of the missing factor be undertaken immediately when such a bleed is suspected—even before confirming the presence of the bleed with diagnostic imaging.

Textbook of Hemophilia, Third Edition. Edited by Christine A. Lee, Erik E. Berntorp and W. Keith Hoots.

Box 62.1 High-risk hemorrhagic events for acute morbidity or mortality in hemophilia A or B. From [6] Hoots WK. Emergency care issues in hemophilia, treatment of hemophilia monograph no. 43, World Federation of Hemophilia, November 2007.

Central nervous system hemorrhage
Intracranial hemorrhage
Paraspinal hemorrhage
Soft-tissue hemorrhage predisposing to airway impingement
Retropharyngeal hemorrhage following mandibular molar extraction leading to hemorrhage along facial planes
Neck hematoma associated with dissection
Tracheal hemorrhage following airway instrumentation
Large tongue hematoma
Gastrointestinal bleeding
Hematemesis from esophageal injury or ulceration of gastric or duodenal mucosa
Hemorrhage from ruptured esophageal varix (varices)
Hematochezia or melena from bleeding telangiectasia polyps, etc.
Ruptured abdominal organ or capusular hematoma of abdominal viscus
Splenic rupture, kidney capsular rupture, liver laceration
Hematoma of bowel wall
Ruptured appendix
Ruptured pelvic or abdominal pseudotumor
Acute compartment syndrome
Hematoma impingement of nerves, vasculature of extremities
Hemorrhage in or around the eye
Hyphema
Vitreous hemorrhage
Hematoma following orbital fracture

Box 62.2 Guidelines for acute management of severe hemorrhage in hemophilia A and B. From [6] Hoots WK. Emergency care issues in hemophilia, treatment of hemophilia monograph no. 43, World Federation of Hemophilia, November 2007.

Assure adequate airway, breathing, and circulation by assessing respirations, pulse, and blood pressure (basic cardiopulmonary resuscitation guidelines)
Attain venous access as expeditiously as possible
Infuse appropriate factor VIIII (hemophilia A) or factor IX (hemophilia B) at a dose calculated to achieve physiologic levels immediately [50 U/kg body weight factor VIII or 100–120 U/kg high-purity factor IX (70–80 U/kg of prothrombin complex concentrate if high-purity factor IX is unavailable), respectively]
Obtain computed tomography scan, ultrasound, or other imaging studies as indicated to ascertain bleeding site/source
Request consultation from appropriate physician consultant for bleeding site, e.g. ophthalmologist for bleeding in/around the eye
Hospitalize
Monitor factor VIII/factor IX levels (for hemophilia A/B, respectively) on a frequent basis to maintain level in the mid-physiologic range
Continue with frequent bolus or continuous clotting factor infusions adjusted according to measured factor VIII/IX plasma levels until the acute bleeding event has resolved. Factor VIII/IX dosing may be adjusted downward as the risk for further bleeding is substantially reduced
Examine the patient following hospitalization to ensure that any sequelae receive appropriate long-term care

An ICH can occur in the subdural space, the epidural/subarachnoid space, or the intraparenchymal tissues [5]. Bleeding at any of these three sites can cause rapid progression of symptomatology such as headache, lateralizing neurologic dysfunction, or even acute-onset loss of consciousness. This results not only from the mass effect of the blood itself but also from the accompanying inflammation which induces brain swelling (Boxes 62.1 and 62.2) [6]. The latter, in the worst-case scenario, can lead to herniation of the brainstem and death. Conversely, rapid replacement with clotting factor concentrates may forestall most or all neurologic sequelae, as long as restoration of physiologic hemostasis is of sufficient duration to allow CNS vessel healing to occur. Even in the latter scenario, the risk for rebleeding at a proximal CNS site may always be higher than prior to the original hemorrhage [7–11]. Further, intraparenchymal hemorrhages in particular can cause symptoms out of proportion to the size of the amount of hemorrhage [12], particularly in young children with hemophilia. This is particularly true when bleeding occurs at a brain locus essential for maintenance of vital organ functioning such as the brainstem.

Since clinical outcome can be related to both the volume of brain injured and the duration of the bleeding-associated inflammation (particularly morbid brain swelling), neurosurgical intervention to evacuate the hemorrhage may save the life of the person with hemophilia and/or preserve his or her long-term neurologic function [11]. This requires adequate hemostasis during and following surgical intervention with sufficient clotting factor replacement (or bypassing activity in the case of a patient with a high-titer inhibitor). Strategies for insuring the adequacy of the hemostasis are discussed elsewhere. For comatose or incapacitated patients, airway protection, appropriate cardiovascular monitoring, and careful maintenance of physiologic intracranial pressure are requisites for an optimal outcome [13,14].

Neonatal central nervous system hemorrhage

An ICH in the newborn occurs most commonly following birth trauma [12]. The use of forceps delivery or vacuum extraction to "facilitate" difficult vaginal delivery is particularly prone to result in ICH among hemophilic neonates [15]. Kulkarni *et al.* in the largest review to date, cite an ICH incidence of 3.58% [16]. Because approximately 30% of male infants with hemophilia represent index cases in a family (because of *de-novo* mutations), all males presenting at birth with diagnosed ICH should be suspected of having a congenital bleeding disorder such as hemophilia A or B. Confirmation with transfontanelle ultrasonography should be done immediately. Concurrently, the neonate should be assessed with a coagulation work-up that includes, minimally, a prothrombin time (PT), activated partial thromboplastin time (aPTT), and platelet count. If the aPTT alone is abnormal, a FVIII (followed by FIX assay should the former be normal) should be performed emergently to direct appropriate replacement therapy [17,18].

Spinal hematoma

Even though the treatment of choice for blood-induced spinal compression is neurosurgical decompression, in patients with hemophilia rapid infusion of clotting factor replacement at the first symptom of pain may obviate the need for surgery. Rapid stanching of bleeding may prevent progression to sensory and motor nerve compromise [19]. In addition, repletion of the missing clotting factor may prevent later spinal deformities when such bleeds occur in young children [20]. In some instances, when unequivocal neural compromise is present, a laminectomy to decompress the cord may be unavoidable. In the latter scenario, a carefully monitored clotting factor replacement strategy, similar to that required for neurosurgery, to treat ICH is mandatory. This treatment should continue for a minimum of 10–14 days, even when laminectomy is avoidable [21]. As with ICH, suspicion that bleeding is compressing the spinal cord requires rapid clotting factor replacement, even before imaging studies to confirm the morbidity are undertaken. Once imaging studies are performed, which verify the presence of blood in the spinal canal, the hemophilic patient needs to be admitted to a critical care unit to insure that hemostasis is adequate for the required duration—even when symptoms rapidly remit.

Clotting factor replacement: recommendations for the treatment of central nervous system bleeds

Three basic principles define strategies for adequate hemostasis replacement therapy for CNS bleeding:

1 Infuse enough FVIII or FIX concentrates for hemophilia A or B, respectively, to achieve a measured recovery of approximately 100%. For patients with inhibitors, dosing is less precise but should aim for the maximum demonstrated safe dose for the respective bypassing agent.

2 Infuse FVIII or FIX often enough to insure that nadir levels are at the low end of physiologic levels (50% minimum for FVIII, perhaps slightly lower for FIX if the patient is older and felt to be at increased risk of deep vein thrombosis).

3 Obtain *in-vivo* measurements of FVIII or FIX levels as frequently as required to ensure that these minimal physiologic levels are consistently achieved.

In patients with hemophilia A, a dose of 50 U/kg FVIII initially then every 8–12 h will typically achieve these levels in a patient with severe disease. If surgery is required, the second dose may need to be given earlier than this because clearance is typically greater because of perioperative hemostatic requirements. Once the clearance has returned to steady state (which may occur after the initial dosing when surgery is not needed), both less frequent and lower dosing may be needed to keep the levels in the physiologic range. There is *no* substitute for measuring the FVIII level to ascertain how to appropriately adjust dosing.

For patients with hemophilia B, dosing will likely need to be product-type specific. When recombinant FIX is infused, an initial dose of 120 U/kg followed by adjusted dosing based on whether or not surgery is needed. Once clearance is close to steady state, dosing frequency will likely need to be every 18–24 h [6]. If high-purity plasma-derived concentrates are administered, a loading dose of approximately 100 U/kg followed by a similar FIX level directed follow-up dosing schedule as with recombinant may be employed. Plasma-derived prothrombin complex concentrates (PCCs) should not be used for managing these patients if either of the above concentrates are available because of a demonstrably greater risk for excess clotting and even disseminated intravascular coagulation. If a PCC is all that is available, an initial dose of 80–100 U/kg is reasonable, but subsequent dosing should be reduced compared with the above recommendations because of the thrombotic risks. Data using these products suggest dosing to achieve nadir levels of 30–40% may provide a safe window that balances bleeding and thrombotic risks [22]. In addition to monitoring FIX levels, platelet count, PT, aPTT, fibrinogen, and a fibrinolytic marker such as D-dimer should be monitored when PCCs are used in this context to monitor for any insidious thrombotic potential.

Alternative strategies for providing hemostatic coverage for patients with CNS hemorrhages, including continuous infusion of either FVIII or FIX, are discussed elsewhere. As with any major surgery or life-threatening event, this alternative has the advantage of more consistent *in-vivo* levels but the potential disadvantage that temporary interruption of the infusion (such as might occur with infiltration of the infusion line) may lead to bleeding. These need to be balanced for each individual circumstance.

The duration necessary to achieve an optimal clinical outcome varies with the injury, whether or not neurosurgery is required, and other confounding factors such as whether the patient has had any antecedent CNS bleeding that may indicate a high predisposition for recurrence. Regardless, the propensity for rebleeding to occur following ICH, for example, appears to be significant. This is particularly true if hemostatic replacement is discontinued prematurely [23]. For this reason, many hemophilia experts advocate a long-term prophylaxis regimen for children and adults who have had a large ICH. This strategy is consistent with observations that neovascularization in areas of the brain affected by hemorrhagic stroke may, for quite some time, result in fragile vessels that may bleed with a minimal insult. The duration of any secondary prophylaxis (distinct from that in individuals already on primary prophylaxis who would presumably return to this regimen once the intensive event-associated replacement therapy is complete) will depend on many factors, such as availability of factor concentrates, severity of injury and associated conditions, patient willingness to adhere to the regimen, and rehabilitative regimens [6].

Neurosurgical management of acute central nervous system events in patients with high-titer inhibitors

Appropriate dosing of bypassing agents for major hemorrhagic events or emergency surgery are discussed elsewhere (FEIBA and rFVIIa). As noted there, an invariably reliable hemostasis for such dire circumstances is problematic when such an antibody against FVIII or FIX is present. Nonetheless, effective hemostasis for both CNS events and the accompanying necessary surgery has been demonstrated in many such circumstances [24]. Establishing a treatment plan prospectively for any high-titer inhibitor patient who may, at some point, incur a brain or spinal cord injury based on his known responsiveness to either bypassing agent is probably a sound strategy. Further, careful serial monitoring of his inhibitor titer may indicate when, if ever, very large doses of either FVIII (hemophilia A) or FIX (hemophilia B) might be utilized initially for a temporarily low titer. The use of these factors in such circumstances before anamnesis occurs allows one to demonstrate an adequate measurable *in-vivo* level for the critical period of time immediately following injury. Once the inevitable anamnesis does occur, bypassing agents can be utilized for the duration of the convalescent period. In rare life-threatening circumstances, a combination of bypassing agents and factor replacement may be required to achieve hemostasis. The risks of combining such agents in such events are justified when all other efforts to stop bleeding has failed.

Noncentral nervous system emergent events

Injury in proximity to the airway

Although CNS injury represents the most commonly observed extreme debility or life-threatening injury state in patients with hemophilia, bleeding that has the potential to lead to airway obstruction may represent the most emergent [17]. Extreme trauma may produce sufficient bleeding to immediately compromise the patency of the trachea. Conversely, the period from injury to acute airway compromise may be long (hours, or even days). However, the evolution to criticality may then be rapid

once the patient begins experiencing dyspnea. This symptom implies significant compromise of the tracheal lumen indicating that further bleeding has the immediate potential to progress to asphyxia. Therefore, hemostatic therapy at this stage may need to be administered concurrently with surgical preparation for tracheostomy. Therefore, there is no substitute for early bleed recognition and rapid replacement to forestall this extreme intervention [25].

Neck injuries or retropharyngeal dissecting hematomas (particularly following molar oral surgery) along facial planes of the neck are the most likely initiating events for tracheal compression from hemorrhage. In rare circumstances, an early sign of a bleeding event with the potential to progress to airway compression is facial swelling [26]. In addition, swelling of the tongue owing to unrecognized injury to the lingual artery may progress to a sufficient mass to block the posterior pharynx [27]. To prevent the risks of oral maxillofacial surgery producing such bleeding in a patient with hemophilia, adequate clotting factor replacement therapy (to normal physiologic levels of approximately 100%) is essential [28]. Accordingly, alternative anesthesia to alveolar nerve block for dental surgery will decrease the likelihood of such events. Clearly, prior consultation between the hemostasis expert and the otolaryngologist is necessary to reduce the risks for morbid bleeding in these circumstances. If airway risks are deemed high or any symptoms of airway compromise are present, anesthesia expertise is also needed.

In addition to traumatic injury, rarely medical conditions can lead to hemorrhage-induced airway compromise. There is at least one recent report of a spontaneous epiglottis hematoma requiring emergent management. [29]. Surprisingly, this hemorrhage was not provoked by a recognizable predisposing event such as *Haemophilus influenzae*-associated epiglottitis.

After the initial dose of clotting factor has been administered to treat the recognized hemorrhage in tissues proximal to the airway, follow-up infusions frequent enough to maintain physiologic levels of FVIII or FIX, respectively, or continuous infusion are required, as is frequent monitoring of the FVIII/FIX level. This should be continued until all neck swelling has resolved and/or the surgical wound shows clear signs of healing. Typically, these life-threatening bleeding episodes will require the patient to be hospitalized in a critical care unit until the risks are controlled and to undergo inpatient hemostatic management for at least 1 week. If the patient was not receiving prophylaxis prior to the injury or surgery, a several-week course of outpatient secondary prophylaxis may be prudent until the wound is completely healed.

Gastrointestinal hemorrhage

Bleeding in hemophilia patients can occur from any gut site from the esophagus to the anus. A review by Mittal *et al.* of 41 episodes of gastrointestinal (GI) hemorrhage in patients with hemophilia cited duodenal ulcer (22%) and gastritis (21%) as the most frequent anatomic sites [30]. Yet, in another 22% no source was identified. In a separate series, Mallory–Weiss syndrome (injury to the mucosa of the esophagus, sometimes related to severe coughing) was cited as a cause of GI hemorrhage in hemophilia patients [31].

When bleeding is from the lower GI tract, as indicated by melena in a patient with hemophilia, clotting factor replacement is almost always required to stop the bleeding, regardless of the source. Accordingly, a vigorous attempt to identify a source using colonoscopy, imaging, or both should follow initial replacement, particularly in adult patients where the risk for colon cancer is not insignificant. Usually when the bleeding is mild or moderate, replacement therapy alone suffices unless an anatomic lesion requiring resection is identified [32]. When the amount of blood loss is copious, providing immediate clotting factor replacement to physiologic levels is crucial; followed when the bleeding fails to stop with the appropriate diagnostic measures. The needed interventional therapy is directed by a gastroenterologist.

Age considerations are also important. In a neonate, melena or hematochezia may represent the initial bleeding event in a *de-novo* presentation of a hemophilia phenotype [33]. By contrast, among adult patients with hemophilia and concomitant hepatitis C infection and cirrhosis, acute bleeding from esophageal varices may be life threatening [34,35]. In this instance, immediate hemostatic replacement therapy may need to be followed by gastroenterologic intervention (e.g. transjugular intrahepatic portosystemic shunt). Once the venous pressure in the varices is reduced by such a procedure, follow-up infusions of physiologic doses of clotting factor will be needed to allow the requisite repair to occur.

On occasion, patients with varices or other manifestations of chronic liver failure will have their hemostatic course complicated by the accompanying deficiencies of other liver-produced clotting factors. Particularly vulnerable to impaired synthesis are the vitamin K-dependent serine proteases II, VII, IX, and X. When these are superimposed on both the hemophilia (in particular FVIII deficiency) and the dilated veins, the patient is at very high risk for life-threatening bleeding. In addition to the above therapeutic strategies, replacement of the acquired deficiencies must be undertaken as well. Replacement with either fresh frozen plasma or prothrombin complex concentrate may be required. The latter must be administered judiciously because of the additional possibility of a concomitant thrombosis risk.

Massive melena rarely has hemophilia as the primary etiology. Vascular lesions such as arteriovenous malformations or bleeding telangiectasias are often the etiologies for such massive blood loss from the lower GI tract [36]. Clotting factor replacement initially allows the necessary interventional diagnostic/ therapeutic procedure to be performed, and follow-up infusions are then needed until healing unassociated with occult GI hemorrhage is achieved. The duration will depend also on whether abdominal surgery is required to remove the source of the hemorrhaging.

Bleeding from organ rupture or hematoma of an abdominal viscus

Evolving intraperitoneal hemorrhage caused by blunt abdominal trauma and associated with massive blood loss can, particularly among patients with hemophilia, lead to exsanguination. Typically, a history of recent trauma is present [36]. Rarely among the hemophilia population, however, are reports of bleeding within a viscus evolving to organ rupture without demonstrable trauma [37,38].

It would appear that the circumstances under which this occurs are very rare. However, mild previous traumatic insults may induce low-grade bleeding that becomes recurrent within the confines of the organ. Encapsulated abdominal organs in which this insidious and progressive hemorrhaging have been described include the spleen, liver, kidneys, bowel wall, and pancreas. When the bleeding does not tamponade, the pressure from the expanding hematoma may become sufficiently high to induce rupture of the capsule and extreme acute blood loss [39]. When the event occurs within the wall of the gut, there may also be the risk of gut obstruction prior to actual rupture. Abdominal pain (or abdominal distension in neonates) [40] may be the only symptom. Certainly, any history of recent abdominal trauma, no matter how mild, in a patient with hemophilia should arouse suspicion, probably justify immediate infusion, and, without quick resolution of the pain, necessitate imaging with ultrasound or computed tomography (CT) to identify the presence of a hematoma.

When the presence of such a hematoma is not suspected or if replacement therapy was of insufficient dose or duration following diagnosis, a real risk for rupture exists. When that happens, blood loss can be very large, shock can ensue, and cardiac arrest can follow quickly. Resuscitation with volume expansion, packed red blood cells, and factor replacement are required invariably, and, in many instances, laparotomy may represent the only mechanism to stanch the bleeding. The latter may be necessary to remove the bleeding organ (e.g. splenectomy) [41,42] or to repair it (liver, kidney, or bowel wall) [37]. Early infusion of clotting factor may pre-empt the expansion of the hematoma and forestall surgery in emergent circumstances [43].

Although hematomas of the psoas and obturator muscles represent fairly common bleeding manifestations among patients with severe hemophilia, rarely is the bleeding sufficient to cause a significant drop in hemoglobin. Typically, the bleeding will tamponade. Nonetheless, bleeding can be significant enough to compress sacral nerves, causing significant pain and immobility [44]. Clotting factor replacement and physical therapy by experts in managing hemophilia patients remain the mainstay of therapy for this bleeding event. Rarely is surgery required unless there is evolution to a pseudotumor.

When an individual with hemophilia experiences a rupture of his appendix, it may be difficult to differentiate from pseudohemophilia, which is a small hematoma of the intestinal wall in the area of the right lower quadrant. Either may be associated with no apparent antecedent trauma [45]. Modern imaging techniques should readily distinguish between the two entities [43]. In either instance early replacement therapy is essential, even if abdominal surgery is not contemplated immediately [40].

Symptoms of nerve compression or compartment syndrome

There is a risk for permanent peripheral neurologic debilitation when hemophilic bleeding in a closed anatomic compartment continues until the vascular or neurologic bundles are compromised. This morbidity, occurring in proximal or distal extremities, is known as a "compartment" syndrome and typically is a consequence of either local trauma or iatrogenically induced bleeding. Examples of the latter include aborted attempts at arterial cannulation or venepuncture (particularly among neonates and small infants). Symptoms begin as swelling and engorgement and, if the bleeding continues into the confined space, progress to paresthesia or even paresis, arterial compression, loss of pulse, and a cold extremity.

As with suspected CNS hemorrhage, early recognition followed by aggressive clotting factor replacement can prevent this evolution of morbidity. In those instances when the injured extremity is clearly cooler and paler than the contralateral one, surgical fasciotomy may be necessary. However, fasciotomies in patients with hemophilia are fraught with risk for protracted bleeding even when prior replacement therapy has been given. Therefore, a good strategy is education of patients about the possibility of a compartment syndrome when closed extremity bleeding is progressing. This recognition must be combined with immediate dosing of factor concentrate to achieve a level of approximately 100% of normal. Thereby, most fasciotomies can be avoided.

Ophthalmologic emergencies

When bleeding occurs in a hemophilia patient's eye (usually following facial or head trauma) [46], this is an extremely emergent event. Bleeding into the anterior chamber (hyphema), vitreous humor, or lens (the rare entity known as hemorrhagic glaucoma) [47–49] jeopardizes vision both acutely and, if of significant magnitude, permanently. Sight can also be compromised by a retinal hematoma forming at the site of a retinal detachment. As with many of the emergent strategies discussed above, a parallel strategy of therapeutic intervention is essential: immediate administration of clotting factor sufficient to raise the *in-vivo* level to 100% *and* urgent assessment by an experienced ophthalmologist. Hospitalization until the clinical situation stabilizes is necessary even if eye surgery is felt not to be indicated. Following discharge from the hospital, collaborative outpatient management by both the ophthalmologist and the hemophilia physician is essential to insure an optimal outcome.

Rare clinical emergencies

Some bleeding events are considered emergent whether or not there is an underlying bleeding disorder. Examples include pericardial bleeding, which can cause life-ending tamponade, or pulmonary hemorrhage of a severity, which can cause severe respiratory distress. In those rare circumstances when these occur in patients with hemophilia, the management complexity increases. The emergency surgery necessary to save the hemophilic individual's life cannot be permitted to exacerbate the bleeding itself because of insufficient concomitant to treatment of the patient's hemophilia.

Rupture of a pseudotumor

Although the presence of a hemophilic pseudotumor does not constitute a hemostatic emergency, rupture of a large one in the pelvis or thigh can lead to massive hemorrhage and shock [50]. Immediate replacement therapy with sufficient FVIII or FIX, respectively, to an *in-vivo* level of 1 U/mL (100%) is required. However, since pseudotumors typically have large volumes of partially clotted blood that has induced significant fibrinolysis, fibrin degradation products may be released, which slow the rate of new fibrin cross-linking. This can predispose to further bleeding even when the FVIII/FIX levels are normal. Laboratory assessment for such secondary fibrinolysis is therefore indicated. When present, concurrent therapy with a fibrinolytic inhibitor such as ε-aminocaproic acid or tranexamic acid may also be needed. Further, surgical resection/evacuation of the remnants the tumor may be needed for healing to occur.

Conclusion

Life-threatening bleeding is uncommon in patients with hemophilia. When such bleeding occurs it is often the result of an injury that would induce severe bleeding even in an individual without an underlying bleeding disorder. For the hemophilic patient, however, restoration of the plasma level of the missing procoagulant (FVIII or FIX) to normal is essential in such circumstances so that other necessary medical interventions to treat the injury do not compound the hemorrhagic state. In terms of priority, only the removal of an acutely injurious agent or cardiopulmonary resuscitation take precedent over clotting factor replacement in an injured individual with hemophilia. This is true regardless of the severity of the hemophilia. Further, initial clotting factor replacement must be followed by recurrent dosing or continuous administration until sufficient healing has occurred. Simultaneous laboratory measurement to insure adequate *in-vivo* levels should be done if at all possible. There also may be special medical management that is required to treat the specific injury or disease state. For these, the expertise of the appropriate medical specialist should be sought. Knowledge of the specialized hemostatic management required in such scenarios and prior discussion of how to proceed in the respective circumstance can help to assure a good clinical outcome when these daunting events do happen.

References

1 Darby SC, Kan SW, Spooner RJ, *et al.* Mortality rates, life expectancy, and causes of death in people with hemophilia A or B in the United Kingdom who were not infected with HIV. *Blood* 2007; **110**: 815–25.

2 Visconti EB, Hilgartner MW. Recognition and management of central nervous hemorrhage in hemophilia. *Pediatrician* 1980; **9**: 127–37.

3 Federici A, Minetti D, Grande C, Gatti L, Mannucci PM. Intracranial bleeding in haemophilia: A study of eleven cases. *Haematologica* 1982; **67**: 747–53.

4 Constantine S, Buckley J, Heysen J. Imaging of the haemorrhagic complications of the haemorrhagic complications of the haemophilias. *J Med Imaging Rad Oncol* 2009; **53**: 13–21.

5 Nuss R, Soucie JM, Evatt B, and the Hemophilia Surveillance System Project Investigators. Changes in the occurrence of and risk factors for hemophilia-associated intracranial hemorrhage. *Am J Hematol* 2001; **68**: 37–42.

6 Hoots WK. Emergency care issues in hemophilia, treatment of hemophilia monograph no. 43, World Federation of Hemophilia, November 2007.

7 Tseng SH. Delay traumatic intracerebral hemorrhage: a study of prognostic factors. *J Formos Med Assoc* 1992; **91**: 585–9.

8 Mamoli B, Sonneck G, Lechner K. Intracranial and spinal hemorrhage in hemophilia. *J Neurol* 1976; **211**: 143–54.

9 Walike JW, Chinn J. Evaluation and treatment of acute bleeding from the head and neck. *Otolaryngol Clin North Am* 1979; **12**: 455–64.

10 Bentacor N, Lavalle E, Vila VM, Johnston E, Borovich B. Intracranial hemorrhage in hemophiliacs. Study of 10 episodes. *Sangre* 1992; **37**: 43–6.

11 Borthne A, Sortland O, Blikra G. Head injuries with delayed intracranial hemorrhage. *Tidsskr Nor Laegeforen* 1992; **112**: 3425–8.

12 Yoffe G, Buchanan G. Intracranial hemorrhage in newborn and young infants with hemophilia. *J Pediatr* 1988; **113**: 333–6.

13 Martinowitz U, Heim M, Tadmor R, *et al.* Intracranial hemorrhage in patients with hemophilia. *Neurosurgery* 1986; **18**: 538–41.

14 DeBehnke DJ, Angelos MG. Intracranial hemorrhage and hemophilia: case report and management guidelines. *J Emerg Med* 1990; **8**: 423–7.

15 Ohga S, Kajiwara M, Toubo Y, *et al.* Neonatal hemophilia B with intracranial hemorrhage. *Am J Pediatr Hematol Oncol* 1988; **10**: 244–8.

16 Kulkarni R, Lusher JM. Intracranial and extracranial hemorrhages in newborns with hemophilia: a review of the literature. *J Pediatr Hematol Oncol* 1999; **21**: 289–95.

17 Bray GL, Luban NLC. Hemophilia presenting with intracranial hemorrhage. *Am J Cardiovasc Dis* 1987; **141**: 1215–17.

18 Pettersson H, McClure P, Fitz C. Intracranial hemorrhage in hemophilic children. *ACTA Radiol* 1984; **25**: 161–4.

19 Myles LM, Massicotte P, Drake J. Intracranial hemorrhage in neonates with unrecognized hemophilia A: a persisting problem. *Pediatr Neurosurg* 2001; **34**: 94–7.

20 Yasouka S, Peterson HA, McCarty CS. Incidence of spinal column deformity after multi level laminectomy in children and adults. *J Neurosurg* 1982; **57**: 441–5.

21 Narawong D, Gibbons VP, McLaughlin JR, Bouhasin JD, Kotagal S. Conservative management of spinal epidural hematoma in hemophilia. *Pediatr Neurol* 1988; **4**: 169–71.

22 Blatt PM, Goldsmith JC, Roberts HM. Prothrombin complex concentrates. *Arch Intern Med* 1978; **138**: 827.

23 Eyster ME, Gill FM, Blatt PM, Hilgartner MW, Ballard JD, McKinney TR. Central nervous system bleeding hemophiliacs. *Blood* 1978; **51**: 1179–88.

24 Negrier C, Hay CM. The treatment of bleeding in hemophilia patients with inhibitors with recombinant factor VIIa. *Semin Thromb Hemost* 2000; **26**: 407–12.

25 Roderick PJ, Robinson AC. Life-threatening oro-pharyngeal bleeding in a haemophiliac with factor VIII inhibitors. *Clin Lab Haemat* 1988; **10**: 217–19.

26 Bogdan CJ, Strauss M, Ratnoff OD. Airway obstruction in hemophilia (factor VIII deficiency): a 28-year institutional review. *Laryngoscope* 1994; **104**: 789–94.

27 Kuhlmann TP, Abidin MR, Neal DA. Computed tomography diagnosis of acute facial swelling in an adult hemophiliac. *Ann Emerg Med* 1989; **18**: 681–3.

28 Chase CR, Hebert JC, Franham JE. Post-traumatic upper airway obstruction secondary to lingual artery hematoma. *J Trauma* 1987; **27**: 593–4.

29 Hishoren N, Varon D, Weinberger JM, Gross M. Airway obstruction and haemophilia A: epiglottis hematoma. *Laryngoscope* 2010; **120**: 1428–9.

30 Mittal R, Spero J, Lewis JH, *et al.* Patterns of gastrointestinal hemorrhage in hemophilia. *Gastroenterology* 1985; **88**: 515–22.

31 Lander E, Pechlander C, Mayr A, Mortl M, Probst A. Mallory–Weiss syndrome in a patient with hemophilia A and chronic liver disease. *Ital J Gastroenterol* 1995; **27**: 73–4.

32 Reish O, Nachum E, Naor N, Ghoshen J, Nerlob P. Hemophilia B in a neonate: unusual early spontaneous gastrointestinal bleeding. *Am J Perinatol* 1994; **11**: 192–3.

33 Lander E, Pechlaner C, Mayr A, Mortl M, Propst A. Mallory–Weiss syndrome in a patient with hemophilia A and chronic liver disease. *Ital J Gastroenterol* 1995; **27**: 73–4.

34 Singh R, Clarkston W, Zuckerman DA, Joist JH, Bacon BR. Transjugular intrahepatic portosystemic shunt for palliation of bleeding esophageal varices in a patient with severe hemophilia A, advanced HIV infection, and cirrhosis. *Am J Gastroenterol* 1993; **88**: 2112–14.

35 Griffin PH, Chopra S. Spontaneous intramural gastric hematoma: a unique presentation for hemophilia. *Am J Gastroenterol* 1985; **80**: 430–3.

36 Nigam K, Hughes RG, Murphy B. Conservative management of splenic rupture in a haemophiliac adult. *J Roy Coll Surg Edinb* 1998; **43**: 57.

37 Brook J, Newnam P. Spontaneous rupture of the spleen in hemophilia. *Arch Intern Med* 1965; **115**: 595–7.

38 Jones JJ, Kitchens C. Spontaneous intra-abdominal hemorrhage in hemophilia. *Arch Intern Med* 1984; **144**: 297–300.

39 Quick AJ. Emergencies in hemophilia. *Am J Med Sci* 1966; **251**: 409–16.

40 Johnson-Robbins LA, Porter JC, Horgan MJ. Splenic rupture in a newborn with hemophilia A: case report and review of the literature. *Clin Pediatr* 1999; **38**: 117–19.

41 Weintraub WH. Nonsurgical therapy of splenic rupture in a hemophiliac. *J Pediatr Surg* 1992; **27**: 1486.

42 Fort DW, Bernini JC, Johnson A, Cochran CJ, Buchanan GR. Splenic rupture in hemophilia. *Am J Pediatr Hematol Oncol* 1994; **16**: 255–9.

43 Terry NE, Boswell WC. Nonoperative management of delayed splenic rupture in a patient with hemophilia B. *J Pediatr Surg* 2006; **41**: 1607–9.

44 Willbanks OL, Willbanks SE. Femoral neuropathy due to retroperitoneal bleeding. *Am J Surg* 1983; **145**: 193–8.

45 McCoy HE III, Kitchens CS. Small bowel hematoma in a hemophiliac as a cause of pseudoappendicitis: diagnosis by CT imaging. *Am J Hematol* 1991; **38**: 138–9.

46 Morsman CDG, Holmes J. Traumatic hyphaema in a haemophiliac. *Br J Ophthalmology* 1990; **74**: 563.

47 Kobayashi H, Honda Y. Intraocular hemorrhage in a patient with hemophilia. *Metab Ophthalmol* 1984–5; **8**: 27–30.

48 Theobald T, Davitt BV, Shields SR. Hemorrhagic glaucoma in an infant with hemophilia, spontaneous hyphema, aniridia, and persistent iris vessels. *J AAPOS* 2001; **5**: 129–30.

49 Lifshitz T, Yermiahu T, Biedner B, Yassur Y. Traumatic total hyphema in a patient with severe hemophilia. *J Pediatr Ophthalmol Strabismus* 1986; **23**: 80–1.

50 Gilbert MS. Characterizing the hemophilic pseudotumor. *Ann NY Acad Sci* 1975; **240**: 311–15.

PART XVIII

Evaluation of hemophilia

CHAPTER 63

Clinical trials and other methodologies

Sharyne M. Donfield and Alice E. Lail

Rho Inc., North Carolina, USA

Introduction

While the clinical needs of people affected with rare diseases vary widely, many of the methodologic and statistical approaches used in the research of disorders will be similar. The challenges of small clinical trials apply not only to the study of rare diseases and individually tailored therapies, but also to unique study populations, e.g. astronauts, those in emergency situations, or persons in isolated environments [1]. The need for the development of innovative designs for small clinical trials in rare bleeding disorders and the equally urgent task of refining and expanding definitions for use in hemophilia research are being addressed by project groups of the Factor VIII/IX Subcommittee [2]. There are direct links between standardization, data quality, and power for analysis. By standardizing definitions and procedures, variability is reduced, precision of estimates is increased, statistical power is increased, and the return for sample size is greater. It's all about power.

Type of study designs

Parallel-group design is the most commonly used randomized clinical trial approach for assigning subjects to a treatment. Subjects are assigned at random to a treatment arm and remain in that intervention until the end of the study. This permits observation of the long-term effects of the treatment, but the design is vulnerable to drop-out and missing values. Randomization is important because it reduces selection bias, is a basis for inference, and can balance factors, both known and unknown, across treatment groups. In small trials, however, there can be an imbalance in randomization. There are many ways of handling this. Factors can be controlled for in the analysis after completion of the study. Randomization can be stratified. For example, if we wanted to balance randomization across severity of hemophilia, then we could stratify the randomization by severity. Finally, an adaptive randomization could be used. One of the most common is that proposed by Pocock

and Simon [3]. This method measures the imbalance for each factor and then assigns a probability of being randomized to a certain treatment group based on the imbalance. Perhaps the biggest drawback to this method is that it can be difficult to implement, as it requires centralized randomization.

A *cross-over study* comparison of treatments or interventions is one in which the subject completes the course of one treatment, has a washout period, then is switched to the other treatment. The order of treatments received is random. A major advantage [4] of use of the cross-over design for studies of rare bleeding disorders is the statistical efficiency: because each subject serves as his own control, the sample size can be greatly reduced relative to a parallel-group design. The disadvantages relate to possible carryover of the effects of the first treatment to the second treatment, thus care must be taken to identify a sufficiently long washout period between administrations of the two treatments.

An *equivalence design* can be used to test whether two therapies are similar to one another within some specified amount [5]. While typically, inferential statistics focus on evaluating differences between two groups, sometimes we want to show that two groups are the same or that one group is not worse than another with respect to some characteristic. To do this, we must first define what we mean by "the same" or "not different." This criterion should be clinically meaningful. The FEIBA Novo-Seven Comparative (FENOC) study, for example, evaluated two bypassing agents used in the treatment of joint bleeding in congenital hemophilia A complicated by inhibitors [6]. A difference in efficacy of no more than 15% at 6 h after treatment was determined to be a clinically acceptable magnitude for equivalence. If the treatments of interest do not meet the criteria for equivalence, it is important to understand that this does not mean that they are (statistically) different. Equally important is to note the distinction between statistically significant and clinically significant. A common belief is that the sample size requirements for an equivalence study or a noninferiority study are greater than those for studies designed to show a difference. This is not necessarily the case: the required sample size might be greater or

Textbook of Hemophilia, Third Edition. Edited by Christine A. Lee, Erik E. Berntorp and W. Keith Hoots.
© 2014 John Wiley & Sons, Ltd. Published 2014 by John Wiley & Sons, Ltd.

less, depending on the specific assumptions made. Figure 63.1 shows examples of possible outcomes for equivalence and non-inferiority studies.

An *adaptive design* uses accumulating data to modify key aspects of the study design as it continues, including re-estimation of the required sample size [7], adding or dropping doses in a dose-finding study, and seamless phase II/III designs [8]. While the concept is quite attractive, these studies raise significant logistical and statistical issues in terms of compiling data, completing interim analyses, and making informed decisions in a timely manner [9].

Epidemiologic studies are observational, nonexperimental, and include cohort (prospective), case–control (retrospective) and cross-sectional (prevalence) studies. The longitudinal, repeated measures design of cohort studies makes them the most powerful of the epidemiologic studies. The strongest are those that are population based, or indeed, a population as is the case of investigations using countries as the units of comparison, e.g. Norway and Sweden [10], to compare outcome by types of treatment (e.g. prophylaxis vs on demand), and Sweden and the Netherlands in studies of prophylactic treatment examining dosing strategy, outcomes, and the economics of treatment [11].

Surveys and registries contain information systematically collected and are excellent tools for surveillance. They are also useful as sampling frames from which to select subjects for more intensive study, and can provide information about rates of occurrence of events for use in study feasibility determination or sample size calculation.

Multicenter and international studies increase the potential for rapid enrollment of study participants, permitting accrual of sufficient numbers to meet sample size requirements. They also increase the generalizability of study findings, i.e. the extent to which the findings apply to other populations [12]. International multicenter studies present significant, but usually surmountable, challenges including language differences, country-specific research standards, as well as practical complications including time zone differences, travel time, and expense, and logistics of data and sample shipping. For international studies to succeed, their objectives must be definable, measurable, and attainable across multiple countries and languages: further support for the international effort to develop consensus definitions for use in hemophilia research [2].

Statistical considerations

Statistical models provide a method for examining the relationships between variables. Models consist of one outcome variable and one or more predictor variables. The predictor variables will include the variable of interest but may also include covariates (confounding or interacting variables). Table 63.1 lists several of the most common types of statistical models. The type of model will vary by the outcome of interest, and each model produces a different output, e.g. means, odds ratios, rate ratios, or hazard ratios. The analogous "nonmodel" test is also shown in Table 63.1.

It is often the case that we are interested in modeling correlated data such as data from cross-over studies, repeated measurements collected in a longitudinal study, or those from brother pairs or related subjects. Because models assume that each observation is independent of the others, and therefore not correlated, it is necessary to control for any correlation in your model. All of the models shown in Table 63.1 can be adapted to control for correlated data.

One last type of model to consider is the zero-inflated model, which is useful for analyzing left- or right-censored continuous

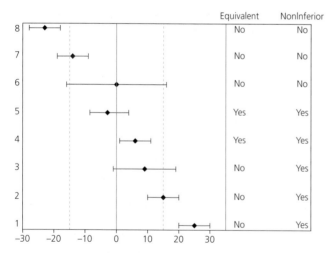

Figure 63.1 The vertical axis shows the line number and the horizontal axis shows the difference in the means. Dashed reference lines show the boundaries at −15 and 15. Lines 4 and 5 are the only two that would meet the definition for equivalence because both the lower and upper confidence intervals are contained within the pre-specified boundaries at −15 and 15. Even though the confidence interval on line 4 does not cross zero, and is therefore a significant difference, it is still considered equivalent because it is contained within the pre-specified boundaries. Lines 1–5 meet the criteria for noninferiority because none of the lower confidence intervals cross the lower boundary.

Table 63.1 The most common types of statistical models.

Model type	Outcome variable	Output	Nonmodel analog
Linear regression	Continuous	Means and slopes	T-test, ANOVA
Logistic regression	Binary category categorical variable (yes/no or disease/no disease)	Odds ratios	Chi-square
Poisson regression	Count data (rare events)	Rate ratios	Chi-square
Cox proportional hazard	Time to event data	Hazard ratios	Kaplan–Meier

data. An example of left-censored continuous data is inhibitory antibodies. Study subjects not having an inhibitor will be below the limit of detection for the assay, while those with an inhibitor will often have log normally distributed titer values. Using a zero-inflated model, one can estimate both the probability of having an inhibitor as well as the mean titer value within the same model.

In general, the use of a continuous variable as an *outcome* provides greater statistical power than the use of a categorical variable (e.g. low/high). This is because there are rarely natural cut points for data and by forcing continuous data such as age or laboratory values into categories, some information is lost. In addition, making decisions as to the appropriate cut point(s) to use to categorize the variable is often quite difficult. Results can vary widely based on where cut points are made. There are a number of opinions as to how best to make the selection [13–15]; however, if there is a cut point that has been traditionally used, it may be worthwhile to categorize a variable to permit comparison with other studies.

A *covariate* is a variable that may have an association with the outcome, either as a variable of direct interest or a confounder. It is sometimes the case that an apparent relationship between the variable of interest and the outcome variable disappears after including a confounding variable in a model. Examples of this in the hemophilia literature include the association between increased risk for development of inhibitors among children exposed to treatment early in life [16] that largely disappeared after adjustment for intensity of treatment [17]; an association between *F8* haplotype and inhibitor risk observed in two cohorts [18,19] that was not apparent after adjustment for type of *F8* mutation in the second study [19]. Determining those confounders that exhibit independence from the variable of interest ensures that the overlap in variance in the fitted model attributed to each predictor is limited. A higher proportion of variance accounted for in the final model improves confidence in the estimates. Choice of covariates provides opportunities to either increase or decrease power, depending on decisions made. An example is the observation that treatment with prophylaxis (variable of interest), per se, was not associated with better test scores on academic achievement tests in a cohort ($n = 126$) of children aged 6 to 12 years with hemophilia because of a high degree of heterogeneity within the prophylaxis category in terms of duration of treatment and compliance with regimen. However, children treated on a regimen of long-term prophylaxis >40% of their lifetime with bleeding rates below the median for the entire group had significantly higher scores in total achievement, mathematics, and reading [20]. Increasing the precision of the predictor decreased the variability, increasing the power of the analysis.

Interactions occur when the variable of interest behaves differently with respect to the outcome variable based on the value of the covariate that you are controlling for. Figure 63.2 shows an example of an interaction. The vertical axis is the outcome and the horizontal axis is the variable of interest. The covariate

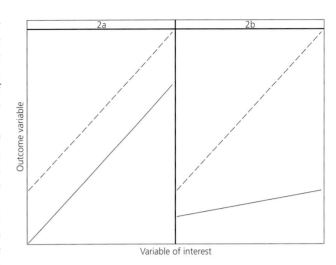

Figure 63.2 Example of an interaction between two variables.

that is being controlled for has two values (e.g. inhibitor/no inhibitor) that are represented by the solid and dashed lines. In the first panel, there is no interaction. The variable of interest behaves the same for both groups of the covariate. As a result, the regression lines are parallel. In the second panel, there is an interaction—the variable of interest does not increase as much in the group represented by the solid line as it does in the other group. The relationship between the variable of interest and the outcome are different for the two values of the covariates. In multicenter clinical trials, the most common type of interaction to test for is a treatment by center interaction. In other words, does the treatment work the same at all the centers that were in the study. Treatment-by-time interactions are also common in both clinical and epidemiologic studies.

Bayesian inference is based on a probability theorem that updates the *prior* probability of a hypothesis with evidence from current data to arrive at the *posterior* probability of the hypothesis. The ability to provide a prognosis for individual patients is one of the reasons why Bayesian reasoning is becoming more popular in clinical trials.

A typical conclusion from a comparison of two hemophilia treatments may be that subjects randomized to treatment A will on average have *x* fewer bleeding episodes compared to those randomized to treatment B. However, it does not imply that the next subject (even if he resembles the average patient) undergoing treatment A will actually have *x* less bleeding episodes. Moreover, neither the *P* value from a significance test of the two treatments nor the confidence interval constructed for the difference between the two can tell how likely it is that a patient on treatment A will have *x* fewer bleeding episodes. In fact, the interpretation of these two frequentist inferential tools defies common conceptions about the conclusions of a clinical trial.

By definition, the *P* value is the probability of observing something as extreme or more extreme than the current result, assuming H_0, the null hypothesis (i.e. treatments A and B have the same efficacy), to be true. Although a small P value, say 0.05, allows us to "reject the null hypothesis" it does not mean that the probability of H_0 is 5% or, equivalently, the probability of the alternative hypothesis (i.e. two treatments differ in efficacy) is 95%. This is because the P value is calculated on the premise that H_0 is true; therefore, it cannot possibly tell us how likely it is that H_0 is true. Similarly, many misconstrue the 95% confidence interval to be the actual values where the treatment difference lies with 95% probability when in reality 95% confidence means that the method used to construct the confidence interval will have, in the long run, 95% accuracy of including the treatment difference under repeated sampling.

In contrast, Bayesian reasoning uses the evidence of the trial to directly infer the plausibility of the null versus the alternative hypothesis. It can calculate the probability that two treatments differ by some pre-specified clinically meaningful difference, and also the predictive probability that a new patient prescribed treatment A will have x fewer bleeding episodes. Furthermore, when a uniform or vague prior distribution is applied to Bayes theorem, the 95% confidence interval can be interpreted as a credible interval where the treatment difference spans with 95% probability. This corresponds to the situation where there is no prior preference of what values the treatment difference will take (i.e. the treatment difference is equally likely from $-\infty$ to ∞), and provides a bridge between the frequentist and Bayesian intervals. When earlier studies document possible treatment differences, the prior distribution can be chosen to cluster around these values to provide a more informed Bayesian analysis of the data. Aside from its advantages in prediction and interpretation, Bayesian inference is naturally suited for interim analyses since Bayes theorem can be repeatedly applied as subject outcomes accrue in the trial, potentially resulting in smaller or more rapidly completed trials. Other benefits include its flexibility to changes in sample sizes, adaptive randomization, and even postprotocol trial modifications like addition or removal of treatment regimens [21].

The main criticism against Bayesian reasoning is the subjectivity involved in constructing the prior distribution as different stakeholders in a clinical trial may very well favor different prior distributions. However, one must not forget that the frequentist approach is also subjective in its choice of α and β, detectable effect size, and study design. Unfortunately, certain preferences (e.g. 5% α, 20% β) have become so popular that some regard them as objective standards, forgetting that a $P = 0.10$ can be "statistically nonsignificant" to one but "showing a trend towards significance" to another. Neither Bayesian nor frequentist approaches will abrogate the necessity of dealing with subjectivity, but the former deals with it explicitly rather than under a facade of objectivity.

Drop-outs and missing data are inevitable in clinical research. Participants may be withdrawn from the intervention because of death, competing risks, safety concerns, lack of efficacy, and personal choice. Statistical procedures are available to address this issue through a procedure called imputation, where an estimated value is substituted for the missing one. Multiple imputation techniques [22,23] involve filling in the missing data with good estimates of what the missing data would have been. Multiple imputation is only valid when the data are missing at random, i.e. not due to a specific reason. There are a number of imputation methods, some techniques more advanced or specific; however, all methods entail a number of "untestable and unverifiable" assumptions that limit their utility [24]. The best defense is to avoid missing data to the degree possible through careful construction of data collection materials, training and performance monitoring of data collectors at the onset and throughout the period of study.

Conclusion

There are many avenues for hemophilia-related research, ranging from basic science to epidemiologic studies and clinical trials, with goals ranging from development of new and better treatments, optimum dose strategies, efforts to identify genetic and environmental contributors to complications, and the best methods for eradication of these, as well as issues related to tailoring treatment from the onset and throughout life. Since by definition the sample sizes in investigations of rare diseases will be small, every opportunity must be taken to maximize the value of each study subject enrolled, from the identification of design and objectives, choice of predictors and outcomes, collection and management of data, through selection of statistical methods for analysis.

The importance of statistician input from study start through conclusion cannot be overestimated. In addition to involvement during the planning phase of an investigation, statisticians are needed to provide interim analyses for data and safety monitoring, reports for sponsors and regulatory agencies, and they have a crucial role in the publication of results in the literature. In addition to helping you get the most from your data, statisticians will be reviewing your manuscripts and applications for research support. Publication and funding decisions are very often based on their recommendations.

Acknowledgments

We wish to thank our Rho, Inc. colleagues for their contributions to this chapter: Henry Lynn, PhD, Karen Kesler, PhD, John Schwarz, PhD, James Rochon, PhD, and Stacey Murphy, MS.

References

1 Evans CH, Ildstad ST (eds.). *Small Clinical Trials: issues and challenges.* Washington DC: National Academies Press, 2001.

2 DiMichele D, Blanchette V, Berntorp E. Clinical trial design in haemophilia. *Haemophilia* 2012; **18**(s4): 18–23.

3 Pocock SJ, Simon R. Sequential treatment assignment with balancing for prognostic factors in the controlled clinical trial. *Biometrics* 1975; **31**: 103–15.

4 Jones B, Kenward MG. *Design and Analysis of Cross-over Trials.* London: Chapman & Hall/CRC, 2003.

5 Blackwelder WC. "Proving the null hypothesis" in clinical trials. *Control Clin Trials* 1982; **3**(4): 345–53.

6 Astermark J, Donfield SM, DiMichele DM, *et al.* A randomized comparison of bypassing agents in hemophilia complicated by an inhibitor: the FEIBA NovoSeven Comparative (FENOC) Study. *Blood* 2007; **109**(2): 546–51.

7 Cui L, Hung H, Wang SJ. Modification of sample size in group sequential clinical trials. *Biometrics* 1999; **55**(3): 853–7.

8 Maca J, Bhattacharya S, Dragalin V, Gallo P, Krams M. Adaptive seamless phase II/III designs—background, operational aspects, and examples. *Drug Inf J* 2006; **40**: 463–73.

9 Gallo P. Operational challenges in adaptive design implementation. *Pharm Stat* 2006; **5**(2): 119–24.

10 Steen Carlsson K, Höjgård S, Glomstein A, *et al.* On demand vs. prophylactic treatment for severe haemophilia in Norway and Sweden: differences in treatment characteristics and outcome. *Haemophilia* 2003; **9**(5): 555–66.

11 Berntorp E, Fischer K, Miners A. Models of prophylaxis. *Haemophilia* 2012; **18**(s4): 136–40.

12 Blumenstein BA, James KE, Lind BK, Mitchell HE. Functions and organization of coordinating centers for multicenter studies. *Control Clin Trials* 1995; **16**(2): 4S–29S.

13 Altman DG, Lausen B, Sauerbrei W, Schumacher M. Dangers of using "optimal" cutpoints in the evaluation of prognostic factors. *J Natl Cancer Inst* 1994; **86**(11): 829–35.

14 Ragland DR. Dichotomizing continuous outcome variables: dependence of the magnitude of association and statistical power on the cutpoint. *Epidemiology* 1992; **3**: 434–40.

15 Suissa S, Blais L. Binary regression with continuous outcomes. *Stat Med* 1995; **14**(3): 247–55.

16 van der Bom JG, Mauser-Bunschoten EP, Fischer K, van den Berg HM. Age at first treatment and immune tolerance to factor VIII in severe hemophilia. *Thromb Haemost* 2003; **89**(3): 475–9.

17 Gouw SC, van der Bom JG, Auerswald G, Ettinghausen CE, Tedgård U, van den Berg HM. Recombinant versus plasma-derived factor VIII products and the development of inhibitors in previously untreated patients with severe hemophilia A: the CANAL cohort study. *Blood* 2007; **109**(11): 4693–7.

18 Viel KR, Ameri A, Abshire TC, *et al.* Inhibitors of factor VIII in black patients with hemophilia. *N Engl J Med* 2009; **360**(16): 1618–27.

19 Schwarz J, Astermark J, Menius E, *et al.* F8 haplotype and inhibitor risk: results from the Hemophilia Inhibitor Genetics Study (HIGS) Combined Cohort. *Haemophilia* 2012; **19**: 113–18.

20 Shapiro AD, Donfield SM, Lynn HS, *et al.* Defining the impact of hemophilia: the Academic Achievement in Children with Hemophilia Study. *Pediatrics* 2001; **108**(6): e105.

21 Berry DA. Introduction to Bayesian methods III: use and interpretation of Bayesian tools in design and analysis. *Clin Trials* 2005; **2**(4): 295–300; discussion 301–4, 364–78.

22 Lavori PW, Dawson R, Shera D. A multiple imputation strategy for clinical trials with truncation of patient data. *Stat Med* 1995; **14**(17): 1913–25.

23 Schafer JL. Multiple imputation: a primer. *Stat Methods Med Res* 1999; **8**(1): 3–15.

24 Verbeke G, Molenberghs G. *Linear Mixed Models for Longitudinal Data.* Berlin: Springer-Verlag; 2000.

CHAPTER 64

Quality of life in hemophilia

Sylvia von Mackensen[1] and Alessandro Gringeri[2]

[1] University Medical Centre of Hamburg-Eppendorf, Hamburg, Germany
[2] Baxter Innovations, Vienna, Austria

Introduction

Hemophilia is a congenital life-threatening disorder characterized by spontaneous and post-traumatic bleeding events in joints, muscles, and other soft tissues; these manifestations, when not prevented, inexorably lead to severe pain, arthropathy, and disability with detriment of quality of life (QoL). The modern management of hemophilia has visibly influenced not only clinical symptoms, orthopedic outcome, and survival of patients but also their perceived QoL [1].

Nevertheless, other concerns continue to challenge hemophilia management: the risk for plasma-derived and recombinant concentrates of contaminating viruses or prions and the risk of development of inhibitory antibodies that still involve about 25% of patients who are exposed for the first time to coagulation factors. Inhibitors often result in an increased number of muscle, joint, and deep-tissue bleeds and an increased risk of disability [2].

All these characteristics of hemophilia care require the absorption of a huge amount of human and economic resources, in a time of ever-increasing fiscal constraints [3, 4]. These staggering costs of care must be considered not only in the context of morbidity and mortality but also of QoL.

Improvement of patient wellbeing and QoL has always been one of the goals of healthcare professionals and is indeed increasingly regarded as one of the most relevant health outcome measure in medicine [5]. Health outcome data are essential to optimize treatments and allocate resources in a cost-intensive chronic disease such as hemophilia where traditional outcome measures such as mortality are no longer influenced by diverse treatment options.

Quality of life

Several definitions ranging from operational to more philosophical approaches are available and well accepted in the international QoL field [6].

Definition of quality of life

A general definition of QoL was provided by the World Health Organization (WHO), which defined QoL as "individuals' perceptions of their position in life in the context of culture and value systems in which they live, and in relation to their goals, expectations, standards, and concerns" [7]. In medicine, the term QoL much more implies how the disease or the treatment is affecting the different aspects of life. Therefore, the term "health-related quality of life" (HRQoL) was created [8]: "Health-related quality of life (HRQoL) is a multidimensional construct pertaining to the physical, emotional, mental, social and behavioral components of wellbeing and function as perceived by the patients and/or observers" [9]. HRQoL is not only influenced by a disease and its treatment but also by personal characteristics such as coping or internal locus of control as well as by living conditions and socioeconomic status.

Issues concerning quality of life

Quality of life assessment is considered an important outcome measure in medicine from an epidemiologic perspective describing the wellbeing and function of patients, from a clinical perspective evaluating treatment intervention effects on wellbeing and from a health economics perspective, where analyses of quality and cost of care are associated.

Quality of life research is based on different theoretical models such as the concept of satisfaction, social comparison approaches, expectation models, as well as the so-called needs models. A widely used utility measure is the patient preference measure assessing the importance attributed to different health status conditions. One of the most important issues in QoL assessment is the direct perception of patients. It is well known that observers overestimate some aspects of QoL of patients, whereas psychologic aspects are often underestimated. It is recommended to use self-rated measures (so-called subjective measures) in which the patient is directly asked about his/her assessment of health and wellbeing [10]. Other-rated measures, or "proxy" measures, are used in young

Textbook of Hemophilia, Third Edition. Edited by Christine A. Lee, Erik E. Berntorp and W. Keith Hoots.
© 2014 John Wiley & Sons, Ltd. Published 2014 by John Wiley & Sons, Ltd.

children or patients unable to answer (e.g. mentally impaired patients). In this case, parents or other caregivers related with the patient should be asked. Since there is only a moderate concordance between self- and parent-reported QoL, both assessments are required when possible [11], especially in adolescents who are increasingly involved in their own health-care decisions [12].

Instrument characteristics

Quality of life assessment must be differentiated according to measures for adults and measures for children. The assessment of QoL in children with chronic conditions has increased in the last years, but it is still in need of development for the majority of pediatric health conditions. QoL assessment in children should involve the parents perception of children's QoL as well as the rating of their own QoL, including perceptions of the child's siblings. These instruments for children should be especially developed considering age groups and developmental status. In small children, the parents' reports of children's well-being are necessary, while in grown-up children the comparison between children's and parent's perspectives turns out to be of interest by itself [13].

Development of quality of life instruments

For the construction of a new QoL instrument different steps must be considered: (1) development; (2) translation (for international use); (3) testing; and (4) norming [14]. An instrument should be developed by specifying measurement goals and by generating items by focus groups (e.g. healthcare professionals and patients). Subsequently, items should be pretested and patients should be asked about how they understood each single item (cognitive debriefing). After item review and reduction, the questionnaire can be pilot-tested in order to examine its feasibility. In international studies the questionnaire must be translated into the respective languages following internationally recommended translation rules [15] with forward and backward translations. Different approaches for the international scale development include: (1) a sequential approach, in which the instrument is originated in one country and then translated into other languages; (2) a parallel approach, in which the instrument is developed in parallel in different countries with common dimensions and items; and (3) a simultaneous approach, in which the items are identified nationally and then translated into English [16]. It is important in the comparison of QoL across different countries, that instruments were cross-culturally equivalent [17].

The questionnaire must then be *psychometrically tested* with respect to reliability, validity and responsiveness. *Reliability* is an indicator of the reproducibility of an instrument and refers to how consistently and accurately test scores measure a construct. It can be examined with the internal consistency coefficient (Cronbach's α), an indicator of the extent to which the items are interrelated; longitudinal consistency is usually measured with the test-retest reliability, based upon analysis of correlations between repeated measurements, or with the intraclass correlation coefficient (ICC) . *Validity* testing examines whether an instrument measures what it intends to measure. Construct validity gives information about the theoretical relationship of the items to each other and can be measured by the following: *convergent validity* (comparing new items with other similar well-established questionnaires; moderate to high correlation coefficients are expected); *discriminant validity* (comparing new items with other well-established questionnaires assessing different aspects; low correlation coefficients are expected); and *known groups validity* (differentiating clinical subgroups of patients; detecting expected differences). *Responsiveness* is the ability of a scale to detect changes over time and therefore can be tested only in longitudinal studies. Finally, the questionnaire should be *normed* [18], through the application of a scale to a representative sample of the national population in order to obtain information about age, gender, and other influencing comparators. Guidelines on the development of QoL questionnaires have been published [16,19].

Recently, the US Food and Drug Administration (FDA) has recommended that HRQoL instruments be developed according to specific guidelines which are published [20]. According to the guidance of the FDA and the European Medicines Agency (EMA), patient reported outcome (PRO) instruments must be based on an appropriate and clearly defined framework: these require documentation of patient interviews, literature reviews, and expert clinical opinion in order to support the concepts, domains and their associations, and based on patient involvement [21].

Measures of quality of life

For the assessment of QoL, individual measurements such as interviews and psychometrically constructed questionnaires have been developed in the past 30 years. They are represented by one-dimensional measures that assess just one dimension of QoL (e.g. index, summary) and multidimensional measures that assess several dimensions of QoL. Instruments also differ regarding their purpose of use, ranging from diagnosis of the individual patient in a specific clinical context versus outcome assessment in prospective observational studies, controlled clinical trials, or epidemiologic studies [6]. Early on, only generic instruments were available for the assessment of QoL. In recent years a significant number of disease-specific measures have been developed.

Generic instruments

Generic instruments can be used irrespective of a specific disease in patients with different conditions or in general population. A short description of the most frequently used generic questionnaires is provided in the following sections, categorized by instruments for children versus those for adults.

Generic instruments for adults

The *Medical Outcomes Study 36-Item Health Survey (SF-36)* [22] is the most widely used generic questionnaire, translated and validated in several languages. The SF-36 consists of 36 items covering eight dimensions of general health status, namely physical functioning, role-physical, bodily pain, general health, vitality, social functioning, role-emotional, and mental health. Two summery scores can be derived: a physical component score (PCS) and a mental component score (MCS) [23].

The *Sickness Impact Profile (SIP)* [24] is another measure assessing the perceived health status and consists of 136 items.

With the *Nottingham Health Profile (NHP)* [25] emotional, social, and physical distress is assessed. The questionnaire consists of 38 items pertaining to the dimensions covering sleep, pain, emotional reactions, social isolation, physical morbidity, and energy level.

The *EuroQol (EQ-5D)* [26], which has been validated in many languages, asks five questions about mobility, self-care, usual activities, pain/discomfort, and anxiety/depression, followed by a global question concerning the actual health status, providing a *composite utility score*.

The *World Health Organization Quality of Life assessment Questionnaire (WHOQoL)* [27] assesses the respondent's perception and subjective evaluation of various aspects of life. The WHOQOL consists of six domains (physical, psychologic, level of independence, social relationships, environment, spirituality/religion/personal beliefs) with over 100 measurement items. A short-form version with 16 items has also been developed.

Generic instruments for children

For the assessment of QoL in children, several instruments have been developed as well. Most of these measures have been only validated on a national level.

One of those instruments that has been validated in different languages is the *Child Health Questionnaire (CHQ)* [28], which assesses QoL in children from the parent perspective. It consists of several subdimensions such as "general health perceptions," "physical functioning," and "mental health."

Another psychometrically tested instrument translated in more than 27 languages is the *KINDL* questionnaire [29], originally developed for the assessment of QoL in the general pediatric population in Germany. The KINDL is available as a self-administered and as a proxy version for three age groups (4–7, 8–12, and 13–16 years of age) and consists of 24 items pertaining to six dimensions (physical function, psychologic wellbeing, self-esteem, family, friends, and school) and an additional chronic generic dimension [30].

The *PedsQL* has been developed in the United States [31] and is translated in over 40 languages [32]. The PedsQL consists of 23 items and is available as self- and parent-report forms for four age groups (2–4, 5–7, 8–12, and 13–18 years).

The European *KIDSCREEN* instrument has been simultaneously developed in several languages and is validated in over 20 000 children [33]. The KIDSCREEN consists of 52 items pertaining to 10 dimensions of children's and adolescents HRQoL (KIDSCREEN-52). In addition a shorter version consisting of 27 items and five scales (KIDSCREEN-27) and a short index of global HRQoL (KIDSCREEN-10) were developed. These KIDSCREEN instruments are available as self-report versions from the age of 8 years and proxy versions. Currently, all three versions are available in 29 languages [34].

The European chronic generic measure *DISABKIDS* focuses on the experience of having a chronic illness [35] and is available in seven different languages [36]. It can be completed by children/adolescents from the age of 8 years and by parents. The DISABKIDS instrument tool set includes the following modules: DISABKIDS Chronic Generic Measure—long form (DCGM-37), DISABKIDS Chronic Generic Measure—short form (DCGM-12), and DISABKIDS Smiley Measure (for younger children aged 4–7 years). Condition-specific modules are available for asthma, arthritis, cerebral palsy, cystic fibrosis, dermatitis, diabetes, and epilepsy.

Disease-specific instruments

Although generic instruments allow a comparison of the investigated patient population with other patient groups or with the general population, they are not able to provide a clear pattern of symptoms or impairments related to a specific disease and are not sensitive enough to treatment consequences. For this reason disease-specific measures are especially developed for the assessment of QoL in patients with a specific health condition, such as cancer, metabolic disease, or cardiovascular disease, as well as respiratory, neurologic, psychiatric, rheumatologic, conditions, and so on [37,38]. Only in the last decade disease-specific QoL instruments have been developed for children and adults with hemophilia in different countries [39,40].

Hemophilia-specific instruments for children

The first hemophilia-specific questionnaire *Haemo-QoL* was developed for hemophilic children and their parents with a parallel approach in six European countries (Germany, France, Italy, Spain, the Netherlands, UK) [41]. The initial development of the questionnaire used parents' assessment of children's QoL as well as clinical expert consensus on relevant dimensions. The Haemo-QoL is available as a self-administered questionnaire for children of three age groups (4–7, 8–12, and 13–16 years of age) as well as respective proxy versions for their parents. The questionnaire was validated in 339 children from 20 European centers [42]. The psychometric structure of the questionnaire showed acceptable psychometric properties for the three age group versions as well as the accompanying parent forms. Different versions exist for various study purposes (long versions, short versions, and index version) [43]. The Haemo-QoL has been translated into several languages [44,45] and has been linguistically validated in 34 languages [46], which can be downloaded from the Haemo-QoL website (www.haemoqol.org). Further languages are currently under development.

Another hemophilia-specific questionnaire for children is the *Canadian Hemophilia Outcomes—Kids Life Assessment Tool (CHO-KLAT)*, which includes the perspectives of children with hemophilia [47]. The CHO-KLAT is available for children 5–18 years of age and includes parents- and self-report forms. The questionnaire consists of 35 items and has a single summary score representing overall QoL based on questions regarding: treatment, physical health, family, future, feeling, understanding of hemophilia, other people and friends, and control over your life. Psychometric testing in 52 children revealed good to very good values for test-retest reliability and inter-rater reliability and showed good convergent validity, but no discriminant validity [48,49]. Additional languages such as Dutch, French, German, Spanish, and Mandarin Chinese are available [50,51].

The *QoL questionnaire for young patients* was developed in the US and is only available as a proxy instrument for parents of hemophilic children aged 2–6 years [52]. The questionnaire consists of 39 items pertaining the following nine domains: "somatic symptoms," "physical functioning," "sleep disturbance," "stigma," "social functioning," "fear," "resentment/reaction," "energy level," "mood/behaviour," and "restrictions." The questionnaire has been validated in 103 parents of hemophilic children and 249 parents of healthy controls and psychometric characteristics revealed good values for reliability in terms of internal consistency as well as moderate values for convergent and discriminant validity.

Hemophilia-specific instruments for adults

The first hemophilia-specific QoL questionnaire for adults is the *A36Hemofilia-QoL*, which was originally developed in Spain [53]. It consists of 36 items assessing nine domains ("physical health," "daily activities," "joint damage," "pain," "treatment satisfaction," "treatment difficulties," "emotional functioning," "mental health," and "relationships and social activity"). The A36Hemofilia-QoL has been validated in 121 adult patients and psychometric characteristics were acceptable in terms of reliability (internal consistency, test-retest) and validity (concurrent and discriminant) [54]. The questionnaire has been translated for use in several languages (e.g. Czech, Croatia, Danish, English, Iranian, Norwegian, Polish, Sesotho, Swedish, and Tagalog) [55]. However, psychometrics for the translated versions is currently only available for few languages.

The *Haem-A-QoL* [39] was originally developed in Italy, which consists of 46 items pertaining to 10 dimensions ("physical health," "feelings," "view," "sport and leisure time," "work and school," "dealing," "treatment," "future," "family planning," and "relationship") and a total score. The questionnaire has been validated in 233 adult hemophilia patients and showed quite good reliability values in terms of internal consistency and test-retest reliability as well as for validity (convergent, discriminant). The Haem-A-QoL has been linguistically validated up to now in 61 languages [46], further languages are currently translated. The Haem-A-QoL has a core instrument with 27

shared items with the pediatric Haemo-QoL that allows a comparison between HRQoL of adults and children. A specific version of the Haem-A-QoL has been developed for elderly patients (Haem-A-QoL$_{Elderly}$). The Haem-A-QoL$_{Elderly}$ instrument consists of 63 items pertaining to 11 dimensions and showed good psychometric characteristics in terms of reliability and validity [56].

The *MedTap questionnaire (Haemo-QoL-A)* was developed in the US, Canada, Spain, and Germany [57]. The questionnaire consists of 41 items pertaining to six dimensions ("physical functioning," "role functioning," "worry," "consequences of bleeding," "emotional impact," and "treatment concerns") and four independent items. The Haemo-QoL-A questionnaire was validated in 221 adult hemophilia patients and showed in the psychometric testing good to excellent values for reliability in terms of internal consistency and test-retest reliability. Validity was good for concurrent and discriminant validity. The Haemo-QoL-A questionnaire was translated in the frame of the European ESCHQoL Study enrolling 21 European countries [58] and cross-cultural validations for further languages are ongoing [49].

The *Hemolatin-QoL* [59] was developed for Latin-American countries (Spanish and Portuguese languages). Preliminary version consists of 47 items pertaining to nine dimensions ("pain," "physical health," "emotional functioning," "social support," "activities and social functioning," "medical treatment," "mental health," "satisfaction with condition," and "general wellbeing") and one single item for "general health". The preliminary version was applied to a larger sample of patients with hemophilia from seven Latin-American countries in order to identify the best items [60]. The psychometric study is in progress, and the final version is expected to be available in 2014.

Choice, use, and interpretation of quality of life measures

Due to the multiplicity and diversity of instruments, physicians are uncertain which of the existing hemophilia-specific instruments are to use. The choice should be based on *study-related* (such as age group of patients, aim and design of the study) and *instrument-related issues* (such as feasibility, psychometric characteristics, aspects covered) [61]. When choosing a measure one must keep in mind the kind of investigation planned. In fact, generic instruments can measure general health status in different patients' populations ("cross-illness comparison") and can allow comparison with the general population. Disease-specific measures can study specific problems of a selected cluster of patients. These measures are more sensitive than generic measures: a greater sensitivity allows detecting small changes and makes these measures suitable for the assessment of a specific treatment intervention over time ("within-subject comparison"). The choice of a specific instrument relies upon its validation in the respective country, the reported sensitivity and even the number of items included. Moreover, the choice of a specific measure depends on the areas and dimensions mainly investigated by the instrument. In fact, health outcomes of a therapeutic intervention, namely efficacy and benefits, cannot always be predicted and/or measured, since the effects of an intervention cannot completely be foreseen. Another approach that can help to select an appropriate instrument is to link existing hemophilia-specific instruments to the International Classification of Functioning, Disability and Health (ICF) [62], which was developed by the WHO [63]. Furthermore, the ICF helps to identify not only impairments, but also restrictions and barriers of the target population [64].

Recently, it has been recommended to include HRQoL assessment not only in observational, but also in clinical trials (CT), especially when the following criteria are met: [65]: HRQoL is a main endpoint (e.g. when a patient is serious ill or in palliative care), when different treatments with equivalent efficacy exist (e.g. new treatment could confer HRQoL benefits), when a treatment with small clinical benefit might adversely affect HRQoL, or when a treatment with short-term efficacy results in a high overall failure rate. In hemophilia HRQoL is mainly included as secondary outcome in clinical trials. It would be helpful to include HRQoL assessments as primary outcome, especially in prophylaxis studies in hemophilia. Longitudinal studies in HRQoL assessment in hemophilia patients are scarce; therefore the sensitivity of most hemophilia-specific HRQoL instruments has not yet been tested. Interventional studies in hemophilia patients should include also HRQoL assessment. HRQoL assessments done in conjunction with randomized clinical trials (RCT) may help to elucidate cause-and-effect relationships.

In order to interpret HRQoL data precisely, knowledge of the content, scoring, reliability, and validity of a questionnaire is important. Different methods for the interpretation of HRQoL data are available [66]. *Distribution-* and *anchor-based* interpretation are distinct approaches: *distribution-based strategies* use the statistical distribution of results (e.g. means, standard deviations, statistical tests of differences or changes over time, effect size), while *anchor-based strategies* relate HRQoL levels or changes to clinical status or to other meaningful criteria [e.g. life events, global rating (MID), disease conditions, changes with therapy]. A content-based interpretation involves examining the content of general health measures, using qualitative and quantitative descriptions of scales and their anchors. In contrast to these approaches, *construct-based* interpretation examines the relationship between or among scales, while *criterion-based* interpretation uses information about how scale scores relate to external variables in order to establish their meaning. *Norm-based analysis* involves calculating scores for a large population-based sample and using these norms to examine how the study group deviates in HRQoL. *Interpretation based on the Standard Error of Measurement (SEM)* is a proxy to evaluate clinically meaningful change; estimated by multiplying the standard deviation of the scale by the square root of 1 minus its reliability coefficient.

Most of the HRQoL data in hemophilia are interpreted based on their statistical distribution. Only one study reported so far about minimal important differences (MID) in HRQoL data [67]. Several studies used construct-based interpretation of their HRQoL data comparing hemophilia-specific and generic instruments. Criterion-based interpretation is often deployed related to orthopedic status and disease severity. Norm-based data are up to now only available for generic instruments such as the SF-36. Several studies in hemophilia patients compared the target population with the general population. Norm data for the disease-specific instruments are still lacking.

Quality of life research in hemophilia

Recently, there has been a growing interest in the assessment of QoL in the field of hemophilia. However, the first publications on QoL and hemophilia mentioned QoL only as a condition of the patient, which was considered important. Only few studies assessed QoL with validated instruments [63]. In these studies it was mainly stated that for example prophylactic treatment or home therapy is improving the QoL of hemophilic patients, but without measuring QoL. Literature reviews in which QoL assessments were cited, have primarily utilized mainly generic instruments [68,69,70].

Results from generic instruments
Results in adult hemophilia patients
One of the first studies was conducted in 935 Dutch hemophilia patients and showed that hemophiliacs did not differ from the general population in the view of their own QoL [71]. By contrast, in Canada hemophilia patients showed significantly more limitations in their QoL compared to the general population [66].

In another study on clinical outcomes and resource utilization associated with hemophilia care in more than 1000 European patients on prophylactic treatment, QoL was better, assessed by the SF-36, compared to patients on on-demand treatment [72]. Miners *et al.* [1] found in their study, in which SF-36 and EQ-5D were administered to 249 British hemophiliacs, that patients with severe hemophilia reported poorer levels of QoL. They suggested that early primary prophylaxis might increase the QoL in these patients. A French study in 116 patients with severe hemophilia showed that physical function and social relation were acceptable, whereas QoL scores in the pain dimension of the SF-36 were low [73]. Another study that administered the SF-36 to 150 Finnish patients with bleeding disorders showed that QoL levels were correlated with the clinical severity [74]. In a Spanish study in 70 patients using the SF-36, QoL was negatively affected by severe orthopedic impairment related to hemophilia [75]. This was confirmed in Italy as well for inhibitor patients [76]. In a Canadian survey of mild, moderate, and severe hemophiliacs the Health Utility

Index Mark 2 (HUI-2) and Mark 3 (HUI-3) was used. Hemophiliacs reported a greater burden of morbidity than the general population, being associated linearly with the severity of hemophilia [77]. QoL is often assessed after treatment as it was done by Schick *et al.* in 11 hemophilia patients after knee arthroplasty, using the SF-12, WOMAC, and Knee Society Score [78]. Even though several publications report psychologic issues in hemophilic patients with human immunodeficiency virus (HIV), only a few assessed QoL with appropriate instruments [79]. More impairments were found in the HRQoL domains "general health" and "vitality" of the SF-36 in hepatitis C virus (HCV)-infected hemophilia patients [80]. Elander *et al.* found that the intensity of pain had the main influence on physical QoL assessed with the SF-36, while negative thoughts about pain had the main influence on mental QoL [81]. Early prophylactic treatment (at the age of ≤3 years) was shown to positively impact on adult patients' HRQoL, assessed with the SF-36, compared to patients starting prophylaxis later on [82]. Moreover, patients having started later prophylaxis had reduced bone mineral density which was highly correlated with impairment in the physical domains of HRQoL [83]. A study assessing HRQoL in patients with inhibitors during prophylaxis with an activated prothrombin complex concentrate (aPCC) or on-demand treatment revealed that in good responders (≥50% reduction in bleeding events), HRQoL was significantly improved during prophylaxis, assessed with the SF-36 compared to on-demand treatment [84]. Another study conducted in Germany demonstrated that reduced physical scores in the SF-36 correlated with older age, presence of HIV and target joints [85]. An Italian case–control study of elderly hemophilia patients (≥65 years) showed not only impairments in health status and daily activities, but also significantly more emotional problems compared to controls. Hemophiliacs reported depression more frequently and had a lower health-related QoL assessed with the EQ-5D and the WHOQOL-Bref [86].

Results in pediatric hemophilia patients

The HRQoL in children (*n* = 27) with severe hemophilia was first investigated by Liesner *et al.* in the UK in 1996 [87]. Prophylaxis significantly decreased the average number of bleeds compared to prior prophylaxis and families reported an improved health perception. In a multicenter study concerning the effects of two prophylactic treatment regimes, 128 children with hemophilia from Sweden and the Netherlands were investigated including QoL measures [88]. Clinical scores and QoL were similar in both prophylactic groups. High-dose prophylaxis increases treatment costs significantly; however arthropathy could only be slightly reduced after a follow-up of 17 years. In a study of 140 American children with hemophilia, Shapiro *et al.* found that those with few bleeding events had higher physical functioning scores assessed by the Child Health Questionnaire (CHQ) and were similar to the general population [89].

An Iranian study showed that children with a congenital bleeding disorder (aged 2–15 years) have a better dental health situation in primary dentition and a similar oral health-related QoL, assessed with the OHR-QoL, compared to children without congenital bleeding disorders [90].

Results on health economics and quality of life

Only recently has the relationship between health economics and QoL been examined in hemophilia patients using for example the standard gamble technique [91] or the quality-adjusted life years approach (QALYs) [1]. Szucs *et al.* found in their study regarding socioeconomic impact of hemophilia treatment involving 50 German hemophiliacs significant differences between hemophiliacs and healthy men concerning limitations in physical activities, pain, and general health scores as assessed by the SF-36 [92]. In a huge European study in more than 1000 patients with hemophilia, it was shown that prophylaxis was associated with higher costs but better QoL scores as measured by the SF-36 [4]. In an Italian study in 56 hemophilic patients combining QoL (SF-36) and utility assessment (EQ-5D), low scale values were found in the general health perceptions and higher scale values in social functioning [93]. Another Italian study (COCIS) involving 52 Italian hemophilic patients with inhibitors prospectively evaluated cost of care and QoL [3]. HRQoL measured with the SF-36 questionnaire was similar to that of patients with severe hemophilia without inhibitors. In comparison to other diseases, physical functioning was similar to that of patients with diabetes on renal dialysis, whereas mental wellbeing was comparable to that in the general population. This study showed that aggressive management of hemophilia complicated by inhibitors required high amounts of resources but provided a satisfactory QoL. As far as bleeding frequency in inhibitor patients is concerned, a reduced number of bleeding events due to secondary rFVIIa prophylaxis was found to be associated with improved HRQoL across countries, as assessed by the EQ-5D [94]. The comparison of intermediate-dose versus high-dose prophylaxis in severe hemophilia patients revealed that clinical outcome (e.g. bleeding, joint status) was slightly inferior in the intermediate-dose group although social participation and QoL assessed with the EQ-5D were similar compared to the high-dose group [95].

In a cost–utility analysis in six hemophilic children with inhibitors Eckert *et al.* included the Child-Health Questionnaire (CHQ) for the assessment of QoL and the EQ-5D for utility valuation [96]. HRQoL improvements were observed in several important areas as perceived by both patients and their families and were associated with incremental increase in cost per QALY.

Results from disease-specific instruments

In a Dutch study, 31 patients with severe hemophilia were investigated including a generic QoL instrument (SIP) and a disease-specific instrument, the Arthritis Impact Scale (AIMS) [97]. This questionnaire is an arthritis-specific measurement, but not a QoL measure in the precise sense. Physical health components of the Dutch AIMS and the SIP were significantly correlated; in contrast, there were no correlations for the psychosocial component between the D-AIMS and the SIP. Another arthritis-specific questionnaire (CHAQ: Children's Health Assessment Questionnaire) was used in a Dutch study, in which hemophilic children ($n = 39$) on prophylactic treatment were compared to their healthy peers; no significant differences were found. Although 90% of the hemophilic children had no disabilities in activities of daily living (ADL), 79% reported that the disease impacted on their lives [98].

Results in pediatric hemophilia patients

The HRQoL in pediatric patients with hemophilia was shown to be satisfactory. In one study, young children reported the highest impairments in the Haemo-QoL dimension "family" and "treatment", whereas older children had higher impairments in the social dimensions, such as "perceived support" and "friends" [99]. The Haemo-QoL questionnaire also showed that the initial burden induced by prophylaxis in younger children is highly compensated by improvements in HRQoL in older children, as indicated by impaired scores in the dimension "feeling" in smaller children and improved scores in the dimension "school and sport" in older children [99]. Using psychosocial determinants of QoL such as coping, locus of control, life satisfaction, and social support, it was apparent that QoL is dependent not only on clinical but also on psychosocial characteristics [100]. These psychosocial predictors varied across countries, although life satisfaction and social support explained the highest proportion of variance [101]. In the European ESCHQoL Study, significant differences in QoL were found across different regions according to factor consumption per capita: the study showed worse QoL in regions with a low factor consumption per capita (<2 IU) compared to regions with a higher factor consumption per capita (≥2 IU) [102]. In a paper by Bradley et al., differences and similarities among the European Haemo-QoL and the Canadian CHO-KLAT have been described [103].

A study assessing the impact of sport on clinical and HRQoL outcomes and physical performance in children aged 6–17 years living in the UK reported that children participating in sports had a significant better physical performance and HRQoL, assessed with the Haemo-QoL, than boys who did not [104].

Results in adult hemophilia patients

Italian adult hemophilia patients on continuous replacement therapy reported worse QoL compared to patients on on-demand treatment, which can be explained by the deteriorated clinical situation of these patients [105]. Up to 64% of the variance of HRQoL in German adult patients assessed with the generic SF-36 and the hemophilia-specific Haem-A-QoL could be explained by physical performance measured with the HEP-Test-Q [106] indicating that physical activity and sports is beneficial for HRQoL [107].

In a German study the impact of a specific aqua-training on patients' clinical outcomes, physical performance, and HRQoL was investigated [108]. Patients showed significant improvements in their physical performance compared to patients not attending the aqua-training over a 12-month period, but did not show improvements in their HRQoL, assessed with the SF-36 and the Haem-A-QoL.

A US study showed that switching from prophylactic treatment to on-demand treatment resulted in an increased number of bleeds and a worsened HRQoL, assessed with the Haemo-QoL-A, in late teens and early adults with severe hemophilia A [109]. In a Spanish prospective study, QoL and musculoskeletal assessment was compared 12 months after switching from on-demand treatment to secondary prophylaxis in severe adult hemophilia A patients. Patients on secondary prophylaxis showed a significant improvement in their QoL assessed with the A36Hemofilia-QoL while the musculoskeletal assessment remained similar or was slightly improved [110].

Future developments

A questionnaire for the assessment of HRQoL in patients with von Willebrand disease has been developed in Italy [111]. It has been translated into different languages (Danish, English, Finish, Norwegian, Portuguese, Russian, and Swedish in the frame of the Wilcome Study) and is currently being validated in Germany in the context of the Wil-QoL Study [112] and will be validated in the frame of the French WiSH-QoL study [113].

Currently, a disease-specific questionnaire for hemophilia patients with inhibitors (INHIB-QoL) for different age groups (adults, adolescents 13–17 years old, and parents of young children aged up to 12 years) is being validated [114]. The INHIB-QoL aims to quantify the impact of relative merits of different treatment regimens on hemophilia patients with inhibitors.

No specific instrument for women with bleeding disorders or hemophilia carriers exists currently [115]. Such an instrument could potentially provide insight into the specific problems of these women related to their disease.

Conclusion

In hemophilia, modern management has been successful in improving the clinical symptoms, orthopedic status, and the survival of patients. More recently, these aims have broadened to include the more comprehensive wellbeing and HRQoL of patients with hemophilia [1]. QoL assessment has become more utilized in the field of hemophilia research in the last decade, allowing the assessment of patient's perception of the overall effect of hemophilia care.

The hemophilia-specific questionnaires described here have been psychometrically tested and validated, some of them cross-culturally, but they still need to be implemented in international studies (observational, clinical). This is consistent with the recommendations of the Health Related Quality of Life Expert Working Group of the International Prophylaxis Study Group (IPSG) and further work is needed in order to confirm the psychometric properties of these instruments, especially regarding specificity and responsiveness [39]. Before choosing a QoL instrument, it is important to consider aim, design, type of patients, and scientific intention of the study. When possible, the patient should always be the individual to whom the QoL instrument is administered. Other observers do provide valuable additional information, but their perception is not identical to that provided by the patient directly. Only methodologically sound instruments should be used combining generic and disease-specific questionnaires to allow measurement of intervention effects and comparison of QoL of the target population with the general population or other chronic diseases. Comprehensive strategies for interpretation of hemophilia-specific questionnaires and their results should be applied [65, 116]. Divergences among the measures should be investigated based on clinically significant and MID [117].

Moreover, QoL should be included in CTs evaluating the effects of different treatment options, or in product licencing studies or gene therapy trials. Benefits of different treatment strategies can be assessed by asking the patient how his well-being has improved due to his treatment. Based on cross-cultural QoL assessment, healthcare systems or hemophilia care resources can be compared among countries aiming to provide adequate care and to harmonize different healthcare services.

Finally, QoL questionnaires should be part of medical armamentarium for the global assessment and care of patients with hemophilia in order to detect their specific healthcare needs and QoL [61].

Disclosure

AG has been appointed as co-author to this chapter when employed at the Department of Clinical Sciences and Community Health, Università degli Studi di Milano, Milan, Italy, as Associate Professor of Internal Medicine. Presently, he is employed at Baxter Innovations GmbH, Vienna, Austria as Medical Director, Global Medical Affairs Hemophilia.

References

1 Miners AH, Sabin CA, Tolley KH, Jenkinson C, Kind P, Lee CA. Assessing health-related quality-of-life in individuals with haemophilia. *Haemophilia* 1999; **5**(6): 378–85.

2 Gouw SC, van den Berg HM, Oldenburg J, *et al.* F8 gene mutation type and inhibitor development in patients with severe hemophilia A: systematic review and meta-analysis. *Blood* 2012; **119**(12): 2922–34.

3 Gringeri A, Mantovani LG, Scalone L, Mannucci PM. Cost of care and quality of life in hemophilia complicated by inhibitors: the COCIS Study Group. *Blood* 2003; **102**: 2358–63.

4 Schramm W, Royal S, Kroner B, *et al.*, for the European haemophilia economic study group. Clinical outcomes and resource utilization associated with haemophilia care in Europe. *Haemophilia* 2002; **8**: 33–43.

5 Cella DF, Tulsky DS. Measuring quality of life today: methodological aspects. *Oncology* 1990; **4**(5): 29–38.

6 Spilker B. *Quality of Life Assessment in Clinical Trials.* New York: Raven Press, 1996.

7 Orley J, and the WHOQOL-Group. The Development of the WHO Quality of Life Assessment Instruments (the WHOQOL). In: Orley J, Kuyken W (eds.) *Quality of Life Assessment. International Perspectives.* Berlin: Springer-Verlag, 1994: 41–57.

8 Guyatt GH, Feeny DH, Patrick DL. Measuring health-related quality of life. *Ann Intern Med* 1993; **118**(8): 622–9.

9 Bullinger M. Quality of life-definition, conceptualization and implications—a methodologists view. *Ther Surg* 1991; **6**: 143–9.

10 Bowling A. *Measuring Health. A Review of Quality of Life Measurement Scales.* Milton Keynes: Open University Press, 1991.

11 Rajmil L, Lopez, AR, Lopez-Aguilà S, Alonso J. Parent-child agreement on health-related quality of life (HRQoL): a longitudinal study. *Health Qual Life Outcomes* 2013; **11**: 101.

12 Sattoe JNT, van Staa A, Moll HA for On Your Own Feet Research Group. The proxy problem anatomized: Child–parent disagreement in Health Related Quality of Life reports of chronically ill adolescents. *Health Qual Life Outcomes* 2012; **10**: 10.

13 Eiser C, Morse R. A review of measure of quality of life for children with chronic illness. *Arch Dis Child* 2001; **84**: 205–11.

14 Juniper E, Guyatt GH, Jaeschke R. How to develop and validate a new health-related quality of life instrument. In: Spilker B (ed.) *Quality of Life and Pharmacoeconomics in Clinical Trials.* Philadelphia: Lippincott-Raven, 1996: 49–56.

15 Acquadro C, Jambon B, Ellis D, Marquis P. Language and translation issues. In: Spilker B (ed.) *Quality of Life and Pharmacoeconomics in Clinical Trials.* Philadelphia: Lippincott-Raven, 1996, 575–85.

16 Bullinger M, Anderson R, Cella D, Aaronson N. Developing and evaluating cross-cultural instruments from minimum requirements to optimal models. *Qual Life Res* 1993; **2**: 451–9.

17 Hui C, Triandis HC. Measurement in cross-cultural psychology: a review and comparison of strategies. *J Cross-Cultural Psychol* 1985; **16**(2): 131–52.

18 Guyatt GH, Feeny DH, Patrick DL. Measuring health-related quality of life. *Ann Int Med* 1993; **118**: 622–9.

19 Beaton DE, Bombardier C, Guillemin F, Ferraz MB. Guidelines for the process of cross-cultural adaptation of self-report measures. *Spine (Phila Pa 1976)* 2000; **25**(24): 3186–91.

20 Food and Drug Administration (FDA). Guidance for industry: patient-reported outcome measures: use in medical product development to support labeling claims: draft guidance. US Department of Health and Human Services FDA Center for Drug Evaluation and Research; US Department of Health and Human Services FDA Center for Biologics Evaluation and Research; US Department of Health and Human Services FDA Center for Devices and Radiological Health. *Health Qual Life Outcomes* 2006; **4**: 79.

21 Bottomley A, Jones D, Claassens L. Patient-reported outcomes: assessment and current perspectives of the guidelines of the Food and Drug Administration and the reflection paper of the European Medicines Agency. *Eur J Cancer* 2009; **45**(3): 347–53.

22 Ware JE, Sherbourne CD. The MOS 36-item short-form health survey (SF-36). I. Conceptual framework and item selection. *Med Care* 1992; **30**: 473–83.

23 Ware JE, Snow KK, Kosinski MA. *SF-36 Health Survey: Manual and Interpretation Guide*. New England: Health Institute, New England Medical Center, 1993.

24 Bergner M, Bobbit RA, Carter WB, Gilson BS. The Sickness Impact Profile: development and final revision of a health status measure. *Medical Care* 1981; **19**: 787–805.

25 Hunt SM, McKenna SP, McEwen J, Williams J, Papp E. The Nottingham Health Profile: subjective health status and medical consultations. *Soc Sci Med* 1981; **15A**: 221–9.

26 Kind P. The EuroQol Instrument: an Index of Health-related Quality of Life. In: Spilker B (ed.) *Quality of Life and Pharmacoeconomics in Clinical Trials*. Philadelphia: Lippincott-Raven, 1996, 191–201.

27 Power M, Harper A, Bullinger M. The World Health Organization WHOQOL-100: tests of the universality of Quality of Life in 15 different cultural groups worldwide. *Health Psychol* 1999; **18**(5): 495–505.

28 Landgraf I, Abetz L, Ware JE. *Child Health Questionnaire (CHQ): A users manual*. Boston: the Health Institute Press, 1997.

29 www.kindl.org/english/language-versions/

30 Ravens-Sieberer U, Bullinger M. Assessing the health related quality of life in chronically ill children with the German KINDL. First psychometric and content-analytic results. *QoL Res* 1999; **7**: 399–408.

31 Varni JW, Seid M, Rode CA. The PedsQL: measurement model for the pediatric quality of life inventory. *Med Care* 1999; **37**: 126–39.

32 http://www.pedsql.org/translations.html/

33 The KIDSCREEN Group Europe. *The KIDSCREEN Questionnaires—Quality of life questionnaires for children and adolescents*. Lengerich, Germany: Pabst Science Publishers, 2006.

34 http://www.kidscreen.org/english/language-versions/existing-language-versions

35 The DISABKIDS Group Europe. *The DISABKIDS Questionnaires—Quality of Life Questionnaires for Children with Chronic Conditions*. Lengerich, Germany: Pabst Science Publishers, 2006.

36 http://www.disabkids.org/language-versions

37 Bowling A. *Measuring Disease. A review of disease-specific quality of life measurement scales*. Buckingham: Open University Press, 2001.

38 Saleck S. *Compendium of Quality of Life Instruments*. Toronto, Canada: John Wiley & Sons, 2004.

39 von Mackensen S, Gringeri A. Quality of life in haemophilia. In: Preedy VR, Watson RR (eds.) *Handbook of Disease Burdens and Quality of Life Measures*, Vol. 3. Heidelberg: Springer, 2009: 1895–920.

40 Bullinger M, Globe D, Wasserman J, Young NL, von Mackensen S. Challenges of patient-reported outcome assessment in hemophilia care—a state of the art review. *Value Health* 2009; **12**(5): 808–20.

41 Bullinger M, von Mackensen S, Fischer K, *et al*. Pilot testing of the Haemo-QoL quality of life questionnaire for haemophiliac children in six European Countries. *Haemophilia* 2002; **8**(Suppl. 2): 47–54.

42 v. Mackensen S, Bullinger M, the Haemo-QoL Group. Development and Testing of an Instrument to assess the Quality of Life of

Children with Haemophilia in Europe (Haemo-QoL). *Haemophilia* 2004; **10**(Suppl. 1): 17–25.

43 Pollak E, Mühlan H, v. Mackensen S, Bullinger M, the Haemo-QoL Group. The Haemo-QoL Index: developing a short measure for health-related quality of life assessment in children and adolescents with haemophilia. *Haemophilia* 2006; **12**(4): 384–92.

44 Mercan A, Sarper N, Inanir M, *et al*. Hemophilia-Specific Quality of Life Index (Haemo-QoL and Haem-A-QoL questionnaires) of children and adults: result of a single center from Turkey. *Pediatr Hematol Oncol* 2010; **27**(6): 449–61.

45 Tantawy AA, Mackensen SV, El-Laboudy MA, *et al*. Health-related quality of life in Egyptian children and adolescents with hemophilia A. *Pediatr Hematol Oncol* 2011; **28**(3): 222–9.

46 von Mackensen S, Campos IG, Acquadro C, Strandberg-Larsen M. Cross-cultural adaptation and linguistic validation of age-group-specific haemophilia patient-reported outcome (PRO) instruments for patients and parents. *Haemophilia* 2013; **19**(2): e73–83.

47 Young N, Bradley C, Blanchette V, Wakefield C, Barnard D, McCusker P. Development of a Health-Related Quality of Life Measure for Boys with Hemophilia: the Canadian Hemophilia Outcomes-Kids Life Assessment Tool (CHO-KLAT). *Haemophilia* 2004; **10**(1), 34–43.

48 Young NL, Bradley CS, Wakefield CD, Barnard D, Blanchette VS, McCusker PJ. How well does the Canadian Hemophilia Outcomes-Kids' Life Assessment Tool (CHO-KLAT) measure the quality of life of boys with haemophilia? *Pediatr Blood Cancer* 2006; **47**(3): 305–11.

49 Young NL, Wakefield C, Burke TA, Ray R, McCusker PJ, Blanchette V. Updating the Canadian Hemophilia Outcomes-Kids Life Assessment Tool (CHI-KLAT Version 2.0). *Value Health* 2013; **16**(5): 837–41.

50 Young NL, St-Louis J, Burke T, Hershon L, Blanchette V. Cross-cultural validation of the CHO-KLAT and HAEMO-QoL-A in Canadian French. *Haemophilia* 2012; **18**(3): 353–7.

51 Wu R, Zhang J, Luke KH, *et al*. Cross-cultural adaptation of the CHO-KLAT for boys with hemophilia in rural and urban China. *Health Qual Life Outcomes* 2012; **10**: 112.

52 Manco-Johnson M, Morrissey-Harding G, Edelman-Lewis B, Oster G, Larson P. Development and validation of a measure of disease-specific quality of life in young children with haemophilia. *Haemophilia* 2004; **10**: 34–41.

53 Arranz P, Remor E, Quintana M, *et al*., and the Hemofilia-QoL Group. Development of a new disease-specific quality-of-life questionnaire to adults living with haemophilia. *Haemophilia* 2004; **10**: 376–82.

54 Remor E, Arranz P, Quintana M, *et al*., in representation of the Hemofilia-QoL Project Group. Psychometric field study of the new haemophilia quality of life questionnaire for adults: The Hemofilia-QoL. *Haemophilia* 2005; **11**: 603–10.

55 http://www.proqolid.org/instruments/hemophilia_specific_health_related_quality_of_life_questionnaire_a36_hemofilia_qol_r?fromSearch=yes&text=yes

56 von Mackensen S, Gringeri A, Siboni SM, Mannucci PM; and the Italian Association of Haemophilia Centres (AICE). Health-related quality of life and psychological well-being in elderly patients with haemophilia. *Haemophilia* 2012; **18**(3): 345–52.

57 Rentz A, Flood E, Altisent C, *et al*. Cross-cultural development and psychometric evaluation of a patient-reported health-related

quality of life questionnaire for adults with haemophilia. *Haemophilia* 2008; **14**(5): 1023–34.

58 Schramm W, Gringeri A, Ljung R, *et al.* and the ESCHQOL Study Group. Haemophilia care in Europe: the ESCHQoL study. *Haemophilia.* 2012; **18**(5): 729–37.

59 Remor E, and the Hemolatin-QoL Group. Hemolatin-QoL: Desarrollo de una medida específica para la evaluación de la calidad de vida en pacientes adultos con hemofilia en America-Latina: el Hemolatin-QoL. *Rev Int Psicol* 2005; **39**(2): 211–20.

60 Remor E. Psychometric field study of the HemoLatin-QoL, evidence for 297 adult patients living with hemophilia in Latin American countries. *Haemophilia* 2008; **14**(Suppl. 2), 152 (Abstract 29 PO 15).

61 Gringeri A, v. Mackensen S. Quality of life in haemophilia. *Haemophilia* 2008; **14**(Suppl. 3): 19–25.

62 Riva S, Bullinger M, Amann E, von Mackensen S. Content comparison of haemophilia specific patient-rated outcome measures with the international classification of functioning, disability and health (ICF,ICF-CY). *Health Qual Life Outcomes* 2010; **8**: 139.

63 World Health Organization (WHO). *International classification of functioning, disability and health.* ICF. Geneva: WHO, 2001.

64 Krasuska M, Riva S, Fava L, von Mackensen S, Bullinger M. Linking quality-of-life measures using the International Classification of Functioning, Disability and Health and the International Classification of Functioning, Disability and Health-Children and Youth Version in chronic health conditions: the example of young people with hemophilia. *Am J Phys Med Rehab* 2012; **91**(13 Suppl. 1): S74–83.

65 Gotay CC, Moore TD. Assessing quality of life in head and neck cancer. *Qual Life Res* 1992; **1**(1): 5–17.

66 Marquis P, Chassany MD, Abetz L. A comprehensive strategy for the interpretation of quality-of-life data based on existing methods. *Value Health* 2004; **7**(1): 93–104.

67 Walsh M, Macgregor D, Stuckless S, Barrett B, Kawaja M, Scully MF. Health-related quality of life in a cohort of adult patients with mild hemophilia A. *J Thromb Haemost* 2008; **6**(5): 755–61.

68 Fischer K, van der Bom JG, van den Berg HM. Health-related quality of life as outcome parameter in haemophilia treatment. *Haemophilia* 2003; **9**(Suppl. 1): 75–81.

69 Szende A, Schramm W, Flood E, *et al.* Health-related quality of life assessment in adult haemophilia patients: a systematic review and evaluation of instruments. *Haemophilia* 2003; **9**: 678–87.

70 Remor E, Young NL, von Mackensen S, Lopatina EG. Disease-specific quality-of-life measurement tools for haemophilia patients. *Haemophilia* 2004; **10**(Suppl. 4): 30–4.

71 Rosendaal FR, Smit C, Varekamp I, *et al.* Modern hemophilia treatment: medical improvements and quality of life. *J Intern Med* 1990; **228**: 663–40.

72 Royal S, Schramm W, Berntorp E, *et al.* Quality-of-life differences between prophylactic and on-demand factor replacement therapy in European haemophilia patients. *Haemophilia* 2002; **8**: 44–50.

73 Molho P, Rolland N, Lebrun T, *et al.* Epidemiological survey of the orthopaedic status of severe haemophilia A and B patients in France. The French Study Group. *Haemophilia* 2000; **6**: 23–32.

74 Solovieva S. Clinical severity of disease, functional disability and health-related quality of life. Three-year follow-up study of 150 Finnish patients with coagulation disorders. *Haemophilia* 2001; **7**: 53–63.

75 Aznar J, Magall M, Querol F, Gorina E, Tusell J. The orthopaedic status of severe haemophiliacs in Spain. *Haemophilia* 2000; **6**: 170–6.

76 Scalone L, Mantovani LG, Mannucci PM, Gringeri A, and the COCIS Study Investigators. Quality of life is associated to the orthopaedic status in haemophilic patients with inhibitors. *Haemophilia* 2006; **12**(2): 154–62.

77 Barr RD, Saleh M, Furlong W, *et al.* Health status and health-related quality of life associated with hemophilia. *Am J Hematol* 2002; **71**: 152–60.

78 Schick M, Stucki G, Rodriguez M, *et al.* Haemophilic: arthropathy: assessment of quality of life after total knee arthroplasty. *Clin Rheumatol* 1999; **18**: 468–72.

79 Bussing R, Johnson S. Psychosocial issues in hemophilia before and after the HIV crisis: a review of current research. *Gen Hosp Psychiatr* 1992; **14**: 387–403.

80 Posthouwer D, Plug I, van der Bom JG, Fischer K, Rosendaal FR, Mauser-Bunschoten EP. Hepatitis C and health-related quality of life among patients with hemophilia. *Haematologica* 2005; **90**(6): 846–50.

81 Elander J, Robinson G, Mitchell K, Morris J. An assessment of the relative influence of pain coping, negative thoughts about pain, and pain acceptance on health-related quality of life among people with hemophilia. *Pain* 2009; **145**(1–2): 169–75.

82 Khawaji M, Astermark J, Berntorp E. Lifelong prophylaxis in a large cohort of adult patients with severe haemophilia: a beneficial effect on orthopaedic outcome and quality of life. *Eur J Haematol* 2012; **88**(4): 329–35.

83 Khawaji M, Astermark J, Von Mackensen S, Akesson K, Berntorp E. Bone density and health-related quality of life in adult patients with severe haemophilia. *Haemophilia* 2011; **17**(2): 304–11.

84 Gringeri A, Leissinger C, Cortesi PA, *et al.* Health-related quality of life in patients with haemophilia and inhibitors on prophylaxis with anti-inhibitor complex concentrate: results from the Pro-FEIBA study. *Haemophilia* 2013; **19**(5): 736–43.

85 Pollmann H, Klamroth R, Vidovic N, *et al.* Prophylaxis and quality of life in patients with hemophilia A during routine treatment with ADVATE [antihemophilic factor (recombinant), plasma/albumin-free method] in Germany: a subgroup analysis of the ADVATE PASS post-approval, non-interventional study. *Ann Hematol* 2013; **92**(5): 689–98.

86 Siboni SM, Mannucci PM, Gringeri A, *et al.*, for the Italian Association of Haemophilia Centres (AICE). Health status and quality of life in elderly persons with severe hemophilia born before the advent of regular replacement therapy: a case control study. *J Thromb Haemost* 2009; **7**(5): 780–6.

87 Liesner RJ, Khair K, Hann IM. The impact of prophylactic treatment on children with severe haemophilia. *Br J Haematol* 1996; **92**: 973–8.

88 Fischer K, Astermark J, Van-Der-Bom J, *et al.* Prophylactic treatment for severe haemophilia: Comparison of an intermediate-dose to a high dose regimen. *Haemophilia* 2002; **8**: 753–60.

89 Shapiro A, Donfield S, Lynn H, *et al.* Defining the impact of hemophilia: the Academic Achievement in Children with Hemophilia Study. *Pediatrics* 2001; **108**: E105.

90 Salem K, Eshghi P. Dental health and oral health-related quality of life in children with congenital bleeding disorders. *Haemophilia* 2013; **19**(1): 65–70.

91 Naraine V, Risebrough N, Oh P, *et al.* Health-related quality-of-life treatments for severe hemophilia: Utility measurements using the Standard Gamble technique. *Haemophilia* 2002; **8**: 112–20.

92 Szucs TD, Offner A, Schramm W. Socioeconomic impact of hemophilia care. Results of a pilot study. *Haemophilia* 1996; **2**: 211–17.

93 Trippoli S, Vaiani M, Linari S, Longo G, Morfini M, Messori A. Multivariate analysis of factors influencing quality of life and utility in patients with haemophilia. *Haematologica* 2001; **86**: 722–8.

94 Hoots WK, Ebbesen LS, Konkle BA, *et al.* Novoseven (F7HAEM-1505) Investigators. Secondary prophylaxis with recombinant activated factor VII improves health-related quality of life of hemophilia patients with inhibitors. *Haemophilia* 2008; **14**(3): 466–75.

95 Fischer K, Steen Carlsson K, Petrini P, *et al.* Intermediate-dose versus high-dose prophylaxis for severe hemophilia: comparing outcome and costs since the 1970s. *Blood* 2013; **122**(7): 1129–36.

96 Ekert H, Brewin T, Boey W, Davey P, Tilden D. Cost–utility analysis of recombinant factor VIIa (NovaSeven) in six children with long-standing inhibitors to factor VIII or IX. *Haemophilia* 2001; **7**: 279–85.

97 de-Joode E, van-Meeteren N, van-den-Berg H, de-Kleijn P, Helders P. Validity of health status measurement with the Dutch Arthritis Impact Measurement Scale 2 in individuals with severe haemophilia. *Haemophilia* 2001; **7**: 190–7.

98 Schoenmakers M, Gulmans V, Helders P, van-der-Berg H. Motor performance and disability in Dutch children with haemophilia: a comparison with their healthy peers. *Haemophilia* 2001; **7**: 293–8.

99 Gringeri A, v. Mackensen S, Auerswald G, *et al.* for the Haemo-QoL Study*. Health status and health-related quality of life of children with haemophilia from six west European countries. *Haemophilia* 2004; **10**(Suppl. 1): 26–33.

100 Bullinger M, v. Mackensen S, the Haemo-QoL Group. Quality of life in children and families with bleeding disorders. *J Pediatr Haematol Oncol* 2003; **25**: 64–7.

101 Bullinger M, von Mackensen S. Psycho-social determinants of quality of life in children and adolescents with haemophilia—a cross-cultural approach. *Clin Psychol Psychother* 2008; **15**: 164–72.

102 Bullinger M, Gringeri A, von Mackensen S. Quality of life of young patients with haemophilia in Europe. *Bundesgesundheit Gesundheitsforsch Gesundheit* 2008; **51**(6): 637–45.

103 Bradley CS, Bullinger M, McCusker PJ, Wakefield CD, Blanchette VS, Young NL. Comparing two measures of quality of life for children with haemophilia: the CHO-KLAT and the Haemo-QoL. *Haemophilia* 2006; **12**: 643–53.

104 Khair K, Littley A, Will A, von Mackensen S. The impact of sport on children with haemophilia. *Haemophilia* 2012; **18**(6): 898–905.

105 von Mackensen S, Scalone L, Ravera S, Mantovani L, Gringeri A, for the COCHE Study Group. Assessment of health-related quality of life in patients with haemophilia with the newly developed Haemophilia-specific Instrument (Haem-A-QoL). *Value Health* 2005; **8**: A127 (Abstract PHM5).

106 von Mackensen S, Czepa D, Herbsleb M, Ziezo R, Hilberg T. Quality of life and subjective physical performance in adult haemophilia patients. *Haemostaseologie* 2008; **28**(Suppl. 1): S118–19.

107 von Mackensen S. Quality of life and sports activities in patients with haemophilia. *Haemophilia* 2007; **13**(Suppl. 2): 38–43.

108 Von Mackensen S, Eifrig B, Zäch D, Kalnins J, Wieloch A, Zeller W. The impact of a specific aqua-training for adult haemophilic patients—results of the WATERCISE study (WAT-QoL). *Haemophilia* 2012; **18**(5): 714–21.

109 Manco-Johnson MJ, Sanders J, Ewing N, Rodriguez N, Tarantino M, Humphries T, TEEN/TWEN Study Group. Consequences of switching from prophylactic treatment to on-demand treatment in late teens and early adults with severe haemophilia A: the TEEN/TWEN study. *Haemophilia* 2013; **19**(5):727–35.

110 Aznar JA, Garcia-Dasi M, Perez-Alenda S, *et al.* Secondary prophylaxis vs. on-demand treatment to improve quality of life in severe adult haemophilia A patients: a prospective study in a single centre. *Vox Sang* 2013 (in press).

111 Von Mackensen S, Federici A. Quality of life assessment in patients with von Willebrand's disease: development of a first disease-specific instrument (VWD-QoL). *Haemostaseologie* 2007; **1**: 126.

112 Von Mackensen S, Moorthi C, Auerswald G. Assessment of health-related quality of life in VWD patients—results of the VWD-QoL pilot study. *Haemophilia* 2010; **16**(Suppl. 4): 139 (Abstract 31P27).

113 Von Mackensen S. Quality of life issues in von Willebrand. LFB Symposia at the World Federation of Hemophilia Congress, 2012. *Thromb Haemost* 2013; 11–13.

114 Von Mackensen S, Riva S, Khair K, *et al.* Development of an inhibitor-specific questionnaire for the assessment of helath-related quality of life in haemophilia patients with inhibitors (INHIB-QoL). *Value Health* 2013; **16**(3): A196: PHS63.

115 von Mackensen S. Quality of life in women with bleeding disorders. *Haemophilia* 2011; **17**(Suppl. 1): 33–7.

116 Osoba D, Bezjak A, Brundage M, Zee B, Tu D, Pater J, and the Quality of Life Committee of the NCIC CTG. Analysis and interpretation of health-related quality-of-life data from clinical trials: basic approach of the National Cancer Institute of Canada Clinical Trials Group. *Eur J Cancer* 2005; **41**: 280–7.

117 Wyrwich KW, Bullinger M, Aaronson A, Hay, RD, Patrick DL, Symonds T. The Clinical Significance Consensus Meeting Group. Estimating clinically significant differences in quality of life outcomes, *Qual Life Res* 2005; **14**(2): 285–95.

CHAPTER 65

The economics of hemophilia treatment

Katarina Steen Carlsson[1] and Erik E. Berntorp[2]
[1]Lund University and the Swedish Institute for Health Economics, Sweden
[2]Skane University Hospital, Sweden

Introduction

Health economics is the application of economic theory and method in the analysis of questions concerning people's health. There are two fundamental conditions in all economic analyses. The first is that resources in terms of labor (human capital) and equipment, energy, and raw materials (capital) are scarce with respect to people's needs. That is, there are not enough resources to meet all needs and choices are necessary. The second is that resources can be used in alternative ways. Using the economic formulation of choice of resources use within healthcare does not contradict medical decision making or ethical considerations, but should be seen as complementary. The economic analysis contributes with a systematic comparison of cost of resources and consequences of resource use. Table 65.1 lists the key concepts for health economic analyses.

Health economic methods and the economic perspective

The health economic problem may be formulated in terms of the choice between relevant alternatives with the purpose of obtaining as much health and welfare as possible with respect to resources used. Health economic questions concern individual health-related behavior and view the healthcare system as a system of production; they also address problems about insurance against healthcare costs and loss of income as a consequence of illness or injury; distributional and equity aspects are also raised, as well as the consequences of globalization on health.

Health economic research, like all other economic research, applies an individualistic perspective. The typical economic model strives to formulate the decision-making problem in terms of an agent (e.g. an individual, a company, an organization, an authority) with the aim of maximizing something good (e.g. health or wealth) or minimizing something bad (e.g. costs). The decision is however subject to constraints. To achieve better health or more wealth, the agent has to put in effort in terms of time and/or money. A theoretic economic model then explores how the agent can achieve the optimal solution, that is, the best possible outcome given the restrictions.

The starting point is that the sum of all reactions to events by single actors and political actions will have consequences for both the single actor and for society as a whole. For example, the primary interest of economic analyses is *not* to find out the reaction of the single individual to more information on the negative consequences of tobacco smoking, to a tax increase on cigarettes, or to the prohibition of smoking in public places. The primary research question concerns the *joint effect* on public health, on the economic situation of families, and on the expenditure of the social insurance system.

In economic theory, abstract models are used to describe the main features of the situation to be analyzed and the assumptions that make it possible to study the phenomena or behaviors of interest. One basic assumption for economic models is that agents (e.g. patients or professionals, firms, organizations) are rational. By rationality, economists mean that the agent acts as if he or she strives toward an apparent goal with the purpose of reaching this goal to the greatest possible extent. The economic perspective has a strict individualistic basis from which it follows that it is not possible to determine what would be rational for someone else. Nevertheless, some types of behavior may seem irrational—someone who smokes too much or exercises too little, for example, given the amount of knowledge regarding the impact of lifestyle factors on health. Economic models are not conditioned on all individuals (or even one) striving toward maximum health. The basic premise for health economists is that other things in life may generate meaning and pleasure, and that individuals therefore make trade-offs between health and other desirable goals. These goals will vary between individuals. For example, the behaviors and values of peer groups are important for teenagers and smokers derive pleasure from the cigarette while smoking. For single individuals, economists usually assume that the goal is to obtain as much utility or wellbeing as possible in life. The firm/corporation

Textbook of Hemophilia, Third Edition. Edited by Christine A. Lee, Erik E. Berntorp and W. Keith Hoots.
© 2014 John Wiley & Sons, Ltd. Published 2014 by John Wiley & Sons, Ltd.

Table 65.1 Key health economic concepts in alphabetical order.

Term	Description
Cost	Value of resource use (see also opportunity cost)
Cost-efficiency	Cost of a treatment strategy in relation to its effect/outcome
Direct costs	Value of total resource use within the healthcare system and in other sectors because of illness or injury. Restricted to costs based on resource use within outpatient and inpatient care and of pharmaceuticals in studies applying a healthcare sector perspective. Included in societal costs
Dominant strategy	Term in economic evaluations. A treatment alternative that renders better outcomes and has lower cost than the comparisons, or that is equally effective but costs less
Incentive	Motivation. Factors that describe the conditions under which individuals and other agents acts. May be financial (e.g. remuneration to doctors, nurses, or hospital departments for produced care or the price a patient pays for a healthcare visit)
Indirect cost	Value of lost production as a consequence of illness or injury that may concern the ill person themselves or family and friends. In practise, the valuation of lost production is often restricted to the person with the illness or injury. Included in societal costs
Incremental cost-efficiency ratio (ICER)	Term within health economic evaluations. Denotes the ratio of the difference in cost to the difference in effect for the two alternatives under comparison (see Equation 1)
Intangible cost	Cost in terms of reduced quality of life as a consequence of illness
Opportunity cost	A principle to value resource use building on the assumption that all resources have (at least) one alternative use. Choosing one alternative implies forgoing the value that could be obtained with an alternative use. The opportunity cost measures the highest valued alternative use of the resource. The identification of the opportunity cost depends on the decision situation
Quality-adjusted life-year (QALY)	An index measure that weighs changes in life-years gained (quantity) by the morbidity (quality) of life in those years
Societal cost	Sum of direct, indirect, and intangible cost in society as a result of an illness or injury

is assumed to strive toward as much profit as possible, and a hospital toward low cost for the healthcare provided for the general public; politicians toward as many votes from their constituency as possible; and public authorities toward a bigger organization.

Agents are, however, restricted in their actions and cannot usually reach all their goals. For the hospital, this means that if the needs of the general public are to be satisfied, costs must not be reduced beyond certain limits. A firm must consider the conditions for production, wages, and other production costs as well as the price at which the goods or services will sell. The individual is constrained by time (24 hours per day) and by his or her income and other economic resources. There may also be rules that constrain the agent's actions, e.g. the doctor's prescription to obtain certain drugs.

The goal and questions in health economic analyses cover a vast area. However, the most common economic studies within the medical field represent comparative evaluations of alternative treatment strategies and descriptive studies of costs of illness.

Health economic analyses in practise

The past decade has seen an increasing number of authorities and government bodies within the healthcare arena in Europe and North America where health economic evaluations are an integrated part in the decision-making process. Two examples of national agencies using health economic analysis are the National Institute for Health and Clinical Care Excellence (NICE; www.nice.org.uk) in the UK and the Dental and Pharmaceutical Benefits Agency (TLV; www.tlv.se) in Sweden. NICE was established in the UK in 1999 with an aim to reduce variation in the availability and quality of National Health Service treatment and care. NICE publishes guidance to support healthcare professionals and others to make sure that the care they provide is of the best possible quality and offers the best value for money. TLV was established in Sweden in 2002 with the mandate to decide whether a pharmaceutical product should be subsidized based on its cost-efficiency. In practise, the TLV influences the Swedish healthcare market since drugs that cannot provide evidence on cost-efficiency at the price demanded by the producer will not be subsidized. Nonsubsidized drugs may still be sold on the Swedish market provided they have received approval by the Medical Products Agency, but the lack of public subsidy will, in practise, often imply that the drug is withdrawn from the market. Other examples of countries with government bodies using input from health economic evaluations include Canada, Scotland, the Netherlands, Belgium, and Denmark.

Health economic evaluation

A health economic evaluation is a systematic comparison of costs and consequences for two or more relevant treatment alternatives. In hemophilia, examples of such treatment alternatives include plasma-derived versus recombinant factor concentrates, alternative regimens for providing replacement therapy [1,2], immediate surgery compared with watchful waiting for the patient with arthrodeses, and individual patient education programs versus education in groups. The minimum for an economic evaluation is two alternatives, but more than two alternatives may be relevant for clinical decision-making, and then pair-wise comparisons will be performed. For the health economic evaluation, it is necessary to combine health economic and clinical expertise in the formulation of the relevant problem and the characterization of each treatment alternative.

Perspective

Health economic evaluations may be conducted using different perspectives. If the analysis concerns the allocation of resources within a given healthcare budget, the evaluation may take a healthcare sector perspective. The comparison of costs and consequences will then include direct costs that accrue within the healthcare sector and outcome measures of relevance (e.g. reduced number of hospitalizations or bleeds, or patient outcomes such as health-related quality of life). Costs in an evaluation from the health sector perspective will then include all costs for the healthcare provider. These may include the cost of contact with doctors, nurses, and physiotherapists; the hospital days due to hemophilia treatment; and treatment provided because the patient has hemophilia, including factor concentrates and other pharmaceuticals and infusion aids. Resource use and the cost that falls on other sectors are not considered.

Analyses from the societal perspective consider costs and consequences of the treatment alternative that may occur within the health sector and within other sectors of society. Decisions in the health sector have consequences for the family, community care, employers, and so on. To illustrate the difference, we use an example where a program aiming at reducing the length of stay in hospital after hemophilia surgery is compared to usual care. An economic evaluation with a health sector perspective would then focus on the cost side by measuring the number of hospital days for patients in the program, the costs for patients receiving usual care, and, when applicable, potential subsequent outpatient visits following surgery. Assuming that the program is successful in reducing length of stay, the conclusion would be that it is cost saving as long as outpatient visits do not differ.

An economic evaluation with a societal perspective would investigate the consequences of early discharge from hospital for the family, community care, employers, and so on. An evaluation using a societal perspective would then measure the cost of family caregivers being absent from work to care for the patient as well as services by community care. Adding increased costs in other sectors would reduce the expected savings compared to an analysis from the more limited health sector perspective.

Three methods for economic evaluation

A health economic evaluation is a comparison of (at least) two treatment alternatives. There are three alternative tools for systematic analyses of costs and consequences for the comparison of healthcare programs:
- Cost-effectiveness analysis (CEA).
- Cost–utility analysis (CUA).
- Cost–benefit analysis (CBA).

Table 65.2 summarizes the information needed for each type of analysis, and how results are interpreted for each of the three methods. Common for all three methods is that costs are measured in monetary terms, but the methods differ in terms of how consequences are measured.

In a CEA, consequences are measured in natural units, for instance life-years gained or bleeding episodes avoided [1,3]. Bleeding episodes avoided is a relevant outcome measure within hemophilia care, but it is disease specific and cannot be meaningfully used in comparisons with treatments in other hospital departments. Life-years gained may be applicable for many diseases with risk of fatality, but it may not be sensitive in catching differences in quality of life.

For allocation of resources within the health sector, the analyst needs outcome measures that are not tailored for disease-specific groups. Health economists have developed a preference-based index denoted quality-adjusted life-years

Table 65.2 Characteristics of three alternative methods for full economic evaluation.

Method	Cost	Consequence	Recommendation for decision-making	Tool for priority setting
Cost-effectiveness analysis (CEA)	Resource use measured in monetary terms (e.g. Euro, dollar, pound)	Single-dimension consequences measured in physical units. For example, life-years gained, reduction in number of bleeds per year, or reduction in pain from start of bleed	Choose the alternative with the lowest cost per unit gained	Enables comparisons between treatment alternatives with the same relevant outcome dimensions
Cost–utility analysis (CUA)	Resource use measured in monetary terms (e.g. Euro, dollar, pound)	Consequences measured in quality-adjusted life-years (QALYs), which simultaneously measure reduced morbidity (quality gains) and reduced mortality (quantity gains)	Choose the alternative with the lowest cost per QALY gained	Enables comparisons between treatment alternatives within different parts of the healthcare sector using common outcome
Cost–benefit analysis (CBA)	Resource use measured in monetary terms (e.g. Euro, dollar, pound)	Consequences measured in monetary terms (e.g. Euro, dollar, pound)	Choose the alternative with the biggest net benefit (sum of benefits – sum of costs)	Enables comparisons between alternatives in different sectors of society

(QALYs) [4]. Over the last decade, QALYs have become a well-established tool for health economic evaluations used by authorities such as NICE and TLV.

The CUA measure consequences by QALY using standardized instruments such as the EQ-5D [5] or SF-6D [6]. Drummond *et al.* provide a well-written introductory textbook on the methods for these evaluations [7]. Health economic evaluations in hemophilia using CUA have been published from Canada [1] and the UK [8].

The result from CEA and CUA are presented as a ratio of pair-wise comparisons of differences in cost to differences in effect. This ratio, the incremental cost-effectiveness ratio (ICER), may be used to rank treatment alternatives within a given healthcare budget. Equation (1) presents the ICER schematically for two alternative treatments, A and B:

$$ICER = \frac{Costs_A - Costs_B}{Effects_A - Effects_B} \tag{1}$$

where $Costs_A$ and $Costs_B$ are the cost of treatments A and B, respectively, and $Effect_A$ and $Effect_B$ are the effects associated with treatments A and B, respectively.

A special case of CEA and CUA would be when the two alternative treatments under consideration achieve the same outcome to the same extent, e.g. pharmaceuticals containing the same active substances but sold under different brand names. In this case, the denominator of the ICER is 0 and a comparison of costs of the alternatives would suffice. Such a cost-minimization analysis is considered as a partial evaluation since it examines only costs in practise.

The third method for economic evaluation (the CBA) measures both cost and consequences in monetary units (e.g. Euros, dollars, pounds). Using a common metric, results are expressed as net benefits, and a treatment alternative, where the sum of benefits exceeds the sum of costs, is then worthwhile. Techniques to elicit people's willingness to pay for nonmarket goods and services have been developed, hence the concept of willingness to pay (WTP) (see Bateman *et al.* for a comprehensive overview of stated preference techniques including WTP [9]). Health economic evaluations applying WTP have been published from the US [10], evaluating the treatment of von Willebrand disease, and from Sweden [11,12], evaluating the treatment strategies for severe hemophilia.

Study design and data

The appropriateness of the design of evaluation by CEA, CUA, or CBA depends on the characteristics of the economic problem and on data availability. Economic evaluations may rest on patient-level data, either observational data collected directly for the purpose of the evaluation or piggy-backed on a clinical trial.

While data from a randomized controlled trial (RCT), have high internal validity, the external validity and generalizability to a typical population with, for instance, severe hemophilia may be limited due to strict inclusion and exclusion criteria used in the RCT. Another limitation of RCTs is that the limited duration of follow-up may fail to capture important consequences [13]. For chronic diseases like hemophilia where treatment is life-long and outcomes such as arthropathy may develop gradually, observational data from high-quality patient registries provide essential information for economic evaluations. Recent years have seen important developments in statistical methods for handling selection bias and issues of confounding when using observational data to make causal inference. Nevertheless, collaboration between economists and clinicians in designing the study, extracting data, and interpreting the results is a prerequisite.

Health economic evaluations often use decision-analytic modeling, for instance Markov model cohort simulation and individual-based Monte Carlo microsimulation (examples in hemophilia are discussed in [1,8,14,15]). Decision-analytic models conceptualize the decision-making problem using a set of health states and transitions between these states. A model may then merge information from several sources, expanding prognoses for costs and/or outcomes for longer time horizons. Models are a useful tool when few data exist on new treatments, for instance when there is still uncertainty regarding real world implementation of new treatments. Decisions regarding the choice of treatment must still be made and health economic models assist healthcare decision makers by describing costs and outcomes of alternative strategies given current knowledge including smaller case studies and assumptions.

For example, health economic analyses of alternative treatment strategies for hemophilia patients who have developed inhibitors to factor VIII concentrate may serve as an illustration of choice of design strategies. Until recently, there were no larger scale trials on inhibitor treatment from which economic data had been retrieved. Three publications used decision-analytic modeling to compare the two alternative hemostatic agents used in the treatment of patients with inhibitors: activated prothrombin complex concentrate (aPCC) and recombinant factor VIIa (rFVIIa) [16–18]. The comparison concerned treatment with the two alternative bypassing agents during one bleeding episode, but the conclusions were ambiguous.

Scientific journals demand that the assumptions and the structure of the model are clearly reported, enabling re-estimations using other data on costs and effects or changing the assumptions to fit other clinical settings. Figure 65.1 shows an example of the decision tree visualizing the model structure used by You *et al.* for analyzing the cost-effectiveness of bypassing agents [19]. The first head-to-head trial of the two alternative bypassing agents, the FENOC study, was published by Astermark *et al.* [20]. The clinical data were also used for a piggy-back cost-effectiveness analysis where patient-rated outcomes were used for measuring effect: treatment effectiveness, bleeding stopped, and pain reduction [21], and the results reported as ICERs (see Equation 1 above) for aPCC compared with rFVIIa.

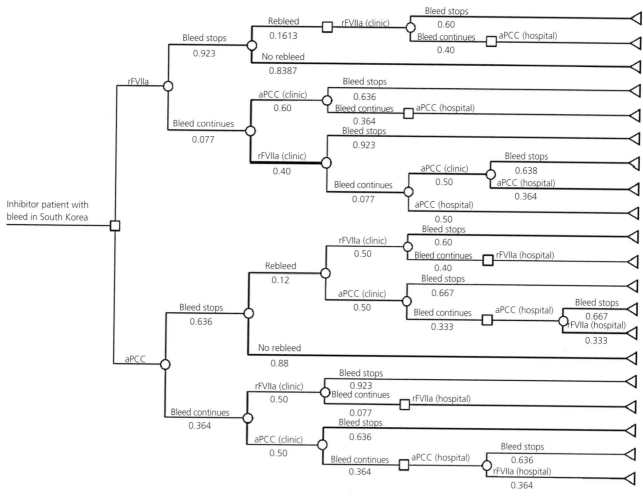

Figure 65.1 Decision-making model structure. aPCC, activated prothrombin complex concentrate; rFVIIa, recombinant factor VIIa. Reproduced from [19] with permission.

The analysis also showed the role of prices on resource use for the cost-effectiveness results and the ICER.

Research design based on observational data has the advantage that it may capture the variation of actual patients and in the daily clinical work. However, comparisons between alternative treatment strategies may not be feasible based on observational data where differences in treatment will depend on differences in patient characteristics and need for treatment. Conversely, protocol-based trial data may be well suited for comparisons when patients are randomized to the alternative treatment strategies. The drawback is that the trial situation may entail strict inclusion and exclusion criteria and may have study-driven compliance limiting the generalizability on a large scale. Decision-analytic modeling is attractive since it enables sensitivity analysis and easy adaptation when new results on efficacy, efficiency, and cost are available, but is sensitive to assumptions. In conclusion, the alternative designs all have their place in supplying decision-makers with information, and sometimes the combination of studies provides the clear picture.

Conclusion

The starting point for all economic analyses is that resources are scarce with respect to people's needs and that resources will always have alternative uses. The scarcity of resources may be especially evident in healthcare, and therefore tools to make systematic considerations of the costs and consequences of the available treatment alternatives are an important input in decision-making. This chapter provides an overview of the economic scientific perspective, methods for economic evaluations of healthcare programs (cost-effectiveness, cost–utility, and cost–benefit analyses), and discusses data availability and choice of study design.

References

1 Risebrough N, Oh P, Blanchette V, Curtin J, Hitzler J, Feldman BM. Cost-utility analysis of Canadian tailored prophylaxis, primary

prophylaxis and on-demand therapy in young children with severe haemophilia A. *Haemophilia* 2008; **14**: 743–52.

2 Steen Carlsson K, Hojgard S, Glomstein A, *et al.* On-demand vs. prophylactic treatment for severe haemophilia in Norway and Sweden: differences in treatment characteristics and outcome. *Haemophilia* 2003; **9**: 555–66.

3 Miners AH, Sabin CA, Tolley KH, Lee CA. Assessing the effectiveness and cost-effectiveness of prophylaxis against bleeding in patients with severe haemophilia and severe von Willebrand's disease. *J Intern Med* 1998; **244**: 515–22.

4 Tsuchiya A, Dolan P. The QALY model and individual preferences for health states and health profiles over time: a systematic review of the literature. *Med Decis Making* 2005; **25**: 460–7.

5 EuroQol Group. A standardised instrument for use as a measure of health outcome, 2014. Available at: http://www.euroqol.org/

6 Brazier JE, Roberts J. The estimation of a preference-based measure of health from the SF-12. *Med Care* 2004; **42**: 851–9.

7 Drummond MF, Sculpher MJ, Torrance GW, O'Brien BJ, Stoddart GL. *Methods for the Economic Evaluation of Health Care Programmes*, 3rd edn. Oxford: Oxford University Press, 2005.

8 Miners A. Revisiting the cost-effectiveness of primary prophylaxis with clotting factor for the treatment of severe haemophilia A. *Haemophilia* 2009; **15**: 881–7.

9 Bateman IJ, Carson RT, Day B, *et al. Economic Evaluation with Stated Preference Techniques: a manual.* Cheltenham: Edward Elgar, 2002.

10 Eastaugh S. Willingness to pay in treatment of bleeding disorders. *Int J Technol Assess Health Care* 2000; **16**: 706–10.

11 Steen Carlsson K, Höjgard S, Lethagen S, Lindgren A, Berntorp E, Lindgren B. Willingness to pay for on-demand and prophylactic treatment for severe haemophilia in Sweden. *Haemophilia* 2004; **10**: 527–41.

12 Steen Carlsson K, Höjgard S, Lindgren A, *et al.* Costs of on-demand and prophylactic treatment for severe haemophilia in Norway and Sweden. *Haemophilia* 2004; **10**: 515–26.

13 Fischer K, Grobbee DE, van den Berg HM. RCTs and observational studies to determine the effect of prophylaxis in severe haemophilia. *Haemophilia* 2007; **13**: 345–50.

14 Fischer K, Pouw ME, Lewandowski D, Janssen MP, van den Berg HM, van Hout BA. A modeling approach to evaluate long-term outcome of prophylactic and on demand treatment strategies for severe hemophilia A. *Haematologica* 2011; **96**: 738–43.

15 Miners AH, Sabin CA, Tolley KH, Lee CA. Cost-utility analysis of primary prophylaxis versus treatment on-demand for individuals with severe haemophilia. *Pharmacoeconomics* 2002; **20**: 759–74.

16 Joshi A, Stephens J, Munro V, Mathew P, Botteman M. Pharmacoeconomic analysis of recombinant factor VIIa versus APCC in the treatment of minor-to-moderate bleeds in hemophilia patients with inhibitors. *Curr Med Res Opin* 2006; **22**: 23–31.

17 Odeyemi IA, Guest JF. Modelling the economic impact of recombinant activated Factor VII compared to activated prothrombin–complex concentrate in the home treatment of a mild to moderate bleed in adults with inhibitors to clotting Factors VIII and IX in the UK. *J Med Econ* 2002; **5**: 119–33.

18 Putnam K, Bohn R, Ewenstein B, Winkelmayer W, Avorn J. A cost minimization model for the treatment of minor bleeding episodes in patients with haemophilia A and high-titre inhibitors. *Haemophilia* 2005; **11**: 261–9.

19 You C, Lee S, Park S. Cost and effectiveness of treatments for mild-to-moderate bleeding episodes in haemophilia patients with inhibitors in Korea. *Haemophilia* 2009; **15**: 217–26.

20 Astermark J, Donfield S, DiMichele D, *et al.* A randomized comparison of bypassing agents in hemophilia complicated by an inhibitor: the FEIBA NovoSeven Comparative (FENOC) Study. *Blood* 2007; **109**: 546–51.

21 Steen Carlsson K, Astermark J, Donfield S, Berntorp E. Cost and outcome: comparisons of two alternative bypassing agents for persons with haemophilia A complicated by an inhibitor. *Thromb Haemost* 2008; **99**: 1060–7.

PART XIX

Comprehensive care and delivery of care

CHAPTER 66

Hemophilia databases

Charles R.M. Hay

Manchester Royal Infirmary, Manchester, UK

Introduction

Bleeding Disorder Databases of one sort or another have now been established in most developed countries [1–6]. These databases vary in their scope and purpose, from long-standing and multipurpose national and international databases such as the UK National Haemophilia Database (NHD), the CDC Universal Data Collection, PedNet and the European Haemophilia Adverse Event System (EUHASS) to registries formed to address limited and disease-specific questions, such as the European Acquired Haemophilia (EACH) Registry. There are many challenges to be overcome in starting and maintaining a bleeding disorder database, including the difficulty of obtaining long-term funding and commitment from clinicians and patients and the limitations imposed by the need to comply with data protection legislation. This chapter gives a brief overview of the benefits of setting up such a database, how it may be organized and the approaches which may be used to overcome the difficulties involved.

Functions of a national bleeding disorder database

Bleeding disorder databases have three possible basic functions: healthcare planning, epidemiologic research and pharmacovigilance. Databases collect patient demographic and observational data relevant to healthcare concerns which are specific to bleeding disorders such as the prevalence and severity of the disease, the prevalence and incidence of factor VIII/IX inhibitors, viral infections, treatment intensity and, increasingly, treatment outcomes. Improvement in hemophilia treatment and the impact of new medical interventions, such as prophylaxis or the use of antiviral therapy may thus be assessed over time by clinicians and healthcare providers. The dataset collected requires regular review and amendment to address new research questions and to address the changing needs of the health service and suppliers. The dataset currently collected by the UK NHD may be viewed on www .UKHCDO.org.

Healthcare planning

The extent to which databases can serve these functions will depend upon the completeness and accuracy of the data held, the extent of the dataset collected and the timeliness of the data collection and reporting. Where clinical service provision for patients with bleeding disorders is poorly developed, even basic disease prevalence data may be useful for planning purposes. Where hemophilia services are already very well developed, however, healthcare planning requires timely, complete and relatively comprehensive data, since the focus in such a healthcare system has usually shifted from providing a basic service to optimizing the quality and distribution of care, cost-control, financial planning and the measurement of clinical outcome. Healthcare providers are very focussed on hemophilia care because of the extremely high cost of the treatment and the inexorable, 7–10%, annual increase in treatment cost, which they wish to understand better. This focus will only increase as healthcare systems come under increasing financial pressure.

Hemophilia databases have potentially a very important role in analyzing the causes of this growth in treatment cost and in helping to optimise treatment and justify current treatment practises. In the UK, the NHD also had a central role in national procurement of clotting factor concentrates [7], monitoring the national contract and benchmarking individual hemophilia centers, i.e. comparing their factor usage and clinical outcomes. The principal results of our annual report may be viewed on www.UKHCDO.org. Disease monitoring is also important. Adverse events are reported as they arise and the patient group monitored for events related to HIV, HCV, and vCJD. The NHD processed this data and presented it to Healthcare Commissioners and The Health Protection Agency on a quarterly basis.

Textbook of Hemophilia, Third Edition. Edited by Christine A. Lee, Erik E. Berntorp and W. Keith Hoots.

© 2014 John Wiley & Sons, Ltd. Published 2014 by John Wiley & Sons, Ltd.

Research

Research is an important function of any disease database but, increasingly, carefully validated and comprehensive datasets, collected by protocol are required for useful research to be conducted within a reasonable time frame. Some databases attempt a complete data collection from all patients in their country (UK, Canada, Australia, Germany, and Italy) whereas others collect only from a selection of participating centers, e.g. US Universal Data Collection System, EUHASS, and PedNet. Reports of data collected only from interested centers may be prone to selection bias.

The collection of treatment data may enable the efficacy of different treatment regimens to be evaluated, but only if adequate outcome data is also collected. The collection of mortality data makes it possible to investigate the natural history of the disease and to assess the effect of improvements in care on mortality from bleeding and to evaluate the effect of treatment complications, such as inhibitors HIV and hepatitis C on life expectancy. This data has also been used by patient groups campaigning for compensation.

Both longitudinal cohort analyses and case-control comparisons of database data have been used to explore the natural history, treatment, and complications of bleeding disorders [8,9]. The database is an important research resource for the whole of its parent organization. For some questions either the complication rate may be too low (e.g. risk factors for inhibitors in previously treated patients), or the sample size too small (e.g. differences in immunogenicity of different factor VIII concentrates) for individual databases to provide a definitive answer to the scientific question posed [10]. In the future such circumstances may make it necessary for databases to collaborate and aggregate anonymous data to achieve adequate statistical power.

Pharmacovigilance

Market research and pharmacovigilance also require real-time data collection and rapid reporting. Regulators are increasingly concerned with safety issues, such as the development of factor VIII inhibitors, for which traditional safety and efficacy licencing studies are statistically under-powered. This is a generic problem for all products used for rare diseases, because large scale trials are impractical in these conditions for reasons of cost and lack of study subjects. Regulatory licencing studies lack the statistical power to determine whether new products are more immunogenic than previously marketed concentrates. For that reason, new factor VIII and XI concentrates will necessarily be licensed on condition that extended postmarketing surveillance is conducted. These studies are expensive and difficult to recruit to. National databases already collect reports of adverse events in real-time and so may have an important part to play in conducting future postmarketing surveillance studies. NHD have already conducted such studies and have reported data for licencing purposes for several products now [11]. The weakness of such data at present is that it is not collected to GCP/FDA standards with source data verification. Its strength is the large sample size and the independence of the data collection from the manufacturer in question.

Problem of funding

Most bleeding disorder databases were started by groups of enthusiastic clinicians using short-term grants from a funding body or from one or more of the manufacturers. Often a point is reached when the data collected is no longer adequate to address either healthcare planning or current research needs. At this point, the database must either develop and expand or close. This is challenging and requires a lot of commitment and money. Industry, government or healthcare providers may provide the necessary finance, but only if they can be persuaded of the utility of the data collected. It may be argued that the cost of setting up and running such a database is a very small proportion of the high cost of the treatment being monitored and that the data may help health commissioners or industry to plan. Public funding may be associated with a high level of bureaucracy and accountability, however, and such funding bodies may directly or indirectly influence the direction that the database may take and the type of data collected. Perhaps counterintuitively, unrestricted grants from industry usually leave the database policy makers with greater freedom to take the database in the direction that they want. Funding may be short term and linked to specific projects, however. There is no single model for funding such a database and most continue to struggle to fulfil long-term aims with short term funding. A recent survey showed that although the Italian Database was funded by industry, EUHASS, the UK NHD, and the US Universal Data Collection, Canadian, Australian, and German Databases were all at least part-funded by government agencies. This probably provides the most stable source of funding.

Governance issues

Even though databases collect observational data only and do not conduct interventional clinical trials, they nevertheless exist in an increasingly tightly controlled regulatory environment. Ethical approval for databases is not mandatory in many jurisdictions but is recommended. Databases also have a duty to put in place appropriate mechanisms to ensure strict data security and to comply with the Data Protection Act of the UK. Finally, all databases require an oversight committee as a governing body to review the running of the database, to consider requests for data, to direct database policy and to produce research from the database. These are discussed in greater detail below.

Data security

Modern databases collect and store all their data electronically. Data security is designed into such systems at a high level.

Access to the database should be password protected, with timed lockouts. Registered users with a password and username may log onto the database to interrogate it or enter data into a holding database, but may view named data on patients from their own center only and aggregate anonymous data from the rest of the country, for benchmarking comparison. Electronic communications with the database should be encrypted using a 126-bit encryption key. The UK Database is also protected from the web by the firewalls of the NHS net. Named patient data is only communicated within this safe envelope and only using an encrypted link. All reports are anonymized.

No copies of the database or part of the database are permitted outside the database building. Daily backups are stored in a fireproof safe. The data is held on a fileserver housed in a secure, temperature-controlled server hotel within the NHS-net. The database area is always locked when unattended. The office is largely "paperless."

Annual inspections by the "Caldecott Guardian" are requested by the Database to document secure data handling and compliance with the Data Protection Act (DPA) 1998 and the Caldecott Guardian's report is published on our website (www.ukhcdo.org) to demonstrate our compliance to the outside world.

Data Protection Act and consent

Data protection legislation must be considered and complied with when setting up a disease register. The DPA 1998 of the UK was introduced to tighten up data protection and to harmonize with existing European Union legislation (view on: http://www.opsi.gov.uk/Acts/Acts1998/ukpga_19980029_en _1). The Act concerns all "named" data, which is defined as data linked by any identifier linking the data back to the patient's name or record. Patients have to give consent for their data to be included in a database of named data. In the UK, this does not currently have to be written consent and an "opt out" approach is widely used. Patients are sent a patient information leaflet every 5 years (also on our website: www .UKHCDO.org) and informed of their rights under the DPA 1998 so that they may have their data deleted or not included if they wish. Few patients have opted out. We have over 24 000 patient records in the UK NHD and these patients are circulated every 5 years.

Data protection legislation has been harmonized to a high-degree in the European Union (EU), and very similar legislation exists in North America and elsewhere. Nevertheless, local variations in interpretation of the law have caused considerable problems and delays in setting up databases in some countries. Even for existing databases the cost of addressing data protection legislation and the risk of patient nonparticipation was widely perceived to be a threat to future activities of such databases [12–14]. Explicit written consent may become the norm in the future, but the danger to databases of such an approach derives not just the enormous effort required from medical and nursing staff to obtain such consent but also because the commonest reason for failure to obtain consent is failure return the form rather than active refusal to participate. Participation in the Canadian Stroke Registry, for example, was reduced to 39% following the need for written consent [14].

Anonymous or named database?

Most databases, including the Canadian CHARMS database and the Italian Database, have anonymized their data by using a patient code or number [4]. Anonymization may ease some of the problems obtaining consent. However, in some administrations the identification code may qualify as a patient identifier under the definition used by the DPA, since the code has to be traceable back to the hemophilia center and the patient to avoid duplicate entries for patients attending more than one center. Anonymization can also limit the extent to which the patient data may be analysed geographically and used for administrative and planning purposes.

The UK NHD has been a named database since its inception. The possibility of anonomyzing the database was carefully considered by UKHCDO when the DPA 1998 came into force in 2000, but it was felt that the advantages of maintaining a named database far outweighed the effort required to obtain the patient's implied consent. Furthermore, it would have been impossible for us to conduct some of our healthcare planning functions for the Department of Health for England without recording multiple patient identifiers. The distribution of finance for the rollout of recombinant factor VIII and IX and the modeling of the National Procurement for clotting factor concentrates required the NHD to have data including the patient's name, NHS number GP practise code annual factor usage, brand, and unit cost. This is also required to benchmark outcomes from individual centers and map treatment by healthcare administrative region.

Database oversight committee

Many, but not all hemophilia databases are run under the umbrella of their national hemophilia treaters organization. All databases should be directly supervised by an oversight or steering committee which meets regularly and reports back to their parent organization and to other stakeholders. This oversight committee will determine database policy and direction, regularly review the dataset, oversee the organization and running of the database and produce research and reports from the data. All the stakeholder groups should be represented on this committee. The oversight committee for the UK NHD, for example, includes the Vice Chair and Chair of UKHCDO, the Chairs of all the UKHCDO working parties, a software engineer, and representatives from the Haemophilia Nurses Association, the Data Managers Forum and the Haemophilia Society, a patient, and two Healthcare Commissioners. There is also input from the Department of Health.

Technical specification, design, and staffing

The philosophy behind the organization of the UK database is to maximize data collection whilst minimizing duplication of effort from the hemophilia centers. We only want to collect data once. Hemophilia centers around the world already collect a great deal of data, partly for clinical management and partly for financial administration. Although this data may be of interest for research, pharmacovigilance and national planning, it may be held on computer systems not compatible with or inaccessible to the national database. Indeed, neither the US Universal Data Collection System nor the Canadian Databases are networked to all centers.

To circumvent this problem in the UK and to recruit support from Health Commissioners, we developed a fully integrated software system which fulfils both administrative and research functions. This consists of four fully integrated and connected modules: Haemtrack, the Haemophilia Centre Information System (HCIS), the National Haemophilia Database (NHD) and the on-line reporting system. Haemtrack is a home therapy module which is used by the patient to send bleed-level data on home therapy and home stock control to the hemophilia center and NHD using a personal computer, tablet, phone-app, or (least favored) paper. We aim to retrieve this data in real time as far as possible and the system is endorsed and mandated by the Health Commissioners. The HCIS accepts Haemtrack data and other clinical and administrative treatment and adverse event data, joint scoring, virology, etc. Adverse event data is uploaded to the NHD as they occur and other data, including Haemtrack data, are uploaded quarterly into the NHD. The NHD produces quarterly and annual reports and special reports on request. Much of this anonymized data may be viewed on line by commissioners for contract monitoring and planning purposes. Data need therefore only to be keyed in once and may be exported to the national hemophilia database semiautomatically.

The flow of data through the HCIS system is illustrated diagrammatically in the figure. New diagnoses and adverse events such as new inhibitors, death, or viral infection are reported as they arise through the secure network. All UK Hemophilia centers are networked to the national hemophilia database, even those lacking an HCIS system. Data is imported into a holding database from the HCIS quarterly. After verification and resolution of supplementary enquiries the data is imported from the holding to the main database and incorporated. The data is then analysed and reports issued to stakeholders. The organization of the different elements of the system and flow of data are illustrated in Figure 66.1.

Patient home treatment data including reason for treatment, bleed details including position and outcome, batch number, and dose may be imported either manually or electronically using the Haemtrak system. This is an electronic patient information system sponsored by Baxter to replace the Advoy system,

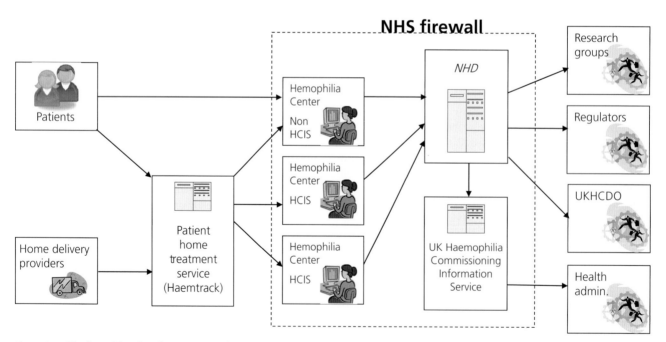

Figure 66.1 The flow of data from home-care suppliers and patients through Haemtrack to hemophilia centers, most of which use the Haemophilia Centre Information System (HCIS). Hemophilia centers upload adverse events as they occur and all other data quarterly to the National Haemophilia Database (NHD). NHD processes and cleans this data and makes it available to hemophilia centers, health commissioners, public health bodies, the Department of Health, research groups, regulators, and industry. Data provided to non-NHS bodies is anonymized. Only the Haemtrack component exists outside the NHS-net, separated from the world wide web by a firewall, and within which all communications are encrypted. UKHCDO, UK Haemophilia Centre Doctors' Organisation.

which was recently withdrawn from the UK. Similar systems have been developed in other countries.

Most databases use a robust server program which will accommodate simultaneous multiuser access such as SQ-server or Oracle. The Data is stored on large fileservers with a data and power backup ensuring that hard-drive failure does not lead to loss of data. The constant task of chasing data and verifying it is labour intensive despite the support of an impressive hardware and software infrastructure. The staff also provides logistic support for the specific research projects for individual groups of investigators.

The future

The HCIS will be networked so that all participating hemophilia centers in the UK may administer their centers and collect their data directly using two centralized fileservers working in tandem rather than a server in their own hospital. Improvements in band width and speed within the health service have made this advance possible. This will reduce the cost of running the system, improve reliability, and make it easier to get smaller centers using the HCIS system. It will also give the national database access to far more data accumulated as it is entered.

The future is also likely to see hemophilia databases maturing and developing stronger relationships with healthcare commissioners, industry, and regulators since these databases will become the natural source of data for healthcare planning, outcome evaluation, and pharmacovigilance. Databases will also become a powerful tool for large scale epidemiologic research and the evaluation of treatment outcomes. This requires long-term planning and commitment.

References

1 Evatt BL. World Federation of Hemophilia guide to developing a national patient registry. World Federation of Haemophilia, 2005. Available at: http://www.wfh.org/2/docs/Publications/Diagnosis_and_Treatmen/Registry_Guide_2005.pdf

2 Hay CRM. The UK Haemophilia Database: a tool for research, audit and healthcare planning. *Haemophilia* 2004; **10**(S3): 21.

3 Walker I. The Canadian Hemophilia Registry. *Haemophilia* 2004; **10**; 21–2.

4 Walker I, Pai M, Akabutu J, *et al.* The Canadian Hemophilia Registry as the basis for a national system for the monitoring of the use of factor concentrates. *Transfusion* 1995; **35**: 548–51.

5 Iorio A, Oliovechio E, Morfini M, Mannucci PM, on behalf of the Association of Italian Hemophilia Centre Directors. Italian Registry of Haemophilia and Allied Disorders. Objectives, methodology and data analysis. *Haemophilia* 2008; **14**: 444–53.

6 Soucie JM, McAlister S, McLellan A, Oakley M, Ying S. The Universal Data Collection Surveillance System for Rare Bleeding Disorders. *Am J Prev Med* 2010; **38**(4S): S475–81.

7 Hay CRM. purchasing factor concentrates in the 21st century through competitive tendering. *Haemophilia* 2013; **19**: 660–7.

8 Hay CRM, Palmer B, Chalmers E, *et al.* Incidence of factor VIII inhibitors throughout life in severe hemophilia A in the United Kingdom. *Blood* 2011; **117**(23): 6367–70

9 Gouw SC, Van der Bom JG, Ljung R, *et al.* for the PedNet and Rodin Study Group. Factor VIII Products and Inhibitor Development in Severe Hemophilia A. *N Engl J Med* 2013; **368**(3): 231–9.

10 Hay CRM, Palmer BP, Chalmers E, *et al.* on behalf of UKHCDO. The incidence of factor VIII inhibitors in severe haemophilia A following a major product switch in the UK: a prospective cohort study. *Blood* 2014 (in preparation).

11 Hay CRM, Bjerre J, Dolan G, on behalf of UKHCDO. Real-life use of high and standard initial doses of activated recombinant Factor VII (rFVIIa) in patients with haemophilia A and B with inhibitors—data from the UKHCDO/NHD registry. *Haemophilia* 2014, in press (abstract) (in preparation).

12 Baker RI, Laurenson L, Winter M, Pritchard AM. The impact of information technology on haemophilia care. *Haemophilia* 2004; **10** (Suppl. 4): 41–6.

13 Verity C, Nicoll A. Consent, confidentiality and the threat to public health surveillance. *Br Med J* 2002; **324**: 1210–13.

14 Tu JV, Willison DJ, Silver FL, *et al.* Impracticability of informed consent in the registry of the Canadian Stroke Network. *N Engl J Med* 2004; **350**; 1414–21.

CHAPTER 67

Comprehensive care and delivery of care: the developed world

Christopher A. Ludlam[1] and Cedric R.J.R. Hermans[2]

[1] University of Edinburgh and Royal Infirmary, Edinburgh, Scotland
[2] St-Luc University Hospital, Brussels, Belgium

Introduction

Although access to safe and sufficient clotting factor concentrates is fundamentally important, this alone is not sufficient to provide optimal care to patients with hemophilia. Because of its rarity and complexity, hemophilia was recognized as early as the 1950s to require the development of specialist care. The wideranging needs of people with hemophilia and their families are indeed best met through the coordinated delivery of comprehensive care by a multidisciplinary team of healthcare professionals. Comprehensive care of hemophilia addresses the treatment and prevention of bleeding, the long-term management of hemophilic arthropathy and other complications of bleeding, the management of significant complications of treatment (the development of inhibitors and transfusion transmitted infections), and the psychosocial support and education required to manage the bleeding disorder [1]. Comprehensive care therefore requires collaboration between several specialists as well as a core team (usually a hematologist, laboratory staff, nurses, physiotherapist, and social worker).

The delivery of a high-quality comprehensive service to patients with hemophilia and other bleeding disorders depends upon defined standards and a network of hemophilia centers. In the UK, the Haemophilia Doctors' Organisation (UKHCDO) is an example of an organization that has grown from a small beginning to a larger collaboration of doctors who have been able to lead effectively the developments in care and set standards to improve the lives of those with hemophilia [2]. To help recruitment and training of physicians in the specialty, a European curriculum for thrombosis and hemostasis has been developed [3]. Similarly, patients have organized themselves into national societies, for example the UK Haemophilia Society (www.haemophilia.org.uk), and these have been very effective in patient advocacy. Many other countries have similar organizations, e.g. the National Haemophilia Foundation in the USA

(www.hemophilia.org). These national societies have been drawn together into the World Federation of Haemophilia (WFH), which has promoted hemophilia care particularly effectively in developing nations (www.wfh.org). It has encouraged international collaboration between designated specialist centers of expertise (WFH International Training Centers) and countries with developing services.

The comprehensive care model has been one of the most successful public health programs in many developed countries, resulting in significantly improved health for patients with hemophilia as well as producing a reduction in healthcare utilization [4]. The improved outcomes in morbidity and mortality when comprehensive care occurs within a hemophilia treatment center setting are well established [5].

The first part of the chapter outlines the overall framework within which national hemophilia services should be provided as has recently been set out by the European Association for Haemophilia and Allied Disorders (EAHAD; www.eahad.org) in the document *European Principles of Haemophilia Care* [6]. To illustrate how these principles have developed in detail to provide services, the arrangements in the UK are described in some detail as they offer one national model which has worked effectively over the past 40 years [7]. The second part summarizes international networking and collaborative initiatives recently implemented across Europe (EUHASS and EUHANET) and the major role the WFH has played in promoting comprehensive care globally.

European principles of hemophilia care

The EAHAD document, *European Principles of Haemophilia Care* describes the essential components of a national comprehensive care hemophilia service under 10 recommendations (Box 67.1). These emphasize the necessity for coordination of

Textbook of Hemophilia, Third Edition. Edited by Christine A. Lee, Erik E. Berntorp and W. Keith Hoots.
© 2014 John Wiley & Sons, Ltd. Published 2014 by John Wiley & Sons, Ltd.

Box 67.1 European Principles of Haemophilia. Adapted from Colvin BT et al., Haemophilia 2008; **14**: 361–74.

National hemophilia coordinating organizations with supporting local organizations
National hemophilia patient registry
Provision and maintenance of comprehensive care centers (CCCs) and hemophilia treatment centers (HTCs)
Partnership in the delivery of hemophilia care
Access to safe and effective concentrates at optimum treatment levels
Access to home treatment and delivery
Access to prophylactic therapy
Access to specialist services and emergency care
Management of inhibitors
Education and research

the services, and the first recommendation states that this can best be accomplished by having a national committee to include all stakeholders to oversee and plan national services. The second, and almost as important, recommendation is that there should be a confidential national registry of all patients. By knowing the number and severity of patients with congenital bleeding disorders, it becomes possible to start to plan the service and especially ensure the provision of therapeutic materials. The third recommendation relates to ensuring that comprehensive care hemophilia centers and hemophilia centers are established within an appropriate network; the exact arrangements will depend upon the distribution of patients and geographic factors. The other recommendations relate to details of service provision at the centers, e.g. monitoring of adverse therapeutic events, home therapy, and arrangements for prophylaxis. The *European Principles of Haemophilia Care* is now being used in Europe as a framework for service development throughout the continent especially in countries with less well developed nationally coordinated arrangements. It has proved useful to advocates to take to national government health departments when campaigning for improvements in services. To promote acceptance of the 10 principles of care within the European community, it has been presented to, and well received by, members of the European Parliament. The level of service provision within different countries in Europe compared to the recommendations set out in the principles of care has recently been audited by two studies; one by physicians and the other patients' organizations [8,9].

Arrangements for hemophilia care in the UK

Over the past 60 years, the UK's hemophilia service has evolved in response to advances in medical knowledge and provision of therapeutic materials and is now one of the most carefully defined and audited national clinical services in the country.

Since 1950, there has been a national UK approach to delivery of hemophilia care and a summary of its history has been set out in the previous edition of the *Textbook of Haemophilia* [2].

The professional responsibility for the hemophilia service has been led by UKHCDO (UKHCDO.org). This organisation was established in 1969, includes all doctors who work in hemophilia centers and it provides oversight and guidance for developments in the service. Within the UK, there are currently 24 comprehensive care centers (CCC) and 41 hemophilia centers for a population of approximately 60 million. The arrangements in the UK are very similar to those set out in the European Principles of Haemophilia Care and are set out in the UK National Service Specification (haemophiliaalliance.org).

In England, at the time of writing, there are major changes taking place in the way health services are to be provided in future. As provision for hemophilia is complex and specialized, it will be overseen nationally by the newly established NHS Commissioning Board which will receive advice from a Clinical Reference Group for Haemophilia. Over the past 20 years, Scotland, Wales, and Northern Ireland have developed a degree of devolution from the UK government in London and their health services are arranged a little differently although they all aim to provide services to the standards set out in the Service Specification.

UKHCDO National Register of Patients

Since 1969, the UKHCDO has maintained a confidential national register of patients with heritable bleeding disorders (as well as acquired hemophilia and von Willebrand disease). Hemophilia centers regularly inform the database which patients have been treated and the amount of and type of products received. It also records whether the patient has an inhibitor, the human immunodeficiency virus (HIV) status, and whether the genetic mutation is known. From time to time, additional requirements for information are added either to form part of the ongoing permanent record or for specific research of other projects. These arrangements allow very accurate assessment of the national use of coagulation factor concentrates [10], and a record of the side-effects or treatment.

UKHCDO working parties develop guidelines

One of the other important responsibilities of UKHCDO is to establish short-term working parties, which develop guidelines to inform practise, set standards (against which the quality of the service can be audited), and undertake research. Copies of the guidelines are available at www.ukhcdo.org. The most widely read is the Guidelines on Therapeutic Products which is updated approximately every 3 years [11].

The UK Haemophilia Society

The UK Haemophilia Society is an organization of patients and their families which provides support for those with heritable bleeding disorders (www.haemophilia.org.uk). It is a well-organized and effective pressure group which encourages improvements in service provision. It has a major educational responsibility and publishes highly regarded information booklets.

The Haemophilia Nurses Association

The UK Haemophilia Nurses Association (HNA) has approximately 150 members who care for patients and families with inherited bleeding disorders in hospital and at home. Communication, support, training, and education is delivered to nurses and other allied healthcare professionals via our on-line professional development site www.haemnet.com which also welcomes international nursing and allied healthcare input.

The Haemophilia Chartered Physiotherapists Association

The Haemophilia Chartered Physiotherapists Association brings together those with skills in developing the musculoskeletal system, and thus helps to prevent bleeds and minimizing their detrimental effects when they do occur. Although a much smaller group than the nurses, it has been well organized nationally and has developed and published a very useful recent guide.

Social work support

Social work support is critical both to help a family adjust to a new member with hemophilia and to assist those who develop relationship (and financial) difficulties as a result of their hemophilia or the consequences of its treatment, e.g. HIV. In the UK, hemophilia social workers collaborated nationally to sustain and develop their expertise and services. With the move away from hospital-based social work services to the community, it has been harder to maintain an active professional grouping, and the amount of support overall which social workers can provide has regrettably declined.

Laboratory scientists

Laboratory scientists provide the critical diagnostic services essential for hemophilia centers. Those with an academic scientific background as clinical scientists are employed primarily in research and development and more recently in ensuring that the latest advances in genetic techniques are available to benefit hemophilia families. As this has become one of their primary responsibilities, they have collaborated to establish the UK Haemophilia Genetic Laboratory Network and through this grouping have developed effective guidelines and standards for hemophilia genetic services (www.ukhcdo.org). Biomedical scientists, with a more technical focus on the laboratory service, are members of the Institute of Biomedical Scientists (IBMS) which is a large umbrella organization for scientists in all branches of pathology (www.ibms.org).

The Haemophilia Alliance

One of the challenges of hemophilia care is to ensure that the multidisciplinary team works collaboratively within the hospital and community and to provide as seamlessly as possible the range of appropriate services. To continue to develop this integrated service the professional organizations outlined above, along with the patients' Haemophilia Society, have come together to form the umbrella organization the UK Haemophilia Alliance. This has developed and published a model for comprehensive care for hemophilia in its Service Specification (www.haemophiliaalliance.org.uk).

Comprehensive hemophilia care in the UK

One of the guiding principles in designing arrangements for providing care for those with hemophilia and their families is that all individuals, wherever they live, should have access to the full range of services and specialties that make up comprehensive care for hemophilia. Whilst the majority who live near a CCC will be able to access these directly, those living more remotely who attend their local hemophilia center may need to be referred to the most convenient CCC for some of the more specialist aspects of clinical or laboratory service.

The Haemophilia Alliance Service Specification

The Service Specification of standards for hemophilia care was compiled by a multidisciplinary team representing the Alliance's constituent professions and the Haemophilia Society (www.haemophiliaalliance.org.uk). The standards were based on guidelines, which had been previously issued by the individual professional groups. It thus brought together into one document a description of the standards for a coordinated service for patients and their families, and in doing so provided an invaluable resource both for users and funders of the services as well as those in the hospitals providing the care. The contents of the report are listed in Box 67.2.

Service standards and delivery

This section of the document sets out in detail the components of the system which need to be provided [12–14]. The range of services which a CCC should provide is set out in Box 67.3. To provide these, it will often be necessary to have network

---

Box 67.2 National Service Specification for Hemophilia.

Target patient group
Methodology
Service objectives
Service standards and delivery
Quality standards
Treatment recommendations
Carrier detection, genetic counseling, and antenatal diagnosis
Outcomes
Service arrangements
Purchase of coagulation factor concentrates
Record-keeping and data collection

Box 67.3 Functions that must be able to be carried out by comprehensive care centers.

Coordination of the delivery of hemophilia services—in both the hospital and the community—while liaising with affiliated hemophilia centers and appropriate community agencies

A 24-h advisory and response service for hemophilia centers, general practitioners, dental surgeons, hospital doctors, patients, and families

Delivery of a comprehensive care program for patients with hemophilia; there must be at least 40 severely affected patients with hemophilia under the care of the center

A home-therapy program for patients with severe hemophilia, including the administration of prophylactic therapy where appropriate

Home treatment training programs, including home and school visits where appropriate

Provision of coagulation factor concentrates, for both hospital treatment and home-therapy programs

A diagnostic and reference laboratory service, performing a full range of laboratory tests for the diagnosis and monitoring of inherited and acquired disorders of hemostasis

Counseling for patients and their families

Social work support and welfare advice

Genetic counseling and diagnosis, in conjunction with specialized laboratories

Physiotherapy

Specialist operative and conservative dentistry

Specialist rheumatologic and orthopedic follow-up and intervention

Provision of obstetric and gynaecologic support for the clinical management of hemophilia carriers and women with von Willebrand disease

Specialized services for patients with HIV and hepatitis, including support groups

Family support groups

Participation in clinical trials

Participation in clinical and laboratory audit, external and internal quality control, with submission of results to commissioning authorities

Participation in research and development

Educational programs for medical and nursing staff, biomedical scientists, and related paramedical personnel

Educational programs for patients and their families concerning all aspects of home therapy and community care

---

arrangements with specialists, e.g. orthopedic surgery. The details of these networks will depend on how the other specialists provide their services locally and of the arrangements between CCC and the local hemophilia centers.

The Service Specification also emphasizes the importance of the establishment of a regional hemophilia network which comprises those who commission and fund the service as well as those who provide and use it. This regional network should oversee the coordinated service provided by CCCs and hemophilia centers to promote strategic planning and implementation of the service specification. These regional networks are at different stages of evolution in the UK, with some areas having well-developed arrangements whilst others are still being established.

Quality standards

The Service Specification sets out standards for data collection, laboratory performance, and clinical protocols (as set out by UKHCDO, HNA, and HCPA).

Treatment recommendations

This section of the Service Specification covers in some detail the framework for treatment, prophylaxis and home therapy, arrangements for children, and clinical review, and includes the importance of patient participation in the care process and record-keeping. Advice is given on management of inhibitors, immune tolerance, acquired hemophilia, von Willebrand disease, and rarer coagulation defects including inherited platelet disorders (www.ukhcdo.org).

Carrier detection, genetic counseling, and antenatal diagnosis

With the widespread ability to readily identify the individual mutation causing hemophilia in a family, this is now a recommended part of the assessment of hemophilic individuals. This has led in the UK to a re-examination of the arrangements for genetic counseling and the establishment of local genetic registers and genetic laboratory facilities at some CCCs as set out in the UKHCDO guidelines [15].

Outcomes of hemophilia care

There is increasing interest in being able to assess the outcome of hemophilia therapy, particularly as treatment is difficult, potentially hazardous, and expensive. Outcome measurements are difficult to quantify. One important aim of treatment is prevention of joint damage and its progression, but this needs to be assessed over many years. Such studies are very time-consuming and expensive and for this reason a number of surrogate measures of effectiveness of treatment have been suggested, e.g. regular magnetic resonance imaging scanning or clinical assessment of joints. Others include number of breakthrough bleeds per year in those on prophylaxis or days missed from school or work. This is a developing area of hemophilia care and one in which socioeconomic evaluation is being increasingly applied and for which appropriate tools are being developed [16].

Audit

Over the past 15 years in the UK, it has become increasingly important to demonstrate objectively, by external review, the quality of medical services. Prior to the audit visit, questionnaires are sent to a random selection of 30 patients registered at the center, which are returned anonymously to the auditors. Three auditors, a hemophilia physician, a nurse, and a patient visit the center for a day and review the clinical and laboratory facilities against the standards in the Service Specification. They also comment on whether recommendations in the previous audit have been implemented. Following their visit, a report is compiled and returned to the CCC and copies to the UKHCDO chair.

European networking initiatives

Cooperation and networking of hemophilia centers across Europe has been instrumental in implementing international registries and pharmacovigilance program and should play a key role in developing a system for certification of the delivery of hemophilia care in Europe.

The PEDNET (European Paediatric Network for Haemophilia Management) is a collaboration of 23 pediatricians from 16 European countries that provides an infrastructure for clinical research and management of children with hemophilia. The members of the group are responsible for the care of a substantial number of children with hemophilia in Western Europe. Annual workshops serve as a platform for informal discussion on important topics to improve quality of care by promoting information exchange about clinical practise and research [17]. Patients with congenital hemophilia A and B born after 1 January 2000 are eligible for enrolment in the PEDNET Haemophilia Registry. Baseline and follow-up assessments are obtained from all patients [18]. Using the PEDNET data, the RODIN study recently produced evidence on the effect of patient and treatment characteristics on the occurrence of inhibitors among patients with hemophilia [19].

EUHASS (European Haemophilia Safety Surveillance) (www.euhass.org) is a pharmacovigilance program to monitor the safety of treatments for people with inherited bleeding disorders in Europe. The EUHASS project has been running since 2008 and involves 80 centers from 26 European countries caring for almost 30 000 persons with bleeding disorders. Participating hemophilia centers report new adverse events that occur in their patients and these include allergic reaction, infections transmitted by concentrates, inhibitors, thromboses, malignancies, and deaths. Since the start of the project, more than 750 events have been prospectively reported. The ultimate aim of this project is to support improvements in patient safety by creating a European network for the monitoring and communication of health information and treatment safety data.

EUHANET (European Haemophilia Network) (www.euhanet .org) was recently set up as a new project aimed at establishing a network of hemophilia centers to work together on a number of related initiatives to improve the care of European citizens with inherited bleeding disorders. There are five associated partners: European Haemophilia Consortium (EHC), European Association for Haemophilia and Allied disorders (EAHAD, University Medical College Utrecht, Medical Data Solutions and Services Ltd (MDSAS), and Fondazione IRCCS Ca' Granda in Milan. There are 420 known hemophilia centers in Europe whose size and services offered vary enormously. EUHANET will develop a system for certification of the delivery of hemophilia care in Europe. During the first year of the project, criteria defining two levels of hemophilia care will be defined through extensive consultation. Treatment centers will then be invited to apply for certification and their level of service will be assessed according to which criteria they satisfy. The Haemophilia Central website (www.haemophiliacentral.org) will include information on guidelines, clinical information on all inherited bleeding disorders, location of hemophilia centers, details of clotting factor concentrates, database of active clinical trials, a news service, and a service for affected individuals to ask questions.

World Federation of Haemophilia and comprehensive care training

At a global level, the WFH International Haemophilia Training Center (IHTC) fellowship program has been providing intensive specialized multidisciplinary training since its inception in 1969. Fellows undergo 6–8 weeks of training at a WFH designated training center. Post-fellowship, the network of fellows provides an important base for many other WFH development program. Since the beginning of the programs, hundreds individuals covering all medical disciplines have been awarded fellowships to train at one of the 28 recognized training centers. The WFH HTC twinning program provides more extensive comprehensive care training. Twinning is a formal, two-way collaboration between developing and developed HTCs [20]. In 2010, there were 38 twinned HTCs. Twinning often serves as the catalyst for development of a national program [21].

Future developments in provision of hemophilia care

Over the past 20 years, factor VIII and other concentrate use has risen steadily at approximately 5% per annum, and there is no sign of this rate declining; it may in fact accelerate with increased use of prophylaxis, especially in adults. The cost is rising faster than the increase in use by factor VIII unitage with the move from plasma-derived to the more expensive recombinant concentrates. It is likely that the introduction of long half-life products will increase expenditure further although the ability by Bayesian techniques to predict trough levels during prophylaxis may allow more efficient use of concentrates and mitigate the higher costs. This financial pressure will make the gathering of outcome data to justify the increased use of concentrates more urgent. There will be an increasing focus on treatment and immune tolerance of those with inhibitors.

Patients are seeking increasing information about their condition: with developments in reliable genetic diagnostic tests to identify carriers, there is a need for more input of time for counseling both affected individuals and family members. The aspiration that all patients should have access to the full range of comprehensive care services, wherever they live, will best be brought about with networking arrangements between CCCs and hemophilia centers. To be effective, these arrangements will need to be formalized.

Overall life expectancy and quality of life among persons with hemophilia have increased in recent years. Older hemophilic patients now face aging comorbidities that are common in the general male population, such as cardiovascular or metabolic diseases, prostate hypertrophy, and hepatic, prostate, and other cancers. The prevalence of cardiovascular disease and incidence of vascular events among older hemophilic patients can be expected to increase and hemophilic patients may become prone to some cardiovascular risk factors, warranting preventative measures. The treatment of long-term complications of hepatitis C virus infection such as liver cirrhosis and hepatic cancer can be expected to be required in a large portion of the older hemophilia population for some years to come. Appropriate antiviral treatment and close monitoring for possible disease advancement will constitute an important part of routine medical care, and special considerations may be appropriate in conjunction with invasive procedures, chemotherapy, or radiotherapy. At the moment, hard data on which to base the management of these conditions are largely lacking, but can be expected to increase dramatically in the coming decades. In the meantime, the aging population of hemophilia patients should be offered the same comprehensive healthcare offered to the general population, which may require a restructuring of healthcare delivery [22].

As ever, there will be a need to be mindful of the potential side-effects of therapy whether infectious pathogens in the concentrates or inhibitors arising secondary to their use. Those who provide hemophilia care have found the past challenging and in future it will be necessary to respond proactively to an unpredictably changing environment.

References

1 Bolton-Maggs PH. Optimal haemophilia care versus the reality. *Br J Haematol* 2006; **132**(6): 671–82.

2 Ludlam C. Comprehensive care and delivery of care: the developed world. In: Lee C, Berntorp E, Hoots W (eds.) *Textbook of Haemophilia*. Oxford: Blackwell Publishing, 2005; 359–65.

3 Astermark J, Negrier C, Hermans C, *et al.* European curriculum for thrombosis and haemostasis. *Haemophilia* 2009; **15**(1): 337–44.

4 Evatt BL. The natural evolution of haemophilia care: developing and sustaining comprehensive care globally. *Haemophilia* 2006; **12** (Suppl. 3): 13–21.

5 Soucie JM, Nuss R, Evatt B, *et al.* Mortality among males with hemophilia: relations with source of medical care. The Hemophilia Surveillance System Project Investigators. *Blood* 2000 15; **96**(2): 437–42.

6 Colvin BT, Astermark J, Fischer K, *et al.* European principles of haemophilia care. *Haemophilia* 2008; **14**(2): 361–74.

7 Spooner R, Rizza C. Development of a national database to provide information for the planning of care of patients with congenital blood coagulation defects. In: Rizza C, Lowe G (eds.) *Haemophilia and Other Inherited Bleeding Disorders*. London: Saunders, 1997; 433–53.

8 Fischer K, Hermans C. The European Principles of Haemophilia Care: a pilot investigation of adherence to the principles in Europe. *Haemophilia* 2013; **19**(1): 35–43.

9 O'Mahony B, Noone D, Giangrande PL, Prihodova L. Haemophilia care in Europe: a survey of 19 countries. *Haemophilia* 2011; **17**(1): 35–40.

10 Rizza CR, Spooner RJ, Giangrande PL. Treatment of haemophilia in the United Kingdom 1981–1996. *Haemophilia* 2001; **7**(4): 349–59.

11 Keeling D, Tait C, Makris M. Guideline on the selection and use of therapeutic products to treat haemophilia and other hereditary bleeding disorders. A United Kingdom Haemophilia Center Doctors' Organisation (UKHCDO) guideline approved by the British Committee for Standards in Haematology. *Haemophilia* 2008; **14**(4): 671–84.

12 UK Department of Health. Provision of haemophilia treatment and care. Health circular HSG (93) 30. London: HMSO.

13 UK Department of Health. Organisation of haemophilia centres. Health circular HC (76) 4, 2013. London: HMSO.

14 UK Ministry of Health. Health memorandum. Arrangements for the care of persons suffering from haemophilia and related disorders, 1968. London: HMSO.

15 Ludlam CA, Pasi KJ, Bolton-Maggs P, *et al.* A framework for genetic service provision for haemophilia and other inherited bleeding disorders. *Haemophilia* 2005; **11**(2): 145–63.

16 Schramm W, Royal S, Kroner B, *et al.* Clinical outcomes and resource utilization associated with haemophilia care in Europe. *Haemophilia* 2002; **8**(1): 33–43.

17 Donadel-Claeyssens S. Current co-ordinated activities of the PEDNET (European Paediatric Network for Haemophilia Management). *Haemophilia* 2006; **12**(2): 124–7.

18 Chambost H, Ljung R. Changing pattern of care of boys with haemophilia in western European centres. *Haemophilia* 2005; **11**(2): 92–9.

19 Gouw SC, van der Bom JG, Ljung R, *et al.* Factor VIII products and inhibitor development in severe hemophilia A. *N Engl J Med* 2013; **368**(3): 231–9.

20 Giangrande PL, Mariani G, Black C. The WFH Haemophilia Centre Twinning Programme: 10 years of growth, 1993–2003. *Haemophilia* 2003; **9**(3): 240–4.

21 Poon MC, Luke KH. Haemophilia care in China: achievements of a decade of World Federation of Hemophilia treatment centre twinning activities. *Haemophilia* 2008; **14**(5): 879–88.

22 Dolan G, Hermans C, Klamroth R, Madhok R, Schutgens RE, Spengler U. Challenges and controversies in haemophilia care in adulthood. *Haemophilia* 2009; **15**(Suppl. 1): 20–7.

CHAPTER 68

Comprehensive care and delivery of care in hemophilia: the developing world

Alok Srivastava and Auro Viswabandya
Christian Medical College, Tamil Nadu, India

Introduction

The management of patients with hemophilia, particularly those with severe disease (factor activity <1%), is more complex than replacement of factor concentrates alone. Since the clinical impact of the severely compromised hemostasis is felt from a very early age, and the fact that optimal curative treatment still eludes this condition, these patients develop many complications that require involvement of a variety of healthcare personnel. Comprehensive care promotes physical and psychologic health and quality of life while decreasing morbidity and mortality [1]. These include the following:

- Early recognition of the condition and accurate diagnosis by the primary physician before any serious complication occurs due to hemorrhage.
- Consultation with a specialist physician/hematologist to plan the management of the individual including a plan for factor replacement therapy and other supportive measures.
- Counseling of the family on the implications of coping with this diagnosis and its socioeconomic impact. This usually involves a nurse or a social worker.
- Involvement of a physical therapist, psychiatrist, and an orthopedic specialist to manage the almost inevitable musculoskeletal complications.
- A dentist for dentition-related complications which are not uncommon.
- An appropriate molecular genetics laboratory for carrier detection and prenatal diagnosis, if needed.
- Infectious disease specialists and hepatologists to cope with the legacy of viral infections with human immunodeficiency virus (HIV) and hepatitis C virus (HCV) from factor concentrates used in the 1980s among many adult patients.
- A psychologist to take care of long-term psychosocial aspect of a chronic incurable disease.
- Inhibitors to factors VIII and IX develop in a proportion of these patients and require special management.

Such an approach to the management of people with hemophilia is termed "comprehensive care" [2,3]. The actual delivery of such care to a person with hemophilia and his family requires a healthcare system and other supportive mechanisms. Patients ideally should be seen by all core team members at least yearly (children every 6 months) for a complete hematologic, musculoskeletal, and psychologic assessment, and to develop, audit, and refine an individual's comprehensive management plan [1,4]. This chapter describes the special considerations required in providing comprehensive care to people with hemophilia in developing countries.

Developing world and its problems with hemophilia care

Of the estimated 400 000 people with hemophilia in the world, about 80% live in developing countries reflecting the overall distribution of population in the world in 143 of the 191 member states of the World Health Organization [5]. As opposed to a per capita gross domestic product (GDP) of nearly $30–40 000 in developed countries, the per capita GDP in developing countries varies from less than $1000 for about 40% of these people (low income), to $1000–4000 for another 40% (lower middle income) and $4000–12 000 for the remaining 20% (upper middle income) [6]. The expenditure on health in these countries is usually between 1 and 3% of GDP, most of which goes toward maintaining infrastructure. The limited healthcare budget under these circumstances is therefore often directed toward nutritional deficiencies and infectious diseases (high-volume, low-cost conditions) rather than hemophilia or other hereditary bleeding disorders (low-volume, high-cost conditions). While there is no doubt that limitation of resources impacts very significantly on the ability of countries in the developing world to spend on hemophilia care, the other most important factor in this regard is the attitude of the people and their government

Textbook of Hemophilia, Third Edition. Edited by Christine A. Lee, Erik E. Berntorp and W. Keith Hoots.
© 2014 John Wiley & Sons, Ltd. Published 2014 by John Wiley & Sons, Ltd.

toward healthcare in general and hemophilia in particular. Within the social and economic diversities of these countries, examples abound of countries with similar per capita GDP spending very differently on health. In recent years, directed expenditure on hemophilia care has significantly increased in most of these countries.

Comprehensive care and delivery of care

Providing comprehensive care to people with hemophilia in developing countries requires a few core components to be established [7]. These include:

1 Appropriate medical infrastructure.
2 Identification and registration of people with hemophilia.
3 Selection of appropriate models of care (protocols and products).
4 Educating patients and families about hemophilia care.
5 Improving social awareness of hemophilia and promoting advocacy.
6 Developing a program for delivery of care.

Establishing appropriate medical facilities

There should be at least one center in each country that can provide comprehensive care according to international standards. Therefore, it is essential to identify and train physicians who are committed to the field of hemostasis. They can then help train others in the country. More emphasis should be placed on the management of bleeding disorders, indeed hematology in general, in the medical curriculum in developing countries. Annual workshops held in different regions, to emphasize various aspects of hemophilia care, can significantly improve the understanding and skills of the care providers. In this regard, programs of the World Federation of Hemophilia (WFH) such as the International Hemophilia Training Centers fellowships, center twinning program, and workshops have been very useful in the rapid transfer of information and expertise [8,9]. Other training options also exist through professional societies and individual institutions.

The number of care centers required in each country will depend on the geographic distribution of the patient population. The facilities at each center will vary according to the level of expertise and infrastructure available (Table 68.1). Detailed guidelines should be prepared for the management of these conditions in a way that is appropriate and practical for each country. It would be best to integrate these services with the existing healthcare system, if possible, so that the diagnostic and clinical facilities at these centers will be useful for patients with other bleeding disorders as well.

While the treatment of hemophilia is extremely expensive, prevention is not. This is an aspect of hemophilia care that needs particular emphasis in developing countries. With the knowledge of the genetics of hemophilia and utilizing current techniques of molecular biology highly accurate carrier

Table 68.1 Establishing facilities at different levels of care for people with haemophilia in developing countries.

Level of clinical care	Facilities available
Primary care center	Provision of basic care to patients with diagnosed bleeding disorders
	Storage and administration of therapeutic products
	Participation in appropriate clinical audit.
Treatment center	All facilities mentioned above along with laboratory service for screening tests for the diagnosis of bleeding disorders. Facilities for assays and screening for inhibitors, if possible
	Physiotherapy
	Counseling and advisory services
	Advice on home therapy, where appropriate
Comprehensive care center	All facilities mentioned above and 24-h clinical service capable of handling emergencies and advising other centers.
	Laboratory facilities for assays of factor levels and inhibitors.
	Specialist service for surgeries, infectious diseases and social issues
	Rehabilitation services
Reference center	All facilities mentioned above and Reference laboratory for evaluation of atypical cases and rarer bleeding disorders
	Genetic evaluation, carrier detection and antenatal diagnosis
	Training of members of the comprehensive care team
	Maintain national registry
	Conduct data analysis and clinical audit
	Formulation of national policies
	Research that is appropriate for the country

Level of laboratory	Tests available
Coagulation laboratory	Blood film, platelet count, clot retraction, bleeding time, prothrombin time (PT), activated partial thromboplastin time (APTT), thrombin time (TT), correction studies with "control" and factor VIII and factor IX deficient plasma from appropriately screened patients and inhibitor screening, qualitative test for factor XIII
Comprehensive coagulation laboratory	All tests mentioned above and factor assays (VIII, IX, I, II, V, VII, X, XI) inhibitor assays, platelet function tests, von Willebrand factor (vWF) activity
Reference coagulation laboratory	All tests mentioned above and vWF multimers, vWF antigen, factor IX antigen, genotypic analysis, carrier detection, prenatal diagnostic tests and evaluation of rarer coagulation disorders
	Coordinate external quality assessment program
	Appropriate research

detection and prenatal diagnosis can be established cost-effectively in many of these countries [10].

It is also important that, together with help for establishing diagnostic and treatment facilities, concepts of quality management in all aspects of the work involved be emphasized. A system of clinical audit should also be developed. All laboratories should be encouraged to participate in at least one external quality assessment program [11].

Identification and registration of people with hemophilia

In developing countries from which data is available, the proportion of the estimated number of people with hemophilia identified varies between 10 and 80%. Overall, only about 30% of people with hemophilia estimated to exist in these countries (based on gene prevalence data) have been identified [12]. Inadequacy of healthcare facilities, lack of adequate knowledge of bleeding disorders among primary-care physicians, and poorly developed hematology services, particularly with respect to diagnosis of bleeding disorders contribute to the fact that the majority of people with hemophilia in these countries remain undetected or inadequately diagnosed [7].

The challenge of identifying affected people and making an accurate diagnosis of hemophilia in developing countries requires multiple strategies: educating healthcare personnel; increasing awareness in society; establishing laboratories capable of performing tests of hemostasis, with appropriate quality control of these tests; and monitoring of these services for their impact on hemophilia care.

The importance of creating a national registry of people with hemophilia cannot be overemphasized. This is the only way to chart out the demography of people with hemophilia in any country, document their clinical status, and monitor their progress over a period of time to assess the efficacy of the care program.

Selecting appropriate models of care
Protocols for treatment

Factor replacement therapy in hemophilia is often based on following convention rather than evidence for optimum protocols. In situations without significant constraints on resources, the guiding principle is to use high doses that guarantee efficacy, albeit at an extremely high cost. In developing countries, this approach is impractical and requires a prudent selection of protocols that are most cost-efficient since more than 90% of the cost of hemophilia care is the purchase of factor concentrates. Therefore selecting suitable protocols for use in each country becomes critical [13].

The three main indications for factor replacement in hemophilia are:
- Prevention/treatment of hemarthroses.
- Surgery.
- Immune tolerance therapy.

Prevention/treatment of hemarthrosis

The predominant cause of morbidity in hemophilia is the damage resulting from repeated bleeding into joints. It has been the aim of therapy to establish a standard where damage to the joints, clinically and radiologically, can be completely prevented. Prophylactic administration of clotting factor concentrates

prevents bleeding and joint destruction and should be the goal of therapy to preserve normal musculoskeletal function [14–16]. Prophylactic replacement of clotting factor concentrate has been shown to be useful even when factor levels are not maintained above 1 U/dL at all times [16,17]. This has been achieved by prophylactic replacement of factor concentrates 2–3 times/week at 25–40 IU/dose. The effectiveness of this approach in preserving joint integrity has been established with long-term follow-up data from Sweden [18]. Effectiveness has also been shown from long-term follow-up data from the Netherlands where a moderate prophylactic dose of factor concentrate 2–3 times/week at 15–30 IU/kg is used. Effectiveness of prophylactic factor support has also been proved in multiple randomized trials [15,16]. Unfortunately, the annual cost of such therapy, currently at US$100–300 000/person has been so high that it has been difficult even for countries with developed economies to adopt it universally [15]. Therefore other models of prophylaxis perhaps using lower doses need to be explored. This is now being done in several developing countries. Some of the initial data is promising [19,20]. Until optimal dosing is possible in developing countries, the aim of replacement shifts from maintaining perfect joint integrity to maintaining good joint function that will allow the person to remain functionally independent. This can usually be achieved with smaller doses of factor concentrate. Out of necessity and not out of choice, people with hemophilia in developing countries and their physicians have to accept this fact [21].

Prophylaxis in the classic way has generally been considered feasible only after availability of about 3 IU/capita of the national population is achieved. This model is predicated on an assumed target dose of 25–40 IU/kg for each prophylactic infusion. It is possible that lower doses may also be effective or at least better than on-demand therapy. With many developing countries moving in to the 1–3 IU/capita range of usage of clotting factor concentrates [12], other models of prophylaxis need to be considered until the optimal doses are worked out and availability improves in these countries. A hypothetical situation is therefore described below. Based on the usually quoted number of five people with hemophilia/100 000 populations, a country of 10 million people will have about 500 people with hemophilia. If they have access to even 1 IU/capita, then they have 10 million units of concentrate available. This would amount to about 20 000 IU every year for each person with hemophilia. If the average weight of young children (<10 years) is taken to be about 25 kg, the children can be given a prophylaxis of 250 IU (∼10 IU/kg) two times a week, they would require about 25 000 IU for the year. It is very likely that this regimen will be better than on-demand therapy and should be attempted. Depending on the availability of concentrates over 1 IU/capita suitable regimen for prophylaxis can be worked out increasing the dose and frequency while all the time documenting bleeding and musculoskeletal outcome until what is acceptable to the community is achieved. Where continuous prophylaxis is not practical, for patients with repeated bleeding, particularly into target joints, short-term prophylaxis for 4–8 weeks can be used to interrupt the bleeding cycle. This may be combined with intensive physiotherapy or synoviorthesis [22,23].

The actual amount of factor replacement for joint bleeding in developing countries is variable. The limited data available suggest that the total quantity of factor concentrate used varies from about 2–30 000 IU/person annually [24]. Some of these hemophilia centers that use factor concentrates in the intermediate range report preservation of reasonable joint function and functional independence. However, this is not backed by data on long-term orthopedic outcome. Therefore it would be useful to longitudinally evaluate a large number of patients with emphasis not only on their clinical and radiologic scores but also on their functional status. Such data could help establish the dose that maximizes the cost–benefit ratio.

The other important aim is to prevent chronic synovitis. Synovium becomes inflamed and friable after repeated bleeding and it leads to its hypertrophy. Repeated bleeding does cause articular damage, muscle atrophy, and subsequent loss of motion. The goal of therapy is to quiesce the inflamed synovium as quickly as possible and to preserve joint function. It can be achieved through regular physiotherapy, short courses of factor infusion, and a course of nonsteriodal anti-inflammatory drugs (NSAIDs) (COX-2 inhibitors), which will reduce inflammation. Synovectomy should be considered if chronic synovitis persists with frequent recurrent bleeding not controlled by other means. It can be done either by chemical, surgical, or radioisotope method. Synoviorthesis using radioactive isotopes is highly effective, has few side-effects, and can be done in an outpatient setting. A single dose of clotting factor is often sufficient for a single injection of isotope and regular physiotherapy postinjection is advised to help the patient regain strength, proprioception, and normal functional use of the joint [25,26].

A prospective study was carried out to assess the correlation between clotting factor concentrate use and musculoskeletal outcome among 10 centers from developing countries. However, there was wide variation in the use of clotting factor concentrate among centers and most patients were treated with episodic (on demand) rather than prophylactic therapy. Surprisingly, there was not much difference between the bleed frequency, musculoskeletal and functional outcome between different centers irrespective of the amount of clotting factor concentrate use (MUSFIH study, unpublished data). This is so far the only study looking prospectively at the correlation between the use of clotting factor concentrates and musculoskeletal outcome.

Surgery

Large quantities of factor concentrates are needed for people with hemophilia undergoing surgery. When factor concentrates are used at the usually recommended dosage for intermittent bolus infusions, most major surgical procedures require about 1000 IU/kg per procedure [27]. With continuous infusion of factor concentrates, this can be reduced to about 400–500 IU/kg per procedure [28]. In situations of extreme resource constraints, lower doses, aimed at maintaining 30–40% trough levels in the first 2–3 days, followed by 20–30% in the next 3–4 days and 10–20% levels during the subsequent days, can reduce factor usage to about 300 IU/kg per procedure even with intermittent infusion protocols for major surgical procedures, not including joint replacement surgery [29].

Immune tolerance therapy

There is a perception that the incidence and prevalence of inhibitors in developing countries is lower than that reported in the developed world although there are limited data to support this. Extremely large quantities of factor concentrates are required for immune tolerance therapy for people with hemophilia who develop persistent high-titer inhibitors. The optimal dose remains to be defined and varies. Usually about 50–200 IU/dose, 2–3 times/week is administered for several months [30]. Though stopped prematurely, the International ITI study, a multicenter prospective randomized study looking at high dose (200 IU/kg/day) vs low dose (50 IU/kg/day 3 times/week) in patients with high-titer FVIII inhibitor did not find any difference in overall success of the two protocols [31], though breakthrough bleeds were higher in the lower dose protocols. Success of ITI varies between 60 and 80% depending on protocol used [32]. Very little data are available on such therapy from developing countries. In Turkey, four out of seven patients underwent successful immune tolerance therapy with 25 IU/kg factor VIII three times weekly over 1–4 months [33,34]. This is encouraging data but needs to be attempted on larger numbers of patients. Unfortunately, most centers in developing countries are unable to offer such treatment for lack of resources.

Products for treatment

The greatest challenge for those attempting to provide care for people with hemophilia in developing countries is the provision of factor concentrates in adequate quantities for replacement therapy. Availability and cost determine the choice of products for factor replacement in developing countries unlike developed countries where safety and purity are the predominant considerations. Different models and possibilities exist and each country needs to choose its options carefully [35].

Importation of factor concentrates

Importation of the required quantities of safe virus-inactivated factor concentrates of a suitable purity from the international market is an option. The advantage of this approach is that safe factor concentrates can be immediately made available to people with hemophilia. With the use of recombinant factor concentrates in developed countries, safe plasma derived concentrates are now available at about US$ 0.30–0.40/IU. Unfortunately even at this price, they remain out of reach of most people with hemophilia in developing countries. The recent introduction of a large number of newer clotting factor concentrates, some with improved function, such as longer half-lives, may allow the classic factor concentrates to become more available and affordable in other parts of the world.

The other important concern is that as more people with hemophilia become identified in these countries, there will not be enough plasma-derived concentrates with current levels of production to meet the needs of people with hemophilia worldwide. There is need therefore for different levels of self-sufficiency in plasma and plasma products in developing countries.

Local self-sufficiency of plasma and factor concentrates

There are two separate issues here as follows.

1 Self-sufficiency in plasma: This is certainly desirable, and requires improving and expanding blood transfusion services so that adequate quantities of safe plasma can be collected. Such plasma could be used as fresh frozen plasma or cryoprecipitate initially, with viral inactivation, if possible, until other options become available. If enough plasma can be collected, then fractionation can be considered.

2 Self-sufficiency in fractionation: Two options exist for fractionation of locally collected—contract fractionation outside the country at a suitable facility or establishing infrastructure for fractionation locally. Though a variety of factors need to be considered including volume of plasma available, quantity and purity of factor concentrates required and the resources available for choosing between these options, it may be best for smaller countries to opt for contract fractionation and those with large populations to choose the latter option.

Perhaps the best option is a combination of these two approaches. Initially, a country could import modest quantities of factor concentrates that can provide the existing people with hemophilia with a safe therapeutic option while trying to establish a good transfusion service for collecting large quantities of plasma. As plasma collection increases, fractionation could be done either locally or on contract at a distant site to different levels of purity as deemed appropriate and factor replacement practises could change accordingly. Such an approach is also likely to be more acceptable for governments that may prefer to use their resources to support local industry rather than paying to import factor concentrates.

There have been a few examples of plasma fractionation facilities in developing countries in the past. Brazil, Cuba, Thailand, and South Africa have been able to produce small quantities of low/intermediate purity virus-inactivated products in modest plasma fractionation plants in the past that has served their needs to some extent [36]. In South Africa, the needs of about 1500 people with hemophilia using about 12 000 IU each annually at that time had been almost entirely met from these manufacturing units. Large quantities of factor concentrates and other plasma products are fractionated at multiple facilities in China [36]. While developing countries

attempt to establish facilities for fractionation, the overriding principle should be attention to ensure that current good manufacturing practises are followed with regard to quality of plasma and viral inactivation. It should also be noted that almost none of the examples mentioned above have been able to sustain and provide significant quantities of clotting factor concentrate to their own countries. This is therefore a challenging task.

Educating patients and families about hemophilia

While this is extremely important everywhere, it is even more so in situations where care is inadequate. A knowledgeable patient can actually help prevent iatrogenic complications of hemophilia that are not uncommon under these conditions. Facilities should be established for adequate counseling and education about the disease for families with individuals diagnosed to have hemophilia. Apart from information related to the principles of managing this condition, they should also be made aware of the support systems available to cope with it socially and financially. Written information should also be provided to them. It would be very useful if, at the time of diagnosis and registration, an information booklet in the local language is given to each patient and their family. This would not only provide essential information immediately, but would also compensate to some extent for lack of proper counseling facilities at the center where the diagnosis was made. It could later be supplemented by discussions regarding specific problems.

Improving social awareness and advocacy

Increasing social awareness of hemophilia is important for two reasons. First, it helps identify more people affected by this condition as families with individuals who may have hemophilia seek medical attention. Second, it also helps in creating social support for the cause of hemophilia, which can play a crucial role in improving care for people with hemophilia. Both the print and visual media can be used to achieve this.

Experience has shown that getting support from government for hemophilia care requires strong advocacy groups. Establishing a vibrant and well-informed national organization that represents all people with hemophilia in a country and advocates their cause is extremely important for this. The WFH also has major programs to assist in this process.

Developing a program for delivery of care

Two models currently exist in many developing countries. The first involves support from the government and a program of care integrated with national healthcare facilities. The level of support from government and insurance agencies varies in different countries. The second is a situation where there is no significant support for people with hemophilia from the government and most of the care is provided by a parallel system of healthcare involving private hospitals and other nongovernmental organizations.

The data collected by the WFH through its global survey confirms that countries with successful programs for hemophilia care have support from their national healthcare systems. These are countries with GDP in the middle- and low-middle income groups and strong patient advocacy groups. Conversely, countries with the lowest GDP and insignificant patient advocacy have extremely inadequate or absent organized care for hemophilia [37]. Lobbying for support from the health budget of the country therefore becomes crucial for successful implementation of such programs and improving awareness of hemophilia and its management are crucial aspects of establishing care and its delivery.

Conclusion

The majority of people with hemophilia in the world continue to have inadequate care due to paucity of resources and lack of knowledge. Varying conditions that prevail in developing countries make it difficult to recommend an ideal model for the delivery of hemophilia care. It is possible, though, to define the basic requirements that are necessary to achieve this as described in this chapter. The details will depend upon local circumstances and each country will need to choose the model best suited for its purpose. However, in the last decade, mainly due to the efforts of the WFH and the cooperation of many governments, significant progress has taken place in improving hemophilia care in developing countries. If this momentum is sustained, indeed accelerated, then the quality of life of people with hemophilia in developing could vastly improve in the next decade.

References

1 Srivastava A, Brewer AK, Mauser-Bunschoten EP, *et al.* Treatment Guidelines Working Group on Behalf of the World Federation of Hemophilia. Guidelines for the management of hemophilia. *Haemophilia* 2013; **19**(1): e1–47

2 Kasper CK, Mannucci PM, Boulyzenkov V, *et al.* Haemophilia in the 1990s: Principles of treatment and improved access to care. *Semin Thromb Haemost* 1992; **18**: 1–10.

3 Berntorp E, Boulyzenkov V, Brettler D, *et al.* Modern treatment of haemophilia. *Bull WHO* 1995; **73**: 691–701.

4 de Moerloose P, Fisher K, Lambert T, *et al.* Recommendations for assessment, monitoring and follow up patients with haemophilia. *Haemophilia* 2012; **18**(3): 319–25.

5 United Nations. Human development report, 2003. Geneva: United Nations Development Program.

6 World Bank. World Bank report, 2000.

7 Srivastava A. Delivery of haemophilia care in the developing world. *Haemophilia* 1998; **4**(Suppl. 2): 33–40.

8 Giangrande PL, Mariani G, Black C. The WFH Hemophilia Center Twinning program: 10 years of growth, 1993–2003. *Haemophilia* 2003; **9**: 240–4.

9 Carman CJ. Developing and maintaining of hemophilia programs in developing countries. *Southeast Asian J Trop Med Publ Health* 1993; **24**(Suppl. 1): 46.

10 Jayandharan G, Shaji RV, Chandy M, Srivastava A. Identification of factor IX gene defects using a multiplex PCR and CSGE strategy – a first report. *J Thromb Haemost* 2003; **1**: 2051–4.

11 Preston FE. Laboratory diagnosis of hereditary bleeding disorders: external quality assessment. *Haemophilia* 1998; **4**(Suppl. 2): 12–18.

12 World Federation of Hemophilia. World Federation of Hemophilia report on the annual global survey, 2011.

13 Srivastava A. Factor replacement therapy in haemophilia – Are there models for developing countries? *Haemophilia* 2003; **9**: 391–7.

14 Astermark J, Petrini P, Tengborn L, *et al.* Primary prophylaxis in severe haemophilia should be started at an early age but can be individualized. *Br J Haematol* 1999; **105**: 1109–13.

15 Marilyn J. Manco-Johnson, Thomas C. Abshire, Amy D. Shapiro, *et al.* Prophylaxis versus episodic treatment to prevent joint disease in boys with severe hemophilia. *N Engl J Med* 2007; **357**: 535–44.

16 Gringeri A, Lundin B, Mackensen SV, *et al.* ESPRIT Study Group. A randomized clinical trial of prophylaxis in children with hemophilia A (the ESPRIT Study). *J Thromb Haemost* 2011; **9**(4): 700–10.

17 Petrini P. What factors should influence the dosage and interval of prophylactic treatment in patients with severe haemophilia A and B? *Haemophilia* 2001; **7**(1): 99–102.

18 Nilsson IM, Berntorp E, Lofqvist T, Pettersson H. Twenty-five years' experience of prophylactic treatment in severe haemophilia A and B. *J Intern Med* 1992; **232**: 25–32.

19 Wu RH, Luke KH, Poon MC, *et al.* Low dose secondary prophylaxis reduces joint bleeding in severe and moderate hemophilia children: a pilot study in China. *Haemophilia* 2011; **17**: 70–4.

20 Tang L, Wu R, Sun J, *et al.* Short-term low-dose secondary prophylaxis for severe/ moderate haemophilia A children is beneficial to reduce bleed and improve daily activity, but there are obstacle in its execution: a multi-centre pilot study in China. *Haemophilia* 2013; **19**(1): 27–34.

21 Srivastava A. Choice of factor concentrates for haemophilia: A developing country perspective. *Haemophilia* 2001; **7**: 117–22.

22 Kavakli K, Aydogdu S, Taner M, *et al.* Radioisotope synovectomy with rhenium186 in haemophilic synovitis for elbows, ankles and shoulders. *Haemophilia* 2008; **14**(3): 518–23.

23 Luchtman-Jones L, Valentino LA, Manno C, and Recombinant Therapy Workshop Participants. Considerations in the evaluation of haemophilia patients for short-term prophylactic therapy: a paediatric and adult case study. *Haemophilia* 2006; **12**(1): 82–6.

24 Srivastava A, Chuansumrit A, Chandy M, Duraiswamy G, Karabus C. Management of haemophilia in the developing world. *Haemophilia* 1998; **4**: 474–80.

25 Thomas S, Gabriel MB, Assi PE, Barboza M, Perri ML, Land MG, *et al.* Radioactive synovectomy with Yttrium90 citrate in haemophilic synovitis: Brazilian experience. *Haemophilia* 2011; **17**(1): e211–16.

26 van Kasteren ME, Nováková IR, Boerbooms AM, Lemmens JA. Long term follow up of radiosynovectomy with yttrium-90 silicate in haemophilic haemarthrosis. *Ann Rheum Dis* 1993; **52**(7): 548–50.

27 Rickard KA. Guidelines for therapy and optimal dosages of coagulation factors for treatment of bleeding and surgery in haemophilia. *Haemophilia* 1995; **1**(Suppl. 1): 8–13.

28 Martinowitz U, Schulman S, Gitel S, Horozowski H, Heim M, Varon D. Adjusted dose continuous infusion of factor VIII in patients with haemophilia A. *Br J Haematol* 1992; **82**(4): 729–34.

29 Srivastava A, Chandy M, Sunderaraj GD, *et al.* Low dose intermittent factor replacement for post-operative haemostasis in haemophilia. *Haemophilia* 1998; **4**: 799–801.

30 DiMichele D. Immune tolerance therapy dose as an outcome predictor. *Haemophilia* 2003; **9**(4): 382–6.

31 Hay CR, Dimichele DM. The principal results of the International Immune Tolerance Study: a randomized dose comparison. *Blood* 2012; **119**: 1335–44.

32 Mariani G, Siragusa S, Kroner BL. Immune tolerance induction in hemophilia A: a review. *Semin Thromb Hemost* 2003; **29**(1): 69–76.

33 Kavakli K, Gringeri A, Bader R, *et al.* Inhibitor development and subsititution therapy in a developing country: Turkey. *Haemophilia* 1998; **4**: 104–8.

34 Chuansumrit A, Pakakasama S, Kuharthong R, *et al.* Immune tolerance in a patinet with haemophilia A and high titre inhibitors using locally prepared lyophilized cryoprecipitate. *Haemophilia* 2000; **6**: 523–5.

35 Bird A, Isarangkura P, Almagro D, Gonzaga A, Srivastava A. Factor concentrates for haemophilia in the developing world. *Haemophilia* 1998; **4**: 481–5.

36 World Federation of Hemophilia. Third global forum on the safety and supply of hemophilia treatment products, 22–23 September, 2003, Budapest, Hungary. *Haemophilia* 2004; **10**: 290–4.

37 Evatt BL, Robillard L. Establishing haemophilia care in developing countries: Using data to overcome the barrier of pessimism. *Haemophilia* 2000; **6**: 131–4.

CHAPTER 69

Comprehensive care and delivery of care: the global perspective

Mark W. Skinner[1] and Alison M. Street[2]

[1] Institute for Policy Advancement, Washington DC, USA
[2] Monash University, Melbourne, Australia

Introduction

With proper diagnosis, management, and care, people with bleeding disorders can live perfectly healthy lives. Without treatment, the reality is that many will die young or, if they survive, suffer joint and other tissue and organ damage that leaves them with permanent disabilities.

Worldwide, 1 in 1000 men and women live with a bleeding disorder [1]. Only about 25% of people with hemophilia receive adequate treatment [2]. The percentage is far lower for those with von Willebrand disease (VWD) and the rarer bleeding disorders.

Children in low-income countries are at great risk of dying young. World Federation of Hemophilia (WFH) Global Survey [3] data suggest that as the economic capacity of a country decreases, the ratio of adults to children also decreases (Figure 69.1).

The improved outcomes in morbidity and mortality when comprehensive care occurs within a hemophilia treatment center (HTC) setting are well established [4]. Even in "low" resourced countries, where treatment is typically not immediately and consistently available and patients are at increased risk of suffering severe and permanent disability and early death, there are benefits with the introduction of comprehensive care [5].

Many people with inherited bleeding disorders, particularly those living in countries with emerging economies, still have insufficient access to diagnosis and care. This issue is our greatest challenge.

Role of the World Federation of Hemophilia in global development

The vision of the WFH has been to achieve "treatment for all" patients with inherited bleeding disorders, regardless of where they live. Treatment for all is the foundation upon which the WFH global development strategy is built. It means provision of:

1 Proper diagnosis, management, and care by a multidisciplinary team of trained specialists.
2 Safe and effective treatment products, available for all people with inherited bleeding disorders.
3 Expanded services beyond hemophilia, to those with VWD, rare factor deficiencies, and inherited platelet disorders.

The healthcare development work of the WFH is carried out in collaboration with its national member organizations (NMOs) and a dedicated group of medical and lay volunteers. It is based on a comprehensive development model that aims to achieve sustainable comprehensive care and treatment for all. The WFH is achieving its goal to develop sustainable care through country-specific as well as global programs and activities [6].

We can demonstrate the global impact of the WFH Development Model (WFH Model) and significant progress through its systematic approach using data from the WFH Global Survey. Figures 69.2 and 69.3 demonstrate the increase over time in the number of patients identified with bleeding disorders and the availability of clotting factor concentrates (CFC).

Introduction of comprehensive care

Given the complexity of managing bleeding disorders, one of the core steps to improving outcomes is the introduction of comprehensive care. To optimize treatment, care for patients with bleeding disorders should be provided in a specialized HTC, where hematologists, nurses, orthopedists, physical therapists, psychologists, social workers, dentists, laboratory technicians, and others come together as a specialized multidisciplinary care team to look comprehensively after each patient's unique care needs. When an HTC provides the full range of facilities for the diagnosis and management of inherited

Textbook of Hemophilia, Third Edition. Edited by Christine A. Lee, Erik E. Berntorp and W. Keith Hoots.
© 2014 John Wiley & Sons, Ltd. Published 2014 by John Wiley & Sons, Ltd.

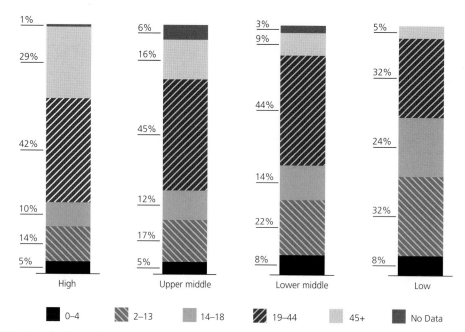

Figure 69.1 Hemophilia A age distribution for country groups based on World Bank economic rankings. Based on 2009 World Bank Gross National Income (GNI) rankings in US dollars (low income $US995 or less, lower–middle income $US996–3945, upper-middle income $US3946–12 195, and high income $US12 196 or more). Data from [3].

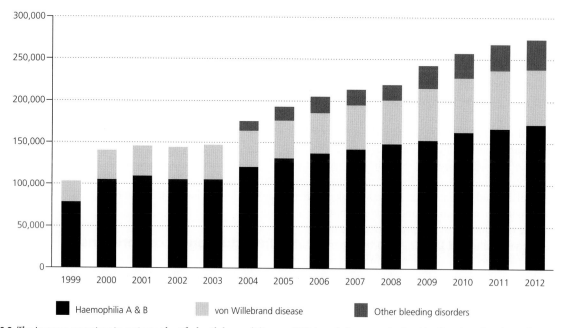

Figure 69.2 The increase over time in patients identified with hemophilia, von Willebrand disease, and other bleeding disorders (rarer factor deficiencies and inherited platelet disorders) contain data from the history of the WFH Global Survey. Data from [3].

bleeding disorders it is referred to as a hemophilia comprehensive care center (HCCC). Data from the WFH Global Survey also indicate that the ratio of full HCCC compared to basic HTC declines as the economic ranking of a country declines.

Because care for these patients is very specialized, life long, and affects many other areas of the patient's physical and mental health, it is best met through a patient-centered multidiscipli-

nary team approach (Figure 69.4). Comprehensive care ensures that the unique treatment needs of a patient are met to maintain health, including physical, emotional, psychological, social, and educational aspects.

The comprehensive care model (also described in modern healthcare parlance as a model of chronic disease management) has been one of the most successful public health programs in

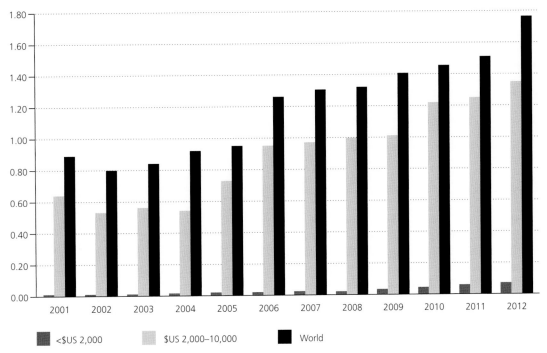

Figure 69.3 The availability of clotting factor concentrates (units of factor VIII per capita) in countries with <$US2000 gross domestic product (GDP), countries between $US2000 and $US10000 GDP and worldwide. Data from [3].

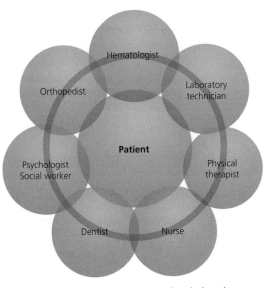

Figure 69.4 Illustration of the patient-centered multidisciplinary team approach of the comprehensive care model.

Box 69.1 Benefits of using the World Federation of Hemophilia (WFH) development model in promoting comprehensive care.

- Studies show that mortality and hospitalization rates of persons with haemophilia decrease when they are treated in a hemophilia treatment center
- A multidisciplinary comprehensive care team develops and maintains the necessary experience to provide appropriate treatment
- Prompt treatment leads to more effective use of replacement therapy, which can actually decrease the cost of treating specific bleeding episodes
- Resources, such as hospitals, diagnostic laboratories, and emergency services, are similarly used more appropriately
- Proper patient education and implementing timely, preventive care and exercise programs help strengthen joints and muscles preventing initial and recurrent bleeding episodes.
- Carrier detection and genetic counseling helps identify risk of having a child with haemophilia.

many developed countries. In hemophilia, its adoption has resulted in significantly improved health for patients with hemophilia as well as producing a reduction in healthcare utilization. Improved outcomes in morbidity and mortality when comprehensive care occurs within an HTC setting are well established [7]. Even in "low" resourced countries, where treatment is typically not immediately and consistently available and patients are at increased risk of suffering severe and permanent disability and early death, there are benefits with the introduction of comprehensive care [8].

The WFH has long promoted the delivery of care for patients with inherited bleeding disorders through specialized centers using the comprehensive care model. There have been two joint WFH meetings with the World Health Organization (WHO), first in 1990 to discuss "Prevention and Control of Haemophilia" from which a Memorandum was published [9] including among a list of recommendations, "that each country should set up and fund a network of specialized haemophilia centres where patients can be diagnosed and treated with an integrated multidisciplinary approach." The topic for the second WFH–WHO meeting in 2002 was "Delivery of Treatment for Haemophilia" and the

---

Box 69.2 Key points in developing and delivering comprehensive care

- Provide and coordinate services for both inpatient and outpatient care of patients and their families
- Initiate, provide training for, and supervise home therapy with clotting factor concentrates (where available)
- Educate patients, families, and other caregivers including health professionals about benefits of the comprehensive care system
- Collect data and where possible conduct research (Practise note: To promote and undertake research, it must be performed in an ethical manner according to the codes of good clinical practise)

Box 69.3 Benefits of a national patient registry

- Centralizes all relevant diagnostic and clinical patient information
- Establishes disease prevalence and the geographic location of patients
- Allows monitoring of trends in health and provides comprehensive surveillance systems for treatment-related adverse events
- Allows analysis and audit of standard of care and measureable clinical outcomes
- Enables identification of resources needed and facilitates priority setting for improved outcomes
- Informs and improves the tendering process for purchase of replacement products
- Facilitates the establishment of better communication networks between all interested parties

---

recommendations as to delivery of treatment were that it be dispensed from a treatment center, integrated into the existing healthcare system, where patients should be listed on a registry. There should be protocols for dosing of CFC and follow-up which are recorded as progress details (now commonly referred to as clinical outcome analysis) and regular research and development conducted to establish optimal treatment guidelines which are quality assessed (evidence based) [10].

The WFH promotes these practises through many training activities and has published a Fact Sheet on the Structure and Functions of Comprehensive Hemophilia Treatment Centres [11]. The WFH Guideline on Management of Hemophilia [12] and the European Principles for Haemophilia Care [13] both provide additional guidance on the implementation and management of comprehensive care programs.

Building justification for comprehensive care through surveillance and data collection

Quantifiable results contained in national registries facilitate the measurement of the effectiveness of healthcare programs. Using data collected from national patient registries, the impact, trends, and significant progress achieved through a systematic development approach can be demonstrated.

The WFH recommends the development of national patient registries through collaboration between national patient organizations, healthcare professionals, treatment centers, and ministries of health [14]. Registries are beneficial for patients and their quality of life, to doctors and nurses for the identification of changing care needs, and to public health authorities for better projection and management of care requirements and resources.

Basic registry data, such as increases in the number of patients diagnosed or the life expectancy of people with bleeding disorders, are useful in evaluating the worth and success of various development programs to improve care within countries. The need to have a an auditable outcomes system becomes more and more important as ministries of health want to measure the

outcomes of investing resources into hemophilia and other bleeding disorders.

All countries have a limited amount of resources to spend on healthcare, allocated according to what they assume are the highest priorities. A properly designed registry of patients with inherited bleeding disorders that tracks utilization as well as clinical outcomes (including complications of treatment) will allow analysis to inform future health planning. Resources should be used to achieve visible results. This is important for two reasons. First, successful healthcare outcomes (such as reduced days of hospitalization or absence from school) will increase the engagement and enthusiasm of the affected population and their clinicians; and second, the successes will demonstrate to the health authorities the usefulness of this program. Data obtained from a centralized registry are invaluable in identifying those resources with the highest priorities for successful outcomes.

To fully understand the outcomes of care, continual monitoring is important to be aware of trends or changes. Examples of these data elements include the incidence and prevalence of infections with blood-borne viruses (e.g. human immunodeficiency or hepatitis C viruses), the number of patients with joint disease or the degree of joint disease in the patients, the number of patients that have inhibitors, liver disease, are hospitalized, or die. This information is critical in identifying the changing experiences and needs of the patients, identifying particular problems that need to be addressed, as well as assessing and documenting the effect that changes in healthcare delivery have made for the population.

Introducing and developing national care programs

Through many years of experience, the WFH identified six essential elements for a stepwise model to introduce and develop a national care program. The elements of the WFH Model are integrated and interdependent (Table 69.1). The WFH Model is

Table 69.1 World Federation of Hemophilia Development Model steps for developing a national hemophilia care program by essential element. Development steps do not necessarily denote chronological order. Situations may vary by country. Data from [17].

Government support	Care delivery	Medical expertise	Treatment products	Patient organization	Data collection and outcomes research
Objectives					
• To obtain government support for national hemophilia care program within the health system	• To provide accurate diagnosis and appropriate treatment		• To obtain the best quality blood products in sufficient quantity at an affordable cost • Develop and improve regulatory knowledge	• To develop a strong patient organization for advocacy and education	• To set good and efficient data collection system within health services with contribution of all key players • To develop the ability to track and report patient health outcomes through surveillance, enhanced data collection and outcome analysis • To conduct basic descriptive studies on bleeding disorders
Development steps					

• No government support or interest in hemophilia care
• Government recognition of main HTC as a reference center
• Some level of government involvement in hemophilia care
• Limited central or regional government resources allocated for hemophilia care
• Official government commitment to hemophilia care
• Government contributes substantial financial support for hemophilia care
• Hemophilia is a line item in a country's annual healthcare budget
• Government is a key partner in sustainable national hemophilia care program
	• Isolated doctor in major city works with no resources
	• Basic treatment is possible in hospital(s) in major city
	• Regular hematology outpatient clinic with follow-up offered
	• Creation of a core team within hospital that forms the basis of a full HTC
	• Core team within hospital (HTC) has a medical patient registry & treatment guidelines/protocols
	• Additional HTCs with core teams for children and/or adults in major cities
	• Coordinated network of designated HTCs with national treatment protocols
	• Full comprehensive hemophilia care team is formed in the major HTC(s)
	• Basic teams formed in other areas/regions
	• Established sustainable national hemophilia care program
		Laboratory diagnosis
		• Basic laboratory diagnostic ability
		• Basic screening tests (bleeding time, platelet count, coagulation test)
		  ○ PT
		  ○ APTT
		  ○ TT
		• Internal quality control
		• Factor assays
		• Participation in EQAS
		• VWD assays and Inhibitor detection
		• Molecular genetic detection/DNA mutation detection and carrier detection/prenatal diagnosis
		
		Medical treatment
		• Basic medical knowledge in hematology (includes pediatricians and general practitioners)
		• Doctor specialized in hematology
		• Hematologist(s) assigned to hemophilia care
		• Key hematologist(s) trained in hemophilia
		• Specialized hemophilia core team (hematologist, nurse, physiotherapist, orthopedist, lab technologist)
		• Education provided to patients
		• Home care available for patients
		• Specialized comprehensive care team (social worker, dentist, psychologist, infectious diseases specialist, genetic counselor)
		• Education offered to general medical community
			• Local production of:
			  ○ whole blood
			  ○ plasma
			  ○ FFP
			  ○ cryoprecipitate
			  ○ freeze-dried cryoprecipitate
			• Combination of local production of cryoprecipitate and/or FFP and some purchase of plasma-derived factor concentrates:
			  ○ less than 0.2 IU per capita of concentrates
			  ○ between 0.2 and 0.5 IU
			  ○ between 0.5 and 1 IU
			  ○ between 1 and 2 IU
			• Proper national tender system in place
			• Examine feasibility of contract fractionation of plasma-derived concentrates
			• Examine feasibility of local fractionation of plasma-derived concentrates
			• Purchase of plasma-derived concentrates (>2 IU per capita)
			• Examine feasibility of combined purchase of plasma-derived and recombinant concentrates
				• Organization formed by a nucleus of patients
				• Organization structured, recognized/registered with a constitution
				• Organization holds regular meetings with a core group of volunteers and educates patients and families in major city
				• NMO patient registry
				• Organizes activities including:
				  ○ educational services
				  ○ fundraising
				  ○ training
				  ○ membership
				  ○ volunteer recruitment
				  ○ advocacy
				  ○ budgeting
				• Outreach to other regions of the country to identify new patients
				• Regional chapters are formed
				• National organization follows a strategic plan
				• National organization is a partner in national hemophilia care program
					• No demographic data on people with bleeding disorders
					• Data collected by doctors at some hospitals and/or patient organizations
					• Basic registry of all patients with hemophilia in hospitals or patient organization
					• Basic registry of all patients with bleeding disorders in hospitals or patient organization
					• Registry of all identified patients with bleeding disorders based on accurate diagnosis and detailed medical information
					• Ministry of Health central registry with mandatory reporting and real-time data entry
					• Collate and analyse information on quality of life for people with bleeding disorders
					• Design and conduct observational studies on bleeding disorders
					• Participate in multinational/multicenter comparative research on people with bleeding disorders

APTT, activated partial thromboplastin time; FFP, fresh frozen plasma; HTC, hemophilia treatment center; NMO, national member organization; PT, prothrombin time; TT, thrombin time; VWD, von Willebrand disease.

equally applicable to economically developed and developing countries. When such interventions are implemented, patients can expect to live longer, healthier, and more productive lives. The six essential elements of the WFH Model are as follows:

1 Achieving government support for a national program (Government Support).
2 Improving the care delivery system (Care Delivery).
3 Ensuring accurate laboratory diagnosis and appropriate treatment (Medical Expertise).
4 Increasing the availability of treatment products (Treatment Products).
5 Building a strong national patient organization (Patient Organization).
6 Tracking and reporting patient health outcomes (Data Collection and Outcomes Research).

The WFH Model for the stepwise development of national hemophilia care programs aspires to success and leverages the critical interdependence of government, funders, clinicians, and patients' commitment to optimizing human and financial resources and clinical outcomes. The model emphasizes these interrelationships in developing and resourcing care delivery, through improving medical expertise, making treatment product available, enhancing patient organization capacity, and collecting clinical data including clinical and social outcomes and costs. It is helpful in negotiating with government and other funders, to recognize that they are familiar and supportive of disease management (DM) program concepts and that comprehensive care for patients with inherited bleeding disorders is an early and successful model of this type.

Whatever the level of funding for a national or regional care program, its maintenance or growth can be achieved only by mutual commitment and trust of all parties and provision of credible, locally relevant data. The selection of the data elements required needs to be agreed by all parties and resources allocated to its collection, audit, and analysis.

Future challenges

Through continuing research, clinical tools and knowledge are further evolving to allow treatment delivery to be tailored and personalized, recognizing individuals' different needs and responses to treatment, rather than by using a more formulaic approach. Concepts such as personalized prophylaxis, the identification of individuals at risk of developing an inhibitor, and health indicators unique to women with bleeding disorders are moving into clinical practise. Accurate and comprehensive data will further inform and accelerate these advances and optimize their utility in clinical care.

WFH volunteers and staff also show great interest and commitment to discussion and promotion of emerging issues of comprehensive care delivery, such as early introduction of low-dose prophylaxis where replacement product supply is constrained, as well as support for wide engagement in

clinical effectiveness review and health technology assessment studies [15].

In some parts of the world, there are challenges in recruiting young clinicians to the field of hemostasis compared with practise in malignant disorders or stem cell therapies. Fortunately, there are many new and exciting scientific and clinical frontiers in bleeding and thrombotic disorders to promote to bright and enthusiastic young colleagues, aside from remuneration issues.

The broadened mandate of WFH to deliver care to all patients with inherited bleeding disorders, not only to those with hemophilia, has brought challenge as well as opportunity to both clinicians and patients. Inclusion of patients who previously had no large organization to whom to turn for education and support, many of whom are women, extends diagnostic capacity and clinical service profiles of HTCs.

A more extensive discussion of developing models of hemophilia care was presented as a State of the Art Paper for the WFH World Congress in Paris, July 2012 [16].

Acknowledgment

The authors gratefully acknowledge the support of Elizabeth Myles, WFH Chief Operating Officer for her review and assistance with this chapter.

References

1 Skinner MW. WFH: Closing the global gap—achieving optimal care. *Haemophilia* 2012; **18**: 1–12.
2 Bolton-Maggs PH Optimal haemophilia care versus the reality. *Br J Haematol* 2006; **132**: 671–82.
3 World Federation of Hemophilia (WFH). Report on the Annual Global Survey 2012. Montreal, QC, Canada: World Federation of Hemophilia, 2013.
4 Soucie JM, Nuss R, Evatt B, *et al.*, and the Hemophilia Surveillance System Project Investigators. Mortality among males with hemophilia: relations with source of medical care. *Blood* 2000; **96**: 437–42.
5 Skinner MW. Building our global family—achieving treatment for all. *Haemophilia* 2010; **16**(Suppl. 5): 1–10
6 World Federation of Hemophilia (WFH). Development Programs http://www.wfh.org/en/page.aspx?pid=792
7 Soucie JM, Nuss R, Evatt B, *et al.* and the Hemophilia Surveillance System Project Investigators. Mortality among males with hemophilia: relations with source of medical care. *Blood* 2000; **96**: 437–42.
8 Skinner MW. Building our global family—achieving treatment for all. *Haemophilia* 2010; **16**(Suppl. 5): 1–10.
9 World Health Organization (WHO). Prevention and control of haemophilia: memorandum from a joint WHO/WFH meeting. *Bull WHO* 1991; **69**: 17–26.
10 World Health Organization (WHO). Delivery of Treatment for Haemophilia. Report of a WHO/WFH/ISTH meeting, London, UK, 11–13 February 2002. Geneva, Switzerland: WHO, 2002.

11 World Federation of Hemophilia (WFH). *Structure and Functions of Comprehensive Hemophilia Treatment Centres. WFH Fact Sheet 7*. Montreal, Canada: World Federation of Hemophilia, 2011.

12 Srivastava A, Brewer AK, Mauser-Bunschoten EP, *et al.* and the Treatment Guidelines Working Group The World Federation Of Hemophilia. Guidelines for the management of hemophilia. *Haemophilia* 2013; **19**: e1–e47.

13 Colvin BT, Astermark J, Fischer K, *et al.* European principles of haemophilia care. *Haemophilia* 2008; **14**: 361–74.

14 Evatt B. *Guide to developing a national patient registry*, Montreal (Que): World Federation of Hemophilia, 2005.

15 Berntorp E, Astermark J, Baghaei F, *et al.* Treatment of haemophilia A and B and von Willebrand's disease: summary and conclusions of a systematic review as part of a Swedish health-technology assessment. *Haemophilia* 2012; **18**: 158–65.

16 Street A. Developing models of haemophilia care. *Haemophilia* 2012; **18**(Suppl. 4): 89–93.

17 World Federation of Hemophilia (WFH). WFH Development Model. http://www1.wfh.org/docs/en/Programs/Development_Steps_EN.pdf

Subject Index

Notes: Page number in *italics* refer to figures and those in **bold** to tables. Coagulation factors are abbreviated to 'F' in subentries and von Willebrand disease and von Willebrand factor to VWD and VWF respectively.

abdominal viscus hematoma 467–468
ABO blood group, von Willebrand disease 143, 357
abortion, spontaneous 440, 441
acetabular hemorrhages 183
acetaminophen (paracetamol) 147, 160, 269
N-acetylgalactosamine 12
acetylsalicylic acid 147
acquired hemophilia (AH) 87–94
  associated disease states 87, 88–89
  autoantibody inhibitor eradication 92–93
  clinical manifestations 88, 89
  drug-induced 89
  epidemiology 87
  laboratory diagnosis 89–90
  pregnancy 88–89
  prevalence 87
  relapse rates 93
  residual FVIII activity 88
  treatment 90–92
acquired von Willebrand syndrome 387
activated factor V (FVa) 403–404
activated factor VII (FVIIa) 4, 325, 413
  recombinant *see* recombinant activated factor VII (rFVIIa)
activated factor VIII (FVIIIa) 5, 9, 24
activated factor XI (FIXa) 429
activated factor XIII (FXIIIa) 437, 447
activated FXIII-A$_2$ (FXIII-A$_2$*) 437
activated partial thromboplastin time (aPTT)
  acquired hemophilia 89–90
  age effects 143
  children 141–142
  coagulation inhibitors effects 312
  determination 312–313
  FVII deficiency 416
  FVIII deficiency 312
  FIX deficiency 312
  FX deficiency 422
  FXI deficiency 312, 313, 432
  internal quality control 311–312
  limitations 328
  neonates 133
  prolonged 312
  prothrombin deficiency 400
  reagent sensitivity 312, 313, **313**
  reference ranges 312
activated protein C 6

activated prothrombin complex concentrates (aPCCs)
  acquired FIX inhibitors 112
  acquired hemophilia 90, 91
  concomitant rFVIIa infusion 110, 216
  enhanced 194
  FVIII inhibitors, acute bleeds treatment 79–80, 81, 82
  perioperative management 214, **214**
  plasma-derived 109–110
  postoperative management 214
  prophylaxis 72
    clinical trials evidence 74–75
    immune tolerance induction 73, 73–74
    monitoring 75
    on-demand treatment *vs.* 75
  side effects 81, 213
  standardization 325
  surgery 213
  tranexamic acid and 216
  see also individual products
acute coronary syndromes 157
acute lymphocytic leukemia, radiosynovectomy-induced 230
ADAMTS13 355, *356*, 357, **359**, 372
adeno-associated virus vectors 288–289, 291, 295
  FIX-R338A 304
  future developments 295
  liver transduction 292
  neutralizing antibodies to 288, 294–295
  problems identified/solved 292–294, **293**
  trials 292–294, **294**
adenoidectomy 201–202
adenoviral vectors 287, 301
adolescence 150–153
  behavioral changes 150, 151
  brain development 150
  compliance 151
  heavy menstrual bleeding 345
  hemophilia-related issues 151
  individualized dosing 125, *125*, 126
  prophylaxis 151
  psychosocial progression/regression 150, *151*
  sport participation 151
  transitional care 151–152, **152**
ADP receptor defect **143**
Advate **166**, 166–168
  clinical trials 167, 169
  continuous infusion 205, 207, *208*
  inhibitor development 169
advocacy 512
afibrinogenemia 142, **448**, 448–449
  clotting times 448
  genetics/molecular biology 448–449

prophylaxis 449
  therapy 449
  women 448
agarose gel electrophoresis 372
aging hemophilia patients *see* old age medicine
AHF-Kabi 393
airway injury 466
alanine aminotransferase (ALT) 266, 269
albinism, oculocutaneous 139
albumin, recombinant 192–193
albumin fusion 192–193
allergic reactions
  FIX inhibitors 69, 104, 108
  FIX replacement 108
  fresh frozen plasma 175
Alphanate 391, 392
ε-aminocaproic acid (EACA)
  dental surgery 201
  desmopressin and 388
  FVIII inhibitors, acute bleeds management 81
  major surgery procedures 200
  α2-plasmin inhibitor deficiency **455**
  plasminogen activator inhibitor 1 deficiency **455**
amniocentesis 340
amyloidosis 424–425, 450
analgesics 147, 159
anaphylaxis
  F9 gene deletions 103
  FIX inhibitors 104
anemia
  acquired hemolytic 89
  iron-deficiency 337, 338, 363, 416, **454**
angina pectoris 157
animal models, FVIII inhibitors 43–44
ankle
  arthrodesis 224, 250
  arthropathy 237, 249
  joint bleeding 224
  replacement 224
  synoviorthesis *229*
antenatal diagnosis 339, 456, 505
antepartum hemorrhage 348
anticoagulant inhibitors **4**
anticoagulant proteins **4**
anticoagulant receptors **4**
antifactor VIII antibodies *see* factor VIII inhibitors
antifibrinolytics
  bypassing agents and 216
  dental surgery 201
  desmopressin and 388
  endoscopy 201
  FVIII inhibitors, acute bleeds treatment 81
  FXI deficiency 433

Textbook of Hemophilia, Third Edition. Edited by Christine A. Lee, Erik E. Berntorp and W. Keith Hoots.
© 2014 John Wiley & Sons, Ltd. Published 2014 by John Wiley & Sons, Ltd.

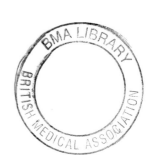